Paediatrics and Child Health

*A Handbook for Health Professionals
in the Third World*

**Edited by H. M. Coovadia
and W. E. K. Loening**

1992
Oxford University Press
Cape Town

OXFORD UNIVERSITY PRESS
Walton street, Oxford OX2 6DP, United Kingdom

Oxford New York Toronto
Delhi Bombay Calcutta Madras Karachi
Kuala Lumpur Singapore Hong Kong Tokyo
Nairobi Dar es Salaam Cape Town
Melbourne Auckland Madrid

and associated companies in
Berlin Ibadan

PAEDIATRICS AND CHILD HEALTH
A HANDBOOK FOR HEALTH PROFESSIONALS IN THE THIRD WORLD

ISBN 0 19 570731 1

Third Edition 1992
2nd Impression 1995
© Oxford University Press 1984

Oxford is a trademark of Oxford University Press

Cover design by Tony Mays

Published by Oxford University Press Southern Africa,
Harrington House, Barrack Street, Cape Town, 8001, South Africa

Set in $9\frac{1}{2}$ on $11\frac{1}{2}$ pt Times by Peter Newman, OUPSA, and Three's Company, Cape Town
Reproduction by Three's Company
Printed and bound by Clyson Printers

Contents

Acknowledgements

We thank the following for permission to reproduce copyright material:

American Academy of Pediatrics
   Lubchenco, L.O., Intrauterine Growth Charts, in *Pediatrics,* vol. 37, no. 3 (March 1966), p. 403.
Ballière Tindall
   Godfrey *et al.*, 'Peak Expiratory Rates in Normal Children', in *British Journal of Diseases of the Chest,* vol. 64, no. 15 (1970).
Blackwell Scientific Publications Ltd.
   Buckler, J.M.H., *A Reference Manual of Growth and Development,* Oxford, 1979.
   Tanner, J.M., *Growth at Adolescence,* 2nd edn., Oxford, 1962.
The C.V. Mosby Company
   Dubowitz *et al.*, in *Journal of Paediatrics,* vol. 77, no. 1 (1970).
Denver Developmental Materials Inc.
   Denver developmental screening test.
Pro-Ed
   'ELM scale score sheet', from Coplan, J. *Developmental and Behavioural Paediatrics,* Texas, 1983.
Thomson Publications (SA) (Pty) Ltd.
   'Typhoid fever and its management with special reference to childhood', in S.A. *Journal of Hospital Medicine,* vol. 2, no. 10 (Oct. 1976), pp. 556-60.
W.B. Saunders Company
   'Developmental characteristics related to adolescent health care needs', in *Essentials of Paediatrics,* Philadelphia, 1990.
World Health Organization, Geneva
   Road-to-health chart and Mortality data *(Fig. 3.4).*

List of authors

ADHIKARI, Professor M., F.C.P. (Paeds) S.A., M.D. (Natal).
Associate Professor, Department of Paediatrics and Child Health, University of Natal, Durban.

ALLWOOD, Doctor C., B.A. M.B.Ch.B. (U.C.T.), M.Med Psychiatry, F.F. (Psych) S.A.
Principal and Head, Department of Psychiatry, Baragwanath Hospital and University of Witwatersrand, Johannesburg.

BEATTY, Professor D. W., M.B.Ch.B (U.C.T.), F.C.P. (Paeds) S.A., M.D. (Cape Town).
Professor and Head, Department of Paediatrics and Child Health, University of Cape Town.

BONNICI, Professor F., M.B.Ch.B, M.Med (U.C.T.), F.C.P. (Paeds) S.A.
Professor, Department of Paediatrics and Child Health, University of Cape Town, and Head of Endocrine and Diabetes Unit, Groote Schuur Hospital, Cape Town.

CHOTO, Doctor R.G., M.D., F.Z.I.M.L.S.
Lecturer and Consultant, Department of Paediatrics and Child Health, University of Zimbabwe, Harare.

COOVADIA, Professor H.M., M.Sc. (Birmingham), M.D. (Natal), F.C.P. (Paeds) S.A.
Professor and Head, Department of Paediatrics and Child Health, University of Natal, Durban.

CRONJE, Professor R.E., M.B.Ch.B (Wits), M.D. (Pretoria), F.R.C.P.E. (Edinburgh).
Professor and Head, Department of Paediatrics and Child Health, University of Pretoria.

FERNANDES, Doctor C.M.C., M.B.Ch.B, F.C.S. (S.A.).
Acting Head, Department of Otorhinolaryngology, University of Natal, Durban.

GIE, Doctor R. P., M.B.Ch.B. (Stellenbosch), L.K.I. (Paeds), M.D. (Paeds).
Senior Specialist, Department of Paediatrics and Child Health, University of Stellenbosch.

HADLEY, Professor G.P., M.B.Ch.B (St. Andrews), F.R.C.S. (Edinburgh).
Professor and Head, Department of Paediatric Surgery, University of Natal, Durban.

HANSEN, Professor J.D.L., D.Sc. (Hon), M.D. (Cape Town), F.R.C.P. (London), D.C.H. (London)
Emeritus Professor of Paediatrics and Child Health, University of Witwatersrand, Johannesburg.

HESSELING, Professor P., M.B.Ch.B., M.Med (Paeds), M.D.
Professor and Head, Department of Paediatrics and Child Health, University of Stellenbosch.

HILL, Doctor I.D., M.B.Ch.B., M.D. (U.C.T), F.C.P. (Paeds) S.A., M.B.Ch.B.
Senior Lecturer, Department of Paediatrics and Child Health, University of Cape Town.

HOUSEHAM, Professor K.C., M.B.Ch.B., M.D. (U.C.T), F.C.P. (Paeds), D.C.H. (S.A.).
Professor and Head, Department of Paediatrics and Child Health, University of Orange Free State, Bloemfontein.

JENKINS, Professor T., M.B. B.S. M.D. (London), M.R.C.S. L.R.C.P. D.R.C.O.G. (London), F.R.S.S.A.F.
Professor and Head, Department of Medical Genetics, South African Institute of Medical Research and University of Witwatersrand, Johannesburg.

KROMBERG, Professor J.G.R., B.A. (Social Work), M.A. Ph.D. (Wits).
Associate Professor, South African Institute of Medical Research and University of Witwatersrand, Johannesburg.

LEVIN, Professor S.E., M.B.Ch.B. (Wits), F.R.C.P. (Edinburgh), D.C.H. R.C.P.S. (Eng.).
Professor of Paediatric Cardiology, Department of Paediatrics and Child Health, University of Witwatersrand, Johannesburg.

LOENING, Professor W.E.K., M.B.Ch.B (U.C.T), F.C.P. (Paeds) S.A.
Stella and Paul Loewenstein Professor of Maternal and Child Health, Department of Paediatrics and Child Health, University of Natal, Durban.
MOODLEY, Doctor M., M.B.Ch.B. (Natal), F.C.P. (Paeds) S.A., M.R.C.P. (U.K.).
Principal Specialist/Senior Lecturer, Department of Paediatrics and Child Health, University of Natal, Durban.
NAIDOO, Doctor J.A., M.B.Ch.B., M.Med (Paeds) (U.C.T.).
Principal Specialist/Senior Lecturer, Department of Paediatrics and Child Health, University of Natal, Durban.
NATHOO, Doctor K.J., M.B.Ch.B., D.C.H. M.R.C.P.
Senior Lecturer and Consultant, Department of Paediatrics and Child Health, University of Zimbabwe, Harare.
NEL, Professor N., B.Sc. Diet, Diploma Hospital Diet (Pretoria).
Professor, Dietetics and Home Economics, University of Natal, Pietermaritzburg.
OWEN, Professor C.P., B.D.S. (Eng.), M.Sc. Dent (S.A.) M.Ch.B. (S.A.).
Professor, Department of Prosthetic Dentistry, University of Western Cape.
PETERS, Professor A.L., M.B.Ch.B. (U.C.T.), M.Med (Ophth) (Natal).
Professor and Head, Department of Ophthalmology, University of Natal, Durban.
PETTIFOR, Professor J.M., M.B.Ch.B., Ph.D. (Wits), F.C.P. (Paeds) S.A.
Professor and Chief Paediatrician, Baragwanath Hospital, Johannesburg.
ROSS, Ms F.M., B.Sc. (Natal), Diploma Hospital Diet (Pretoria), M.S. Nutrition Ed. (Columbia).
Dietician, Department of Dietetics and Home Economics, University of Natal, Pietermaritzburg.
ROTHBERG, Professor A.D., B.Sc. (Wits), M.B.Ch.B. (Wits), D.C.H. F.C.P. (Paeds) S.A., Ph.D. (Wits).
Professor and Head, Department of Paediatrics and Child Health, University of Witwatersrand.
SCHULZ, Professor E.J., M.B.Ch.B., D.P.H., M.Med (Derm) (Pretoria).
Professor and Head, Division of Dermatology, Department of Medicine, University of Witwatersrand.
THEJPAL, Doctor R., M.B.Ch.B., F.C.P. (Paeds) S.A.
Lecturer, Department of Paediatrics and Child Health, University of Natal, Durban.
WESLEY, Professor A.G., M.D. (U.C.T.), F.R.C.P. (Edinburgh), D.C.H. (London).
Associate Professor, Department of Paediatrics and Child Health, University of Natal, Durban.
WEINBERG, Professor E.G., M.B.Ch.B. (U.C.T.), F.C.P. (Paeds) S.A.
Associate Professor, Head of Allergy Service, Red Cross War Memorial Children's Hospital, Cape Town.
WITTENBERG, Professor D.F., M.B.Ch.B. (U.C.T.), F.C.P. (Paeds) S.A., M.D. (Natal).
Associate Professor, Department of Paediatrics and Child Health, University of Natal, Durban.
VAN NIEKERK, Doctor C.H., M.D. (U.C.T.), F.C.P. (Paeds) S.A., D.C.H. (S.A.).
Medical Director Roussel Lab.

Foreword

Over the last two decades we have seen an enormous change in the direction of health care. Unfortunately across the world in both developed and developing countries, we have come to realize that health care has become unbalanced. Too much emphasis has been placed on the 'doctor-orientated curative care' often provided so well by the 'disease palace' *(Fig. 1)*.

WHICH OPTION ?

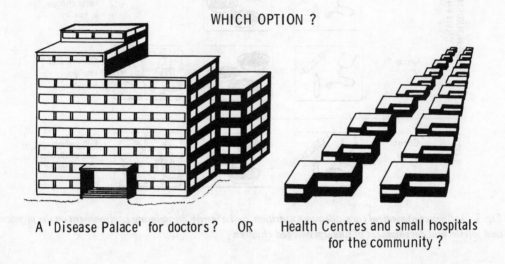

A 'Disease Palace' for doctors?   OR   Health Centres and small hospitals for the community ?

Fig. 1   Large hospitals are favoured by doctors, politicians, and the patients who can gain access to them. They have little effect on the health of most people in less developed countries

Hospitals are required for many of the severe illnesses of childhood, but a better understanding of disease and its prevention should mean that resources spent in health centres and community programmes would do more to reduce the overall mortality than continuing to pour such extensive resources into large hospitals.

We have also come to realize that health services play only a small part in the total development of the child. My own views on the subject were altered when I visited a project in Cali, Colombia, South America. There the families of sixty children in three different groups were offered a variety of resources, none of which was currently available to them *(Fig. 2)*.

The study showed that children who received only health care showed no improvement in their physical or intellectual growth. The second group who, in addition to health care, received a full and adequate diet, managed to catch up physically with the élite control group from the same area. However, they showed little change in their intellectual levels. The third group was offered a loving and stimulating environment in addition to health care and an improved diet, and they caught up almost one hundred per cent with the élite in their society.

Health workers need to realize that one of the most important prerequisites for an improvement in the health of children is an adequate and suitable diet.

In northern Europe, an important aspect of this diet is considered to be breast-feeding for at least the first twelve months, if at all possible. To this, appropriate foods should be added, determined by the growth and needs of the child. However, children, particularly in less affluent communities, are frequently

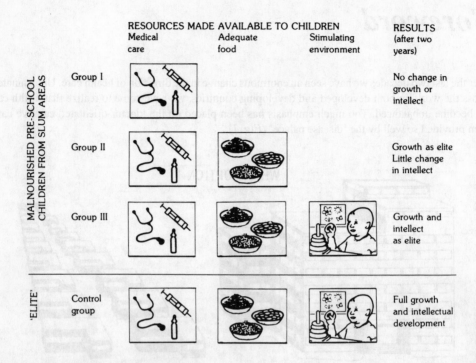

Fig. 2 Influence of medical care, adequate nutrition, and a loving, stimulating environment on the physical and intellectual development of underprivileged children

ill, and unless the preventative measures and the simple resources necessary for primary health care are made available, they cannot derive the full benefit of a good diet. Finally, it must be emphasized that all children should grow up in the most loving and stimulating environment that their parents can provide, with support from the community in which they live.

This book, written from the Durban School of Paediatrics, brings out the special needs of the majority of children living in southern Africa. In the development of any nation the paediatricians have a special responsibility, as governments look to them for guidance in the development of the health and potential of the children, the future of any country. In southern Africa the problems are particularly acute, but this book, written from a background of many years of experience, gives useful guidance concerning the overall needs of child health.

DAVID MORLEY
Emeritus Professor of Tropical Child Health
London University

Preface

This book has enjoyed considerable popularity among medical students and is extensively used by health personnel throughout southern Africa. Now that South Africa is emerging from political and social isolation, it is hoped that this edition will gain wider acceptability in Africa and elsewhere in the developing world.

The format has been improved, and all chapters have been thoroughly revised to keep abreast of recent advances in medicine, thus providing information that is both up-to-date and easily accessible. There are 17 new authors; 14 chapters have been written afresh, and the remainder completely reworked. We have refined the presentation in order to further our original aim of providing a textbook for undergraduate students which encourages a problem-oriented approach to dealing with children's diseases. In a wide-ranging handbook such as this it is not possible to give in-depth coverage of all paediatric problems. We have therefore concentrated on those aspects which are most relevant for developing countries, and for southern Africa in particular. We hope that tutors will guide students deftly through the more detailed sections of the text, and that health professionals in the field and in practice will continue to find this work a helpful reference.

We are appreciative of the support from our many authors, and grateful for the patience of our publishers.

H.M. COOVADIA
W.E.K. LOENING
July 1992

1

History-taking and physical examination of the child

Children are not men or women; they are almost as different creatures, in many respects, as if they never were to be the one or the other; they are as unlike as buds are unlike flowers, and almost as blossoms are unlike fruits.

W.S. LANDOR, 18TH CENTURY ENGLISH POET

Introduction

Paediatrics is the study of growth and development of the child from the moment of conception through to adolescence. It also embraces the science and art of the prevention, diagnosis, and treatment of the diseases of childhood, whether these disturbances be physical, mental, or emotional. Paediatrics deals with all the changes in size, form, and complexity of function that constitute growing up.

Health professionals dealing with children must continually be aware of the many differences between newborn and young infants as compared to the older infant, child, or adolescent. These differences are due to:

- function of various organs
- degree of immunity to diseases
- responses to the effects of disease
- drug dosages and tolerance of drugs
- mental and motor ability, etc.

With age, the rate of change tends to slow down, but the change continues throughout childhood: childhood *is* change.

Age periods of childhood

It should always be borne in mind when obtaining a history and/or physically examining children that babies 1 minute old differ from babies 1 hour old; they in turn differ from babies 1 day old or 1 week old, and from children 1 year or 5 years or 15 years old. To enable doctors to help children to the best of their ability, they need to understand the differences that occur with age, and how these affect the basic processes of disease. Children of different ages may be exposed to different hazards, and may respond differently to the same hazard.

Childhood can be divided into a number of age periods (defined in Chapters 2 and 3).

Neonatal period

During this period the child is extremely vulnerable, and most childhood deaths occur during the neonatal period or during the first year of life. Certain problems and conditions are only present during the neonatal period, viz., hyperbilirubinaemia due to ABO blood group incompatibility, hyaline membrane disease, etc.

Infancy and toddler period

This is a time of extremely rapid physical, mental, and emotional growth and development. Organ systems mature rapidly, and the infant has better control of various physiological and biochemical functions. This is also the period in which the child is very vulnerable to nutritional deficiencies. The extremely rapid growth makes adequate dietary intake extremely important, and any deficiency in intake will result in undernutrition or frank malnutrition.

The pre-school child

The pre-school period follows the same general trends as infancy: physical growth is at a slower rate, mental development is progressing steadily, and emotional patterns are becoming more fixed.

During infancy the environment of the child is restricted to the home. In the pre-school period the child enters a new world: the neighbourhood — the local homes and fields, the supermarket, shops, and perhaps the nursery school or kindergarten.

1

Only infants exceed the pre-school child in their capacity to invite accidents. Most accidents involving infants occur in the home, but those involving the adventurous pre-school child occur outside the home to an ever-increasing degree. The frequency of traffic accidents involving children rises as children get older. Increasing contact with people also means an increasing contact with infectious agents, and pre-school children are vulnerable to the common infectious diseases. This age group therefore has a relatively high incidence of infections of the respiratory and gastrointestinal tracts, compared to the other age groups.

The school child

The school years are generally the healthiest, as the child has passed through the potential danger period of the early years involving infections and accidents, and has probably been exposed to a variety of pathogenic agents and acquired immunity to some of them. School children are relatively free of disease. They continue to have their share of respiratory tract infections, but usually handle them well. However, certain diseases to which they were not as susceptible earlier in their childhood may now appear, such as rheumatic fever and acute glomerulonephritis.

Many psychological problems encountered in this age group centre on schooling problems and learning difficulties.

Adolescence

This is a period when major physical, cognitive, and psychosocial growth and change occur. It is the time when sexual maturation occurs, and the body takes its final adult form. Major causes of death in this age group are accidents, poisoning, violence, and motor vehicle accidents.

Clinical problem-solving

A health professional solves problems that people have as a result of some malfunction of their body or mind. In this context all of her actions are directed towards this goal, no matter how simple the activity, how mundane the task, or how routine the procedure. If she is treating patients, she is solving problems.

The clinical problem-solving process can be seen as a directional flow from data to action *(see*

Fig. 1.1). In this simplified flow diagram, the clinician collects data, forms explanations for their presence, tests formulations, and decides upon a course of action. Shown as clearly separate stages in the diagram, the process actually blends into one in practice: hypotheses are formed as data are collected, testing may occur before formulation of the final hypothesis, and clinical action is sometimes taken before solution of the 'problem'.

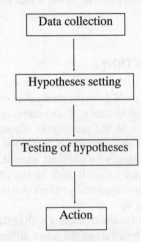

Fig. 1.1 Flow diagram of the clinical problem-solving process

In solving clinical problems, the clinician uses a variety of sources of information or data. Some information comes from the patient's voluntary expression of what he senses, feels, or observes. Some is obtained by questioning the patient to elicit non-voluntary responses. Other information comes from the clinician's store of knowledge, from sources available to her, or is derived from the examination of the patient. Information may also come from clinical, laboratory, radiologic, or other tests.

These data do not exist as separate entities but are part of a whole, and each bit represents a small portion or sample of the total information available. One of the first principles in clinical medicine is that these bits of information called 'clinical data', are all linked to the individual in totality. As more information is gathered, the relevance or otherwise of these linkages will become apparent. If a coherent pattern emerges, a diagnosis is made.

The fundamentals of clinical problem-solving and diagnosis are:

- skilful history-taking
- careful physical examination with keen powers of observation
- judicious selection of appropriate laboratory and other technical procedures, and
- a good analytical mind.

The paediatric history

Introduction

None of the above-mentioned fundamentals of clinical problem-solving outranks the importance of obtaining a complete and thorough history. The diagnosis may be established on this alone in a large proportion of cases, yet more errors are made because of inadequate history-taking and superficial examination than due to any other cause. The ability to *listen* is the most important of the skills and attitudes necessary in good data collection. Much important information is lost, misunderstood, incomplete, or misinterpreted due to the inability of doctors to listen.

There is a tendency among clinicians to hurry through the history-taking, to get on with the physical examination, and to depend unduly on laboratory procedures and other special investigations. A good history should be seen as the launching pad to the diagnosis.

The ability to obtain a good paediatric history and to conduct a thorough physical examination is not only basic to the diagnosis of disease, but is also essential in the evaluation of the normal child. The latter applies especially to the child who has only a slight deviation from the norm, but still falls within the normal range for her age.

The perceptive individual will also find history-taking an excellent opportunity to evaluate parent-child relationships, and attitudes towards disease and possible hospitalization. A history will also reveal the degree of co-operation between the parents in the management of the child's illness, as well as other factors which may contribute to an understanding of the sick child within the family setting.

The attitude and manner of the interviewer should always be friendly, dignified, courteous, and uncritical. One hears too often of 'ignorant, uneducated' parents. Doctors, particularly, should remember that their cultural, educational, and social backgrounds are often very different from

those of the patients they treat, and this imposes a special responsibility on them to be sympathetic, considerate, and accommodating in their approach. No two informants are alike: one is educated, articulate and accurate, while another is less educated and can barely give a clear account of his problem. One is calm, another is frantic. One is sensibly co-operative, another is inhibited, and yet another is garrulous and irrelevant. Part of the task of a health professional is to understand people and to appreciate why they act as they do.

Elements of a complete history

In some respects history-taking in the paediatric patient is similar to that with adults. Patients with similar physical or diagnostic problems, be they children or adults, can all be approached in a similar way to obtain:

- general information, which includes the name, age, birth date, sex, and race of the patient
- the present illness
- the main complaint
- a systematic review of other organ systems
- details of any treatment and response to treatment, and
- details of change in condition.

Details of the history which pertain more to the paediatric age group, and which should be specifically obtained include:

- the pregnancy and mother's health during pregnancy
- events of labour and delivery
- the condition of the baby in the neonatal period
- growth and development
- immunizations
- diet and feeding history
- previous diseases and whether sequelae occurred
- previous history, including previous operations or hospitalizations
- the child's emotional development and adjustment
- family history, and
- social history.

Perinatal health

Prenatal history

The doctor should enquire about the pregnancy, all previous pregnancies, and the health of the

3

mother during these pregnancies. Maternal illnesses acquired before or after conception may affect the child, and thus the history should include data on any infections, illnesses, vaginal bleeds, or toxaemia that occurred during pregnancy. Results of serology tests as well as the blood group of the mother should be recorded.

Birth history

The duration of the pregnancy, the ease or difficulty and duration of labour should be noted. It is also important to know whether the delivery was spontaneous, forceps-assisted, or whether a Caesarean section was performed. The place and date of birth, birth weight, difficulty in initiating breathing, and Apgar scores are also pertinent.

Neonatal history

Important information which should be obtained includes the presence of cyanosis, difficulty in establishing feeds, convulsions, blood transfusions, medications, nursing in an incubator, and the length of stay in the nursery. A history of jaundice must be specifically elicited, together with the age of onset, duration, and treatment given, e.g., exchange transfusion, phototherapy, etc.

Growth and development

Growth and development are the distinguishing features of infancy and childhood as compared to adulthood. It is therefore important to assess physical parameters such as height, weight, and head circumference. Perusal of the child's Road-to-Health Card should provide serial information. The sequential acquisition of each of several milestones is an integral part of this process, and therefore the history should be appropriate to the child's age, as the developmental milestones occur at specific periods, e.g., at the age of one year the baby should be able to say a few words besides 'mamma' and 'dadda'. Accordingly, pertinent developmental milestones must be recorded *(see Chapter 2)*. For a school-age child the grades and marks achieved in school should be noted.

Immunization history

A record of immunizations should be obtained from the Road-to-Health Card. It is important to list those immunizations that have been given, and whether any adverse reactions occurred to them. The dates and number of immunizations must be noted.

Diet and feeding history

This is especially important in the small baby and infant. Important aspects that should be recorded include whether the baby was breast or bottle fed, and how well the baby took the first feed. Details concerning the use of vitamins, iron, and the introduction of solid foods are also important.

In a child with feeding difficulties or a nutritional problem, detailed facts must be obtained about the date of the onset of the problem, methods used in feeding, types of formula or feeds used, the interval between feeds, weight changes, and any other relevant data. Twenty-four hour dietary recall is the best way of obtaining an accurate reflection of the child's food intake.

Previous diseases and hospitalization

The history of each past disease should include the date of onset, symptoms, diagnosis, course, complications, and sequelae. If the child was hospitalized, the diagnosis for the illness should be established, and the results of any surgery determined. All accidents, injuries, and poisonings should be included.

Family history

Many illnesses or disorders run in families or are inherited. In no other division of medicine is the family history as important as in paediatrics. All medical conditions present in blood relatives, which may by their presence or absence have an effect on the health of the child, should be recorded.

Social history

Social factors frequently modify and influence health and illness. The environmental circumstances which may affect the physical and emotional well-being of the patient should be documented. The occupations of the mother and father, housing, access to clean water, school, and play facilities are relevant. These points are crucial in the comprehensive evaluation of disease among disadvantaged children.

The paediatric physical examination

Introduction

It is a striking fact that few doctors miss diagnoses because of ignorance; errors are caused by careless omission of simple procedures and failure to examine patients fully.

There are many physical differences which a health professional accustomed to examining adults might consider abnormal in a child; there are also variations within a group of children which must alert the examiner to the range of what is considered 'normal'. The professional skilled at diagnosis in children is one who is aware of these variants, and makes allowances for them in formulating a final diagnosis.

Most observed variations can best be explained by differences in growth rates of organ systems as they occur from infancy to adolescence. For example, lymphoid tissue is relatively well developed in infancy, becomes maximally expanded during pre-school and school ages, and regresses to small, adult proportions at puberty. The genital system, on the other hand, is infantile at birth, and remains so until puberty.

The findings on physical examination of a child have a special significance which does not apply to adults. The record of an examination represents a brief moment in time in a child's life, because the child is continually growing, developing, and rapidly changing. Therefore, apart from assessing an acute illness, the occasion should always be used to establish a baseline for determining whether a child is growing and developing normally (i.e., according to reference growth charts). The single examination is also useful for determining apparently insignificant variants, so that their importance may be adequately assessed.

It is extremely important to follow the rate of change of the child at each subsequent examination. Evaluating the rate of growth and development, and indeed the rate of progression of difficulties or anomalies, far surpasses the value of a single examination.

Approach to the patient

Every health professional has a number of ways to establish rapport with a child. With an older child, co-operation may be gained by complimentary remarks, suitable conversation with the patient, or a discussion of mutual interests. The pre-school child may be reassured and distracted by interesting objects such as toys. For the infant, one may sometimes have to resort to measures such as sugar-feeding to induce co-operation. Although bribery of any kind is normally deplorable, a timely jelly baby may result in an everlasting bond between the patient and the doctor!

Newborns and infants up to 6 months of age do not often exhibit apprehension on being examined. The group of children who show anxiety and lack of co-operation are those aged between 1 and 4 years. Depending on the emotional maturity of the child, this age range may be extended (in the case of overly-dependent children), or reduced (for those who are more independent and sociable).

The examination is usually performed while the parent is present. If the child is frightened, anxious, or clings to the parent, sending the parent out of the room usually frightens the child even more.

The value of observation

Frequently a tentative diagnosis can be made simply by observing the child while in the mother's arms or as he walks or stands in the room. For instance, much can be learned by remaining seated and observing the mentally retarded child in action, or watching the cerebral palsied child move about the room. With hyperkinetic children it is important to permit them to roam around the consulting room in their often ceaseless, uncontrolled, and driven behaviour; the diagnosis is made by simply observing their actions, and may then be confirmed by further examination. The inexperienced practitioner often makes the mistake of starting palpation, percussion, or auscultation before thorough inspection, and may thereby miss the obvious in searching for the obscure.

Inspection also gives an excellent opportunity to assess the neuromuscular status and developmental level of the small child, as diagnostic techniques for this purpose are based largely on observation. One evaluates the child's abilities in the four fields of developmental progress: motor, language, personal–social, and adaptive.

Conduct of the physical examination

The physical examination begins as soon as the patient enters the room. A glance will uncover much detail about the child: whether the child seems well, sick, malnourished, pale, cyanosed, jaundiced, or shows any other visible abnormalities. Furthermore, the child's attitude towards the parent and the health professional, and the disposition of the parent towards the child and the clinician reveal much about the emotional balance of the child and the parent–child relationship.

There is no 'routine' physical examination of a child. Each examination is individualized. The order of examination is often determined by the child rather than by the doctor.

In general, one begins a physical examination without instruments and gradually introduces the necessary equipment. The examination is usually performed in the position which is most comfortable for the patient. An infant or severely ill child, or a child who is co-operative, may be conveniently examined in the supine position. However, a 6-month-old may have just learned to sit and be eager to demonstrate this ability, in which case the examination should be done chiefly with the patient in the sitting position. Likewise, some children might prefer standing or assuming unusual positions during the consultation, and these preferences should be respected as long as they are compatible with a thorough examination. Children with respiratory distress usually prefer a sitting or prone position.

In the examination of young, apprehensive children, it is a great mistake to remove them immediately from their mother's arms. Much of the examination can be done well with the mother holding the child on her lap or standing close by. When it is necessary to place a small child on the examining couch, the mother should be permitted to stand nearby within sight of the patient. Some children feel reassured as long as they do not see the person examining them. The small child may be held in the mother's arms with his head on her shoulder and the clinician can conduct part of the examination by remaining behind the child.

Regardless of how patient one is, an obstreperous or frightened patient may reject all attempts at examination and will continue to be upset; frequently even such children can be fully examined in their mother's arms. This is the position of preference for many 1 to 3-year-olds. If the patient clings to the mother, the back and extremities may be examined in this position, and the remainder of the procedure can be done later with the patient on his back. It is unsatisfactory to examine the abdomen of a child who is on his mother's lap.

If the mother is helping to restrain the patient, she should be told to hold his hands, rather than the arms. Occasionally it may be necessary to restrain the patient in order to examine the ears or mouth. This may be done by placing the infant's arms under his back, so that his weight rests on his palms. The head may be restrained by either the examiner or mother.

If the child is not upset when the examination begins, it may prove worthwhile initially to examine the site of suspected pathology. For example, if the history indicates the presence of a heart problem, a gentle approach and auscultation of the heart may permit evaluation of a murmur before the child begins to struggle and cry. The same would be true for a suspected abdominal mass.

Naturally, if the presenting complaint indicates a painful region, such as an inflamed joint, examining it first would be an error. The same would be true for inspection of oral or pharyngeal lesions, as this is the most dreaded part of the examination to the child. Furthermore, if a child has a deformity, it is not kind to focus on it initially.

Most practitioners with experience of children know that the sight of instruments may frighten the child, so they begin by examining the lower leg of the child as he sits on the mother's lap. The purpose is not really to examine the leg, but simply to make the first physical contact at a rather remote spot and to make it as gently as possible to allay apprehension. It helps to avoid looking directly in the child's eyes. If the child does not become frightened, one then goes on to examine other areas.

The chest or abdomen should be examined next; inspect, palpate, percuss, and auscultate these areas. Percussion usually worries small children more than auscultation, and should be delayed until auscultation is complete.

The rest of the examination follows, in whatever order seems easiest. It is usually convenient to examine the head, eyes, face, and neck, and then last of all the ears, nose, and throat. The genitalia, femoral region, and anus can be examined at any stage in boys and young girls, but these areas are examined last in older girls.

Blood pressure measurement, measurement of length or height, head circumference, and testing of the mass reflexes conclude examination in the younger child. In the older child, blood pressure and other measurements are determined first, and then the examination may proceed systematically from the head downwards as for an adult. While performing the examination it often helps if the clinician allows the patient to play with the instruments she uses.

When co-operation is desired for more difficult procedures such as examination of the throat, the patient should be told firmly what he is to do rather than be asked to do something. Before any frightening or painful procedure is performed, the patient should be told what is going to be done and what is expected of him.

During each examination the child should be completely undressed so that the entire body may be examined. If the room is cool, or if the patient is modest or frightened, only part of the clothing is removed at any one time. Children exhibit varying degrees of modesty, and this should be respected regardless of age. Notwithstanding any reluctance, a complete physical examination *must* be done, and this will require inspection and examination of the various parts. If the child objects, this can still be done tactfully, exposing one part after another. Obviously the best examination is done when all the clothing is removed except for the underwear.

The successful health professional caring for children must obtain genuine pleasure from examining and dealing with children. She should be friendly and unhurried, and proceed with the examination with interest, patience, skill, and confidence.

Organ systems

It is outside the scope of this text to describe fully the examination of children and their different organ systems. Only specific features that pertain to children will be mentioned.

General appearance

The general appearance of the child may reveal much more than obvious or subtle physical findings. When first seeing a child observe him carefully: does he look well or ill? does he appear comfortable or uncomfortable? is he breathing easily or with difficulty, and so on.

A statement of the general appearance should describe the various aspects of the child, and should document whether he appears well or is in acute distress, chronically ill, alert, comatose, delirious, lethargic, dull, bright, responsive, hostile, or co-operative. The use of descriptive terms should start the examiner off on the road to a proper diagnosis. Note is also made of the interaction between the patient and his parents during the examination.

Individuals caring for children are fortunate in that their patients, unlike adults, rarely fabricate. Regardless of what the mother says, the experienced professional knows that a child does not simulate disease.

Skin

The skin may be examined as a whole, or as each part of the body is exposed. However, regardless of the method adopted, the condition of the skin of the entire body should be noted at each examination. If skin lesions are found, their distribution, colour, and character should be noted.

Cyanosis or jaundice should always be noted. **Cyanosis** is bluish discoloration of a normally pink area. Peripheral cyanosis is most easily detected in the nail beds, whereas in central cyanosis the nail beds as well as the mucous membranes of the mouth are discoloured. It is caused mainly by pulmonary disease or congenital cyanotic heart disease. It should be remembered that visible cyanosis is not a good estimate of the degree of oxygen desaturation, except when the total amount of haemoglobin is between 80 and 100% desaturated.

Jaundice is a yellowish discoloration of the sclerae, the skin, or the mucous membranes: it is best seen in natural light and may be entirely missed in artificial light. It is visible in the newborn when the total serum bilirubin exceeds 90 mmol/l and in the older child when it exceeds 40 mmol/l. It is caused by cellular or obstructive liver disease, or haemolysis.

Pallor or paleness should be noted. In darkly pigmented children it is most easily detected in the nail beds, conjunctivae, oral mucosa, or tongue, all of which are normally reddish-pink. Pallor should never be considered an accurate estimate of haemoglobin concentration. Pallor of the nail beds may be due to hypoproteinaemia, a low haemoglobin concentration, or shock.

The skin is felt for **tissue turgor** and **oedema.** Loss of tissue turgor is one of the reliable estimates of dehydration. Skin turgor is best determined by pinching the patient's abdominal wall skin and subcutaneous tissues between the thumb and index finger, squeezing, and then allowing the skin to fall back into place. Normally the skin appears smooth and firm and, when released, returns into place immediately without residual marks. The skin loses its elasticity and remains suspended and creased for a few seconds in children with poor tissue turgor. This may not occur in obese infants. The skin, especially over the legs, normally feels firm. Little subcutaneous tissue will be felt in malnourished children, and the skin feels thin and loose in children with chronic diseases and malnutrition.

Hair should be its natural colour. In malnutrition it may be paler, lustreless, red or grey, easily broken, thinner, and lacking crinkle.

Head

Shape, bossing *(see Fig. 1.3)*, craniotabes, and the fontanelles (whether open or closed, either prematurely or normally) should be noted. Premature closure of the saggital suture in craniostenosis causes a boat-shaped, scaphocephalic skull; and closure of all sutures, a small skull with proptosis *(see Fig. 1.4)*.

The anterior fontanelle remains open to 18 months, closing prematurely in microcephaly and craniostenosis, and remaining open for longer than normal in hydrocephalus, rickets, and cretinism. Bulging of the fontanelle *(see Fig. 1.5)* occurs with crying or straining, but in the relaxed child such bulging is an extremely important sign, and suggests raised intracranial pressure due to

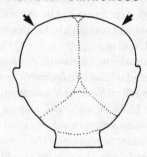

Fig. 1.2   Normal skull with parietal eminences

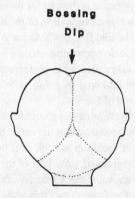

Fig. 1.3   Skull with bossing

meningitis, encephalitis, brain tumour, subdural haematoma, etc. A tense, bulging fontanelle is best noted if the patient is in the sitting position. It is most easily elicited by bringing down the palm of the hand shaped to the curve of the skull, and feeling the bulge of the fontanelle above the level of the surrounding bone. Running the hand from behind forwards also gives the feel of a full fontanelle above the level of the cranial bones. A depressed anterior fontanelle suggests dehydration.

Craniotabes is best found in the temporoparietal or parieto-occipital region, away from suture lines. Firm pressure causes the bone to dip with a snapping sensation like a ping-pong ball being pressed. It is normally felt in prematures, and is present in rickets, hydrocephalus, and congenital syphilis.

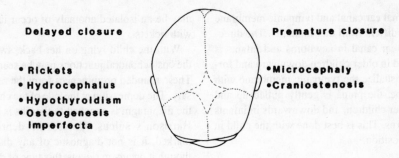

Delayed closure

- **Rickets**
- **Hydrocephalus**
- **Hypothyroidism**
- **Osteogenesis Imperfecta**

Premature closure

- **Microcephaly**
- **Craniostenosis**

Fig. 1.4 The anterior fontanelle

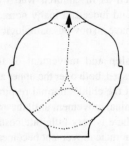

Fig. 1.5 A bulging fontanelle

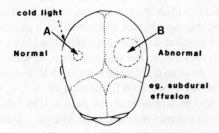

Fig. 1.6 Transillumination of the skull

Transillumination of the skull in small babies and infants in a darkened room will demonstrate abnormal collections of fluid which may lie away from the fontanelle, as in hydranencephaly. A small light of high intensity, preferably cold, is best *(see Fig. 1.6)*.

Auscultation of the skull may reveal a bruit, which may be due to an arterio-venous fistula or a vascular cerebral tumour. Care should be taken to ensure that the bruit is not conducted from the neck.

Face

The appearance of the face may be typical in many disorders, e.g., cretinism, hyperteliorism, mongoloid slanting of the eyes in Down's syndrome, depressed or abnormal nasal bridge, and any tics or habit spasms.

Eyes

Squint, infections, cataracts and conjunctival haemorrhages may be seen. Dryness of the conjunctiva or cornea, keratomalacia, Bitot's spots, and corneal scars occur in children with vitamin A deficiency.

Nose

Discharge can be either mucopurulent or a blood-stained watery discharge of congenital syphilis. The patency of the nasal passages must also be ascertained.

Mouth and throat

The lips, gums, teeth, tongue, and palate must be examined, paying special attention to the soft palate, to exclude a localized cleft. Examination of the throat is often resented by smaller children. Proper and secure immobilization of the head is essential, and a bright light should be used to visualize the oropharynx and tonsils. Koplick spots on the buccal mucosa in measles, herpes ulcers of the tongue, and gingivitis must be noted. Tonsillar exudate — which demands exclusion of diphtheria — also occurs in infectious mononucleosis and moniliasis. Retropharyngeal abscess forms a swelling of the posterior pharyngeal wall which is always unilateral.

Ears

Abnormalities in the shape, size, and position of the pinnae should be noted, as well as any discharge from the ear. The technique of examination

9

of the external ear canal and tympanic membrane in children differs from that in adults. The direction of the ear canal in newborns and infants is upward, and in older children downward and forward. To visualize the tympanic membrane with the otoscope, the pinna is gently pulled up and back in older children, and downwards in infants and newborns. This is best done with the child in the prone position.

Neck

Neck stiffness should always be excluded in all acutely ill children. If present, the Brudzinski and Kernig signs should be elicited. Neck stiffness is demonstrated with the palm of the hand in the nape of the neck, so that minimal muscular spasm can be detected in the small or weak child; this can be missed if the head is flexed from the occiput. Free movement of the neck may be limited by inflamed lymph glands, muscular spasm (trauma), joint disease (rheumatoid arthritis), bony disease, or apical lobar pneumonia.

This is also a good opportunity to feel for lymph nodes in the submental, tonsillar, cervical (deep and superficial), and supra-clavicular regions. Systematic examination of all lymph nodes in other regions is essential.

Chest

Many disease states can be diagnosed by simply looking at the chest. Sometimes it is difficult to do more than observe the hyperactive or crying patient. It may be necessary, depending on the child's attitude, to listen to the chest first, before the child starts to cry, and then to proceed with the other parts of the examination.

The standard methods used in adults in examination of the chest, viz., inspection, palpation, percussion, auscultation, eliciting of vocal fremitus, etc., are applied to children. In the premature infant, the rib cage is thin and the chest may collapse with each inspiration. In infancy the chest is almost round, the anteroposterior diameter equalling the transverse diameter. As the child grows older, the chest normally expands in the transverse diameter.

A funnel-shaped chest, characterized by sternal depression, may be a congenital anomaly. Pigeon chest, in which the sternum protrudes anteriorly, may be an isolated anomaly or occur in children with rickets.

With the child lying on her back, swellings at the costochondral junctions may be seen and felt. These rounded prominences form the rachitic rosary. The depression at the side of the chest where the diaphragm is attached to the ribs is known as Harrison's sulcus. Unless the depression is marked, it is not diagnostic of any disease. Although it occurs in rickets, this type of depression is also found in children with chronic pulmonary disease, as well as in children who were born prematurely, and indeed in many normal young children who have no obvious pathological disturbances.

The expansion and movement of the chest should be assessed, both over the upper and lower lobes. Most of the child's normal respiratory activity is abdominal movement until the age of 6 or 7 years, and there is very little intercostal movement. Later, thoracic movement becomes responsible for air exchange. A note should be made as to whether movement of the intercostal spaces is restricted to one side. There is less movement on the involved side with pneumonia, hydro- or pneumothorax, an obstructive foreign body, or atelectasis, and increased movement on the opposite side of the chest in these conditions.

It is important to note asymmetry. The precordium may bulge in cardiomegaly, whether congenital or acquired. In pneumothorax or a localized chest disease the chest may flatten.

The respiratory system

The **type and rate of breathing** should be recorded. A newborn child, especially the premature, will normally have Cheyne-Stokes type of breathing. Respiratory rate is obtained by watching, palpating or auscultating the chest and counting for 1 minute. In young children, accurate respiratory rates are obtained only during sleep. The rate of respiration (breaths/min) varies from 30–50 at birth, 16–20 at six years of age, and 14–16 at puberty. Children with rapid respiratory rate or tachypnoea usually have respiratory distress or severe infection such as pneumonia, while children with a normal respiratory rate are usually free of respiratory difficulty, but not necessarily free of underlying lung disease, e.g., tuberculosis.

The shallow tachypnoea must be distinguished from the deep, rapid excursions of Kussmaul breathing of metabolic acidosis.

The **position of the trachea is** an important sign of mediastinal shift in the child. It should be elicited by sitting the child up, extending the head, and placing the index finger over the centre of the manubrium in the suprasternal notch, at right angles to the line of the chest, and locating the trachea with the tip of the finger.

Palpation is performed in children by placing the palm of the hand lightly but firmly on the chest and feeling with the palm and fingertips. The entire chest is palpated. Tactile fremitus is easily determined by palpating the chest wall in children who are crying, or in children who can co-operate by speaking. Fremitus, when obtainable, is usually felt over the entire chest as a tingling sensation. Decrease in vocal fremitus suggests the presence of airway obstruction, or may indicate pleural effusion. Fremitus is a poor sign for distinguishing pneumonia, atelectasis, or space-occupying lesions in childhood.

Percussion of the chest should be done last, as it may frighten the child. The chest wall in children is thinner and the muscle smaller: the chest seems more resonant in children than in adults, and it is much easier to get accurate information by percussing the chest of a child than of an adult. If percussion is too vigorous, vibrations over a large area may obscure localized areas of dullness. A decreased percussion note or dullness will normally be found over the scapulae, the diaphragm, the liver, and the heart. Localized areas of decreased resonance, dullness, or flatness may be found in children with consolidation of the lung, such as pneumonia; with lung collapse — atelectasis; or with accumulation of fluid in the pleural space, such as pleural effusion or empyema.

Hyperresonance of the chest is due to an increase in the amount of air in the chest. It is found most commonly in children with emphysema, and is usually accompanied by a lowered diaphragm in cases of asthma or bronchiolitis. Localized hyperresonance may also indicate the presence of free air in the chest, as occurs with pneumothorax or a foreign body acting as a ball valve. Air in the stomach may give an area of localized hyperresonance in the left lower chest anteriorly.

During **auscultation** one listens for breath sounds and adventitious sounds. Because of the small size of the child's chest, and to localize pathological findings, the small bell stethoscope should be used for auscultation in children. The stethoscope should be warmed before use and it must be pressed firmly against the chest wall, or artefacts will be heard. The entire chest, including the axillary areas, should be auscultated.

Breath sounds may seem louder in children than in adults, because of the thin chest wall. Breath sounds in a child are almost all bronchovesicular or even bronchial in nature. Bronchial breathing is due to lobar pneumonia, or other causes of consolidation. Decreased breath sounds indicate decreased air entry, and are found in children with bronchopneumonia, atelectasis, pleural effusion, and pneumothorax.

Stridor is a harsh sound made by air passing through an obstruction of the upper airways from the glottis to the bifurcation of the trachea, and is most commonly heard in croup (infective laryngotracheobronchitis). Generally it is heard better at the mouth than in the chest during auscultation, with the bell of the stethoscope over the mouth. It is usually inspiratory, with chest wall and sternal recession during inspiration.

Wheezing is a softer and higher-pitched sound made by obstruction to smaller peripheral bronchi and bronchioles, as in asthma and bronchiolitis. It is louder at the chest than the mouth, and more marked on expiration than inspiration. Expiration is also prolonged.

Cardiovascular system

Certain basic information must be part of every examination of the heart. This includes rate, rhythm, size, shape, quality of sounds, murmurs, thrills, femoral pulses, and blood pressure. Observations of the heart made in the routine examination should record the presence of precordial bulging — a sign of cardiomegaly — and visible cardiac impulse and its location. The cardiac impulse may be seen in normal children or in the thin or excited child.

External jugular vein distension, with the body inclined to 45 °, can only be looked for in the older child. In the younger child the neck is too short.

Pulse rate is obtained in young infants either by palpation of the femoral artery or auscultation of the heart, and in older children by palpation of the radial artery. The normal pulse rate in children varies from 70–170/min at birth to 120–140 shortly after birth. Rates of 80–140 at 1 year, 80–130 at 2 years, 80–120 at 3 years, and 70–115 after 3 years are within normal limits. Increased pulse rate may reflect anxiety during examination, fever (from whatever cause), restricted exercise tolerance due to congenital or acquired heart disease, and other systemic diseases. The pulse rate is usually increased by 10–12 beats/min for each 1$C of fever. Both radial pulses should be felt; in small children the brachial artery is often more easily felt. The femoral pulses are also felt; radio-femoral delay indicates coarctation of the aorta.

The **apex beat of the heart** is detected by palpation. It is the position most lateral and lowest at which an impulse can easily be palpated. After the age of 7 years this is normally at the 5th intercostal space in the midclavicular line. Before this age it is in the 4th intercostal space, just to the left of the midclavicular line. The apex impulse may be difficult to feel in children of less than 2 years of age, or in children with pericardial effusion, heart failure, or air trapping as in asthma.

Vibratory thrills and pericardial friction rubs may also be palpated. Thrills at the apex are more easily felt with the child on the left side, and basal thrills with the child sitting up.

Percussion dullness to the right of the sternum in the 3rd or 4th intercostal space usually indicates right-sided heart enlargement.

Auscultation of the heart is performed in a similar manner to auscultation of the lungs. The entire precordium is auscultated, with special reference to the valve areas, as in adults.

The quality of **heart sounds** is important. Splitting of the second sound is best heard in the pulmonary area, and is common in normal children. The split widens on inspiration. A third heart sound is common in children, and is best heard at the apex, with a longer interval between the second and third sound, and usually with differing intensities and qualities. It is occasionally difficult to distinguish the third heart sound from the gallop rhythm which indicates heart failure. Occasionally, the three beats of the gallop can be felt on

palpation whereas the normal third heart sound can never be felt as an impulse.

A **venous hum** is a continuous, low-pitched murmur heard at the root of the neck, originating in the internal jugular vein. A hum is usually louder when the patient is sitting, disappears when lying down, and can be stopped by pressure over the internal jugular vein. It usually radiates downward, has no pathological significance, but must be distinguished from a murmur.

To determine the significance of **murmurs** is one of the most difficult diagnostic problems in the physical examination of a child. Many children have murmurs without heart disease — innocent physiological murmurs — and occasionally newborn infants or older children may have severe heart disease with no murmurs, e.g., myocarditis. Murmurs heard in systole are: early systolic, late systolic, or throughout systole (pansystolic). Diastolic murmurs may be heard early (protodiastolic), mid-diastolic, or late in diastole (presystolic).

The quality of the murmurs is recorded as soft, harsh, blowing, whistling, etc. The intensity of the murmur should be graded:

◆ Grade I murmur is the softest possible murmur, heard only in a quiet room. It is not heard in all positions.

◆ Grade II murmur is the weakest murmur heard in all positions in the normal paediatric outpatients or a ward.

◆ Grade III murmur is a loud murmur but not accompanied by a palpable thrill.

◆ Grade IV murmur is a loud murmur with a palpable thrill.

◆ Grade V murmur is heard with the stethoscope barely touching the chest.

◆ Grade VI murmur can be heard without the stethoscope touching the chest.

Blood pressure measurements in children are frequently overlooked. Forgetfulness or lack of proper equipment is the usual reason given for not obtaining a measurement *(see Chapter 16, Renal Disorders, for details)*.

Abdomen

Frequently the abdomen is examined first, especially in the anxious child. It is impossible to do a thorough examination if the child is crying, or if the abdominal wall is tense.

The **abdominal muscles** are thinner than in adults, and the child normally has a lordotic posture, giving the appearance of a prominent 'pot-belly'.

Veins are rarely visible in small infants with good subcutaneous tissue or in dark-skinned children. Visible but not distended veins are usually seen until puberty in normal children, but are especially noticeable in malnourished children. Distended superficial veins are seen with heart failure, peritonitis, or may be collaterals associated with portal hypertension. Direction of flow of blood in distended veins should be established. Normally blood flows downwards from the veins below the umbilicus, and is usually reversed in children with obstruction of the inferior vena cava or with portal hypertension.

Visible peristalsis can be normal; it may be seen through a thin abdominal wall in marasmic or premature infants. If limited to a fixed area, it suggests intestinal obstruction. In infants up to two months of age, a visible gastric wave or peristalsis which passes from under the left costal margin to the right may indicate pyloric stenosis. Intestinal peristalsis occurs in surgical obstruction, in tuberculous adhesions, and when there is a bolus of worms, etc.

During **palpation** one at first palpates gently and superficially, beginning in the left lower quadrant, and then proceeding to the left upper, right upper, and right lower quadrants. But if a localized site of pain or tenderness is found, this area should be palpated at the end, after the other parts of the abdomen have been palpated. Rigidity of abdominal muscles may be due to a medical cause, i.e., lower lobe lobar pneumonia, but peritonitis and surgical causes must first be excluded. If tenderness in the right iliac fossa (RIF) prevents deep palpation of the posterior abdominal wall, it may be due to appendicitis or iliac lymphadenitis.

Distension of the abdomen is caused usually by air or fluid in the bowel, paralytic ileus, faeces in the colon, organomegaly, or by free fluid of ascites. A distended abdomen with little tympany suggests fluid or solid masses. When one suspects fluid, a fluid thrill and shifting dullness should be tested for.

The **liver** is generally palpable during the first year as a superficial mass with a sharp border 1–2 cm below the right costal margin. It may remain just palpable during childhood without pathological significance, but if more than 2 cm below the costal margin it may indicate such disorders as congestion due to right heart failure, hepatitis, fatty infiltration in kwashiorkor, malaria, bilharziasis, septicaemia, or other infections including tuberculosis. A rapidly enlarging liver is an early sign of right heart failure. It should be palpated along its entire margin, as the lobes may be unequally enlarged. Size, consistency, tenderness, and pulsation should be recorded. The upper border must always be determined by percussion, particularly when there is apparent hepatomegaly, as it may be due to downward displacement by over-distended lungs.

A rapidly decreasing liver size may be diagnostic of acute liver necrosis. A normal liver edge should be sharp and flexible so it can be bent slightly. Fatty infiltration of the liver gives a firm edge, while a hard, rounded edge indicates cirrhosis or malignant disease. An irregular surface suggests cirrhosis. Pulsation of the liver occurs in tricuspid incompetence.

The **spleen** is frequently felt as superficial mass in the left upper quadrant, often laterally in the child, enlarging in the direction of the iliac crest. Its size should be recorded and tenderness noted. Splenic enlargement is found in children with such diseases as septicaemia, many of the common viral infections (e.g., measles, infectious mononucleosis), tuberculosis, malaria, bilharziasis and leukaemia. A very large spleen with little hepatomegaly is seen with portal vein obstruction. Kidneys should be palpated bimanually, noting size and whether cystic.

In **congenital pyloric stenosis** a tumour, (which varies in size from a pea to that of the terminal phalanx of the finger) is best felt with the left hand from the left side of the infant on deep palpation. This mass is usually located at the end of the stomach, anywhere along the edge of the liver, from the costal margin in the midline to the underside of the right lobe of the liver. The sausage-shaped tender mass of intussusception can usually be palpated in the right lower quadrant.

The **bladder** may be seen, as well as palpated, lying above the pubis. If it cannot be emptied, some obstruction must be present. The anus should be examined for a fissure. The testes, epididymis, and especially the hernial orifices must be examined; strangulation of gut in a hernial orifice can occur within the first few days of life.

Musculoskeletal

No examination is complete without making the child walk. The posture and gait should always be evaluated, otherwise a subtle gait abnormality or the weakness of a limb will be missed. Abnormalities of length, size, or shape of limbs should be checked for. Clubbing of the fingers and toes should be recorded.

Central nervous system (CNS)

Examination of the CNS is the same as for adults. Older children co-operate well in testing for sensation if they are asked to close their eyes and point to the site touched with cotton wool. Erroneous estimations of the plantar response arise from too heavy a stimulus. The lightest touch along the outer side of the foot should first be applied, and if no reaction occurs, the intensity should be increased.

Extremities, bones and joints

Clubbing of the fingers in small children is best elicited by looking at the fingers in profile, to see if they are terminally clubbed. **Oedema** is demonstrated by firm pressure over the dorsum of the foot, anterior tibia or lower spine. **Skin rashes** are often difficult to see in pigmented skin; petechiae or purpura are better seen if the skin is stretched.

Various **pellagroid skin lesions** occur in malnutrition. There may be areas of hyperpigmented crazypaving and scaling, leaving depigmentation. Acute, bullous lesions of kwashiorkor can be mistaken for second degree burns. Single palmar crease should be looked for in suspected cases of Down's syndrome. Terminal thickening of the radius is found in rickets.

Rheumatic nodules are better looked for than felt. They are best demonstrated with the elbow, knee, wrist, and ankle at full flexion, with the skin drawn tight over the joint. They may be felt over the occiput.

Muscle wasting reflects protein deficiency. Muscle bulk is assessed by palpation; normally it

is firm, especially if muscles are under tension, whereas fat is soft and flabby. The biceps and pectoralis major are easy muscles to feel between the fingers. Children with kwashiorkor may be grossly fat, with very little muscle to palpate. Muscle power is also decreased in undernutrition. Pulling the child up from prone to sitting posture will test the child's power to lift the head.

Spinal examination requires palpation of the spinous processes, which normally lie in a straight line with cervical, thoracic, and lumbar curvatures. Undue prominence or a gibbus, with sharp angulation or lateral displacement of a spinous process, usually results from tuberculous destruction of a vertebral body. Muscular spasm is always present, and is demonstrable by getting the child to pick up an object off the floor, which he does with a stiff back. Rickets can also cause prominence of spinous processes, but it produces an even curvature in the lumbar region, unlike the sharp angulation found in tuberculous disease. Spina bifida can be felt as two separate body prominences.

Joints are tested for full range of movements. The presence of an effusion is best elicited by fluctuation from one part of the joint to another, from below to above the patella, for example.

Measurements

One of the main characteristics which distinguishes a child from an adult is measurable growth; if failure of growth is noted, some abnormality in physical development of the child should be suspected.

The usual measurements taken at the physical examination include height, weight, blood pressure, temperature, pulse rate, and respiratory rate. For the child under 2 years of age the head circumference is routinely measured at each visit. The measurements of weight, height, and head circumference are also discussed in *Chapter 2*, whilst blood pressure recording is discussed in *Chapter 16*.

Weight

A child should be weighed routinely at least once a month for the first 6 months of life, once every 3 months for the next 6 months, twice a year for the next 3 years, and yearly thereafter. Appropriate entries must be made on each occasion on the child's Road-to-Health Card. Weight should be taken to the nearest 10 g in infants and to the nearest 100 g in older children. Children should be weighed in minimal clothing. The weight of the child should be compared with standard height / weight-for-age charts, i.e., NCHS percentiles, due allowances being made for the normal variations. A single measurement tells little compared to the information obtained from serial measurements, which indicate the rate and direction of growth.

Height

Height or length of the child is measured at each visit. The length is measured in infants and children below 3 years of age, in a lying position, and height in older children in a standing position *(see Chapter 2, section on Techniques of Measurement)*. This measurement, together with weight, is not only a good assessment of the overall growth of the child, but also provides a record of the rate of growth for easy comparison with children of similar age in standard charts, i.e., NCHS* percentiles.
(*National Centre for Health Statistics Growth Charts, 1976. *Monthly Vital Statistics Report*. Vol. 25, No. 3 supp. (HFA) 76–1 120.)

Head circumference

The head circumference is determined routinely in the infant and child up to 2 years of age, and is ordinarily not obtained in children over 2 years. The head is measured with a non-stretchable tape measure at its greatest fronto-occipital circumference, and compared with standard normal values.

Temperature

A satisfactory temperature measurement can be obtained in children under 6 years of age by placing the thermometer in the axilla or groin, putting the arm or leg along the patient's body, and holding the limb against the thermometer for 3 minutes. In general, axillary or groin temperatures are about 1 °C lower than rectal, or 0.5 °C lower than oral temperatures. Oral temperature is suitable in older children. Rectal temperatures are best avoided, due to the real danger of perforating the bowel.

Conclusion

Some of the most common errors in examining children should be mentioned. They include:
- inadequate history-taking
- a history that is not appropriate to the child's age
- failure to observe the child
- inadequate inspection of the various organ systems before starting palpation, percussion, or auscultation
- failure to plot height and weight on growth charts and to measure head circumference in infants and younger children
- failure to determine the blood pressure
- failure to observe the gait
- skimpy neurological examination
- failure to examine the genitalia because of modesty on the part of the patient or reluctance on the part of the health professional.

Although many issues raised in this presentation may appear trivial to the uninitiated, the experienced practitioner who values rapport with children and parents uses all or most of the manoeuvres and approaches discussed.

Examination of the newborn
(Also see Chapter 5, Newborns.)

Introduction

As a general rule newborn babies should be examined on at least three occasions. The first examination is in the labour ward, with a two-fold objective:
- to establish the need for resuscitation, and
- to establish whether the baby is normal.

The second examination is usually within 24 hours of delivery, once the baby has settled down and stabilized. The final examination is on discharge of the infant.

Physical examination

The physical examination of the newborn is conducted very much along the lines discussed earlier in this chapter. There is no need to worry about patient co-operation, as this is non-existent. The baby should be kept warm, and the examiner's hands should be warm and disinfected. The examination can proceed systematically from the head downwards.

The evaluation of the newborn should always be in relation to the history of the pregnancy and the delivery. Detailed history of any illness, infection, or medications taken during pregnancy and delivery should be elicited. Details of the various stages of the labour, progress of the labour, the presenting part, evidence of fetal distress, and the method of delivery should also be obtained.

In the labour ward

The aim of the physical examination at this stage is to determine whether or not the baby needs to be resuscitated. This is assessed by using the Apgar score at one minute and at five minutes after birth *(see Chapter 5, Newborns)*.

It must also be ascertained whether the baby is normal. The examination is restricted to gross physical anomalies, and is therefore simple. Minor abnormalities include abnormal size, shape, and position of the ears; size and shape of the mouth; size of the tongue in relation to the mouth; asymmetry of the chest; and a scaphoid abdomen, indicating perhaps a diaphragmatic hernia. The sex of the infant and any ambiguity of the external genitalia must be noted. The hands and feet must be examined to exclude syndactyly, and the fingers and toes counted to exclude polydactyly. The anus should be inspected and the patency determined in all cases. It is extremely embarrassing to be informed by the mother on the second or third day after delivery that the baby has an abnormality of the anal orifice.

In the nursery

Signs and symptoms of illness are minimal in the newborn, even in the presence of life-threatening illness. The aims of the routine physical examination of the various systems are:

◆ to exclude any abnormalities that may have been missed during the relatively superficial examination done in the labour ward

◆ to assess the baby's gestational age *(see Chapter 5, Newborns)*, and

◆ to make sure that the baby is not acutely ill.

The routine physical examination of the various systems is best performed after the baby has been

fed. Each system should be observed and examined systematically as described previously.

Only by recognizing normal findings can the important abnormalities be identified. It is essential that all findings should be evaluated in terms of normal and abnormal, and it is therefore important to know the normal values for the newborn, as follows:

◆ average weight:

white male	3 400 g
white female	3 000 g
black male	3 200 g
black female	2 800 g

◆ average length: 51 cm (range 46–53 cm)

◆ average head circumference: 35 cm (range 33–37 cm)

◆ respiratory rate: 40–60/min

◆ heart rate: average 120 beats/min (range 80–160/min).

The following findings are almost invariably present in all newborns:

General: The full-term infant is fairly active, with movements of all four limbs, a good tone, pink colour, but often with peripheral cyanosis in the first day or two of life. The skin is covered with a thick, white, cheesy substance — vernix caseosa — which will dry and fall off as a powder after several hours. 'Stork bites' or telangiectatic naevi (fine spider-like naevi) are present over the nape of the neck, the glabella, and the upper eyelids. They are deep pink and flat, blanch easily, and disappear during the first years of life. The mongolian spot is an irregular area of blue-grey slate pigmentation distributed over the sacral and gluteal regions. It may, however, be so extensive as to involve much of the infant's back, and is extremely common in darkly pigmented infants.

Milia are white pin-point spots over the bridge of the nose, chin, or cheeks, and are due to retained sebum. Erythema toxicum are small macules on a red base starting on the second or third day of life and disappearing within a few days. The cause is unknown.

Head: Moulding of the head depends on the type of delivery: asymmetrical moulding of the face may occur as the result of posture during pregnancy; overriding of the sutures of the parietal, frontal, and occipital bones is secondary to the moulding of the skull. Caput succedaneum is oedema of the presenting part of the scalp, secondary to pressure of the pelvic brim, and results in a soft, non-fluctuant swelling of that part of the head. There are six fontanelles at birth. The two most important are the anterior and posterior fontanelles, which should be examined to determine their size and tension.

Mouth, tongue, palate, and teeth: Occasionally babies are born with one or two teeth. Epstein's pearls are small white nodules on the hard palate on either side of the midline. Retention cysts may occur on the gum margins. A partial cleft of the posterior soft palate has to be excluded by palpation.

Eyes: Redness of the conjunctiva and oedema of the eyelids due to chemical irritation are common. Subconjunctival haemorrhages may be seen, particularly if the delivery was difficult.

Respiratory system: The normal respiratory rate is at least 40 breaths per minute. Breathing is quiet, thoracic-abdominal breathing. Expansion is symmetrical and the air entry is good. No adventitious sounds should be heard.

It must be stressed that the **respiratory rate** is the most significant of these signs, as auscultation may be normal in the prescence of signifcant pathology.

Abdomen: Respiratory movements are mostly abdominal, and the liver is usually palpable 2–3 cm below the right costal margin. The tip of the spleen may be palpable in some infants. The lower end of both kidneys can be palpated in thin infants, or with complete relaxation of the abdominal muscles.

Neurological system: There are a number of primitive reflexes that can be elicited in the newborn and young infant *(see Chapter 5, Newborns)*. Abnormal responses include an absent or asymmetric response, or persistence of a reflex after the age at which it usually disappears.

The primitive reflexes are:
- *The grasp reflex* is elicited by placing a finger in either the palm of the hand from the ulnar side, or the sole of the foot, resulting in reflex flexion and grasping of the finger.
- *The rooting reflex* is elicited by stroking the lip with the finger, resulting in the turning of the infant's head to the side of the stimulus.
- *The moro reflex* is elicited by a sudden movement of the head in relation to the position of the

spine. The normal response is extension and abduction of the arms and legs, followed by adduction of the arms and flexion of the elbows and fingers across the chest.
- *Sucking* is usually strong in the term infant and weak in the pre-term.
- *Swallowing* is well co-ordinated with sucking by 35 weeks of gestational age.
- *Deep tendon reflexes* that may be elicited are the brachial, knee, and plantar.

Levels of consciousness may be classified as normal, alert, drowsy, or sleeping. Abnormal states are hyperactivity, stupor, or coma.

Tone is assessed symmetrically as normal, floppy, or increased flexor or extensor tone.

Cranial nerves are assessed by the eye movements, pupillary responses, normal facial movement, swallowing, and a normal cry.

Vision is assessed by the response to following a bright light. Response to a loud noise suggests hearing ability.

Problem-oriented case notes

The conventional method of recording history, physical examination findings, diagnosis, and investigations in patients' case notes is flawed. There is too great an emphasis on diagnosis and differential diagnosis. Attempts are made to fit all signs and symptoms into one diagnosis, and fine nuances of disease expression which deviate from well-known patterns are ignored. The older methods do not pay sufficient attention to the main reasons for the patient seeking medical assistance — namely 'problems'. Often these problems require individual management, e.g., fever, pain in the joints, and skin rash in a child with meningococcal meningitis. If all the problems of the patient are the result of one disease defined by a single diagnosis, the conventional approach may be satisfactory. However, in many cases this is not so, and the child's signs, symptoms, or abnormal laboratory findings cannot be accounted for in one diagnosis. In developing countries, children often present with many problems and multiple diagnoses, all requiring separate management, e.g., marasmus, vitamin A deficiency, septicaemia, candidiasis, and emotional deprivation.

For all the above reasons, problem-oriented case notes are superior to traditional medical records. This approach includes the following:

♦ information gathering
♦ defining problems
♦ assessment/diagnosis
♦ plan of action
♦ progress notes
♦ discharge summary

Information-gathering

Information is obtained through:

♦ history
♦ physical examination
♦ bedside tests.

Taken together these will provide a provisional list of problems (e.g., swelling of eyelids, raised blood pressure, rash, haematuria, and proteinuria), and possibly even allow a tentative diagnosis (acute glomerulonephritis) to be made. More detailed investigations can lead to a complete diagnosis (post-streptococcal glomerulonephritis with hypertension and oedema). In addition to the *routine* aspects of history and physical examination (i.e., screening), the investigator should *direct the enquiry specifically* to problems or diagnoses (e.g., to the character of cough, to the clinical features of chronic liver disease in a child with jaundice).

Defining problems

This definition is based on all the data gathered above and may therefore be very wide-ranging. It can be medical, psychosocial, educational, social; it may be a symptom, sign, or abnormality detected on investigation. The following is not unusual as a list of problems in a single patient:

i. diarrhoea
ii. underweight
iii. convulsions
iv. hypoglycaemia
v. mental retardation
vi. family: single-parent

vii. unemployed mother.

Assessment/diagnosis

This is the process of establishing coherence, or finding a minimum of explanations or diagnoses for a multiplicity of problems detected. In the example given above the most likely diagnosis is acute gastroenteritis in a malnourished child, complicated by anorexia and hypoglycaemic fits. Malnutrition is probably related to cerebral palsy and a socially dislocated family.

Plan of action

This involves investigations and treatment (both curative and rehabilitative).

Progress notes

Progress notes relate to those problems previously identified. For example, in relation to those cited above, comment is called for only as regards problems where there has been 'progress', for example:

i. Diarrhoea — 5–7 watery stools persist.
ii. Hypoglycaemia — Dextrostix® normal for past 24 hours.
iii. Mother seen by social worker.

These notes are specifically problem-oriented, and screening procedures are done only cursorily. Notes include:

♦ history of progress in current problems
♦ physical examination directed to problems; quick screening
♦ laboratory tests
♦ assessment of problems
♦ plan of action for resolving problems.

Discharge summary

This is essential, as it provides an opportunity to make sense of the data and progress, and encourages rational thinking about clinical problems.

C.H. van Niekerk
H.M. Coovadia

2

Growth and development

Growth is a function of several often interrelated factors: genetic, nutritional, psychosocial, and medical. All those involved in child health and development should ensure that growth and development are monitored by means of established tests which screen for deviations from the norm.

◆ Standardized tables or charts are used to assess weight, length or height, skull circumference, and growth velocity.

◆ Normal development in early childhood is assessed according to achievement in the areas of locomotion, fine motor adaptation, language, and personal/social development.

◆ Puberty is the sequence of clearly defined biological stages through which the individual is transformed into an adult.

◆ Adolescence is the period following puberty, during which all the dimensions of growth, development, and maturity are completed.

General principles

The health of the adult is in part determined by his/her health as a child; the growth and development of one generation affects the next generation. The well-being of the child is therefore central to life. Closely related to the health of the child is the health of the mother.

The normal growth, development, and maturation of the healthy child from fetal life to adulthood are continuous and dynamic interrelated processes. They take place in tissues, organs, regions, systems, and in the different physiological and chemical functions of the body at different rates and velocities *(see Fig. 2.1)*. The sequence in which they proceed is largely predictable and similar for all children. These dimensions may vary considerably during intrauterine life, infancy, the toddler period, pre-school childhood, prepubertal and pubertal childhood, adolescence, and adulthood *(see Fig. 2.2)*. Some stages are characterized by sensitive periods with specific requirements, such as adequate nutrition and appropriate

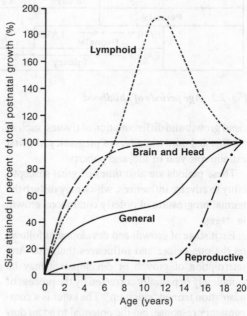

Growth curves of different parts and tissues of the body, showing the four chief types. All the curves are of size attained, and plotted as percentage of total gain from birth to 20 years, so that size at age 20 is 100 on the vertical scale.
Lymphoid type: thymus, lymph nodes, intestinal lymph masses.
Brain and head type: brain and its parts, dura, spinal cord, optic apparatus, cranial dimensions.
General type: body as a whole, external dimensions (except head), respiratory and digestive organs, kidneys, aortic and pulmonary trunks, musculature, blood volume.
Reproductive type: testis, ovary, epididymis, prostate, seminal vesicles, fallopian tubes.

Fig 2.1 Differences in the growth curves of different parts and tissues of the body
(From Tanner, J.M. 1962. *Growth at Adolescence* (2nd edition). Oxford: Blackwell Scientific Publications. Redrawn from Scammon, 1930.)

stimulation to ensure normal progression; other stages are characterized by a slowing down or acceleration of the rate of growth and/or development. Normal progression from one stage to the next can only take place if specific biological, emotional, and social needs are met. These are especially important during vulnerable periods of fetal life and childhood which are characterized by

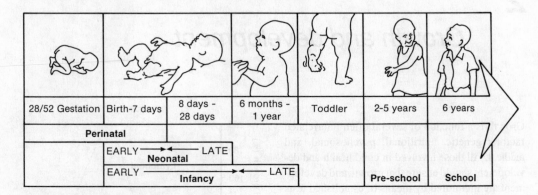

28/52 Gestation	Birth-7 days	8 days - 28 days	6 months - 1 year	Toddler	2-5 years	6 years

Fig. 2.2   Age periods of childhood

rapid growth and differentiation of tissues, such as the first and third trimesters of pregnancy, the first extrauterine year of life, and puberty.

These periods are also times of great susceptibility to adverse influences, which may disturb the normal progression of orderly continuous growth in stages.

Each stage of growth and development follows on the one before and influences the next. Any interruption of growth or development may be completely or partially corrected by the process of adaptation termed 'catch-up'. The latter is a compensatory response, but the potential to adapt during childhood diminishes with recurring insults and with age.

Food and energy for biosynthesis are essential for normal growth. In developing countries, lack of food must be regarded as the major factor which may adversely affect the growth and development of childhood populations. In large families of lower socio-economic status there is a relationship between family size and short stature, possibly because there is less food available. Inter-relationships between various factors must also be considered, e.g., while nutritional deprivation is likely to occur under poor socio-economic conditions, both of these factors will influence outcome. In other words, factors besides food may influence the growth of a child, and emotional, social, and environmental deprivation affect growth and development both directly and indirectly. In situations where siblings have to compete for parental care and love, growth may be adversely affected. Such deprivation is often brought about by circumstances beyond the control

of the mother, which may lead to a vicious cycle comprising a lack of well-being, physical and emotional exhaustion, poverty, and an inability to give proper care to her infant. Factors which inhibit socio-economic development, such as family disruption, unwanted (or too many) pregnancies, poverty, famine, war, and civil unrest may all affect the health of a mother. Under these circumstances her inability to meet the biological, emotional, and social needs of her children may have a profound influence on their growth and development.

Height and secular trend in growth

Height or stature is one of the most heritable traits recognized in people. Given an adequate environment, the height of an individual child bears a significant relationship to his or her genetic background, as exemplified by the height of the parents. Genetic background also influences the rate of maturation, and therefore the length of time required to achieve adult size.

In developing countries, in contrast to developed countries, growth takes place over a longer period, and final height may be attained at a later stage. This is an important factor when comparing the height or stature of childhood populations in developing countries with those in developed countries. This changing growth pattern in the past one or two hundred years is referred to as the *secular trend*. During this period there has been a profound change in the pace of maturation and, to a lesser extent, the ultimate size of individuals in

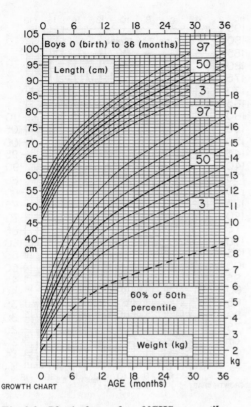

Fig. 2.3 Physical growth — NCHS percentiles.
Boys: birth to 36 months

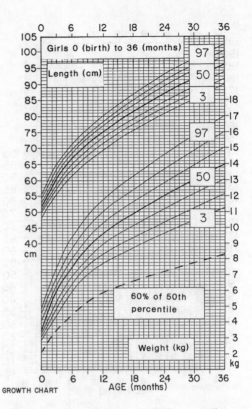

Fig. 2.4 Physical growth — NCHS percentiles.
Girls: birth to 36 months

developed countries. Faster maturation has resulted in greater increments of growth and a larger
size-for- age during childhood, and in an earlier
advent of adolescence and final height attainment.
A century ago the average male did not reach final
height until the age of 23 years; he now reaches it
by 13 to 17 years. These changes can probably be
attributed to a decrease in growth-inhibiting
factors such as poor childhood nutrition, chronic
childhood disease, and genetic outbreeding.

This trend is well illustrated among a section of
socially-advantaged Indian South Africans who
over time have reduced many of the growth-
inhibiting environmental factors prevalent in the
native land of their forefathers and who have
children whose heights and weights are similar to
the NCHS standards.

Chronic states of ill health in childhood may
also affect growth, development, and maturation.
These include:

◆ infections

◆ congenital defects
◆ emotional illness
◆ metabolic abnormalities
◆ endocrine disturbances
◆ disability or handicap.

Their effects depend on both the severity and
duration of such conditions. Acute illnesses, however, do not retard development, and even major
diseases may be followed by a growth spurt.

Definitions and terminology

Growth implies an increase in the size, composition, and distribution of tissues. It is associated
with changes in their proportions, shape, and functions.

The **rate** at which a process takes place is a
record of its measurement at a point in time, i.e.,
age in terms of its relation to a reference standard
for that age.

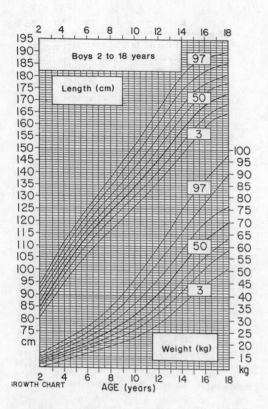

Fig. 2.5 Physical growth — NCHS percentiles. Boys: 2 to 18 years

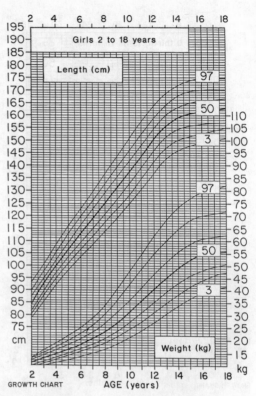

Fig 2.6 Physical growth — NCHS percentiles. Girls: 2 to 18 years

The **velocity** or speed at which the process takes place may be measured over a period of time and is expressed as the rate of change between measurements per unit of time. Rate and velocity are employed for the assessment of the growth of one or more children over a period of time, and its speed at a given age or phase of growth. A growth spurt implies an increase in growth velocity. Growth lag refers to a decrease in the rate or velocity of normal expected growth.

Catch-up growth is a return towards the size that would have been attained if the growth lag had not occurred.

Development is the increases in the complexity of the structures and of their functions which take place in the same age period, and often in a parallel fashion. It is the product of the interaction between the processes of maturation and learning.

Gross motor (locomotion) is the progression of abilities which ultimately enable the child to

assume an upright posture and perform skilled activities while maintaining posture and equilibrium.

Fine motor (manipulation) and adaptive behaviour: Fine motor development refers to a series of skills which develop through a visually guided ability to grasp, use thumbs and fingers accurately, and the transition from unilateral to bimanual manipulation. Adaptive behaviour places these skills in the context of the environment and includes the ability to initiate new experience and to profit from past experience.

Language/communication: Communication refers to the transmission of meaningful symbols. Language is the primary medium of communication, and involves the formalization of thought.

Personal/social: Personal development is assessed on culturally monitored skills of daily living, and social development is behaviour which is

22

in accordance with social expectations. This is acquired through socialization.

A **milestone** is designated by usage as the 'age' at which a specific measurement is achieved, and varies considerably between children. The 'age' may be expressed in terms of the chronological, decimal, height, bone, or mental age.

Records of age

Chronological age is recorded in terms of years and months calculated from the birth date of the individual.

Corrected age is used to adjust for prematurity, particularly in very low birth weight infants (< 1 500 g) born 2–3 months prematurely. In correcting age for prematurity one 'gives back' the number of postnatal weeks required to bring the pregnancy to term, e.g., an infant born after 28 weeks and assessed at 12 weeks chronological age would be evaluated as a term infant (28+12 = 40 weeks corrected age), not as a 3-month-old. Correction is employed for at least the first year in such infants.

Bone age is a measurement of the osseous maturation in long bones (usually the hand and wrist).

Mental age is difficult to define in precise terms, but in essence it is what one child can manage in a large number of tests compared with the average achievements of a large number of children.

Standards

Standards produced for North American children in the form of tables or charts for length/height (stature), weight, and head circumference are preferred (National Centre for Health Statistics Growth Charts, 1976. *Monthly Vital Statistics Report* Vol. 25, No. 3 Supp. (HFA) 76–1120.)

In developing communities they can be used only as a basis for comparison and not for absolute assessment of physical growth. They have been compiled in an area where nutrition is often excessive and obesity, rather than under-nutrition, is a major disorder of childhood. North American children also grow at a faster tempo even than children in other developed countries, for instance Britain. Caution should also be exercised in assessing purely breast-fed infants, who commonly show a reduced growth velocity from birth to 6 months of age when compared with standard growth curves which are based on predominantly artificially-fed infants.

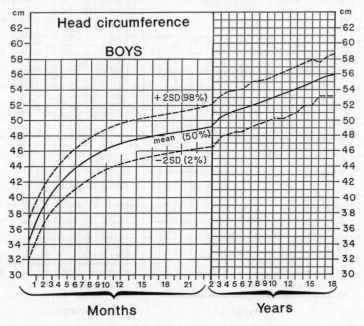

Fig. 2.7   Head circumference — NCHS percentiles. Boys: birth to 18 years

▶ The most important feature of growth charts is that they provide the health professional with a measure to compare and monitor the physical status of childhood populations, or of an individual child, on an ongoing basis.

The Road-to-Health Card *(Chapter 4, Community Paediatrics, Fig. 4.2)* has been introduced on a world-wide basis. One of its most significant assets is that it enables parents as well as health workers to see at a glance whether the child is gaining weight appropriately.

Centiles

There is a wide variation amongst children at any age in length or height, weight, and head circumference, and in the velocity of growth from one age to the next. This variation within the normal range at a given age is expressed conventionally as **centiles** or **percentiles,** i.e., 3rd (or 5th), 10th, 25th, 50th, 75th, 90th and 97th (or 95th), in columns and tables or as lines in charts, for boys and girls separately or combined. The centile lines are primarily designed for the longitudinal study of an infant or child, i.e., sequential study over a period of time. They are referred to as 'distance charts'.

Adapted NCHS charts, to include 3rd and 97th (or 5th and 95th) percentiles for length/height, weight, and head circumference, are given in *Figs 2.3 – 2.9.*

Understanding the meaning of a centile (or percentile) is important. It means that of the population of boys, for instance, from which at a given age centiles and percentiles were constructed for height, out of 100 boys, 3 would have measurements for height under the 3rd centile, 10 under the 10th centile, 50 under the 50th centile, and so on. At the the end of the scale, 97 boys would have measurements below the 97th percentile and only 3 above it. Height has a normal (Gaussian) distribution, and the 50th centile measurement therefore corresponds to the mean height of the population measured.

Velocity charts provide standards to compare the rate of growth. Contrary to longitudinal or distance studies, where an individual child tends to follow the same centile from infancy to adulthood, even the healthy child will not stay on the same velocity centile throughout growth, unless s/he is very close to the 50th. An example of a velocity chart for boys is shown in *Fig. 2.9.*

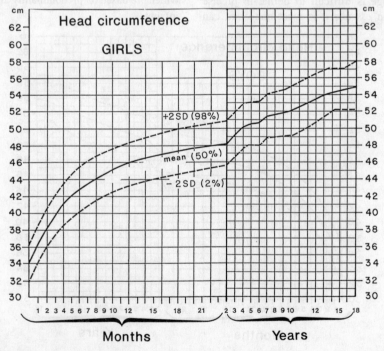

Fig 2.8   Head circumference — NCHS percentiles. Girls: birth to 18 years

Longitudinal and velocity charts and tables may be employed in child health screening programmes:

◆ to identify children in need of care, because of:
 – poor socio-economic and nutritional status
 – ineffective measures to promote family spacing and limit population growth
 – social and cultural attitudes disadvantageous to mother and child, and
◆ to measure:
 – response to management of a child with suboptimal growth
 – effectiveness of intervention programmes attempting to raise the standard of child health care. *(see Chapter 4, Road-to-Health Card, Fig. 4.2.)*

Normal growth patterns

In the normal child, values for height, weight, and skull circumference tend to conform and follow the same percentiles until puberty. Accurate longitudinal measurements plotted on a standard percentile chart are much more informative than single measurements. The influence of family patterns on growth measurements should always be considered in measurements which do not fall between the 3rd and 97th percentiles, but where they tend to follow the general percentile pattern of the standard chart. Reference has already been made to the influence of parental height.

A gross difference between values for the same child, such as a head circumference below the 3rd

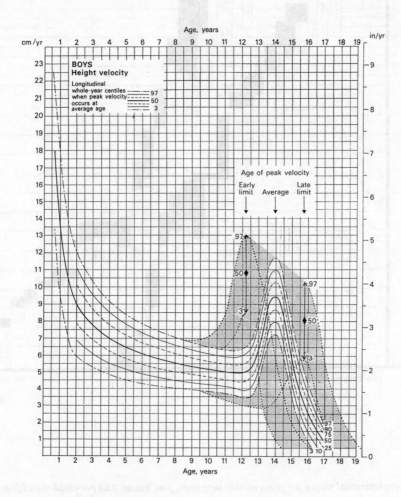

Fig. 2.9 Height velocity centile chart for boys

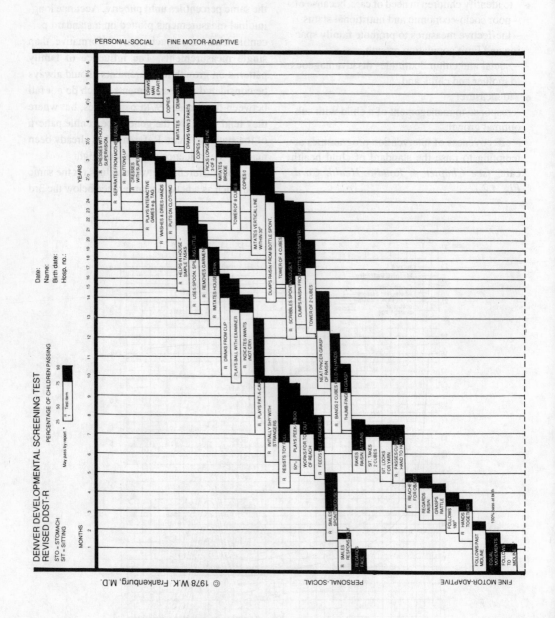

Fig. 2.10 *Developmental stages for gross motor, language, fine motor, and personal-social functions. (Adapted from Denver Developmental Screening Test)*

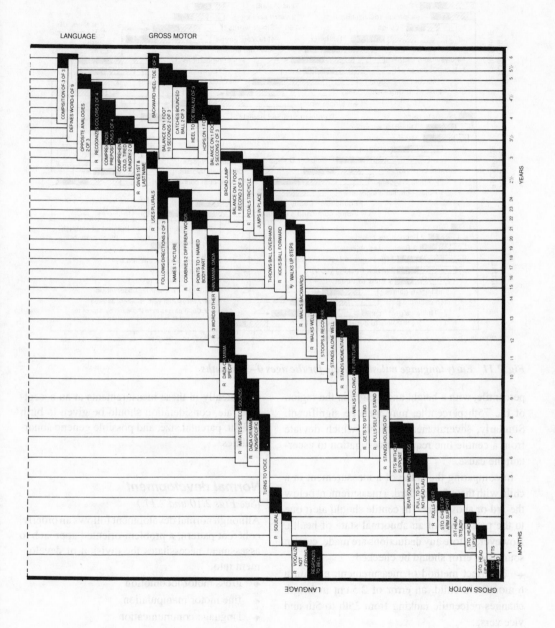

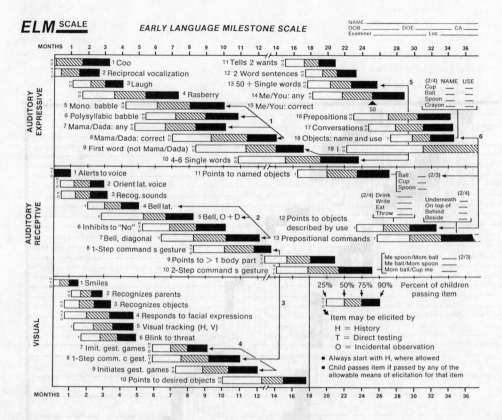

Fig. 2.11 Early language milestone scale for the ages 0–36 months

percentile, with a height and weight in the region of the 75th percentile, may well be significant. Similarly, several measurements which deviate from a centile line require investigation to ascertain the cause.

In comparing the value of a measurement in a child with that of a standard, a measurement below the 3rd or above the 97th centile should alert one to the possibility of an abnormal state of health. However, before any deductions are made, certain sources of error should be checked:

◆ incorrect method of measurement; e.g., in a 6-month-old child, an error of 2.5 cm in length changes percentile ranking from 25th to 5th and vice versa.

◆ incorrect assessment of age, e.g., rounding off 4½ months to 5 months

◆ failure to consider gestational age, i.e., to correct for prematurity.

In a child found to be consistently below the 3rd percentile for weight and height, but who gains

consistently in these measurements at an acceptable rate, consideration should be given to birth weight, parental size, and possible genetic abnormalities.

Normal development
(See Figs 2.10 and 2.11.)

Although normal development follows an orderly, coherent pattern, a problem-oriented approach to assessment necessitates the division of development into:

◆ gross motor/locomotion
◆ fine motor/manipulation
◆ language/communication
◆ personal/social aspects.

Locomotion

The newborn infant assumes a posture of general physiological flexor hypertonus, is relatively hypotonic, and has a number of **primitive reflexes,** e.g., Moro, grasp, placing and stepping, rooting and sucking.

During the first few months of life, apart from a general increase in tone (which may be assessed by noting a decrease in head lag on 'pull to sit'), **extensor facility** develops, which proceeds cephalo-caudally or proximo-distally. When lying prone at 6 weeks the infant can lift his chin off the bed; at 3 months can support himself on his elbows, and by 6 months he supports himself on extended arms. The Landau response (ventral suspension) similarly demonstrates the extensor facility, so that by 6 months there is extension of all joints of the body. Thereafter, the infant has to develop the ability to **break up total patterns of extension or flexion.** For example, before he can sit, he needs to extend his back and at the same time flex his hips.

The primitive reflexes must be suppressed before voluntary movements can commence. For example, the palmar grasp must disappear before the baby can bear weight on his forearms in the prone position; the Moro reflex must go before the postural reactions, which are necessary for sitting, appear; the symmetrical tonic neck reflex must go before crawling can commence; and the placing and stepping must disappear to allow walking.

As the primitive reflexes fade there is a progressive development of **postural reactions.** The *righting reactions* enable the infant to maintain a normal position of the head in space, as well as to align the head, neck, trunk, and limbs. The *equilibrium reactions* are automatic responses to change in posture, and act to restore balance. Once the child has righting reactions in sitting, kneeling, and standing positions, and equilibrium (parachute) responses sideways, forwards, and backwards, he is equipped to walk, and then run, jump, and climb.

Fine motor and adaptive behaviour

In the newborn infant, the **grasp reflex** dominates and the hands are held in a fisted position. By 2 months this should be disappearing, and the hands are open much of the time. Over the next 3 months, **visually guided reaching** matures, so that by 5 months the infant can reach for and grasp an object and then bring it to her mouth. This **mouthing** is an automatic response. At 6 months she is able to

transfer the object to the other hand. Reaching should be equally good with either hand, but until 7 months there is a midline barrier as far as hand use is concerned. This means that the infant is unable to retain an object in each hand simultaneously. By 8 months this becomes possible. Mouthing continues, but is more exploratory in nature.

At 6 months there is a **total (palmar) grasp**. Over the next few months the grasp becomes more **radial.** The child of 9–10 months will isolate and explore with her index finger. At the same time the **pincer-grasp** matures, and by 12 months there is an **apposition** of thumb and terminal phalanx of the index finger. At this stage the infant can usually release an object on request, and mouthing should be infrequent. Children of this age frequently enjoy throwing toys out of the cot. From 15 to 18 months, play becomes increasingly bimanual, and **manipulative skills** develop. These can be tested by block construction, puzzles, and formboards. During the next 3 years, **perceptual skills** and **sensory-motor integration** develop, and lay the foundation for activities required for schooling. Handedness appears after the age of a year, but may change over the next few years.

Language and communication

The newborn infant cries and is able to produce only a few throaty sounds. By 8 weeks he is capable of vowel sounds and vocalizes pleasure. Thereafter, the infant initiates sounds to which his caretakers respond with sensitive timing. This is referred to as 'vocal contagion'. At 20 weeks guttural sounds are produced, and by 32 weeks syllables are combined (babbling), e.g., baba, mama, dada. Soon after this, early concept formation can be demonstrated by 'object permanence'. The infant can retrieve hidden objects such as a block placed under a cup. Gradually the babbling sounds achieve meaning, so that by a year the baby has two to three meaningful 'words'.

Language development slows down for the next few months, but between 15 and 18 months the child shows the beginning of symbolization (inner language) by demonstrating definition by use, e.g., he will show by gesture that he understands the use of a brush, telephone, and so on. This heralds a new acceleration of language development, and by 18 months, two-word utterances

Table 2.1 Developmental characteristics related to adolescent health care needs

Task	Characteristics	Health care needs
	10 to 14-year-olds	
Puberty	Wide variation in rapid physical changes; self-consciousness	Confidentiality; privacy
Independence	Ambivalence	Support for growing autonomy
Identity	Am I normal?; peer group	Reassurance and positive attitude
Thinking	Concrete operational; egocentric; imaginary audience; lack of insight; focus on present	Emphasis on immediate consequences of actions
	15 to 16 -year-olds	
Puberty	Females more comfortable; males more awkward; chronic illness delays puberty	Emotional support for patients who vary from 'normal'
Independence	Limit-testing; noncompliance; 'experimental' behaviours; dating	Consistency; limit-setting
Identity	Who am I?; introspection; global issues	Nonjudgemental acceptance
Thinking	Concrete—formal operational; personal fable; experiments with ideas	Problem-solving; decision-making; education
	17 to 20 -year -olds	
Puberty	Adult appearance; slow change	Minimal needs except in chronic illness
Independence	Ambivalence about real independence, separation from family	Support
Identity	Who am I with respect to others, sexuality, education, job?	Encouragement of identity allowing maximal growth
Thinking	Formal operational; contemplation of future; introspection, commitments	Approach as adult

(From Behrman, R.E., and Kliegman, R. 1990. *Essentials of Peditatrics.* Philadelphia: W.B. Saunders.)

commence. At 2 years he is capable of short phrases and of using pronouns. A 3-year-old has an extensive vocabulary and chats incessantly. Immature articulation is common at this stage, but by 5 years articulation errors have disappeared and the child uses full sentences.

Personal and social development

The important bonding process between mother and child commences soon after birth. By 6 weeks the infant responds to her mother with a smile.

She gradually becomes more sociable, and a 3- to 4-month-old infant smiles and vocalizes freely with strangers. At 6 months she responds to her image in a mirror, usually by patting it. The age of 8–9 months, however, sees the onset of stranger anxiety.

Once on her feet, her world expands and she becomes increasingly explorative. Domestic mimicry commences between 15 and 18 months, as she copies her caretaker's daily activities. A 2-year-old plays alone or in parallel fashion if with other children. Group activities commence after 3 years, and usually involve two to three children. By the age of 5 years, group play is frequent, although the size of the groups remains relatively small (three to five members). However, play is symbolic in that the child identifies herself as someone else, e.g., the farmer, the shopkeeper.

A bottle-fed 3-month-old infant will attempt to hold the bottle. By 6 months she can chew, and by 8 months can drink from a cup if it is held. She can also hold and eat a biscuit. At 15 months she will attempt to use a spoon, but will spill most of the food, whereas by 18 months very little is spilt. At 18 months a cup is handled well.

Soon after she is a year old, the child will help in dressing by pushing her arm into a sleeve. At 18 months she can pull up her pants. A 3-year-old will dress alone, but needs help with buttons. By 4–5 years she can dress without supervision.

An 18-month-old child indicates to her mother that her nappy is wet or dirty. By 24 months sphincter control enables her to be clean and dry by day. Full toilet training is usually achieved by 3 years.

Development is fairly predictable, although it does manifest a wide range of normality.

Adolescence

Early, middle, and late adolescence are characterized by different behavioural and developmental issues *(see Table 2.1)*. The age at which each issue becomes manifest and the importance of the issue will vary widely among individuals, as will the rates of cognitive, psychosexual, psychosocial, or physical development.

Early adolescence: This stage is characterized by maximal somatic and sexual growth. Thinking is focused on the present and on the peer group. Identity is focused primarily on the physical changes, and concern is about normality. Exploratory, undifferentiated sexual behaviour, resulting in physical contact with like-sexed peers, is normal during early adolescence, although heterosexual interests can also develop. Strivings for independence are ambivalent.

Middle adolescence: This can be a most difficult time for both adolescents and the adults who have contact with them. Cognitive processes are more sophisticated. This stage is characterized by experimentation with ideas, consideration of alternative approaches to problems, development of insight, and reflection on personal feelings and those of others. As they mature cognitively and psychosocially, middle adolescents focus on issues of identity not limited solely to the physical aspects of the body. As middle adolescents socialize with peers, experiment sexually, engage in risk-taking behaviour, and develop employment and interests outside the home, they augment their unique, developing identities. As a result of experimental risk-taking behaviour, they may ex-

perience unwanted pregnancies, drug abuse, or motor vehicle accidents. Middle adolescents' strivings for independence, testing of limits, and need for autonomy are maximal, and often distressing to their families, teachers, or other authority figures.

Late adolescence: This period is usually characterized by full formal, operational thinking, including thoughts about the future (educationally, vocationally, and sexually). Late adolescents are usually more committed to their sexual partners than are middle adolescents. Unresolved separation anxiety from previous developmental stages may emerge at this time, as the young person begins to move physically away from the family of origin.

Factors affecting growth and development

Growth and development are products of constitutional and hereditary factors, on the one hand, and of the environment, experience, and circumstances to which the individual is exposed, on the other. The 'nature-nurture' controversy centres on the relative contributions of heredity and environment. However, the issue is resolved when it is considered that nature provides the potential which will be fulfilled, given a favourable environment (nurture)*(see Fig. 2.12)*.

Intrauterine period

During intrauterine life, maternal influences play an important part in the growth of the fetus.

The size of a full-term infant correlates with maternal ◄

◆ size
◆ weight
◆ nutrition
◆ socio-economic status.

Small babies are born to pregnant women who ◄

◆ suffer infections
◆ smoke cigarettes
◆ drink alcohol
◆ have a medical problem, e.g., hypertension; renal, cardiac, or respiratory disease.

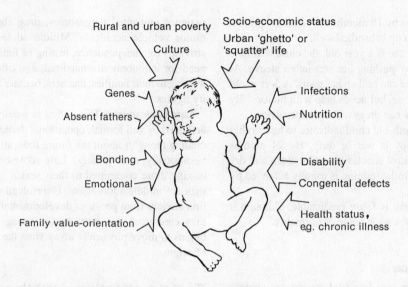

Fig. 2.12 Factors affecting growth, development, and maturation

The smaller babies of primiparous compared to multiparous women, and the known progressive deceleration in the growth rate of twins after 30 weeks of gestation, reflect the restraint placed on late fetal growth by uterine size. The unequal size of monozygotic twins due to pathological lesions of the placenta, such as vascular anastomoses, demonstrates the importance of this structure for intrauterine fetal growth. Male babies are heavier than female babies. This faster later fetal growth rate of the male compared to that of the female takes place mainly in the third trimester, and continues during the first 3–6 months of infancy. From then on there is no appreciable difference in the growth rate of the sexes until the beginning of puberty.

Hereditary and constitutional factors
At conception every human being is provided with a unique genetic and chromosomal composition which is responsible for determining sex, race, and physical characteristics. Genetic inheritance also determines the individual's potential and limitations. Uni-ovular twin studies have indicated that heredity plays a part in personality traits. However, temperament — manifested as the behavioural style of the child — is influenced by child-rearing practices, as well as by the continuous interaction between parents and children.

Postnatal period
The major part of infancy is characterized by a rapid growth rate which becomes increasingly related to the genetic background. The infant at 12 months is more than 50% larger and about three times heavier than at birth. The period of rapid growth is followed during late infancy and the early toddler period by a more consistent growth rate of 5–7.5 cm yearly in the pre-school and pre-pubertal schoolchild. The deposition of fat, which may be striking during infancy, becomes less marked, but increases 2–3 years before the onset of puberty. The latter is associated with striking, increased changes in the growth rate. These are then followed by deceleration, until the cessation in linear growth is reached by 18–21 years of age, with the ossification of the epiphyses of the long bones.

Acquired factors
Nutritional status
Growth is affected by nutrition. Linear growth, expressed as length or height measurement, is a sensitive indicator of the physical health of an infant or child or, collectively, of the health of the children in a community or population. The adequacy of catch-up growth, which follows the correction of the cause of a growth deficiency, will depend on the age of the individual and on the

aetiology, severity, and duration of such a deficiency prior to corrective therapy. Small-for-gestational-age infants due to chronic alcoholism in the mother fail to show catch-up growth, whereas prenatal growth deficiency because of uterine constraint, e.g., twins, usually demonstrates a satisfactory catch-up growth period after birth. When growth deficiency is of postnatal onset, as during infancy due to malnutrition, there may be dramatic catch-up growth following the correction of the infant's nutritional status.

Animal and human studies clearly indicate that malnutrition affects not only physical growth, but also other dimensions (see Chapter 7, Nutritional Disorders).

Health status

The physical and emotional health status of the child and of his family may have a direct or indirect effect on his growth and development. Chronic illness often leads to disability and may result in handicap. In addition, chronic illness is usually accompanied by prolonged or repeated hospitalization. The problems faced by parents of

such a chronically disabled child include uncertainty, chronic sorrow, stigma, and a 'burden of care' which may affect their attitude to the child.

Central nervous system dysfunction, as well as having effects similar to those of any chronic illness, is also often associated with motor and intellectual retardation.

Socio-economic status

Poverty, poor education, and social adversity increase the possibility of having a complication of pregnancy and are associated with an increased risk of low birth weight infants. Many long-term studies have shown that social class can have a major effect on various aspects of a child's growth, performance, and on the incidence of handicap. In addition, social class is of predictive value for different child-rearing styles and practices. Lower-class parents tend to use physical punishment, ridicule, and to emphasize conformity to external standards. Middle-class parents, on the other hand, are more likely to use reason and to stress autonomy and self-direction.

RECOMMENDATIONS FOR PREVENTIVE PEDIATRIC HEALTH CARE

Each child and family is unique; therefore these **Recommendations for Preventive Pediatric Health Care** are designed for the care of children who are receiving competent parenting, have no manifestations of any important health problems, and are growing and developing in satisfactory fashion. **Additional visits may become necessary** if circumstances suggest variations from normal. These guidelines represent a consensus with the membership of the American Academy of Pediatrics through the Chapter Presidents. The Committee emphasizes the great importance of continuity of **care** in

comprehensive health supervision and the need to avoid **fragmentation of care.**

A **prenatal visit** by the parents for anticipatory guidance and pertinent medical history is strongly recommended.

Health supervision should begin with medical care of the newborn in the hospital.

	INFANCY						EARLY CHILDHOOD					LATE CHILDHOOD					ADOLESCENCE[1]			
AGE[2]	By 1 mo	2 mos	4 mos	6 mos	9 mos	12 mos	15 mos	18 mos	24 mos	3 yrs	4 yrs	5 yrs	6 yrs	8 yrs	10 yrs	12 yrs	14 yrs	16 yrs	18 yrs	20+ yrs
HISTORY Initial/Interval	•	•	•	•	•	•	•	•	•	•	•	•	•	•	•	•	•	•	•	•
MEASUREMENTS Height and Weight	•	•	•	•	•	•	•	•	•	•	•	•	•	•	•	•	•	•	•	•
Head Circumference	•	•	•	•	•	•														
Blood Pressure										•	•	•	•	•	•	•	•	•	•	•
SENSORY SCREENING Vision	S	S	S	S	S	S	S	S	S	S	O	O	O	O	O	S	O	O	O	O
Hearing	S	S	S	S	S	S	S	S	S	S	O	O	S3	S3	S3	O	S	S	O	S
DEVELOP/BEHAV[4] ASSESSMENT	•	•	•	•	•	•	•	•	•	•	•	•	•	•	•	•	•	•	•	•
PHYSICAL EXAMINATION[5]	•	•	•	•	•	•	•	•	•	•	•	•	•	•	•	•	•	•	•	•

Key: • = to be performed; S = Subjective, by history; O = Objective, by a standard testing method.

1. Adolescent related issues (e.g. psychosocial, emotional, substance usage, and reproductive health) may necessitate more frequent health supervision.
2. If a child comes under care for the first time at any point on the schedule, or if any items are not accomplished at the suggested age, the schedule should be brought up to date at the earliest possible time.
3. At these points, history may suffice; if problem suggested, a standard testing method should be employed.
4. By history and appropriate physical examination: if suspicious, by specific objective developmental testing.
5. At each visit, a complete physical examination is essential, with infant totally unclothed, older children undressed and suitably draped.

Fig 2.13 Recommendations for preventive paediatric health care

Cultural

Cross-cultural studies have shown variation in developmental patterns. For example, the motor precocity of African infants when compared to those in Europe or America is well documented. This raises the possibility of genetic differences in child development. However, child-rearing beliefs and practices vary markedly from one culture to another. There is evidence to suggest that in the case of precocity among African infants, specific training in certain skills is responsible. In contrast, cultures in which swaddling is practised during the first year are associated with delay in gross motor development.

The child with abnormal growth

When dealing with child in whom abnormal growth has been identified from the history and clinical examination, including measurements of body proportions, the next step is to decide whether the child looks 'normal' or 'abnormal'. The growth and appearance of the child, however, should always be compared to immediate family members.

Disturbed height and growth in the 'normal looking' child may be due to:

♦ extreme variations in normal growth
♦ genetic disorders
♦ environmental causes
♦ systemic or endocrine disorders.

In the 'abnormal-looking' child, dysmorphic syndromes and conditions giving rise to abnormal body proportions should be considered:

	Trunk	Limbs
Hypothyroidism	Normal	Some shortening*
Chondrodystrophy	Normal	Short*
Spondyloepiphyseal dysplasia	Short	Normal

*(affecting metaphyses and epiphyses of long bones)

The next step is to plot the height-age, the height-for-bone-age and the measured height-for-chronological-age on an NCHS chart for the appropriate sex. From these plots, various reasons for the abnormal stature of the child may become apparent (see Table 2.2).

Growth failure in poor communities — protein-energy malnutrition

Children with weights below the 3rd percentile in a developing country should for practical purposes be regarded as being at risk both for morbidity and mortality. In this weight range, they are more likely to have a low serum albumin level, a raised total body water approaching that of a newborn baby, delayed bone age, and are liable to infection. In general, they come from homes with a poor social background. Their bodily reserves to cope with the energy demands of stress (such as measles) are low, and this may lead to kwashiorkor. There is also growing evidence that the child below the 3rd centile may have a diminished IQ and perform less well at school. (Also see Chapter 7, Nutritional Disorders.)

Excess growth in rich communities — obesity

Conversely, in developed countries or in the wealthier socio-economic population groups of developing countries, nutrition may be excessive, resulting in obesity and its associated hazards of hypertension, vascular disease, and increased mortality. The problem, however, is that it may be difficult to detect those infants or children who, unless correctly managed, will become obese adults. There are no generally accepted definitions of obesity in children, except that it is associated with excess fat. Methods used for attempting to classify obesity are all based on relationships between weight and height, or on skinfold measurements, but none is satisfactory. (Also see Chapter 7, Nutritional Disorders.)

Assessment

The basic components for the assessment of physical growth involve measurements of length or height (stature), weight, and head circumference. A number of other standard measurements are also often used by the clinician. They include recording the sizes of the anterior and posterior fontanelles, changes in body proportions, skinfold thickness, mid-upper-arm circumference, eruption of teeth, and physical changes associated with puberty.

A modified schedule of assessment is shown in Fig. 2.13. The complete set of recommendations published by the American Academy of Pediatrics includes additional screening tests and procedures which are beyond the scope of this chapter.

Table 2.2 Growth patterns in the child with small stature

Pattern	Possible causes	Action
Height < 3rd percentile Bone age = chronological age Velocity normal or low-normal	Genetic short stature Dysmorphic syndromes Chondrodystrophies	No investigations
Height < 3rd percentile Bone age = height age Velocity normal	Constitutional delay Mild undernutrition	No investigations Follow-up for 1–2 years or until puberty
Height < 3rd percentile but no, or minimal, deviation Bone age = height age, but both significantly retarded Velocity low-normal or abnormally slow	Extreme constitutional delay Sytemic disease Long-standing undernutrition Mild endocrine deficiencies	Full investigations if the cause is not obvious
Break in the height growth curve	Acquired systemic disease	Full investigation if the cause is not obvious
Height < 3rd percentile Bone age markedly retarded Velocity abnormally slow	Long-standing congenital or systemic diseases or endocrinopathies	Full investigation if the cause is not obvious
Height < 3rd percentile associated with prepubertal slowing Bone age = height age Velocity steady with no acceleration	Non-pathological delayed puberty	No investigations required but follow-up and reassessment
Pubertal delay	General: chronic illness	Appropriate management

In female:
  No breast development by 13 yrs
    or > 5 years between the onset of breast development and menarche
 	
In male:
  No testicular enlargement by 13½ yrs
    or > 5 years between initiation and completion of genital growth
	Physiological:
	  Familial constitutional delay
	Hypothalamo-pituitary:
	  Hypogonadotrophic Hypogonadism
	
	Hypopituitarism (idiopathic, tumour)
	
	Gonadal:
	  Gonadal dysgenesis
	  Klinefelter's syndrome
	  Cryptorchidism
		Full investigation
		
		Refer to an appropriate specialist centre

Techniques of measurement

Length and height are most accurately measured by specially constructed apparatuses. These are expensive, and the following techniques are more commonly employed:

Length

Length is recorded from birth to 2 years using a firm, horizontal board with a fixed vertical head-piece and a sliding vertical footpiece. A scale is fixed along the length of the board. Two observers are required. The infant is measured in the supine position with the ankles gently pulled to stretch the infant, the knees flat, the head against the head-piece and the sliding footpiece in firm contact with the soles of the feet held vertically. The head must be held firmly in line with the body and with the lower orbital border in the same vertical plane as the external auditory canal. The distance between the headpiece and footpiece is recorded. Length and height are measured to the nearest 0.1 cm.

Height or stature

Height is measured with a rule fixed to the wall, with a smooth, sliding headpiece. The position of the child is important: feet together without shoes; back straight, with the occiput, buttocks, and heels lightly touching the measuring rod, head aligned so that the lower rim of the orbit and the auditory canal are in a horizontal plane. The child is told to make herself tall, is stretched gently upward by pressure under the mastoid process, and instructed to relax the shoulders so that they are not shrugged. Care should be taken that the heels are not lifted from the floor. The sliding headpiece is lowered to rest firmly on the head. The distance from the floor to the lower border of the headpiece is meas-ured.

Weight

The weight of the infant or child, naked or with the minimum of clothing, is preferably taken at the same time of day for each recording, and with the same scale. The latter should be checked for accu-racy at regular intervals. Weight is usually taken to the nearest 10 g in infants, or the nearest 100 g in the older child.

Head circumference

Head circumference represents the maximum measurement around the head in the horizontal plane. It is measured with a non-stretchable tape at the maximum point of occipital protuberance posteriorly and above the eyebrow anteriorly. It may be influenced by hair growth, i.e., 1 mm of scalp hair thickness will increase the circumfer-ence by about 6 mm. If hair growth is significant in the measurement, note this on the child's clinic card to make future circumference comparions as accurate as possible.

Anterior and posterior fontanelles

The anterior fontanelle measures approximately 2.5 cm x 2.5 cm at 3 months of age. The size then diminishes, and the fontanelle closes completely sometime between 9 and 18 months. The posterior fontanelle is much smaller, and is closed by the age of 3 months.

Body proportions

The wide differences in rates of growth of different organs at different stages are reflected in the changing body proportions.

Head-to-body size ratio: Dramatic changes in the proportion of the head to the body, due to the early growth of the brain, can be summarized as follows:

The brain at 2 months of fetal life forms 20% of body weight, at birth 12%, at 10 years 6%, and at 16 years 3%.

Upper and lower body segment ratio: The lower segment is measured from the upper level of the pubic ramus to the base of heel on the inner side of the foot. This value is subtracted from the height or length to obtain the upper segment meas-urement, i.e., from the crown of the head to the upper level of the pubic ramus.

The limbs grow faster than the trunk, from early fetal life to mid-puberty. The ratios of the upper segment to the lower segment at different ages are:

birth	1.7 : 1
10 years	1.0 : 1
14 years	0.9 : 1

Thereafter the long bones stop growing and the adult ratio of 1.0 : 1 is reached again.

Arm span

Measurement is from the tip of the middle finger of one hand to that of the other hand, with both shoulders abducted 90 ° and the palms supinated. Normally, arm span equals total height. It is, however, hard to measure accurately, as it combines both arm length and chest breadth.

Skinfold thickness

A skinfold caliper is used to measure the thickness of subcutaneous tissue, which largely reflects fat. It is measured at several sites, but the two most commonly used are the triceps and subscapular areas. The left side of the body is conventionally measured. The triceps skinfold is measured at the midpoint in the mid-posterior line of the left upper arm, between the acromion and the olecranon process, with the arm extended and hanging loosely at the side. This midpoint is determined with the arm bent at a 90 ° angle at the elbow, with the palm up. The subscapular measurement is estimated taking a vertical skinfold directly below the left scapula. The caliper is held in the right hand. A fold of skin and subcutaneous tissue is lifted between the thumb and index finger of the left hand. The jaws of the caliper are applied directly below to enclose this skinfold and the hand then relaxed. The distance between the approximated jaws is read directly from the dial within a few seconds.

Mid-upper-arm circumference

The mid-arm circumference is measured with a non-stretchable tape measure, with the arm hanging loosely at the side. The measure is passed around the circumference of the arm at the same horizontal level as for the measurement of the triceps skinfold thickness. The tape should not be held so tightly as to produce an indentation. The measurement is noted in centimetres. It gives some indication of muscle bulk, but its value in nutritional studies is limited.

Puberty and adolescence

Although the terms 'puberty' and 'adolescence' are often used interchangeably, both denote a specific discrete occurrence. It is thus essential that these terms be defined before normal growth and development at these periods is discussed *(see section on Definitions and terminology, above).*

Puberty

The age range for the onset of puberty has altered considerably over the last 150 years, and secular trends indicate that the onset now occurs considerably earlier than it did at the turn of the century.

Local data are not available, but American studies indicate that puberty normally commences at between $8\frac{1}{2}$ and 13 years in girls, and at between 10 and 15 years in boys. Apart from a sexual variation, the time of onset of puberty may differ between race groups. In the United States, puberty in blacks begins about 6 months later than in Latin Americans. Recent studies by Cameron in South Africa indicate that rural black children have a somewhat later onset of puberty than their urban counterparts.

The physical changes of puberty are preceded by hormonal changes, leading to the appearance of secondary sex characteristics and an increase in growth velocity prior to the final cessation of growth.

Events at puberty can thus be divided into:
◆ hormonal changes
◆ appearance of secondary sex characteristics
◆ change of growth velocity (secondary growth spurt).

Physical changes associated with puberty

Measurement of the changes taking place at puberty is based on the descriptions of Tanner, using standard ratings on a scale of 1 to 5. Variations, such as some degree of transient breast development in the otherwise normal boy, will not be discussed.

Boys

Genital development

Stage 1: Pre-adolescent: The testes, scrotum, and penis are of about the same size and proportions as in early childhood.

Stage 2: Enlargement of the scrotum and testes. The skin of the scrotum reddens and changes in texture. Little or no enlargement of the penis.

37

Stage 3: Lengthening of the penis. Further growth of the testes and scrotum.

Stage 4: Increase in breadth of the penis and development of the glans. The testes and scrotum are larger; the scrotum darkens.

Stage 5: Adult.

Pubic hair

Stage 1: Pre-adolescent: No pubic hair.

Stage 2: Sparse growth of slightly pigmented, downy hair, chiefly at the base of the penis.

Stage 3: Hair darker, coarser, and more curled, spreading sparsely over the junction of the pubes.

Stage 4: Hair adult in type, but covering a considerably smaller area than in the adult. No spread to the medial surface of the thighs.

Stage 5: Adult quantity and type, with distribution of a horizontal pattern and spread to the medial surface of the thighs. Spread up linea alba occurs later and is rated Stage 6.

Girls

Breast development

Stage 1: Pre-adolescent: Elevation of the papilla only.

Stage 2: Breast bud stage. Elevation of the breast and papilla as a small mound. Enlargement of the areola diameter.

Stage 3: Further enlargement and elevation of the breast and areola, with no separation of their contours.

Stage 4: Projection of the areola and papilla above the level of the breast.

Stage 5: Mature stage, projection of the papilla alone due to recession of the areola.

Pubic hair

Stage 1: Pre-adolescent: No hair.

Stage 2: Sparse growth of slightly pigmented, downy hair, chiefly along the labia.

Stage 3: Hair darker, coarser, and more curled, spreading sparsely over the junction of the pubes.

Stage 4: Hair adult in type, but covering a considerably smaller area than in the adult. No spread to the medial surface of the thighs.

Stage 5: Adult quantity and type, with distribution of a horizontal pattern and spread to the medial surface of the thighs. Spread up linea alba occurs later and is rated Stage 6.

Screening tests

Many clinicians use formal screening tests to detect or better define developmental and/or behavioural problems, particularly in the first few years of life. Two commonly used tests are described here.

Denver Developmental Screening Test (DDST)

The 105 items in the DDST were specifically chosen from pre-existing developmental tests for their ease of administration and interpretation. The reliability and validity of the test have been established *(see Fig. 2.10)*.

However, the criteria for passing are set low, which minimizes false positives (labelling normal children as abnormal), but also results in not identifying children with mild — but often significant — developmental problems. Suspect scores must therefore be followed closely.

Speech and language screening

Language screening is important because it is the simplest way to assess an aspect of cognitive development in the early years. A recently developed screening system along the lines of the DDST is the ELM (Early Language Milestone) Scale. This should be used to assess visual, auditory receptive, and auditory expressive communication in the first 36 months *(see Fig. 2.11)*.

A.D. Rothberg

3

Genetics and congenital disorders

Introduction

Genetic and congenital disorders play a major role in the aetiology of neonatal and childhood morbidity and death in the First World. In the Third World, however, they are relatively less important because of the magnitude of environmental factors which threaten the fetus and the infant. These environmental agents include infectious and nutritional diseases, as well as inadequate antenatal and perinatal care. It can be predicted that as health care improves in underdeveloped communities, genetic and congenital disorders will become more apparent. The rational treatment and prevention of these disorders will be possible only if reliable epidemiological data for a particular community are available. It is accepted wisdom to claim that those problems which are common should receive more attention from health planners than those which are rare, as should those with a better prognosis. Doctors, nurses, and other health care workers need to be well-informed on the subject of inherited disorders if they are to help affected patients and the families who care for them. Because of the risks of recurrence, parents of an affected child are entitled to genetic counselling and to information on the steps which may be taken to reduce these risks.

Classification of genetic and congenital disorders

Genetic disorders may be classified in different ways, but probably the most convenient is to arrange them according to their modes of inheritance. There are some which are inherited in strict Mendelian fashion and are said to be due to single gene — *monogenic* or *unifactorial* — inheritance. There are others which are due to the contribution of genes at a number of loci, and which are said to constitute *polygenic* or *multifactorial* inheritance. In addition, there are important chromosomal disorders in which a whole chromosome, or part of a chromosome, may be present as an extra copy or may be missing. The risks of recurrence will depend on the nature of the disorder. There are many congenital abnormalities and dysmorphic states of which the genetics are not yet known, although there are some that are due to specific environmental agents. The health care professional will also be confronted by families with a mentally or developmentally retarded child where there is a strong suspicion of a genetic cause.

Single gene disorders

These conditions together occur in about 10 in 1 000 births. Although most of them follow one mode of inheritance, some may be heterogeneous; retinitis pigmentosa, for example, may be inherited in a dominant, recessive, or X-linked fashion, and there are dominantly and recessively inherited forms of osteogenesis imperfecta and polycystic kidney disease.

Autosomal dominant inheritance

About 1 200 disorders are known to be dominantly inherited. Some, such as polydactyly, may be very mild, while others, such as achondroplasia, are severe, but they are seldom lethal.

In dominant inheritance a parent who carries the defective gene has a 1 in 2 risk of passing it on to his or her offspring (*see Fig. 3.1*). Such a gene manifests its effect in single dose even though it has a normal functioning allelic gene. The risk of 50:50 remains the same for every pregnancy, regardless of the genetic outcome in the previous pregnancy. Male and female offspring are equally at risk, although in some disorders the age of onset and the severity of the defect may be influenced by which parent gave the gene to the child. Some examples of common dominant disorders are shown in *Table 3.1*.

New mutations can be responsible for a dominant condition appearing in a child, and this is usually the case (particularly in the offspring of older fathers) when both parents are normal and

Table 3.1 Common dominantly inherited disorders

Disorder	Clinical features
Achondroplasia	Short-limbed dwarfism
Apert's syndrome	Craniostenosis and syndactyly
Cataracts	Lens opacities – usually bilateral
Ectodermal dysplasia	Hypohidrosis, transparent skin, abnormal and sparse hair, adontia/hypodontia
Haemophilia C (PTC deficiency)	Bleeding disorder
Hypercholesterolaemia	Raised cholesterol levels, myocardial infarction
Huntington's disease	Progressive chorea, dementia, family history
Marfan's syndrome	Tall stature, arachnodactyly, lens dislocation, dilatation ascending aorta
Myotonic dystrophy	Muscle weakness, myotonia, cardiac arrythmias
Neurofibromatosis	Pigmented spots (6 or more), neurofibroma, Lisch nodules
Osteogenesis imperfecta	Skeletal fractures, brittle bones, blue sclerae
Polycystic kidneys (adult type)	Progressive cystic renal enlargement with renal insufficiency
Polydactyly	Extra digits
Porphyria (variegate)	Drug sensitivity, recurrent abdominal pain, CNS signs
Retinitis pigmentosa	Pigmented retinae, night blindness, constricted visual fields
Spherocytosis	Haemolytic anaemia
Tuberous sclerosis	Adenoma sebaceum, seizures, mental retardation
Waardenburg's syndrome	Deafness, heterochromia, white forelock

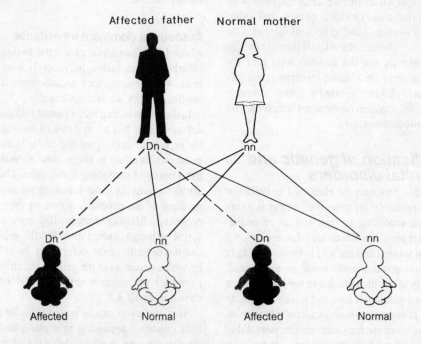

Fig. 3.1 Dominant inheritance

yet the child has a condition which is recognized as a dominantly inherited one. Some dominant conditions have a relatively high new mutation rate (neurofibromatosis is such a condition), and some (such as Huntington's disease) have very low mutation rates. When a child suffers from a condition due to a new mutation, the siblings are not at risk of recurrence, but the affected child's offspring have the usual 1 in 2 (50%) chance of inheriting the mutant gene.

Within a single family in which a dominant gene is segregating, the expression of the gene may vary, with some members manifesting the full-blown syndrome, while others show only a single feature. This phenomenon is called **variable expressivity** of the gene, and it may lead to the condition being difficult to recognize in a particular individual within that family. In Waardenburg syndrome, for example, some individuals will have profound deafness, a white forelock and heterochromia irides, while others will have only one or two of the features.

Penetrance is another important factor in dominant inheritance: in some families key members have the gene but do not show any of its effects. The gene is said to be non-penetrant in such people. The best example in Africa is postaxial polydactyly, which occurs in about 1 in 100 black individuals; it will only be seen in 70 out of every 100 obligatory carrier parents of affected

individuals, and is therefore said to have a penetrance of 70%.

One of the commonest dominant disorders in all populations, as far as is known, is **neurofibromatosis** type 1 (NF1). It occurs in about 1 in 3 000 people, and the clinical features include café au lait patches on the skin (6 or more pigmented spots at least 1.5 cm in diameter in post-pubertal individuals are diagnostic) with neurofibroma and Lisch nodules. Mental retardation, seizures, or malignant changes may occur in about 5–10% of affected individuals, and up to 40% are said to have learning disorders. The penetrance of the gene is high, with most obligatory carriers showing some signs. The offspring of affected females tend to be more severely affected than those of affected males. New mutations are responsible for about 50% of cases. The NF1 locus is situated on chromosome 17, and the gene has recently been cloned. There may be other loci responsible for the disorder in other families.

Autosomal recessive inheritance

Genes for recessive conditions (more than 600 have been identified) are common, and it is estimated that each person may carry four or five of them. They do not have a harmful effect in single dose (the heterozygous state), however, and may have a beneficial or protective effect in some cases (e.g., in the case of the sickle-cell trait, the carrier, when an infant, has a reduced susceptibility to

Table 3.2   Common recessive disorders

Disorder	Clinical features
Adrenogenital syndrome	Ambiguous genitalia, abnormal steroid production
Albinism (oculocutaneous)	Hypopigmentation of skin, hair, and eyes; visual defects
Cystic fibrosis	Malabsorption, failure to thrive, recurrent chest infections
Deafness (some)	Severe bilateral congenital deafness
Galactosaemia	Cataracts, jaundice, vomiting, lethargy in early infancy
Microcephaly (some)	Head circumference < 3rd percentile, mental retardation
Mucopolysaccharidoses (some)	Coarse features, growth and mental retardation, stiff joints
Phenylketonuria	Mental retardation, eczema, seizures, microcephaly
Retinitis pigmentosa (some)	Pigmented retinae, late-onset blindness
Sickle-cell anaemia	Chronic haemolytic anaemia, intermittent pain crises
Spinal muscular atrophy	Hypotonia, weakness, absent deep tendon reflexes
Tay-Sachs disease	Mental retardation, seizures, cherry-red spot on macula
Thalassaemia(s)	Microcytic anaemia, jaundice, hepatosplenomegaly, stunted growth

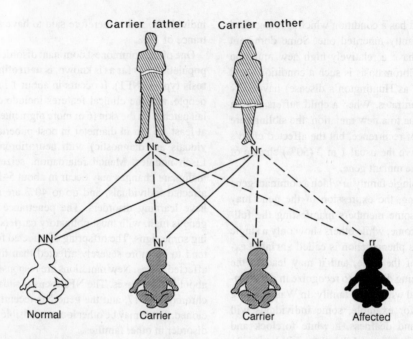

Fig. 3.2   Recessive inheritance

dying from *Plasmodium falciparum* malaria). Recessive conditions only manifest when a child has a double dose (or is homozygous) of the same recessive gene, or else has two deleterious genes even though they are not identical. Females and males are equally affected with these conditions, some of which are listed in *Table 3.2*.

Where both parents are heterozygous for the same genetic mutation, the risks for an affected (homozygous) child will be 1 in 4, and for a heterozygous child 1 in 2 *(see Fig. 3.2)*. If only one parent is a carrier the children cannot be affected with the disorder, but they will have a 1 in 2 chance of being carriers. If both parents are affected (homozygous) all their children will be affected. However, if the disorder is heterogeneous, i.e., caused by genes at different loci (as is the case with the two major types of albinism), then the two affected people will have only unaffected children, although all will be heterozygous at both loci.

Recessive conditions may occur at different rates in different populations. For example, oculocutaneous albinism is the commonest recessive condition in the black South African population, with about 1 in 4 000 babies being affected, whereas only about 1 in 16 000 infants in the white

population has albinism. On the other hand, 1 in 4 000 white infants is born with cystic fibrosis, whereas this disorder hardly ever occurs in black children. The gene for β-thalassaemia has a high frequency in the Indian and Greek populations, whilst the gene for Tay-Sachs disease has a high frequency in Ashkenazi Jewish people.

Consanguineous marriages are generally more likely to produce offspring with a recessive disorder, since the partners have an ancestor in common who might have given them the same gene for a recessive disease. First cousins are given a 1 in 16 risk that their child will be born with a severe recessive disorder. The risks for the children of an uncle-niece mating, which is not uncommon in certain populations in India and Africa, are even higher. Non-specific mental retardation, physical and mental abnormalities, as well as pregnancy loss and neonatal deaths, are also increased in consanguineous marriages.

X-linked inheritance

There are at least 124 genetic conditions which are known to be X-linked. This type of inheritance may occasionally be dominant, but is usually recessive. In the case of the former, females will

Table 3.3   Common X-linked recessive disorders

Disorders	Clinical features
Duchenne muscular dystrophy	Pelvic muscle weakness and deterioration, pseudohypertrophy of calves
Fragile-X syndrome	Mental retardation, large testicles, long facies
Glucose-6-phosphate dehydrogenase deficiency	Haemolytic anaemia, jaundice, haemoglobinuria after exposure to haemolytic agents
Haemophilia A and B	Bleeding diathesis, Factor VIII (A) or Factor IX (B) deficiency
Hydrocephalus (aqueduct stenosis)	Macrocephaly, dilated cerebral ventricles
Incontinentia pigmenti	Bizarre hyperpigmentation patterns, dental anomalies, hair loss
Microphthalmia	Small eyes
Mucopolysaccharidosis (Hurler's syndrome)	Mental and growth retardation, coarse facies, stiff joints
Ocular albinism	Hypopigmentation of the fundus
Retinitis pigmentosa (some)	Retinal pigmentation and degeneration, night blindness, constricted visual fields
Vitamin D-resistant rickets (familial)*	Hypophosphataemia, rickets

* X-linked dominant

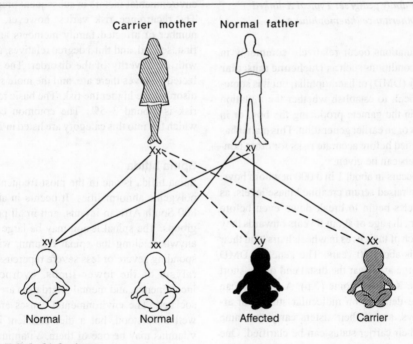

Fig. 3.3 X-linked inheritance

show milder effects of having the gene than do males, and in some cases the condition is lethal in males. However, most of the disorders which have an X-linked mode of inheritance are X-linked recessives, and the female carriers of such a gene

show no signs at all, or very mild signs only (e.g., the slightly reduced Factor VIII levels in some carriers of haemophilia). A list of the common disorders which fall in this group, together with their major clinical features, appears in *Table 3.3*.

In X-linked recessive conditions, if a female is a carrier she will have a 1 in 2 chance of producing a son who is affected, and a 1 in 2 chance of a daughter who is a carrier *(see Fig. 3.3)*. Affected males will have unaffected sons, since they give them their Y chromosome, not their X chromosome which carries the disease-producing gene. All the daughters of an affected male will be obligatory carriers, since they will inherit his X chromosome which carries the mutant gene *(see Fig. 3.4)*.

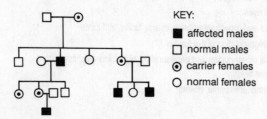

KEY:
■ affected males
□ normal males
◉ carrier females
○ normal females

Fig. 3.4 Family pedigree: Typical X-linked recessive inheritance (haemophilia A)

New mutations occur relatively commonly in X-linked conditions such as **Duchenne muscular dystrophy** (DMD) or haemophilia, but it is sometimes difficult to establish whether the mutation occurred in the gamete producing the boy, or in his mother or an earlier generation. This matter has to be clarified before accurate risks for other family members can be given.

DMD occurs in about 1 in 3 000 newborn boys. They have raised serum creatine kinase levels, as their muscles begin to break down even before birth. From the age of about 8 years onwards they spend much of their lives in wheelchairs, and their life-span is about 20 years. The gene for DMD spans a large area near the distal end of the short arm of the X chromosome (Xp). A deletion can usually be detected on molecular studies in affected boys, and if their sisters carry the same deletion their carrier status can be clarified. One third of cases, however, are caused by new mutations, and in these cases the sisters and brothers are not at risk. *(Also see Chapter 15, Neurological Disorders.)*

Haemophilia A is the commonest form of haemophilia, and is diagnosed in about 1 in 5 000 boys. They have a deficiency of a clotting factor (Factor VIII). New mutations occur in some families, but in most the mother is a carrier and the sisters are therefore at risk of being carriers too. Haemophilia is treated by the infusion of Factor VIII, which is acquired from blood products. In recent years this has given an additional risk of transmitting HIV, the AIDS-causing virus, to affected boys. More mothers are now requesting prenatal diagnosis because of this added risk. *(Also see Chapter 18, Blood Disorders.)*

Polygenic or multifactorial disorders

These disorders are called multifactorial because many factors in addition to defective genes are required to cause them. They are commoner in newborns than the monogenic disorders described above, and in fact occur in about 2% of births. Once a couple has had a child with a multifactorial condition, the recurrence risk is relatively small, due to the different combination of genes and environmental factors in subsequent pregnancies. The recurrence risk varies, however, with the number of affected family members among the first, second, and third degree relatives, as well as with the severity of the disorder. The more affected relatives there are, and the more severe the disorder, the higher the risk. The basic recurrence risk is around 3–5%. The common conditions which fall into this category are listed in *Table 3.4*.

Spina bifida

Spina bifida is one of the most frequently-found polygenic abnormalities. It occurs in about 1 in 800 South African infants, and in all population groups. The spinal lesion may be large or small, anywhere along the spinal column, with corresponding severe or less severe repercussions. Paralysis of the lower limbs, hydrocephalus, incontinence, and mental retardation are often associated. The environmental causes are not yet well understood, but a diet deficient in certain vitamins may be one of them. Vitamin and folic acid supplementation, taken for 3 months prior to and 3 months post conception, appears to reduce recurrence risks, and is advisable in women who have had an affected child. The recurrence risk in high-incidence areas is about 5%, while in low-incidence areas it is only about 2.5–3%. The condition can be detected in fetuses *in utero* by estimating the alpha fetoprotein (AFP) level in the

Table 3.4   Common multifactorial conditions

Disorder	Clinical features
Cleft lip and palate	Facial clefting
Congenital heart disease	Various heart defects
Congenital hip dislocation	Dislocated hips
Diabetes (some types)	Insulin- and non-insulin-dependent diabetes
Hydrocephalus (isolated)	Macrocephaly, dilated cerebral ventricles
Spina bifida, anencephaly	Open neural tube defects
Talipes equinovarus	Clubbed feet

amniotic fluid, and, less reliably, by AFP levels in maternal serum at 16–17 weeks' gestation and by ultrasound scans.

Cleft lip

Cleft lip, with or without cleft palate, is diagnosed in about 1 in 1 000 white infants, but in only about 1 in 5 000 black babies. Although there is quite often a family history and a genetic predisposition, these disorders can be associated with the ingestion of various drugs in early pregnancy. Drugs such as anticonvulsants (phenobarbitone, phenytoin, primidone), retinoic acid, barbiturates, and valium have been implicated, as have alcohol and caffeine.

Congenital heart defects

These can be a feature of rubella embryopathy as well as of uncontrolled maternal diabetes, increased alcohol consumption, lithium, and various anti-epilepsy drugs. The genetic predisposition of mother and fetus, the drug and its dose, and the gestational timing of the exposure all determine the nature of the malformations which occur.

General assessment

Many of these multifactorial conditions consist of isolated malformations. In some cases, however, they are associated with other defects. These cases need careful consideration and evaluation because they may be components of syndromes which have different modes of inheritance and recurrence risks. For example, if cleft lip occurs with other abnormalities such as sparse hair and ectrodactyly (missing digits), then the ectrodactyly-ectodermal dysplasia-clefting

(EEC) syndrome, which is dominantly inherited, may be the correct diagnosis.

Chromosome disorders

Chromosome disorders are very common, and occur in about 6 per 1 000 live births. They may present with full-blown syndromes with serious implications, such as Down's syndrome, or they may be balanced translocations with no clinically-detectable effect. The clinical suspicion of a chromosome disorder should always be confirmed by laboratory analysis. Most chromosome disorders have a low risk of recurrence because they are sporadic, but a few which are inherited will have a high recurrence risk, and these need to be identified. The commonest chromosome disorders are listed in *Table 3.5* with some of their clinical features, although not all affected individuals will have all the features.

Down's syndrome

Down's syndrome is certainly the most widely recognized of the chromosome disorders, affecting about 1 in 700 newborns in all populations. Heart defects cause the death of the child in the first year of life in about 20% of cases. Survivors will have IQs between 30 and 70, and will require stimulation programmes, special schooling, and sheltered employment.

There are three types of Down's syndrome which must be distinguished. The first is the regular Trisomy 21 (occurring in 92% of cases) which has a low recurrence risk of 1%. The second is the translocation type (occurring in about 5% of cases), which is a new mutation in about half the cases and inherited from a balanced translocation

Table 3.5   Common chromosome disorders

Disorder	Clinical features
Trisomy 21 (Down's syndrome)	Hypotonia, epicanthic folds, heart defects, mental retardation
Trisomy 18 (Edwards' syndrome)	Prominent occiput, low-set malformed ears, clenched hands with overlapping fingers, short sternum, rocker-bottom feet, heart defects, profound developmental delay (90% die in first year)
Trisomy 13 (Patau's syndrome)	Cleft lip and palate, polydactyly, scalp defects, clenched fists, microphthalmia, heart defects, mental retardation (50% die in first month)
45X syndrome	Short female, broad chest, (Turner) ovarian dysgenesis, peripheral lymphoedema at birth, webbed neck, coarctation of aorta, usually normal intelligence and lifespan
47,XXY (Klinefelter's syndrome)	Tall male, hypogenitalism, mild mental retardation, behavioural problems
47,XYY syndrome	Tall stature, mild mental retardation
Fragile-X/associated mental retardation (Martin-Bell syndrome)	Enlarged testes, mild to moderate mental retardation, long facies, large ears, (20–30% female heterozygotes mildly mentally retarded)

parent in the remainder. When the mother is the carrier, the recurrence risk is about 10%, and if the father is the carrier it is about 2%. The third type is the mosaic (found in about 3% of cases), in which some cells have the extra chromosome 21 and others have normal chromosomes. In this type the recurrence risk is less than 1%.

The risk of sporadic Down's syndrome due to non-disjunction chromosome 21 is correlated with maternal age: the risk triples between ages 30 and 35 years, and again between 35 and 40. At 35 years the risk is approximately 1 in 300, it is 1 in 100 at 40, and 1 in 25 at 45 years. The influence of paternal age is not clear, but in about 10% of cases the extra chromosome 21 comes from the father. Prenatal diagnosis and selective abortion can be offered to pregnant women over 35 years of age, and in societies where the uptake rate is high, the number of Down's syndrome births has dropped to less than 1 in 1 000.

Hermaphroditism

True hermaphrodites, who have both testicular and ovarian tissue, usually have a 46XX karyotype and ambiguous genitalia. Surgery may be necessary for cosmetic and psychological reasons, an important consideration being the anticipated sexual function of the child when s/he grows to adulthood. True hermaphroditism is not thought

to recur in siblings, but a condition which must be differentiated is congenital adrenal hyperplasia. This condition can cause ambiguous genitalia in a female neonate, is recessively inherited, and is amenable to drug treatment.

Indications for chromosome studies

The main indications for chromosome studies are:
♦   mental retardation of unknown aetiology, especially if associated with dysmorphic features
♦   multiple congenital abnormalities
♦   recurrent spontaneous abortions or still births, or unexplained neonatal deaths (three or more)
♦   ambiguous genitalia
♦   hypogonadism, primary amenorrhoea
♦   family history of chromosome translocation.

Non-genetic congenital abnormalities

Apart from the genetic causes of congenital abnormalities, there are numerous other causes, including prenatal viral infections, *in utero* radiation, and exposure to other teratogenic agents, such as drugs and dietary substances.

Viral infections

Rubella is the most common virus which adversely affects the developing fetus. It results in cataracts, deafness, heart defects, and microcephaly with mental retardation. The fetus is most vulnerable during the first trimester, but an infection in the second trimester may also cause problems.

Cytomegalovirus, as well as toxoplasmosis, can cause microcephaly and mental retardation in the fetus, while congenital syphilis, which is still very important in developing countries, can be associated with facial and other bony abnormalities and keratitis. Exposure of the fetus to the HIV (AIDS) virus can result in immune deficiency, and possibly minor dysmorphic features, and the hepatitis virus may be involved in some cases of biliary atresia.

Radiation
Radiation of the fetus *in utero* often causes much concern. However, the dose has to be high to affect the fetus, and then a spontaneous abortion usually occurs. In the presence of a high dose (at the upper limit of most diagnostic radiation) the risks of malformations, mental retardation, and childhood leukaemias are only increased to about 1 in 1 000. Termination of pregnancy and amniocentesis are, therefore, unwarranted in such cases.

Teratogenic agents
Since thalidomide was taken off the market, the most important teratogenic drugs are warfarin (used in the treatment of rheumatic heart conditions, and in particular when prosthetic heart valves have been inserted), the anticonvulsants, and lithium (used in the treatment of depression). Warfarin can cause bony abnormalities in the fetus, as well as a high fetal and perinatal loss rate, whereas the antiepileptic drugs can cause congenital heart disease, clefting, neural tube defects, mental retardation, and behavioural problems. Lithium has been associated with heart defects in the fetus.

Mothers with a high regular intake of alcohol, and those who have binges at crucial stages of pregnancy, can produce infants with the fetal alcohol syndrome: abnormal facies, reduced somatic and brain growth, microcephaly, mental retardation, and heart defects. The critical level of alcohol cannot be determined, but the full syndrome may only occur with levels which exceed 80 grams per day. Even a small intake, however,

may cause growth retardation, and it is advisable that alcohol be avoided completely during pregnancy. Cigarette smoking can be responsible for infants who are small for date, and should be reduced or preferably avoided in pregnancy *(also see Chapter 5, Newborns).*

In order to prevent possible teratogenic effects on the fetus and congenital abnormalities, all women who are at risk of conceiving should avoid all drugs (that are not absolutely essential), alcohol, and smoking, and should have a healthy, balanced diet at the time of conception and throughout pregnancy.

Mental retardation
(Also see Chapter 30, Psychological and Behavioural Disorders.)

Mental retardation is a common problem, and 1–2% of children may have an IQ of less than 80. The aetiology of mental defects of one sort or another is very varied. In developed countries the monogenic and polygenic conditions are probably responsible for about 22% of mentally handicapped cases, while chromosome abnormalities cause 15% (of which 10% are Down's syndrome), infections, brain damage, and other environmental factors are responsible for 20%, and in about 43% the cause is unknown.

In developing communities, infectious diseases, nutritional deficiencies, poor antenatal care, and birth complications are proportionately more important as causes of mental retardation. Proper emphasis on maternal and child health in developing countries' health services is therefore essential to avoid the morbidity and mental impairment that occur in children where these services are inadequate, or inaccessible to the majority of the population.

Prevention of inherited and congenital disorders
Primary prevention
Primary prevention is a proactive form of prevention in which the behaviour and habits of the couple wanting a baby may be altered to minimize the risks to the child. In this situation a healthy, nutritious diet and good antenatal care is encouraged, together with the avoidance of known teratogens and substance abuse. Couples should plan

their families, prepare themselves and their homes, and take the necessary steps (such as rubella inoculation) at least three months prior to conception. They should also be aware of their family history, and report any abnormalities to their health care practitioner early in the pregnancy so that the need for investigation can be assessed. The couple's ages are also important. In these ways some disorders can be prevented.

Secondary prevention

There are various methods of secondary prevention. Most require investigations during the pregnancy, such as prenatal diagnosis, which may be invasive and risky. Once the results of such investigations indicate that there is an affected fetus, a legal abortion can be offered (in South Africa in terms of the Abortion and Sterilization Act of 1975, which allows for abortion on genetic grounds).

Prenatal diagnosis of fetal defects may be achieved using the following techniques:

Chorionic villus sampling

This may be carried out trans-cervically or transabdominally at 9–11 weeks' gestation. The advantage of this procedure is that an early diagnosis is made using cytogenetic or molecular techniques, and if an early termination of pregnancy is indicated (usually by dilatation and curettage), it can be performed with the minimum psychological sequelae for the mother. The disadvantages are that this is an invasive technique with a 5% risk of miscarriage, that neural tube defects cannot be detected, and a few cases (usually those done earlier than 9 weeks' gestation) have been associated with limb defects in the fetus.

Amniocentesis

This technique, in which an amniotic fluid sample is collected transabdominally under sonar visualization at 13–22 weeks, facilitates chromosome analysis of the fetus as well as the estimation of alpha-fetoprotein for the detection of neural tube defects. The advantage of amniocentesis is that the risk of miscarriage is less than 1%. The disadvantages include the possibility of a late termination, often when the mother has already felt life and may have bonded with the fetus. However, because this technique can now be done by experts in the field as early as 13 weeks, this is usually the method of choice.

Ultrasound scanning

Performed by an experienced person using high-resolution, quality equipment, ultrasound scanning can be used not only to measure fetal biparietal diameters (to detect micro- or hydrocephaly) and to assess gestational dates and fetal growth, but also to measure bone lengths (for achondroplasia, for example), examine vertebrae, and assess heart and kidney defects and limb abnormalities. This is not an invasive technique, but it is expensive, and should therefore be used sparingly and only in suitable at-risk cases.

Fetoscopy

Fetoscopy enables a sample of fetal cord blood to be collected (cordocentesis) when an abnormal scan has alerted the doctor to a problem, but it can usually be performed only relatively late in pregnancy. It carries a high risk of miscarriage (about 10%). Fetoscopy is no longer important for examining the anatomy of the fetus, having been virtually replaced by high- resolution ultrasonography.

Screening programmes

Various screening programmes are available for a variety of disorders:

Maternal serum screening

A sample of the mother's serum can be collected at around 16 weeks' gestation and used to refine her risks for abnormalities in the fetus. This test is sometimes called the 'triple test' because levels of alpha-fetoprotein (AFP), human chorionic gonadotrophin (HCG), and oestriol (E3) are used. If the AFP is raised, the fetus is at an increased risk of having conditions such as a neural tube defect, Turner's syndrome, or some dermatological abnormality. However, a twin pregnancy also gives elevated AFP levels. If the AFP and the E3 levels are reduced and the HCG level is elevated, there is an increased risk that the fetus has Down's syndrome or one of the other trisomies. Since this is only a screening test, with an efficiency of only about 60% (and it has a 5% false positive rate), it is not recommended for high-risk cases. However, it may be useful in detecting those women under the age of 35 years at risk for Down's syndrome, who should be offered an amniocentesis. In the UK, all pregnant woman are being offered the test by the government-funded National Health Service; in South Africa and other developing countries, only those who are able to pay for the test obtain it — such a facility does not constitute a screening programme.

Whole-population screening

The most successful programme has been that available to the Ashkenazi Jewish population, in which about 1 in 20 individuals are at risk of being a carrier of the gene for recessively inherited Tay-Sachs disease. In the USA and South Africa it has been community-based, and couples have the test prior to having their first child. At-risk couples identified in this way usually opt for prenatal diagnosis (and abortion of the affected fetus).

Similar programmes have been developed for diseases such as thalassaemia in Cyprus, where 1 in 6 of the population is heterozygous for the gene. The South African Greek and Indian populations are at high risk for this condition (1 in 10 and 1 in 20, respectively), and couples should be offered testing prior to their first pregnancy. Sickle-cell anaemia can be tested for very easily and cheaply, and such testing is desirable in much of central and western Africa, where the carrier rate may be as high as 1 in 4. South Africa, however, is a low-risk area for sickle-cell anaemia.

Neonatal screening

Neonatal screening for a variety of conditions has been carried out for decades in developed countries. The two best-known conditions are phenylketonuria (PKU) and hypothyroidism. In both conditions the affected infants are seriously handicapped if they are not given appropriate treatment soon after delivery. The cost-effectiveness of these programmes is determined partly by the prevalence of the condition, and partly by the cost of institutional care if the condition is not diagnosed early. PKU seems to be uncommon in people of African or Asian descent, and it may be rare in all South African populations. Congenital hypothyroidism is probably as common among Africans as it is in other populations.

Genetic services for Third World countries

The aims of genetic counselling have been laid down by the World Health Organization. They are to assist the family or the individual in the following ways:

♦ To comprehend the medical facts, diagnosis, prognosis, and management regarding their condition.

♦ To appreciate the genetics of the disorder and the risk of recurrence.

♦ To understand the options for dealing with the recurrence risk.

♦ To choose the appropriate course of action and carry out their choice.

♦ To make the best possible adjustment to the disorder.

Full genetic counselling clinics with a comprehensive service and laboratory back-up may only be available at universities which have medical schools and departments of human genetics. In South Africa, the Universities of the Witwatersrand, Cape Town, Stellenbosch, and Pretoria have such facilities, while smaller clinics are available at hospitals in Durban, Bloemfontein, and Port Elizabeth.

Counselling and information are also provided by the genetics nurses and other staff employed throughout the country by the Genetic Services division of the Department of National Health and Population Development. These nurses do much of the community work required to extend genetic services to outlying and uninformed population groups. Educational leaflets are produced and distributed, and courses of instruction are also provided by the Department.

A lay/medical organization called the Southern African Inherited Disorders Association (SAIDA) is active in some areas of South Africa. It aims to educate people about genetic disorders, to provide support and fellowship for those suffering from inherited disorders (as well as their families), and to encourage research into the diagnosis, treatment, and prevention of such disorders. Affected families can meet similarly-affected families through SAIDA, and thus avoid the isolation so often experienced by those with genetic diseases.

All these services are required in Third World countries, although the emphasis on different aspects might vary — the comfort and support of affected families may be emphasized more than the expensive provision of 'high-tech' laboratories, for example.

A good genetic service would also incorporate a research element. In an underdeveloped community this might include enquiries into the epidemiology of the genetic diseases specific to that community: ascertaining the attitudes to these diseases, and exploring people's religious and cultural views with respect to health and sickness in general. Only after such studies had been completed could priorities be assigned and a relevant and appropriate need-related genetic service be provided.

Conclusion

Five per cent of the population in developed countries will have a genetic disorder by the age of 25 years; and if one includes multifactorial disorders, this figure rises to 65% in a lifetime. In developing countries these figures are less impressive, because of the burden of infections and nutritional disorders which are responsible for the death of as many as 200–300 live-born infants before the age of 1 year. When the infant mortality rate is brought down to perhaps 50 per 1 000 or less, genetic causes of morbidity and mortality will probably become evident and demand some response.

Academic institutions have pioneered genetic services in the developed world and among the wealthy élite in developing countries. With the increasing privatization of health care in South Africa, the laboratory investigations which are an essential component of such services are increasingly being offered by private practitioers. There is a real risk that the public sector will not be able to afford to provide genetic services for the majority of the population — a situation similar to that in many developing countries in Africa and Asia, and even in a First World country like the USA.

In the planning of genetics services for South Africa, the need for equity (equal care for equal need) is obvious: the service must be accessible to the poor, and to those living far from the urban centres with academic institutions. The service must provide a definite benefit to the patient and her family, and not merely add an interesting diagnostic dimension to health care. An effective community network of genetic nurses must be part of the primary health care (PHC) structure, and genetic counselling clinics, access to specialist clinical geneticists, and an efficient laboratory back-up must all be present. Incorporation into the PHC base-unit — with its preventive, promotive, curative, and rehabilitative components — would be desirable, and if the PHC base-unit consisted of a team, then it would be possible to train some of the team members to take on the task of counselling.

It is also possible that genetic services could be integrated into family planning programmes, because appeals to couples to reduce family size or to space their children should be accompanied by efforts to ensure that the children born are born healthy. This would require high-quality antenatal care from early pregnancy, and offering investigations to evaluate the health status of the fetus. Attempts must be made to demonstrate the cost-effectiveness of the service, but this will be difficult in countries which have not been spending significant amounts of money on the care and rehabilitation of children and adults with genetic handicaps.

The first steps in the assault on genetic disorders should be education programmes directed at health care professionals (at both the under- and post-graduate levels of training), and at the public (perhaps at secondary school pupils and women attending antenatal clinics).

Laboratory services will need to be co-ordinated at regional, national, and international levels, because most inherited metabolic disorders are individually rare. The hereditary haemolytic anaemias due to sickle haemoglobin, or the thalassaemias are exceptions, and constitute an enormous burden on the countries in which they are found. Blood transfusion therapy for the thalassaemias can consume an unacceptably high proportion of the health budget, and prevention programmes including carrier detection and prenatal diagnosis become economic necessities if the country is to develop. Thailand is a good example of this particular problem.

At present medical or clinical geneticists are to be found almost exclusively in the First World, where they deal with the proband-related needs of patients and their families. In the future (in both the First and Third Worlds) geneticists will become initiators and health advocates who seek out the public at large to educate, to identify people 'at risk', and to offer 'prospective prevention' on a large scale. When this happens, community genetics will have come of age.

T. Jenkins
J.G.R. Kromberg

4

Community paediatrics

Introduction

The human fetus has the exceptional characteristic of leaving the protective environment of the uterus very early on in its development. Hence, in contrast to animals, the neonate is immature, helpless, and utterly dependent. Furthermore, the human relies to a very limited extent on instinct, as most behaviour is based on learning.

The role of the supportive and protective environment in the development of the child throughout the first five years, when the foundation for the rest of life is laid, cannot be overestimated. Clearly the function of the mother in this respect is paramount: her attitude, knowledge, and skills; her health, and social status are all factors which have a profound effect. In the **preconceptional phase** her attitude to pregnancy and child-bearing, as well as her health in the broadest sense, largely determine when she will fall pregnant and whether she is ready for motherhood.

Throughout **pregnancy** her health is influenced by the food available to her and the use of noxious substances. These in turn have a significant bearing on the development of the embryo and fetus. The detection of risk factors during pregnancy will depend on the availability and utilization of antenatal care.

The **birth process** itself can be markedly influenced by the mother's frame of mind. If, for example, she is in a state of fear, adrenaline-like substances in the circulation are likely to impede efficient uterine contractions.

The **vulnerable neonate** is at the mercy of his mother's care. If she happens to have given birth to an unwanted baby, she is unlikely, for example, to be enthusiastic about breast-feeding; on the other hand, even the most desired baby will fail to breast-feed satisfactorily if the mother lacks the knowledge, skill, and motivation for establishing a process which is in fact quite natural. Furthermore, there will be an appreciable negative effect on both the mother and her baby if she returns to an empty home or to a hostile family after delivery.

Throughout **infancy** it will be the mother who decides on the frequency and type of food to offer her baby and on the need to avail herself of immunization and other valuable preventive/promotive services. She will require determination and motivation to overcome obstacles on the road to her infant's health. She has, for example, to recognize the early features of common health hazards such as dehydration, and to know how to prevent further problems.

The **child's** attainment of full intellectual potential and a stable personality will be determined largely by the quality of home life, cohesion of the family, and level of affective involvement. Welfare of the child depends to a large extent on the interval before the next sibling is born; the shorter the time-span between births, the greater the risk of dying before the 5th birthday.

One overriding factor which will influence the mother's knowledge, attitude, and skills is her educational standard. Literacy has a positive effect not only on all phases of growth and development in the child, but also on the mother's status within her family and in society. Literacy can soften almost any adverse influence that modernization and industrialization might have on the mother and her offspring.

The child and her environment

As nurture rather than instinct is important in development, we need to focus on the environment of the child. This can conveniently be looked at as a series of ecosystems: the micro-, mini- and macro-ecosystem, with the meso-ecosystem bridging the last two.

The **micro-ecosystem** represents the immediate environment which impinges upon the senses of the fetus, neonate, or infant. What does she feel, hear and touch? The family and home provide the **mini-ecosystem.** The bonds between parents and children and amongst siblings, and the quality of interaction between family members play an important role. These will be influenced by cultural and other social factors. The **macro-ecosystem** refers to the community and the locality of the home. Political, social, economic, and cultural factors shape this system. The **meso-ecosystem** is the educational structure which prepares the young child for stepping out from the mini-ecosystem into the world. Child-rearing practices, taboos, customs, and gender attitudes are of primary importance. Early childhood educational facilities, primary and secondary schools, and tertiary institutions are all part of this system.

The role of health professionals in each of these systems can be clearly identified. That role does not necessarily conform to the customary duties of doctors and nurses, but may well demand that professionals be agents for change — agents who endeavour to empower parents and communities to make informed decisions which affect their own and their children's lives. Comprehensive health care is concerned with the quality of life within these different ecosystems, and the interaction between them. Education should provide the necessary knowledge, problem-solving skills, and attitudes to tackle the multiplicity of problems impinging on the health of the mother and child. The community must be able to benefit from the professional's scientific approach and the resources to which he has access.

As the health and well-being of the child is primarily dependent on the immediate environment — the mini-ecosystem — it stands to reason that the mother and her child in their home should form the primary focus of the health care system.

Empowering parents to provide optimal care for their children thus needs to be an important goal for providers of health care.

Evaluation of the health status of the community (community diagnosis)

The health status of the individual is determined largely by the environment — the ecosystems — and is considerably influenced by the health status of the community. Health professionals thus need to have an understanding of the factors that influence the latter. *Table 4.1* lists the indicators of the

well-being of mothers and children, and which in turn are also determinants of the health status of the community.

Mortality rates

An accurate data-collecting system is essential to evaluate the outcome of health care and intervention programmes and to monitor trends. This limb of the infrastructure is often badly neglected, making vital statistics suspect, if not valueless. In many Third World communities children are born and die without any form of registration or notification. The task of obtaining and recording raw data must be in the hands of those working closest to the community. The under-5 mortality rate in particular is an indicator of the outcome of a variety of inputs *(see Table 4.1)*. The high mortality rate in infants is largely accounted for by the vulnerability to infection (due to poorly-developed defence mechanisms), and susceptibility to malnutrition. Between the ages of 1 and 5 years the child in a disadvantaged community is still at great risk of dying from infectious diseases and/or malnutrition.

Table 4.1   Indicators of well-being of mothers and children

Input	Outcome
MCH services	Decreased maternal and perinatal mortality rates
Maternal education	
Vaccination coverage	Decreased infant and under-5 morbidity and mortality
Oral rehydration therapy	Fertility rate
Food availability	Nutritional level improves
Ready access to potable water and sanitation	
Protection against accidents	

The **under-5 mortality rate (U5MR),** i.e., the annual number of deaths of children under the age of 5 years per 1 000 live births, is regarded as the principal indicator of progress towards optimal child well-being.

The **infant mortality rate (IMR)** is the annual number of deaths of infants under the age of 1 year per 1 000 live births. The incidence of low-birth-weight infants and the age and education of the mother are important determinants of IMR. Breast-feeding and appropriate birth-spacing make further significant contributions to survival in the first year.

The **perinatal mortality rate (PMR),** i.e., still-births weighing 500 g or more and deaths during the first 7 days after birth, per 1 000 births, reflects the intrauterine environment and is closely related to maternal morbidity and mortality.

This short period represents a very hazardous phase, when more lives may be lost than during the ensuing 30 years. Health care services which provide antenatal screening, attention to high risk pregnancies, and efficient obstetrical and neonatal care, make substantial contributions to the prevention of wastage of human lives.

PMR is a very useful index for evaluating maternal and obstetric care in the community. The main causes of perinatal mortality are:

- low birth weight (40–75%)
- hypoxic states
- neonatal infections
- congenital malformations.

Morbidity and disease prevalence

For every infant and child death, there are many more episodes of disease and ill-health due to the same causative factors. Thus low birth weight and other significant causes of mortality are responsible for varying degrees of disability. It is obvious from the preceding account that blindness, hearing loss, paralysis, and intellectual stunting are far more prevalent in disadvantaged communities.

After the first 6 months of life, malnutrition begins to make a major contribution to the morbidity pattern, particularly when the infant is not breast-fed: breast milk is the single most effective measure for preventing malnutrition and infection in early infancy.

Morbidity amongst pre-school children is largely determined by interaction within the 'Big Three' of the 'Top Ten'. Characteristically there is multiple pathology which compounds the problem.

Mental health in children has received scant attention in developing communities where the main concern is survival. However, recent surveys have shown that 10–26% of children attending clinics had evidence of mental pathology, which

THE TOP TEN	
The Big Three	
Malnutrition	
Diarrhoea	
Respiratory infection	
Measles	
Whooping cough	
Tuberculosis	In the next decade Aids
Intestinal parasites	will undoubtedly
Malaria	take its place in this list.
Anaemia	
Accidents	

ranged from behavioural disorders to cerebral palsy.

The health of the older child and adolescent is also strongly influenced by the environment. Drug abuse, accidents, and sexually transmitted diseases are the main considerations in this age group. *(see Chapter 30, Psychological and Behavioural Disorders).*

Health care delivery

Large, well-equipped hospitals can easily create the impression of high-quality health care delivery. However, when primary health care does not form the foundation of any health system, the health of the entire community may be seriously undermined.

Primary health care

This was defined by the World Health Assembly at Alma-Ata as: 'essential care based on practical, scientifically-sound and socially-acceptable methods and technology made universally accessible to individuals and families through their full participation, and at a cost that the community and country can afford to maintain at every stage of their development, in the spirit of self-reliance and self-determination. It forms an integral part, both of the country's health system, of which it is the central function and main focus, and of the overall social and economic development of the community'.

Eight activities were included by the Assembly as major concerns of primary health care:

◆ promotion of proper nutrition

◆ provision of adequate supply of safe water

◆ provision of basic sanitation

◆ maternal and child care, including family planning

◆ immunization against the major infectious diseases

◆ prevention and control of locally endemic diseases

◆ education concerning methods of prevention and control of prevailing health problems

◆ appropriate treatment for common diseases and injuries.

In contrast to this, specialization and improved technology have encouraged centralization and a massive drain on national budgets. This is frequently accompanied by a poor peripheral network.

Social, political, and cultural variables will determine the specific type of health system which is appropriate for a particular community.

Factors affecting the quality of care

The care provided by health professionals is determined not so much by their number and qualifications, but rather by their commitment, competence, and by such neglected values as dedication, sense of service, and motivation. Evaluation of the quality of the service is essential. This is based on utilization, compliance, and morbidity and mortality profiles.

Socio-economic status

Socio-economic factors have a profound effect on the health of the individual, the family, and the community. Poverty is not merely the absence of material resources, but can be regarded as a complex syndrome comprising low income; poor housing, water and sanitation; inadequate

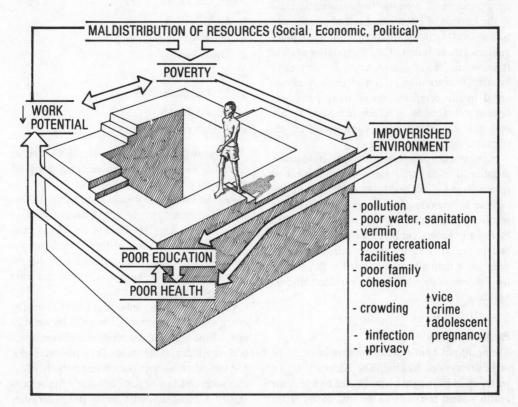

Fig. 4.1 Factors contributing to the persistence of poverty

nutrition; and recurrent disease. The poverty syndrome undermines learning, and therefore also earning capacity, which in turn can lead to family and community violence and a feeling of hopelessness. It is worth noting that the poor are not impoverished by accident, and definitely not by choice. They are, and remain, poor because they lack power and have no seat at the table where the economic cake is cut up.

Environment

The underprivileged generally live in rural areas or high-density urban ghettos. The former are usually deprived of health care facilities and basic needs such as potable water and safe sanitation. There is a dearth of employment opportunities, leading to migratory labour and urbanization with consequent collapse of the extended family system. In urban areas the poor are compelled to congregate in ghettos where housing provides the barest minimum of protection against the elements, and where overcrowding exposes the child to the hazards of infections. Lack of privacy and recreational facilities promote adolescent pregnancies, vice and crime. The underprivileged child thus has far fewer opportunities for formal or informal education, and is considerably disadvantaged in life compared to his more privileged counterpart. Thus the ill-effects of poverty are not only individually damaging, but also collectively reinforce each other *(see Fig. 4.1)*.

Economic development usually means industrialization. This has often had a negative effect on maternal and child health, as evidenced by the decline in breast-feeding, inappropriate weaning practices, poor family support structures, and an increase in adolescent pregnancies, child labour, and pollution. Heavily industrialized countries need to be particularly concerned with environmental deterioration and its adverse effect on child health.

Health policy

The health policy of a country determines the type of health system adopted. The adequacy of the policy must be judged by the degree to which the health system responds to the real needs of the community, and by the state's commitment to the policy. Budgetary allocations are useful indicators in respect of administrative priorities — both within the health budget and in relation to other sectors, such as defence, education, and agriculture.

The policy should provide for mechanisms which protect against an inequitable distribution of resources to those who are most vociferous and have the greatest leverage. It must ensure protection of the most vulnerable and those without the vote. The quality of health services depends not so much on unfettered economic growth as on a commitment to equitable distribution of resources and participation by the community in decision-making.

The care that mothers and children receive in a society gives an indication of its moral values.

Levels of intervention

The UNICEF strategy for a childhood survival and developmental revolution is based on seven elements, viz., GOBI — FFF

♦ growth charts
♦ oral rehydration therapy
♦ breast-feeding
♦ immunization
♦ food supplementation
♦ female literacy
♦ fertility control.

The **growth chart** (Road-to-Health Card) is an essential, inexpensive health record kept by the mother for each child *(see Fig. 4.2)*.

Regular charting of weight is the most valuable method of monitoring health. A flattening of the weight curve suggests inadequate energy consumption, while a drop in the curve is always caused by infection. Take particular care that the weight returns to the normal curve for that child on recovery from an infection.

Oral rehydration methods should be known by every mother. She must be aware of the seriousness of the signs of dehydration and commence oral rehydration at the onset of a diarrhoeal illness. She should use a home-brew in an emergency (e.g. rice water or 1 litre of potable water + 8 teaspoons sugar + 1/2 teaspoon salt), giving 100 ml for every watery stool passed *(see Chapter 11, Gastrointestinal Disorders)*.

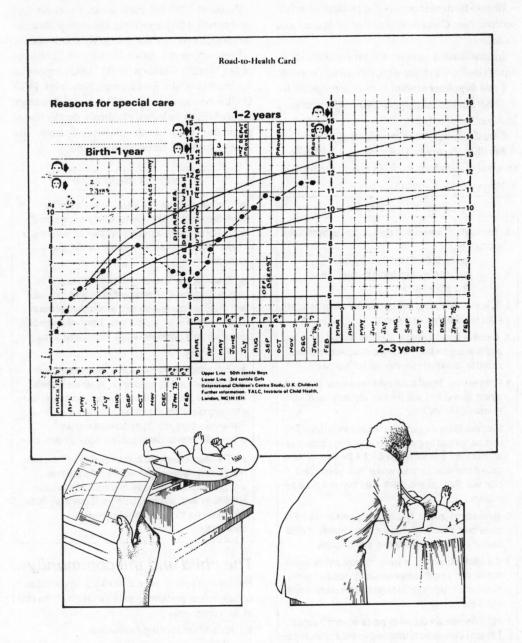

Fig. 4.2   The growth chart (also known as the Road-to-Health Card) *designed for and recommended by the World Health Organization can be suitably adapted to local needs. It is a very useful home-based total health record, which is an important tool in the health care of the child. The reverse side makes provision for personal particulars, birth history, weight chart to the age of 5 years, and the immunization record. The latter can be reinforced by small illustrations of a syringe on the weight chart where the vaccination should be given. (See Tremlett, G., Lovel, H., and Morley, D. 'Guidelines for the design of national weight-for-age growth charts'. From* Assignment Children, *1983, 61/62, pp. 143–175.)*

Breast-feeding increases the chances of infant survival *(see Chapter 6, Feeding of Infants and Toddlers)*.

Immunization against six preventable infections is outlined in *Chapter 8, Infectious Diseases*.

Food supplementation is most appropriate for the undernourished pregnant woman to prevent a low-birth-weight baby.

Female literacy: *See introduction, above.*

Fertility control: The chances of childhood survival diminish appreciably where the birth interval is less than 2 years.

Panel 1:   Facts for life

1. The health of women and children can be significantly improved by:
     spacing births at least 2 years apart
     avoiding pregnancy before the age of 18, and
     limiting births to four.

2. All women should have their pregnancies and births supervised by trained health personnel.

3. Exclusive breast-feeding is the ideal method of feeding infants during the first 3–4 months of life. Additional foods should be introduced when they are 4–6 months old.

4. Children under 3 need to eat 5 or 6 times a day. Their food should be enriched with mashed vegetables and small amounts of fats and oils.

5. Diarrhoea kills by excessive loss of fluid from the body. This must be replaced by giving plenty of the right liquids, such as breast milk, thin porridge, or ORS. If the illness is more serious than usual, a health worker must be consulted. A child with diarrhoea also needs extra food to make a full recovery.

6. Immunization protects against diseases which may kill or cause poor growth and disability. Every woman of child-bearing age should be immunized against tetanus.

7. If a child with a cough is breathing more rapidly than is normal, then a health worker should be consulted quickly. A child with a cold should be helped to drink plenty of fluids and to eat.

8. Many illnesses are caused by germs entering the mouth. This can be prevented by using latrines and washing hands after using the latrine or after any contact with excreta.

9. Illness holds back a child's growth. After an illness a child needs an extra meal every day for at least a week to make up for growth lost.

10. Children should be weighed every month for the first year of life, every 2 months during the second year and every 3 months during the third year. If there is no weight gain, something is wrong.

A recent UNICEF publication, *Facts for Life (see panel)*, provides simple life-saving information which every parent has the right to know.

This section has drawn liberally on 'The State of the World's Children 1991', which reports on the World Summit for Children, New York 1990. On that occasion leaders of 71 nations committed themselves to reducing children's deaths and to protecting their health and development. See Panel 2 for some particular highlights.

Panel 2:   A plan for action

● The essence of the Plan for Action adopted by the World Summit for Children was based on the *new ethic of a first call for children — a principle that the essential needs of children should be given high priority in the allocation of resources*.

● It requires a personal and political commitment of the leaders of nations — a commitment which does not waver with changing circumstances such as economic recession, or even in times of war and civil strife. *There will always be something more immediate — there will never be anything more important*.

● Data collection systems which monitor maternal and child health as carefully as economic growth are essential. Data must be analyzed and publicized as indicators of the well-being of mothers and children *(see Table 4.1)*. Furthermore, there must be mechanisms whereby policy-makers can be alerted rapidly to adverse trends.

● The fallacy of averages must be avoided, as these can hide severely disadvantaged sections of the population, e.g., 75% vaccination coverage may mean 85% for urban and 65% for rural children, or U5MR of 60 may mean 30 for the majority but 150 for pockets of impoverished communities.

The child and the community

Health workers require a working knowledge of certain issues pertaining to the welfare of the child in the community:

◆ legislation relating to children
◆ education
◆ adoption
◆ child abuse
◆ drug dependence.

Legislation: A child care act

Generally a child care act should give the child a degree of protection which is not available to those over the age of 18 years. Every doctor should be familiar with the relevant sections of such legislation, so that the necessary legal steps may be taken to prevent essential care being withheld from any child. The law needs to lay down clearly the circumstances under which a child requires legal protection, and how this can be obtained. Certain people, usually senior social workers and police officers, may be empowered to issue a retention order which requires the child to be confined to a specified place for a defined period. A court enquiry should then be opened within a specified time.

In most instances, these circumstances constitute physical and/or emotional neglect, non-accidental injuries, or some other form of child abuse.

Legislation should provide for the subsequent management of such children, who may be placed:
♦ back in the same family, following suitable reconstruction services
♦ in adoption
♦ in foster care, or
♦ in a suitable institution.

Detailed regulations are required for each of these procedures, which will permit permanent and yet optimal placements to be made as early as possible, to obviate a prolonged stay in an unsuitable environment.

Where parental consent for medical examination and treatment is unobtainable or refused, provision must be made in the law for such care to be made available to a child.

Education
Normal schools
The importance of formal education of the child cannot be overstressed. It must be pointed out that infant mortality, parity, and birth interval are related, *inter alia*, to the mother's education. Furthermore, the most disadvantaged child requires more skilful teaching and therefore higher expenditure, in order to bring the child to the level of his/her more privileged counterpart. The syllabus should be appropriate to needs, yet not overlook the goal of providing equal opportunities for all. The adverse role of malnutrition and other debilitating states in the learning process has been stressed elsewhere *(see Chapter 7, Nutritional*

Disorders). The apathetic, irritable, malnourished child is limited in his capacity to explore and to learn.

It has been recognized that pre-school education is essential, and not simply a luxury.

During the first 5 years of life, the child's mind is at its most receptive. Not only is the ability to absorb maximal during this phase, but the pattern of handling information and of reasoning is established during this stage of rapid development. Greater stress on this aspect of education in overall planning would save much time, money, and unhappiness, and facilitate subsequent learning immeasurably.

Any form of pre-school centre can serve as an entry point into the community for health promotion, where mothers can obtain information and learn skills *(see panel, Facts for life.)*. It also provides an opportunity for screening, as the child with a developmental or specific learning disability can be identified at a stage when corrective teaching will be most beneficial.

Special schools
The proportion of children with varying degrees of disabilities and handicaps requiring special education is relatively high in communities with a deficient primary health care system. Whereas the state should take the responsibility for the education of these children, the cost of establishing and maintaining these special schools is prohibitive. In industrialized countries this type of special school has been largely abolished in favour of integrating the handicapped child into the mainstream education system and providing the teachers with specific instructions to meet these needs. Health professionals have the responsibility of ensuring that these children obtain the most appropriate and efficient support that is available. Accurate data on the prevalence of disabilities and handicaps are an essential preliminary step in determining the country's overall requirements for these children.

In the absence of special schools, rehabilitation field workers who are equipped with basic skills could facilitate and sustain the implementation of programmes designed by relevant professionals. There is a particular need for corrective education (remedial teaching) required by those 5–10% of otherwise-intelligent children who have a specific learning disability. This problem is at times associated with hyperactivity in the Attention Deficit Disorder *(see Chapter 30, Psychological and Behavioural Disorders).*

Informal education

The child learns from day-to-day activities in and around the home far more than from structured teaching. Clearly the child who is nurtured in an enriching environment will be at a great advantage. It is important to stress that sophisticated toys and equipment are not required for this type of learning. A basic requirement is that the parent or child-minder is aware of, and takes an interest in, the needs of the child. Apart from encouraging the child to become engaged in household activities, simple media such as water, mud, wooden blocks, old magazines, and empty containers are of great value. The child's informal education is frequently restricted, as much of the child's drive to explore, experiment, and learn is interpreted as 'naughtiness'.

A great deal can be achieved by providing parents and child-minders with the necessary basic information through clinics, religious groups, women's groups, pre-schools, community centres, radio, and so on.

Adoption

The **procedure** of adoption takes place when a mother abrogates all rights of parenthood and guardianship, and thus consents to her progeny becoming the legal child of a third party. The latter is generally a couple, but in certain situations a single parent may adopt a child. The details of this procedure, which should be laid down in legislation, are primarily in the interests of the child. Legal adoption provides the only avenue of ensuring a secure and suitable family for an unwanted child.

Although the main consideration is the welfare of the child, there is no doubt that the adoptive parents' lives can be immeasurably enriched as the result of an adoption. However, it is hazardous to assume that an insecure marriage will be cemented by virtue of an adoption. This latter motive, as well as that of securing help in the home or sustenance in old age, should be strongly discouraged.

With this in mind, it stands to reason that the **prospective adoptive parents** must be in good health — physically, mentally, and emotionally — and preferably between 25 and 40 years of age. Careful screening by an informed doctor and social workers is necessary.

Precautions must be taken to ensure that the **child** is well. Ideally the pregnancy and birth should be supervised, to avoid perinatal insults to which this type of baby may be exposed. Clearly a detailed examination during the neonatal period is essential. If all significant anomalies have been ruled out, one is then in a position to reassure the adoptive parents that the risk of any inherited disorder is smaller than if they were to have had a child of their own. Serological tests for syphilis, AIDS, and hepatitis should be part of the routine assessment. A medical examination some months after placement of the infant is advisable, before the adoption is finalized.

On the other hand, many couples are prepared to adopt a child with a defect. The implications of this, together with a detailed prognosis, must be put to these prospective 'parents' before such an adoption can proceed.

The **biological parents** obviously also require careful handling. Preferably, the question of adoption is broached early on in pregnancy, so that the necessary emotional adjustments can be made. Wherever possible the father should be drawn into this to engender a sense of responsibility. Not infrequently, mothers of unwanted babies do not avail themselves of antenatal care, and are seen for the first time when in labour. The subject can be raised even at this late hour. It is desirable that the mother gives formal consent for adoption as soon as possible after the birth, without any undue pressure being brought to bear on her. However, some assistance in outlining the issues involved is not out of place. For her there is no ideal solution; giving up the child will naturally result in some mourning and periods of regret. On the other hand, if she opts to keep the baby because she feels guilty or frustrated, she must be made aware of the long-term commitment and sacrifices that parenthood demands.

The **main problems** which arise out of adoption can be avoided by making use of an adoption agency which has experienced social workers and a medical panel at its disposal. No adoption should

be arranged and finalized privately without this assistance, as the risks of subsequent complications are too great. Some of the common problems are:
◆ misconceptions about adoption vs. fostering
◆ maladjustments due to insufficient counselling and subsequent support
◆ attitudes of the community to adoption and illegitimacy; cultural attitudes to biological progeny, etc.

The **role of health professionals** is to suggest adoption whenever the unborn child would appear to be unwanted antenatally, be it in the labour ward or when attending to a neglected child of a pregnant mother. Health professionals are in the best situation to identify the mother who will have difficulty in bonding with and nurturing her child. The gynaecologist or family doctor is ideally situated, when faced with a childless couple who are anxious to have a family, to refer them to a suitable agency.

The number of orphaned and abandoned children is bound to increase during the 1990s, as westernization and AIDS continue to take their toll in the Third World. Adoptive parents will be in great demand, but as few will be economically secure enough to nurture another child, subsidized adoption will have to be given consideration.

Foster care

A child in need of care may be placed in the care of foster parents by a welfare agency. The state may provide a maintenance grant, and the agency should continue to supervise the situation.

Occasionally the child will return to its biological parents, if circumstances have improved as a result of reconstruction services (in the form of counselling and social support structures).

Exploitation of the child and poor emotional bonding are some of the disadvantages of this system.

Child abuse

Customarily this malady has been referred to as 'baby battering'. However, as many of the patients are not battered, and by no means all of them are babies, the term 'child abuse' is preferable. The problem is not uncommon, and is one of great seriousness, with an appreciable rate of morbidity and mortality.

Definition

Child abuse means the infliction, or allowing the infliction, of physical or mental harm on a child, by a person who is responsible for that child. This may be by way of non-accidental injury (NAI), emotional trauma, sexual abuse, neglect and abandonment, or administration of drugs or alcohol.

Prevalence

Most health professionals are reluctant to accept that child abuse occurs in their community. No stratum of society is exempt, although it is far more common among the socio-economically disadvantaged. Accurate statistics on child abuse are very difficult to obtain, as the condition remains under-diagnosed and there is no statutory notification in most countries.

It is remarkable how frequently one encounters suspicious circumstances surrounding trauma when one screens all children under the age of 4 years.

In order to make comparisons with the extent of this problem in other countries, it should be noted that in the United Kingdom it is estimated that two children die of NAI every day; while in the USA, 25% of all fractures in children under the age of 3 are due to child abuse.

Risk factors

The following risk factors contribute to the likelihood of child abuse:
◆ step-child
◆ fostered/adopted child
◆ mental and/or physical defect
◆ one of twins
◆ interference of mother-child bond at birth
◆ prematurity
◆ single, self-supporting parent
◆ teenage mother
◆ socio-economic domestic crisis.

The abuser may be a parent, the parent's lover, a child-minder, a sibling, or a teacher.

Many of the parents who abuse their children have had a disturbed childhood and are themselves survivors of child abuse.

Clinical presentation

As one can seldom make a definite diagnosis of child abuse, the following features should be noted:

History:

♦ implausible (e.g., a fractured limb or skull due to a 'fall from a bed')

♦ inconsistent

♦ delay in reporting the injury

♦ past history of injuries.

Examination: Any marked disparity in the state of hygiene, dress, or nutrition between the mother (or surrogate mother) and the child should be noted. The following are strongly suggestive of NAI:

♦ bruises, whip injuries (parallel or scattered linear abrasions), scars, bite marks, and injuries of varying duration are of particular significance

♦ circumferential injuries of the wrists, ankles, or neck

♦ burns by cigarettes or due to immersion

♦ sub-conjunctival, anterior chamber, or retinal haemorrhage

♦ 'benign' raised intracranial pressure

♦ unexplained impaired consciousness

♦ smell of alcohol

♦ signs suggestive of ruptured abdominal viscera

♦ transverse fractures of long bones or fractures at unusual sites.

Over-zealous and at times brutal corporal punishment by a parent or teacher is one of the most common types of NAI. It is essential to regard this as child abuse and to have each incident followed up, in the hope that the perpetrator may learn alternative modes of discipline.

Diagnosis

It is of utmost importance that all professionals have a high index of suspicion. The diagnosis of child abuse must be considered if some of the above criteria are present. There is obviously no need for definite proof, and one is often required to act on suspicion. Supporting evidence includes a roentgenographic skeletal survey, which can provide evidence of serious trauma in the past.

Bleeding disorders have to be ruled out, but one must bear in mind that the combination of this and NAI may occur, e.g., the author encountered a 2-year-old haemophiliac and a 6-year-old with leukaemia who were subjected to severe non-accidental injuries by their parents.

Management

Notification of child abuse, whether confirmed or suspected, has become mandatory for health professionals in some countries, e.g., South Africa.

A non-judgemental attitude must be maintained. Any attempt to castigate the suspected abuser should be resisted, as it is likely to complicate matters.

Admission to hospital is strongly advisable, to protect the child from further injuries and to undertake the necessary investigations. In many instances this comes as a relief to the abuser, as the injuries are often inflicted impulsively or against better judgement. When the parents refuse admission, legislation should provide the necessary legal cover to enforce the doctor's decision.

A detailed record of the clinical findings must be made, as this may be required for legal proceedings.

Once the diagnosis has been confirmed or is strongly suspected, the parents must be confronted with the implications of the injuries.

Wherever possible a team should be involved, where the social worker, nurse, psychologist, and doctor all play a role. A sympathetic law enforcement officer or lawyer can be of tremendous help in deciding when the abuser should be prosecuted. In many instances a Children's Court Enquiry should be opened. This is largely the responsibility of the welfare agency, but health care workers must provide the necessary professional evidence.

Discharge from hospital should await approval of the social worker, either in the hospital or the outside agency, where available. The main criterion must be the safety of the child. If the home circumstances have not altered substantially, alternative arrangements have to be made. Wherever possible, a definitive plan of action should be mapped out for permanent placement of the child. Repeated moves, involving disruption, and severing of emotional bonds, may result in permanent psychological trauma.

Apart from physical trauma, abused children have generally been subjected to profound **emotional insult**. Those to whom the child looked for love, support, and security have become aggressors and objects of fear. Remedying this situation requires skilled handling under professional guidance, in order to avoid a situation whereby the abused, in turn, becomes a child abuser.

After-care is essential, as the risk factors may still prevail. Defaulting parents should be reported to the Commissioner of Child Welfare.

The **prognosis** for completely restoring the relationships within the family to an acceptable level is often difficult to assess. The following factors suggest a poor outcome, and therefore the need for protection of the child:

- abuse in the parent's childhood
- bizarre, sadistic, or premeditated injuries
- severe neglect associated with physical injuries
- history of minor injuries followed by major trauma
- self-righteous parents obsessed with harsh discipline
- absence of guilt or concern for the child
- low tolerance to stress and high external pressure
- chaotic social life, with little prospect of change.

Neglect and abandonment

This occurs most frequently in unwanted children. Once it has taken place, management becomes difficult and necessitates the involvement of a social worker.

The role of the health professional lies largely in prevention, by:

- identifying the mother–child pair at risk
- promoting bonding during the crucial postnatal period
- providing the community with alternative and acceptable methods of dealing with an unwanted child. These are most effective at key points such as antenatal and well-baby clinics.

The mother who displays little interest in her pregnancy or baby, who is uncooperative during the birth and is loath to breast-feed, can often be identified by the midwife. It is at this stage that the mother must be offered the possibility of adoption or foster placement.

The abandoned child has to be removed to a place of safety until the mother or guardian has been traced and/or adoption or foster care can be arranged. This, regrettably, is a time-consuming procedure, which exposes the child to prolonged institutional care and makes subsequent adoption much more difficult.

The chronically ill or handicapped child is also at risk of being neglected or abandoned. The family must be kept informed, and involved in the therapeutic programme to maintain their interest and prevent emotional withdrawal.

Sexual abuse

This relatively common form of abuse requires special consideration as it is particularly abhorrent and difficult to detect. In most instances the abuser is a male, who may be the father, step-father, or any member of the extended family. The victim is usually a girl, not infrequently of very tender years. Homosexual assaults do occur, but boys are more commonly abused outside the home.

Although the mother may be aware, or have a suspicion, of the practice, she is immobilized by the fear of dissolution of the family. She may herself have been subjected to abuse in childhood and/or be unable to find the necessary inner strength to bring the affair to light. Thus, denial on the part of the mother is not an unusual phenomenon.

The most common modes of presentation are evidence of sexually transmitted diseases, urinary symptoms, genital trauma causing difficulty in walking, and vague psychosomatic complaints.

Gonorrhoea and syphilitic sores are concrete evidence, whilst condylomata accuminata must be regarded with grave suspicion. Late-onset enuresis, urinary tract infection, or dysuria in the absence of infection, should raise the possibility of sexual abuse. Vague lower abdominal pain or unexplained headache may have a similar origin.

Examination of the genitalia can usually be carried out with little difficulty provided it is done sensitively and with tact and patience. Girls under the age of three years are best examined while sitting on their mother's lap with heels well drawn up against their buttocks. Good exposure is obtained on complete abduction of the knees. Bruising and other injuries of the vulva, perineum, or thighs should be carefully noted. The introitus and the hymen must be thoroughly inspected. Sexual penetration causes a midline tear of the hymen. Non-sexual and less forceful penetration increases the size of the hymenal orifice (> 0.7 mm). Careful inspection of the perineum and anus for evidence of sodomy is imperative; viz., bruising, superficial tears, dilated veins, patulous anus. Anal intercourse may be inflicted on girls in association with attempted or successful vaginal penetration.

Specimens of any discharge must be collected on moist sterile swabs for culture and/or microscopy.

Older girls can be examined in a similar way lying supine and appropriately draped. Laxity of the pubo-coccygeal muscle is further evidence of sexual activity. Blood should be taken from every sexually abused child to exclude syphilis and AIDS. A further specimen after 6 weeks is necessary should serology be negative.

Identification of an extra-familial perpetrator should be the responsibility of a specialized unit within the police force.

Management is difficult and calls for the involvement of a social worker and a clinical psychologist. Therapy begins with the disclosure and the first contact with a health professional. It is important that the trust that children naturally have in figures of authority is re-established after the hurt which they have experienced. The specific treatment will depend on the age of the child, the duration of the abuse, the relationship to the perpetrator, and the cultural background of the family. When children have learned to conceal their emotions from early childhood, psychotherapy becomes very difficult. Ideally the family and perpetrator should participate in the process, in the form of group or family therapy.

Drugs and alcohol

These are occasionally given to children to 'keep them quiet'. Unscrupulous child-minders have been known to administer alcohol to their charges to facilitate supervision. The problem may present as a comatose infant with hypoglycaemia due to alcohol intoxication.

Drug dependence

(Drug addiction, drug abuse)

Introduction

Drug dependence must be considered in a wide context, which includes the abuse of alcohol, solvent and glue sniffing, and the smoking of marijuana (cannabis, *dagga*). There are very few children who are not exposed at some time or other to this social disease. The child is particularly vulnerable, as traffickers tend to exploit the young and gullible.

Levels of drug abuse

The child may be involved in drug abuse at three levels:

◆ the infant born to a drug/alcohol-dependent mother enters the world with a profound handicap which, apart from physical and emotional neglect, may present as the fetal alcohol syndrome or drug withdrawal symptoms *(see Chapter 5, Newborns)*

◆ the families of those involved in illicit producing or trafficking of drugs are frequently deprived of adequate education, nutrition, and domestic stability

◆ the child or adolescent deprived of parental love and creative outlets is at risk of falling prey to this social disease.

Aetiological and epidemiological factors

Abusers can be grouped into:

◆ those in search of an exciting experience because their life appears dull

◆ those in search of oblivion because their life lacks any joy or lustre

◆ those in search of a new personality because their life is filled with anxiety and indecision.

In Third World communities, urbanization and industrialization together with migrant labour and high-pressure life-styles have disrupted families and eroded traditions and support structures. The younger generations are, therefore, deprived of stability and have scant resources to fall back on in the face of anxiety, conflicts, and temptations.

Generally males are more frequently abusers, as are those who dwell in urban ghettos. The most important aetiological factors, however, are lack of parental love and understanding, as well as unrealistic expectations.

Clinical features

The drug scene is dynamic, varying with the socio-economic status of the family, the prevailing vogue, and the availability of different types of drug. The characteristics of the dependants are determined by the drug: thus alcohol produces a clinical picture very different from that of solvent-sniffing or the smoking of marijuana. Alcohol and marijuana are used by adolescents, while glue and solvent sniffing is widely practised among younger age groups.

Marijuana in moderate usage causes euphoria, inattentiveness, loss of memory for recent events, increased suggestibility, nausea, and vertigo. Examination shows tachycardia, conjunctivitis, dry mouth, and ataxia. In higher doses depersonalization, hallucinations, and anxiety states may be released. The most significant aspect is that habitual usage may replace social usage in an attempt to evade stress or confrontation. It interrupts the normal psychological growth process, thus preventing emotional maturation. While the abuser is using this escape mechanism, skills for coping with the stresses of everyday life are not developed.

Solvent and glue sniffing: The hydrocarbons in solvents and toluene in glue give rise to euphoria, hallucinations, and vertigo. The practice is not free from serious side-effects. These organic chemicals can cause appreciable liver, kidney, and nervous system damage. Permanent brain damage may occur, with ataxia and personality change, or there may be irreversible peripheral neuropathy.

The diagnosis should be considered when one is dealing with unexplained coma, seizures, ataxia, or behavioural disturbances. Sniffing is frequently the precursor of major drug dependence and is a sign of an emotionally distressed child.

Alcohol: The easy accessibility to alcohol is probably one of the main reasons why alcoholic beverages are abused so frequently. Those who act as models for the child, namely parents and teachers, often contribute to the problem by drinking excessively themselves. Commercial promotion is a further powerful force urging the young to partake of a particular product, with the implied promise of a better life.

The dangers of dependence are no fewer with alcohol than with any of the other substances. As with solvent or glue sniffing, alcoholism in a young patient suggests emotional instability or distress.

The odour of the breath facilitates the diagnosis of the child, if seen within hours of imbibing. The clinical features may resemble those of the all-too-familiar presentation of alcohol intoxication. However, coma ensues earlier in the child and is a high risk in infants. Hypoglycaemia frequently results in coma because of the direct inhibition of gluconeogenesis by alcohol.

Management

Health professionals have an important role to play in both the prevention and treatment of drug abuse. An awareness of the prevalence of drug abuse, as well as the motivations involved, is essential. Prevention depends on community-based programmes which aim to help the dependent individual to associate with a user or non-user who lives in the presence of drugs without becoming dependent on them. This includes the development of social and creative skills and sufficient recreational facilities in an environment where affection, understanding, and encouragement between generations can be fostered. The feeling of personal worth must be engendered, particularly where there is a risk of the individual being submerged in anonymity.

Educational programmes are most rewarding in a younger child, who must be enlightened on the dangers of drug abuse.

Skilled clinical psychologists and/or social workers are essential members of the team. Where these professionals are not available, a suitable member of the nursing profession or the community can be selected and specifically trained to assist in the handling of the individual and the overall problem.

In handling the individual, an authoritarian, judgemental attitude must be avoided. Together with the patient, one can endeavour to establish the causes of anxiety and to find alternatives for meeting emotional needs. This approach has been found to be more successful than attempting to limit usage by a more direct approach. Reducing pressures both at home and at school, at least initially, is advisable.

Specific therapy is rarely available. Supportive measures are important, with the correction of hypoglycaemia and careful monitoring and nursing of the patient with impaired consciousness being paramount.

Neonatal withdrawal syndromes *(See Chapter 5, Newborns.)*

Adolescent pregnancy

Sexual activity amongst teenagers is becoming increasingly prevalent at younger ages in virtually all communities. Amongst factors contributing to this are early physical maturation and changing social norms with increased mobility of youngsters. Social deprivation in overcrowded homes and lack of family cohesion undoubtedly make substantial contributions. Sexual intercourse must be seen as part of adolescent risk-taking behaviour.

The natural consequence of this phenomenon is a rapid increase in the incidence of adolescent pregnancies. Generally contraceptive services, with poor accessibility and availability, are not attuned to the needs of youngsters. On the other hand, many a young girl sees pregnancy as a short-cut to adulthood from a childhood of boredom and misery. Studies have shown that an appreciable number of young girls fall pregnant following sexual abuse or rape. The percentage of unwanted pregnancies amongst girls aged 16 years and under has been found to be 60–80% in Durban, South Africa.

Problems

The problems surrounding this issue are multiple and serious. Due to unfavourable circumstances many of these young girls do not submit themselves to pre-natal supervision, and hence enter childbirth in a high-risk category. Infection, un-controlled pregnancy-induced hypertension, and pre-term labour are common complications. The young mother's parents may reject her, and the father of her child often abandons her, leaving her to enter motherhood ill-prepared and with little or no support.

Whereas health professionals may consider these issues outside their realm, they unquestionably impinge seriously on the life and health of the baby. It is imperative that the mother is armed with the basic knowledge of infant care. Alternatively, the possibility of adoption must be offered to her *(see above)*.

Interventions

Interventions must be considered at many levels, and provide ample opportunity for involvement by health professionals. Life and parenting skills should form an integral part of school curricula. In particular, sex education must be given high priority. Outside the school setting, religious institutions and other social structures can participate in educational camps, and by providing recreational activities. Contraceptive services must be geared to the needs of the adolescent. For the young mother, support groups and 'clubs' are a dire necessity.

Generally, health professionals should remain non-judgemental, whilst not condoning promiscuity. They should promote an understanding that the problem of adolescent pregnancy is a problem of the whole community, and that these large numbers of youngsters should not be allowed to enter premature parenthood by default.

W.E.K. Loening

5

Newborns

Care of the newborn

The first 30 days of life constitute the newborn period. The neonate is in a very vulnerable state during the time when adaptations to extrauterine life take place. This is seen principally in the respiratory and gastrointestinal systems, and in the haemodynamics of the cardiovascular system. The kidneys and liver take on the full excretory and metabolic functions that were shared by the maternal organs during intrauterine existence.

The high-risk pregnancy

There are a number of conditions during pregnancy, labour, and delivery which indicate that serious neonatal problems must be anticipated. Early identification of these conditions is the first step in the prevention of neonatal illness, thus reducing morbidity and mortality. Once a high-risk pregnancy and/or fetus are identified, the progress of labour and delivery are carefully

monitored, and appropriate intervention must follow. Optimal management of these babies requires good communication between those caring principally for the mother and the delivery, and those responsible for the baby. Asphyxia is probably the most common condition following on a high-risk pregnancy, and therefore skilled resuscitation, and correct equipment and drugs are essential. Factors associated with, and which identify, the high-risk pregnancy are outlined in *Table 5.1*.

The high-risk neonate

Morbidity and mortality are appreciably reduced by identifying risk factors both during pregnancy and after birth. The next step is careful observation during the first few days or weeks, depending on the risk factors, and subsequent careful follow-up for long-term complications. Unfortunately, however, the patients who require this are frequently the very ones who are unable to comply,

---

Table 5.1   Factors identifying the high-risk pregnancy

Maternal	Labour and delivery	Fetal
Obstetric:	Maternal hypertension	Oligohydramnios
Elderly primigravida	Maternal hypotension	Polyhydramnios
Anaemia	Maternal sedation	Multiple pregnancy
Poor weight gain, obesity	Prolonged rupture of membranes	Fetal distress (acidosis,
Previous abruptio	Prolonged first or second stage	meconium-stained liquor, abnormal FHR)
Previous assisted delivery	Caesarean section	Growth retardation
Poor obstetric history	Breech	Post-maturity
(stillbirth, > 2 abortions)	Cord compression	Malformations
Previous LBW	Precipitate delivery	
Neonatal death	Pre-term labour	
Illness: diabetes, cardiac, renal	Forceps or vacuum extraction	
Pregnancy-induced hypertention		
Social:		
Age < 16 or > 35 years		
Socio-economic deprivation		
Alcohol consumption		
Smoking		
Child with cerebral palsy		

---

due to poverty and poor access to health care facilities. All babies born from a high-risk pregnancy or labour, as well as those with features outlined in *Table 5.2,* must be considered high risk neonates.

Table 5.2   Factors identifying the neonate at risk

High risk	Medium risk
Pre-term or post-mature	Birth weight 1.5–2.49 kg
Small for gestational age	Clinically stable after
Large for gestational age	resuscitation
Birth weight < 1.5 kg or	Birth trauma
> 4kg	Abnormal CNS signs
Neurological depression	Cold exposure
after resuscitation	Jaundice
Metabolic problems after	Anaemia
birth	Multiple births
Any congenital abnormality	

General

History

The medical history of the neonate aims at identifying preventable conditions which influence morbidity and mortality. These include socio-economic conditions, maternal marital status and age, past obstetric history of abortions, stillbirths, low birth weight, and mode of delivery, neonatal deaths, and congenital abnormalities.

Evaluation of the current pregnancy includes the duration of pregnancy, maternal blood group, syphilis serology, maternal disease such as diabetes, cardiac, renal, and pregnancy-related illnesses (including hypertension, abruptio placentae, placenta praevia), abnormal maternal weight gain, smoking, and substance abuse during pregnancy.

Labour and birth details must include duration of the stages of labour and of membrane rupture, amount and character of liquor, size and appearance of placenta, drugs administered to the mother during labour and delivery, and the need for and extent of resuscitation of the baby.

Initial examination, resuscitation and management in the delivery room

The temperature of the delivery room must be suitable for the baby, i.e., 23–28 °C, and it must be free of draughts. On delivery of the head, the nose and mouth are sucked gently to clear mucus, blood, or meconium. Following a normal delivery the cord is probably best clamped when pulsations have ceased. There is a debate, however, concerning the optimal time, as late clamping results in extra blood volume and problems related thereto, such as polycythaemia. On the other hand, early clamping facilitates rapid resuscitation of the asphyxiated newborn.

The Apgar score *(see Table 5.3)* is determined at 1 and 5 minutes: the 1 minute score indicates the possible need for immediate intervention, and the 5 minute score gives an indication of the long-term prognosis. The score at 10 and 20 minutes is probably equally important. Resuscitation of the asphyxiated neonate is described below.

Once respiration is well-established, a nasogastric tube is passed and the stomach emptied in order to prevent possible aspiration of stomach contents. This procedure has great merit, as it immediately excludes two major congenital malformations, viz. choanal atresia and tracheo-oesophageal fistula.

If the baby is well at delivery the eyes and face are wiped clean, vitamin K 1 mg is given, and the cord is clamped and cut. A rapid examination is performed to exclude cyanosis, pallor, excessive secretions, respiratory distress, jaundice,

Table 5.3   Apgar score

Sign/score	0	1	2
Heart rate	Absent	< 100	> 100
Respiratory effort	Absent	Slow, irregular	Good crying
Muscle tone	Limp	Some flexion	Active movement
Response to nasal catheter	Nil	Grimace or sneeze	Cry
Colour	Pale, central cyanosis	Body pink, extremities blue	All pink

abnormal behaviour and temperature, and major malformations. Early detection of these and appropriate intervention will reduce morbidity and mortality. The baby is then warmly wrapped and handed to the mother for the first feed. After this period of stabilization which lasts 1–2 hours, the first bath is given, when care must be taken to clean the vernix from hair, ears, and skin folds.

Examination of the newborn
A thorough physical examination is carried out at a convenient moment soon after birth, preferably in the presence of the mother. The weight, length, and head circumference must be recorded *(see Chapter 1)*. Care must be taken to avoid hypothermia during the examination. The normal baby need not be re-examined until just before discharge, when the weight and any unusual findings are noted.

BCG and polio immunization are given routinely on discharge from most institutions.

Routine care of the healthy newborn
Healthy newborn babies should not be kept in hospital unnecessarily. However, every baby has to be given some basic care. Following delivery room procedures, the baby should be with the mother to encourage breast-feeding and to promote her observation and caring skills. She must be alerted to her baby's need to be kept warm, and to the danger of infection from contaminated hands. Routine hand-washing or spraying with a disinfectant before handling any baby is very important. The cord must be kept clean and dry by repeated application of an alcohol solution, e.g., chlorhexidine. Attention to the skin folds is essential, as moisture readily permits monilial infection. Clothing must be changed daily, with meticulous washing, rinsing, and drying of garments.

Urine should be passed within the first 24 hours, and stool within 36 hours of birth. The latter is in the form of meconium for 2–3 days, followed by transitional stool which is green to black with milk curds for several days, and thereafter the normal non-offensive soft, yellow, acid stools appear at the end of a week.

The normal infant loses up to 10% of body weight in the first few days, but usually regains this within 10 days. The rate of weight gain thereafter is in the range of 200–300 g per week. The mother must be kept informed regarding the well-being of her baby, her queries and questions handled gently and sympathetically. Breast-feeding difficulties must be anticipated and managed with expertise, to foster the mother's interest and confidence in this form of feeding, and thus to ensure exclusive breast-feeding for the first 4 months.

The process of bonding must be fostered carefully, as a failure to bond may result in maternal rejection and reluctance to breast-feed and cuddle the baby. Lack of maternal co-operation and interest in the baby are features suggestive of rejection. Any indication of this must be handled sensitively. Where facilities exist, professional counselling must be called for, and where indicated, the question of adoption should be raised *(see Chapter 4, Community Paediatrics)*.

While preparing for discharge, the parents should also be advised about routine newborn care, the common signs of illness, the immunization programme, family planning, and regular clinic visits with the Road-to-Health Card *(see Chapter 4)*. The mother must be made fully aware of the merits of this card. Lastly, parents need to be told about the most convenient primary health care facility for continued maternal and child care.

Signs of illness in the neonate
The neonate demonstrates illness by a limited number of non-specific physical signs. Knowledge of these and the ability to evaluate them are important.

Each of these signs is discussed below.

Central cyanosis (i.e., of gums and tongue) usually indicates respiratory insufficiency; occasionally it is due to congenital heart disease. It may also be a manifestation of a convulsion, sepsis, or hypoglycaemia. Peripheral cyanosis indicates a temperature change or hypotension.

Pallor of the face or extremities suggests anaemia, haemorrhage, hypoxia, shock, sepsis, or hypoglycaemia.

Convulsions suggest a central nervous disorder such as asphyxia or meningitis, or they are a non-specific sign of severe illness with circulatory insufficiency.

Apnoea may be the first sign of a convulsion or respiratory disease.

Lethargy can be the result of maternal sedation and analgesia, or it may be due to hypoglycaemia, asphyxia, or infection.

Failure to feed is an important sign, particularly when previous feeds were taken well. Meningitis and other infections must then be considered.

Fever may be environmental, or due to dehydration or infection.

Hypothermia is commonly due to exposure, but severe infection, or central nervous system or circulatory disorders must be ruled out.

Jaundice in the first 24 hours of life is a serious physical sign, indicating either rhesus incompatibility or infection.

Vomiting, particularly when bile-stained, indicates intestinal obstruction, but infection must always be considered *(see also Chapter 28, Surgical Problems)*.

Diarrhoea may be a sign of fat or sugar intolerance, acute gastroenteritis, or a non-specific sign of infection.

Failure to move a limb suggests infection, fracture-dislocation, or nerve injury.

Resuscitation

Delayed onset of respiration is most commonly the result of intrapartum asphyxia. A low 1 minute Apgar score does not necessarily correlate with biochemical evidence of asphyxia, and conversely babies with biochemical evidence of asphyxia may breathe vigorously at birth.

Asphyxia in term babies is the most common cause of neonatal brain damage and is the leading cause of cerebral palsy in the developing world.

Factors causing delay in the onset of respiration at birth are asphyxia, trauma to the brain, and drugs depressing the respiratory centre. Less common causes include profound lung pathology, as in hyaline membrane disease, or meconium aspiration, severe anaemia, and some of the congenital malformations. Occasionally severe immaturity or primary muscle disease is responsible.

Asphyxia may be acute, chronic, or prolonged and low-grade in nature. Intrauterine growth retardation is often associated with partial asphyxia of long standing, as demonstrated by signs of chronic fetal distress.

Although the **clinical manifestations of asphyxia** are in the first instance neurological in nature, which may respond well to resuscitation, less obvious effects on other organs such as the lungs and the kidneys may manifest during the ensuing days. Hypoxia, hypercapnia, and acidaemia resulting from asphyxia cause tissue injury. Clinical manifestations of the cerebral insult are those of hypoxic ischaemic encephalopathy (HIE). Acidaemia in itself affects the myocardium, with a consequent drop in cardiac output. The combination of hypoxia, acidaemia, and hypotension will affect the lungs, kidneys, gut, and liver. Metabolic disturbances such as hypoglycaemia, hyperglycaemia, hypercalcaemia, and inappropriate anti-diuretic hormone secretion may occur. There may also be clotting disturbances resulting in disseminated intravascular coagulation.

Labour ward management of resuscitation

Ideally every birth should be attended by a health professional skilled in neonatal resuscitation. In order to effect rapid and efficient resuscitation, all the necessary equipment must be available and in working order at all times *(see Table 5.4)*. Furthermore, adequate facilities for keeping the neonate warm must be at hand.

The resuscitation procedure is outlined in *Fig. 5.1.*

Table 5.4 Equipment necessary on resuscitation trolley

Laryngoscope — straight blade, plastic, e.g., Penlon®, infant-size, spare batteries and bulbs

Magill's forceps — paediatric size

Endotracheal tubes sizes 2.5, 3.0, and 3.5 mm

Neonatal Ambu-bag® and mask

Suction catheters sizes 8 FG and 6 FG

Umbilical catheters sizes 8 FG and 6 FG — to be used only if peripheral intravenous line is not possible

Feeding tubes sizes 8 FG and 6 FG

Adhesive tape

Dextrostix®

Intravenous fluids 5% dextrose, 5% dextrose in 0.2% saline, 4% albumen

Syringes and needles of different sizes

Blood culture bottles, specimen containers, and tubes

Ampoules of 50% dextrose

Ampoules of 8.5% and 4% sodium bicarbonate

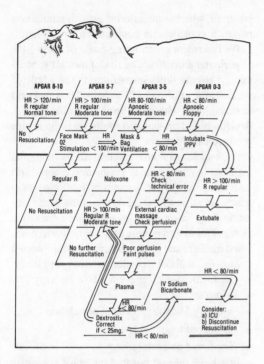

Fig. 5.1 *Flow diagram of resuscitation procedure*
Dosages: Naloxone 0.01 mg/kg; sodium bicarbonate
1 mEq/kg; Dextrose slow infusion of 10% solution.

Immediate intubation with intermittent positive pressure ventilation (IPPV) is essential for the neonate who is floppy, pale, and has a heart rate less than 80 per minute.

Intubation must be preceded by clearing the airway of mucus, blood, or meconium under direct laryngoscopy. The baby must be kept dry and warm during this procedure.

Oxygen is given by mask when the Apgar score is between 3 and 7 (i.e., central cyanosis, heart rate of 100–120, irregular and poor respiratory effort, and some hypotonia). Suctioning of the pharynx is not indicated if there are clear secretions, as irritation by blind, vigorous suction may precipitate laryngospasm, apnoea, and bradycardia *(see also Respiratory Disturbances, below)*.

The infant who does not respond to resuscitation

If the response to resuscitation is poor but the baby is otherwise normal in appearance, technical problems must be excluded. Where there is no air entry, either the oxygen tube is disconnected or the endotracheal tube is kinked or blocked with secretions. In the latter case the tube must be replaced.

Where breath sounds are unequal the tube is probably placed in the right main bronchus and should be withdrawn until breath sounds are symmetrical. Diminished breath sounds and chest movements are probably due to a misplaced endotracheal tube in the oesophagus. In rare instances when too small a tube is used, this needs to be replaced. Unequal breath sounds with a displaced apex beat are due to pneumothorax, which can be confirmed by transillumination and an urgent chest X-ray. An apical intercostal drain must be inserted if the diagnosis is confirmed.

The infant who becomes pink and has a good cardiac output with IPPV, but is unable to maintain respiration after 20 minutes, is suffering from severe asphyxia, drug depression, hypoglycaemia, metabolic acidosis, and/or shock.

Whenever possible a chest radiograph must exclude severe underlying lung disease. Only after all the above conditions have been excluded and drug depression is not a possible contributing factor is it appropriate to discontinue life-support. Neonates with severe asphyxia who have not established sustained respiration after 20 minutes almost always develop signs of severe hypoxic ischaemic encephalopathy, with a poor long-term outcome.

Care following resuscitation

Ongoing care of the infant who required resuscitation is very important. It is necessary to monitor the temperature and blood sugar level, to maintain a clear airway by oropharyngeal suction, to turn the baby regularly, and to give oxygen when necessary. Tube-feeding is advisable until one is certain that oral feeding is quite safe.

Each system should be monitored for signs of asphyxial insult — convulsions, a full fontanelle, and tone and feeding disturbances indicate hypoxic ischaemic encephalopathy (HIE) *(see below)*. The pulse rate, peripheral perfusion, and blood pressure are indicative of cardiovascular function. Abdominal distension, enlarging kidneys, decrease in urine output, and the presence of blood or protein in the urine suggest renal involvement.

Transport of the high-risk patient

(Also see Chapter 28, Surgical Problems.)

Once the high-risk mother or baby has been identified and the immediate needs assessed, the question of transfer to a referral centre arises. Transport of the fetus *in utero* is preferable, but delivery *en route* is hazardous. Active maternal haemorrhage and fetal distress are contraindications until appropriately managed, i.e., intravenous fluids for the former, and oxygen, the lateral position, and beta adrenergics for the latter.

Conditions requiring transfer of the mother before delivery include eclampsia, severe pregnancy-induced hypertension, abruptio placentae, multiple pregnancy, significant maternal disease, and poly- or oligohydramnios.

The referral centre should always be informed before transferring any patient.

With regard to the neonate, the following precautions must be taken:
- ensure a clear airway
- suction and oxygen must be available *en route*
- correct hypothermia and prevent heat loss during transfer; skin-to-skin contact with the mother is most efficient, but at times a transport incubator is preferable
- pass a nasogastric tube
- correct the blood sugar level
- ensure that vitamin K has been given
- if an intravenous line has been established, the drip rate and volume control must be monitored
- appropriate medical information must accompany the patient
- send maternal blood samples in the rare event of the mother not accompanying the neonate.

Low-birth-weight, small-for-gestational-age, and large-for-gestational-age babies

The prevalence of low-birth-weight (LBW) infants is a reflection of the health status of the community. In highly developed countries no more than 7% of births fall into this category, whereas in some underprivileged communities more than 30% of infants weigh less than 2 500 g at birth. The majority of infants in the former group are

pre-term, whereas intrauterine growth retardation makes a considerable contribution to the latter. LBW is a major contributing cause of up to 74% of perinatal mortality. The risk of mortality, however, is twenty times greater during the whole of the first year of life in LBW infants. They also tend to be children who grow up to be malnourished, develop into short-statured adults, and who in turn produce LBW infants.

Poor socio-economic circumstances, maternal malnutrition, adolescent pregnancy, short birth intervals, and physical exertion late into pregnancy are all contributing factors. Low-grade amniotic fluid infection is an established causative factor. This in turn is more prevalent in undernourished mothers and those who practice unprotected coitus (i.e., without a condom) during pregnancy.

The factors which prevent LBW are very few and simple:
- improved health of general population
- improved maternal health
- improved antenatal care.

In a large referral hospital one must anticipate 12–20% of births to be LBW. About 20–25% of these are likely to experience infections. The survival in underprivileged communities can be gauged from *Table 5.5,* where mortality can be seen to be related to birth weight.

Table 5.5 Approximate mortality for African neonates in Durban according to weight groups

Weight (kg)	Mortality (%)
> 2.5	0.5
2.0–2.49	2–3
1.5–1.99	9–10
1.25–1.49	20–25
1.00–1.24	40–45
< 1.00	75–80

Ideally all LBW infants should receive special care. Some need intensive care, but these facilities are rarely available in Third World countries. Apart from efficient primary health care, emphasis should be placed on meticulous routine nursing care, which in itself achieves a great deal for these special infants. Sophisticated monitoring and life-support systems make a negligible contribution to their overall survival, but such equipment is likely

VENTRAL SUSPENSION	HEAD LAG	SCARF SIGN	HEEL TO EAR	POP LITEAL ANGLE	LEG RECOIL	ARM RECOIL	ANKLE DORSI-FLEXION	SQUARE WINDOW	POSTURE	SCORE
				180°	180°	180°	90°	90°		0
				160°	90–180°	90°–180°	75°	60°		1
				130°	<90°	<90°	45°	45°		2
				110°			20°	30°		3
				90°			0°	0°		4
				<90°						5

Fig. 5.2   Neurological criteria for estimating gestational age
(From Dubowitz *et al., Journal of Pediatrics*, 1970: 77)

to make crippling demands on personnel and budget.

Definitions

It is important to recognize three distinct entities, i.e., low birth weight, pre-term infant, and small for gestational age.

Low birth weight is a birth weight of less than 2 500 g.

A **pre-term infant** is one born prior to 37 weeks' gestation.

Small for gestational age (SGA) or **light for date (LFD)** is a birth weight below the 10th centile for that period of gestation.

Large for gestational age (LGA) or **heavy for date (HFD)** is a birth weight above the 90th centile for that period of gestation.

Determination of gestational age

The gestational age is established by the Dubowitz method, using both neurological and external criteria (*Fig. 5.2* and *Table 5.6*). The total score obtained from these criteria indicates the gestational age on the graph in *Fig. 5.3*.

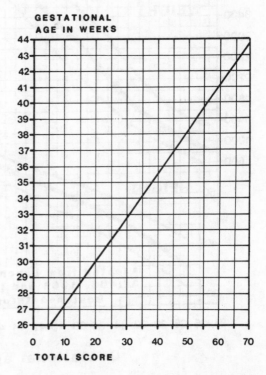

Fig. 5.3   Graph for reading gestational age from total score
(From Dubowitz *et al., Journal of Pediatrics*, 1970: 77)

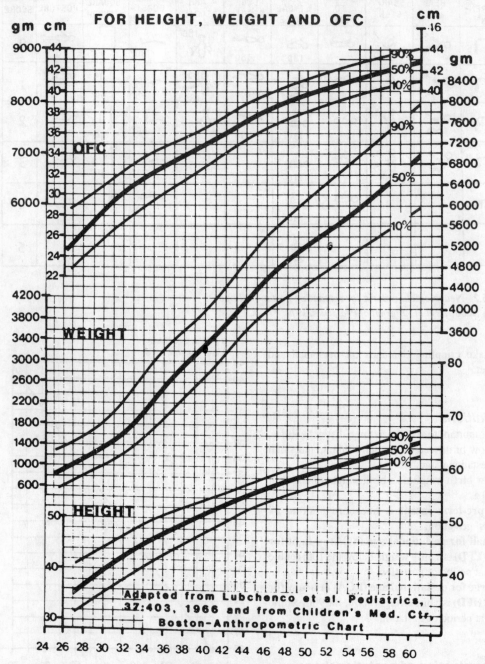

COMBINED INTRAUTERINE-NEONATAL GROWTH CHART FOR HEIGHT, WEIGHT AND OFC

Fig. 5.4 Combined intrauterine growth chart for height, weight, and head circumference (OFC)
(From Lubchenco, L.O., 'Intrauterine growth charts', *Pediatrics*, vol. 37, no. 3, p. 403. Copyright American Academy of Pediatrics)

Table 5.6   External (superficial) criteria for determining gestational age

Sign	0	1	2	3	4
			Score		
Oedema	Obvious oedema hands and feet; pitting over tibia	No obvious oedema hands and feet; pitting over tibia	No oedema		
Skin texture	Very thin, gelatinous	Thin and smooth	Smooth; medium thickness. Rash or superficial peeling	Slight thickening. Superficial cracking and peeling, esp. hands and feet	Thick and parchment-like; superficial or deep cracking
Skin colour (infant not crying)	Dark red	Uniformly pink	Pale pink: variable over body	Pale. Only pink over ears, lips, palms, or soles	
Skin opacity (trunk)	Numerous veins and venules clearly seen, especially over abdomen	Veins and tributaries seen	A few large vessels clearly seen over abdomen	A few large vessels seen indistinctly over abdomen	No blood vessels seen
Lanugo (over back)	No lanugo	Abundant; long and thick over whole back	Hair thinning especially over lower back	Small amount of lanugo and bald areas	At least half of back devoid of lanugo
Plantar creases	No skin creases	Faint red marks over anterior half of sole	Definite red marks over more than anterior half; indentations over less than anterior third	Indentations over more than anterior third	Definite deep indentations over more than anterior third
Nipple formation	Nipple barely visible; no areola	Nipple well defined; aerola smooth and flat; diameter < 0.75 cm	Areola stippled, edge not raised, diameter < 0.75 cm	Areola stippled, edge raised; diameter > 0.75 cm	
Breast size	No breast tissue palpable	Breast tissue on one or both sides < 0.5 cm diameter	Breast tissue both sides; one or both 0.5–1.0 cm	Breast tissue both sides; one or both > 1 cm	
Ear form	Pinna flat and shapeless, little or no incurving of edge	Incurving of part of edge of pinna	Partial incurving whole of upper pinna	Well-defined incurving whole of upper pinna	
Ear firmness	Pinna soft, easily folded, no recoil	Pinna soft, easily folded, slow recoil	Cartilage to edge of pinna but soft in places, ready recoil	Pinna firm, cartilage to edge, instant recoil	
Genitalia male	Neither testis in scrotum	At least one testis high in scrotum	At least one testis right down		
Females (with hips half abducted)	Labia majora widely separated, labia minora protruding	Labia majora almost cover labia minora	Labia majora completely cover labia minora		

From: Dubowitz *et al.* 1970. *Journal of Pediatrics*, Vol. 77, No.1
(Adapted from Farr *et al.* 1966. *Developmental Medicine and Child Neurology.* Vol. 8, pp. 507)

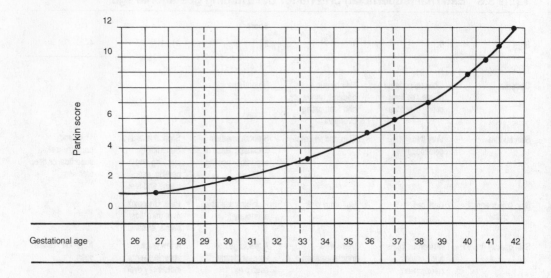

Fig. 5.5 Assessment of gestational age using the Parkin criteria

The appropriate weight for the gestational age is obtained from the Lubchenco Chart *(Fig. 5.4),* which gives intrauterine growth parameters. All those between the 10th and 90th percentile are appropriate-weight-for-age babies (AGA). The ill neonate often has disturbed neurological function,

Table 5.7 Definition and scoring of the criteria for the Parkin score

Skin texture
Tested by inspection and by picking up a fold of abdominal skin between finger and thumb.
0 — Very thin with a gelatinous feel
1 — Smooth and thin
2 — Smooth, medium thickness, irritation rash and superificial peeling may be present
3 — Slight thickening and stiff feeling, superficial cracking and peeling especially on the hands and feet
4 — Thick and parchment-like with superficial or deep cracking

Skin colour
Estimated by inspection when the baby is quiet.
0 — Dark red
1 — Uniformly pink
2 — Pale pink, though colour may vary to very pale over some parts of the body
3 — Pale, nowhere really pink except ears, lips, palms, and soles

Breast size
Measured by picking up breast between finger and thumb.
0 — No breast tissue palpable
1 — Breast nodule palpable on one or both sides
2 — Nodule palpable on both sides, one or both being 0.5–1 cm diameter
3 — Nodules palpable on both sides, one or both being greater than 1 cm diameter

Ear firmness
Tested by palpation and folding of the upper pinna
0 — Pinna soft and easily folded into bizarre positions, does not recoil spontaneously
1 — Pinna soft along the edge and easily folded. Recoils slowly spontaneously
2 — Cartilage felt to edge of pinna, though thin in places. Pinna recoils readily
3 — Firm pinna with definite cartilage extending to periphery, recoils immediately

The total for the Parkin score is converted to gestational age using the chart shown in *Fig. 5.5.*

therefore the neurological criteria of the Dubowitz score become an inappropriate assessment of gestational age. The Parkin score is used for a rapid assessment *(see Fig. 5.5* and *Table 5.7).*

Some notes on techniques of assessment of neurological criteria

(See Fig. 5.2.)

Posture is observed with infant quiet and in supine position. Score O = arms and legs extended; 1 = beginning of flexion of hips and knees, arms extended; 2 = stronger flexion of legs, arms extended; 3 = arms slightly flexed, legs flexed and abducted; 4 = full flexion of arms and legs.

Square window: The hand is flexed on the forearm between the thumb and index finger of the examiner. Enough pressure is applied to get as full a flexion as possible, and the angle between the hypothenar eminence and the ventral aspect of the forearm is measured and graded according to the diagram. (Care must be taken not to rotate the infant's wrist during this manoeuvre.)

Ankle dorsiflexion: The foot is dorsiflexed onto the anterior aspect of the leg, with the examiner's thumb on the sole of the foot and other fingers behind the leg. Enough pressure is applied to get as full a flexion as possible, and the angle between the dorsum of the foot and the anterior aspect of the leg is measured.

Arm recoil: With the infant in the supine position the forearms are first flexed for 5 seconds, then fully extended by pulling on the hands, and then released. The sign is fully positive if the arms return briskly to full flexion (score 2). If the arms return to incomplete flexion or the response is sluggish, it is graded as score 1. If they remain extended or make random movements the score is 0.

Leg recoil: With the infant supine, the hips and knees are fully flexed for 5 seconds, then extended by traction on the feet, and released. A maximal response is one of full flexion of the hips and knees (score 2). A partial flexion scores 1, and minimal or no movement scores 0.

Popliteal angle: With the infant supine and pelvis flat on the examining couch, the thigh is held in the knee–chest position by the examiner's left index finger and thumb supporting the knee. The leg is then extended by gentle pressure from

the examiner's right index finger behind the ankle, and the popliteal angle is measured.

Heel-to-ear manoeuvre: With the baby supine, draw the baby's foot as near to the head as it will go without forcing it. Observe the distance between the foot and the head as well as the degree of extension at the knee. Grade according to diagram. Note that the knee is left free and may draw down alongside the abdomen.

Scarf sign: With the baby supine, take the infant's hand and try to put it around the neck and as far posteriorly as possible around the opposite shoulder. Assist this manoeuvre by lifting the elbow across the body. See how far the elbow will go across and grade according to illustrations. Score 0 = elbow reaches opposite axillary line; 1 = elbow between midline and opposite anterior axillary line; 2 = elbow reaches midline; 3 = elbow will not reach midline.

Head lag: With the baby lying supine, grasp the hands (or arms if a very small infant) and pull him slowly towards the sitting position. Observe the position of the head in relation to the trunk and grade accordingly. In a small infant the head may initially be supported by one hand. Score 0 = complete lag; 1 = partial head control; 2 = able to maintain head in line with body; 3 = brings head anterior to body.

Ventral suspension: The infant is suspended in the prone position, with examiner's hand under the infant's chest (one hand in a small infant, two in a large infant). Observe the degree of extension of the back and the amount of flexion of the arms and legs. Also note the relation of the head to the trunk. Grade according to diagrams.

The pre-term infant

Clinical features

These are well described in the criteria for the assessment of the gestational age, above. The markedly pre-term infant shows very obvious clinical features. It is important, however, to exclude intrauterine growth retardation which might make a greater contribution to the LBW than prematurity. This aspect obviously also needs consideration in the management.

A rapid but superficial impression can be obtained by scrutinizing the breast, nipple development, the plantar creases, and muscle tone.

Complications

The appropriate-for-gestational-age (AGA) pre-term neonate suffers a number of clinical difficulties related to the fact that most organs are functionally and metabolically immature.

Respiratory problems commonly occur due to the immaturity of higher controlling centres, resulting in a periodic pattern of respiration or apnoeic episodes (i.e., 20 seconds or more). The respiratory centre is very sensitive to the effects of hypoxia and maternal sedation, causing respiratory depression. Furthermore, inadequate surfactant results in alveolar collapse and the idiopathic respiratory distress syndrome (IRDS) *(see below)*. Premature labour may be initiated by maternal infection, which can result in pneumonia causing respiratory problems at birth.

Hypoglycaemia occurs with greater frequency in pre-term babies, due to inadequate stores of glycogen. This, in association with poor fat storage, promotes hypothermia. There is difficulty in maintaining the normal body temperature due to the large surface area, poor muscle tone, and inability to shiver.

Hepatic immaturity contributes to the development of neonatal jaundice and a tendency to bleed due to lack of vitamin K-dependent coagulation factors (II, VII, IX and X).

Oedema is a recognized clinical feature of the pre-term infant *(see Miscellaneous Problems, below)*.

Feeding difficulties may pose a significant problem in the care of the premature baby. Adequate sucking and swallowing develop by about 35 weeks of gestation, and thus regurgitation, aspiration, and consequent pneumonia are a constant hazard in more premature babies. Abdominal distension due to a relatively atonic bowel aggravates feeding difficulties and impedes diaphragm movement.

Intraventricular haemorrhage is a constant hazard with pre-term infants, due to the rich network of unsupported capillaries in the germinal matrix. Asphyxia, fluctuations in the blood pressure, and an unstable metabolic status predispose these delicate vessels to rupture, with ensuing peri- or intraventricular haemorrhage.

Immaturity of the immune system results in a predisposition to *Gram-negative infections* in particular. These may present with non-specific physical signs, making the diagnosis difficult. A high degree of suspicion is required to institute the necessary investigations.

Anaemia is a common problem in this group of neonates. The early form arises from exaggerated physiological factors and sluggish erythropoietic response. Late anaemia occurs with rapid growth and depletion of relatively poor iron and folate stores. Vitamin E deficiency may contribute to development of anaemia in a pre-term baby.

Management

Management of the pre-term baby is relatively simple, requiring very basic facilities and careful nursing. This calls for meticulous monitoring of the respiration, heart rate, colour, and temperature.

Maintenance of a normal body temperature is the first and most important step in the management. Great care must be taken to avoid hypothermia, as this in itself diminishes the chances of survival and aggravates other complications. Day and night skin-to-skin contact with the mother has been shown to be very effective both in the prevention and management of hypothermia. More sophisticated equipment can be used where available and necessary.

A normal blood sugar level and the institution of early feeding either orally or by gavage is the next stage of management. Frequent small feeds or continuous nasogastric drip feeds are essential to avoid complications, starting with a total of 50 ml/kg/day and increasing by 25 ml daily to 200 ml/kg/day if tolerated. Intravenous feeding is advisable for the sick pre-term baby, giving 60 ml/kg/day on day 1, and gradually increasing to 150 ml/kg/day provided that there is no oedema. Factors which increase insensible water loss, such as tachypnoea and high ambient temperature (overhead warmer, phototherapy) need to be taken into account.

The airway must be kept clear at all times by correct positioning, and apnoeic episodes must be recognized early for appropriate management *(see Respiratory Disturbances, below)*. The signs of respiratory distress must be similarly noted, and oxygen administered for cyanosis.

Particular attention must be paid to measures which prevent infection. Even mild degrees of jaundice must receive consideration if kernicterus is to be avoided. Haemoglobin levels must be checked serially, starting on the first day.

Once the clinical condition of the infant is stabilized, and life-threatening complications of the first few days of life adequately dealt with, the pre-term baby is observed carefully, with continued precautions against infection being taken. Great patience and considerable time are required to support the mother in establishing breast-feeding. Monitoring the weight gain will assist in evaluating the baby's well-being. The environmental temperature can be decreased gradually, bearing in mind that failure to gain weight is an early sign of undue heat loss. Promoting mother-and-baby contact to establish bonding is an important aspect of pre-term care. The multiplicity of procedures and apparatus are often intimidating for the mother, who will be inclined to withdraw, limiting her involvement with her baby.

The baby is ready for discharge when breast-feeding has been fully established. The suitable weight for discharge should be determined individually, depending to some extent on available health services and conditions at the unit of delivery.

The mother of a pre-term infant should be counselled on the general care and hygiene of her baby, particularly with regard to washing hands, signs of illness, regular clinic attendances, and fertility control.

These aspects must receive particular emphasis in mothers who are at risk, such as the adolescent and those with a poor obstetric history. Wherever possible, home visits should be arranged. The mother and her pre-term baby must be seen by an experienced health worker within a week of discharge.

The management of complications is dealt with in detail in the following section.

Small-for-gestational-age (SGA)/ light-for-gestational-age (LGA) babies

These babies can be classified as symmetrically or asymmetrically growth-retarded. The former implies an early intrauterine insult or other constitutional factors resulting in a small baby with weight, length, and head circumference below the 10th centile. Asymmetrical growth retardation is due to placental factors which cause failure to gain weight, or even loss of weight, on the fetal trunk and limbs, but spare the head.

Common causes of symmetrical growth retardation are genetic abnormalities, chromosomal defects, chronic uterine infection, and teratogenic agents such as alcohol. Asymmetrical growth retardation may be caused by pregnancy-induced hypertension, placental infarction, partial separation of the placenta, poor nutrition of the mother, severe physical exertion late into pregnancy, smoking during pregnancy, and amniotic fluid infection syndrome.

Clinical features

The essential feature common to all these babies is a birth weight below the 10th centile for gestational age. The symmetrically growth-retarded infant may show features of the causative disease, such as a chromosomal defect or intrauterine infection. A high index of suspicion should be maintained for the features of the fetal alcohol syndrome *(see Disorders of Central Nervous System, below)*.

Intrauterine growth retardation (IUGR) of late onset causes loss of subcutaneous fat and minimal or absent vernix caseosa. Facial appearance is one of alertness, with a wizened expression. The skin is thickened and desquamating, with a parchment quality. The muscle tone is generally increased. As the liquor may well have been meconium-stained for some considerable period, the skin and umbilical cord have a dirty green discoloration.

Complications

As the SGA infant may have suffered chronic oxygen and nutritional deprivation *in utero*, the acute stress of the birth process is not well tolerated. The infant is therefore predisposed to a number of clinical problems. **Birth asphyxia** is the most important, and can be detected by monitoring the fetal heart rate during labour and delivery. There is a great risk of **meconium aspiration** both *in utero* and at birth in the term growth-retarded baby, and of **pneumonia** in the pre-term baby. Hyaline membrane disease, in contrast, is relatively uncommon and less severe. **Hypoglycaemia** may occur during the first 48 hours, due to poor glycogen reserves. Temperature regulation is impaired, as fat stores have also been depleted.

Infections occur more readily in the SGA baby, due to suppressed immunity. Furthermore, manifestations of infections are very subtle. Chronic hypoxia stimulates erythropoietin production, resulting in **polycythaemia** and possible complications thereof.

Prognosis

The asymmetrically growth-retarded baby is likely to do fairly well if adequately fed postnatally. The symmetrically small baby appears to have been programmed early *in utero*, and in general does less well. There is a slightly increased risk of cerebral palsy and mental retardation in term SGA infants, and they are at increased risk of manifesting minor neurological disorders. On the other hand, the premature SGA infant appears to have a higher incidence of major handicap than term SGA and AGA premature infants.

Management

The mother with a growth-retarded fetus must be regarded as having a high-risk pregnancy which calls for the best attention available. Early termination of pregnancy should be considered if there is continued evidence of lack of fetal well-being. During labour careful monitoring of the fetal heart will give an indication of the need for oxygen and glucose infusion to the mother. Once again early intervention is called for should there be evidence of acute fetal distress.

During the delivery of a growth-retarded baby, one must anticipate and prevent meconium aspiration, and institute early management which is essential and urgent.

Subsequent observations must be geared to early detection of respiratory distress, of hypoglycaemia by frequent monitoring with Dextrostix®, and of hypothermia by frequent measurement of core temperature.

The neonate with symmetrical growth retardation requires investigation for specific causative factors, and appropriate action.

Feeding is not as problematic in SGA babies as it is in pre-term infants, as they are usually wide awake and take feeds avidly. Supplementary glucose feeds (given by spoon) are advisable during the first few days, to avoid hypoglycaemia. Every effort must be made to ensure adequate nutrition

after discharge, by making the mother aware of the deficit which must be made up and the risks to which the baby is predisposed.

For the rest, the management corresponds to that of the pre-term baby.

The very-low-birth-weight baby (VLBW)

Babies weighing less than 1.5 kg at birth represent a small percentage of live births (1–2%), but they contribute more than 50% to the overall neonatal mortality. Survival rate with tertiary care is about 60%. However, the cost of intensive and high-level care of this group of babies is enormous. Furthermore, the social background is an important consideration for the after-care, as many of these VLBW babies are born to adolescent or other disadvantaged mothers. Often the pregnancy is unplanned, and the babies are frequently rejected. The VLBW baby therefore places a considerable financial and social burden on the community in general.

Prevention

Education and fertility control of the teenager must receive serious consideration. Adequate antenatal care is essential so that early detection and appropriate management of pre-term labour is effected to delay delivery where feasible. Women with threatened labour before 32 weeks of gestation need early transfer, so that optimal conditions for delivery and efficient after-care can be provided.

Immediate problems in the neonatal period

As the homeostatic balance of the VLBW baby is even more precarious than the bigger LBW baby, meticulous attention is essential.

Prompt, skilled **resuscitation** is the single most important determinant of a favourable outcome.

Temperature regulation is critical, as the thermo-neutral range in the smaller baby is narrow, with a marked tendency to hypothermia.

Hypoxia and hyperoxia readily occur in recurrent and prolonged episodes, as tissue levels of oxygen fluctuate widely. Poor respiratory excursion and **apnoea** occur spontaneously and are often induced by handling. The most serious effect

Table 5.8   Swellings of the head

	Caput succedaneum	Vacuum extraction haematoma	Cephalhaematoma	Subaponeurotic haemorrhage
Site	Diffuse over presenting part	Localized at site of vacuum application. Skin and subcutaneous tissue involved	Localized, usually over parietal bones, under periosteum. Extension limited by periosteal adhesion of sutures	Diffuse over whole head underneath cranial aponeurosis
Cause	± Oedema and bruising of presenting part	Oedema ± haemorrhage at vacuum site	Haemorrhage often due to cephalo-pelvic disproportion	Diffuse haemorrhage; sometimes follows vacuum extraction or poorly applied forceps
Onset	Present at birth	Present at birth	Often only detected 6–12 hours after birth. Becomes progressively larger over 1–2 days	May be present at birth; swelling often increases during first 2 days
Distinguishing features	Diffuse. Petechiae over swelling	Usually well-defined. Localized abrasions at periphery of swelling. Overlying skin may be purple	Well-defined. Does not cross suture lines. May be bilateral, but then a groove is present between the two swellings. Skin normal	Diffuse and sometimes massive haemorrhage. Crosses suture lines. Bluish discoloration of upper eyelids or behind ears. Skin normal
Course	Disappears within 48 hours	Subsides within 5–7 days	Persists 6–8 weeks. Centre may become fluctuant	Gradual reabsorption of blood
Complications	Nil	Anaemia, infection, jaundice	Anaemia, jaundice, infection if aspirated. Rarely, underlying skull fracture	Severe anaemia, shock, jaundice
Treatment	Nil	Local antiseptic to abrasions. Treat complications	Usually nil. Observe for complications	Vitamin K. May need urgent blood transfusion

of hypoxia is on the delicate unsupported vessels of the periventricular area, resulting in haemorrhage (see below).

Hyperoxia occurs as a result of over-zealous treatment of apnoeic episodes or hyaline membrane disease, risking injury of the retina (retinopathy) and lung (broncho-pulmonary dysplasia).

The incidence of **hypoglycaemia** is higher in VLBW babies, particularly if feeding is delayed. Similarly, a 10% dextrose infusion may result in hyperosmolality. Fluid and electrolyte balance may be difficult to achieve. The hazards of fluid restriction in these babies are well established. Hypernatraemia, acidosis, hypoglycaemia, and hyperbilirubinaemia are very real hazards unless close attention is paid to early feeding. Monitoring for clinical signs of dehydration and for **biochemical disturbances** is essential to maintain homeostasis.

In the **long term** there are several problems. General health in the first year of life is likely to be affected by frequent infections, particularly of the respiratory tract. The death rate is high due to brain damage or acute respiratory illness. The **sudden infant death syndrome** occurs more often in the VLBW than in the full-term baby. Those who are appropriate for gestational age can be expected to grow at the same velocity as a

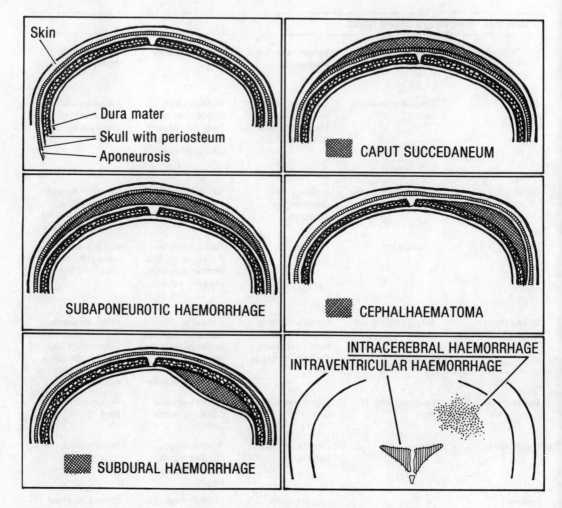

Fig. 5.6 *Caput succedaneum and intra- and extracranial haemorrhage in the newborn*

full-term infant of the same conceptual age. Neo-natal problems cause a delay in regaining the birth weight for 2–3 weeks, but following recovery growth should proceed at the normal rate. Poor growth occurs in the SGA infant, and in those with prolonged undernutrition in the early weeks of life. Visual, auditory, speech, and other neurological deficits must be expected, and actively sought at clinic visits.

The large-for-gestational-age baby (LGA)

The best-known association of LGA babies (those with a birth weight above the 90th centile for gestational age—4.0 kg at term), is maternal dia-betes *(see below)*. Large mothers and those with excessive weight gain during pregnancy can expect to have LGA babies. The Beckwith's syndrome is a much rarer cause, and has associated macroglossia, macrosomia, and small genitalia.

The LGA infant is at risk of peripheral and intracranial birth trauma. As shoulder dystocia is a further possibility, Caesarean section is often indicated.

Management of the LGA baby delivered vaginally includes careful search for cerebral birth trauma, fractured clavicle, or brachial plexus injury. There is a need to monitor the blood sugar level of the infant for the first 36 hours, and maternal diabetes must be excluded.

There appears to be an increased risk of mental subnormality in this group, which is thought to be related to cerebral complications. Caesarean section and careful monitoring of the blood sugar after birth to prevent hypoglycaemia will decrease this risk substantially.

Birth trauma

Minor superficial injuries
Superficial abrasions on the infant's face, scalp, or other parts may be caused by blood sampling, rupture of the membrane by toothed forceps, or scalpel cuts during Caesarean section. Suturing may be necessary to prevent excessive blood loss. These lesions should be kept clean and dry.

Extensive bruising is often seen in the markedly pre-term neonate, particularly following breech delivery. Oedema, bruising, and haematomas may involve the vulva, scrotum, and testes following breech delivery of the baby. These injuries settle in a few days. However, careful examination of the testes subsequently is important, as testicular atrophy may be a rare complication. This extravasation may contribute to hyperbilirubin-aemia.

Subconjunctival haemorrhage often follows difficult delivery. It usually clears spontaneously within a week, requiring no therapy other than reassuring the mother.

Head injuries
Skull **moulding** denotes overriding of the cranial bones due to compression in the birth canal. It does not necessarily imply intracranial injury. The skull bones assume a normal position within a few days.

Swelling of the head is caused by caput succedaneum, vacuum extraction, cephalhaematoma or subaponeurotic haemorrhage, *(see Table 5.8 and Fig. 5.6)*.

Skull **fractures** may be linear, stellate, or depressed. Occasionally there is overlying soft tissue swelling, but rarely intracranial damage. Nevertheless, observation for 36–48 hours for signs of neuropathology is advisable. Depressed fractures are in the nature of a ping-pong ball indentation, and usually require elevation, if only for cosmetic reasons.

Limb fractures
Fractures of the clavicle, humerus, and femur may be substantial during difficult deliveries requiring manipulation. Movements of the affected limb are restricted and very painful. A collar and cuff suffices for the upper limb, whereas femur fractures are allowed to heal on their own. In every case the mother must be warned that a large callus is likely to form.

Nerve injuries
Facial paralysis, either due to forceps application or occurring spontaneously, is characterized by diminished movement of the affected side of the mouth, with or without ability to close the eye on the affected side. The baby may have difficulty in sucking. Treatment consists of keeping the affected eye clean by periodic instillation of sterile saline solution. The baby should be nursed on the unaffected side.

Brachial plexus injury is a serious injury which is usually caused by excessive traction in cases of impacted shoulders or breech delivery. **Erb's palsy** (upper arm paralysis) results from injury to cervical roots 5 and 6. The arm is rotated internally and hangs limply at the shoulder, the elbow is extended, the forearm is pronated, while the fingers are flexed in a 'waiter's tip' position. Wrist action and grasp reflex are normal. **Total arm paralysis** consists of a combination of Erb's palsy and Klumpke's paralysis, which may be associated with phrenic nerve palsy and respiratory embarrassment.

Complete rupture of nerve roots results in permanent lesions. If the paralyses are due to bruising of nerve roots, function returns within several months. Physiotherapy can be given after the first week. For Klumpke's paralysis the wrist and hand are splinted in a position of extension during sleep.

Abdominal viscera
Occasionally a difficult delivery results in rupture of the liver and/or spleen. Large babies are particularly prone to this serious injury. The first sign is usually shock, followed by anaemia and some abdominal distension. An urgent blood transfusion and laparotomy are called for. An additional dose of vitamin K is advisable.

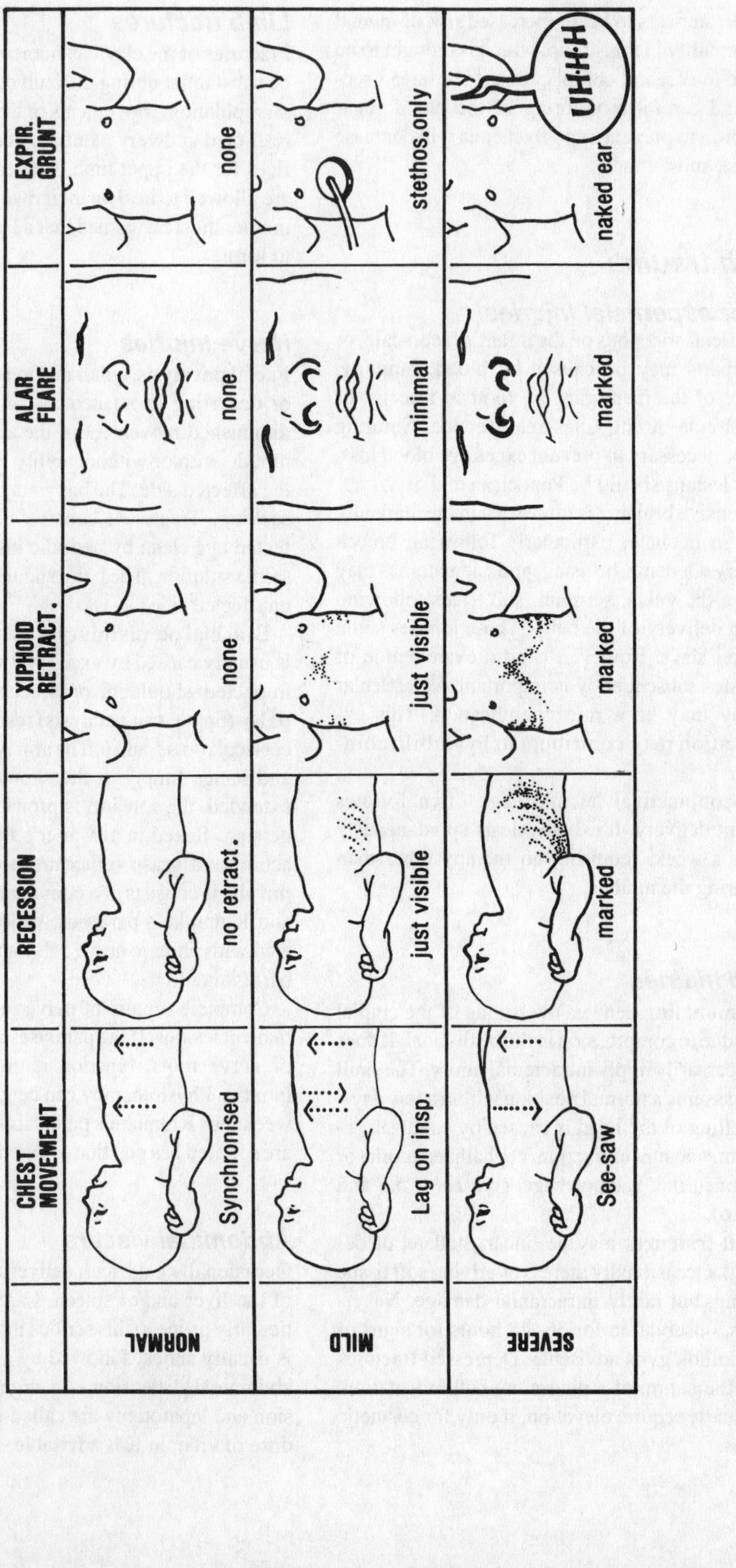

Fig. 5.7 Clinical features of respiratory distress

Table 5.9   Causes of respiratory distress

Pulmonary	Extra-pulmonary	Congenital abnormalities
Hyaline membrane disease	Cold exposure	Pneumothorax
Meconium aspiration	Cardiac failure	Diaphragmatic hernia
Congenital pneumonia	Cerebral damage	Tracheo-oesophageal fistula
Transient tachypnoea	Metabolic disturbances	Lung cysts
Acute pulmonary haemorrhage	Acute blood loss	
	Septicaemia	

Spinal cord injury

This rare injury usually results from traction on the legs in breech delivery. There is flaccid paralysis, with loss of sensation below the level of the lesion, and bladder distension. The prognosis is poor.

Respiratory disturbances

As respiratory problems are a leading cause of neonatal deaths, it is essential to have a clear understanding of the aetiological and preventive factors, and to have the necessary skills for early recognition and efficient management. Furthermore, it is important to recognize that disturbances of almost any of the other systems may manifest as respiratory problems. However, it is not uncommon for newborns soon after birth to have **transient mild respiratory distress**. This is an expression of adaptation from intrauterine to extrauterine conditions. The distress settles within 1–2 hours, and does not warrant investigation.

Disturbances of respiration may be due to problems in almost any system in the body.

Modes of clinical presentation

Cyanosis is most commonly due to pathology of the respiratory tract. Upper airway obstruction may simply be due to secretions or meconium, which are readily relieved by suction. More rarely it is due to a structural abnormality such as choanal atresia. Although parenchymal lung disease is the most common cause of cyanosis, congenital heart disease must be suspected if the cyanosis is not relieved by oxygen *(see Chapter 17, Cardiac Disorders)*.

Stridor indicates an abnormality of the upper airway, such as laryngeal webs or cysts and laryngomalacia. Mass lesions at the base of the tongue may present with intermittent or positional stridor.

Apnoea or poor respiratory effort may be caused by failure or depression of the respiratory centre.

Respiratory distress (RD) *(see Fig. 5.7)* is diagnosed when two or more of the following criteria are present:

- a respiratory rate of 60/min. or more
- the presence of an expiratory grunt
- intercostal and/or sternal recession
- pulmonary crackles
- cyanosis while breathing air.

The causes commonly encountered are listed in *Table 5.9*.

Principles of management of respiratory distress

From the list of causes of respiratory distress it can be seen that it is imperative to have a chest radiograph for an aetiological diagnosis.

Oxygen is administered in a concentration that abolishes cyanosis, and blood gas analysis (if available) should be performed approximately 1 hour after clinical improvement and correction of any metabolic acidosis. A whole blood transfusion is indicated if the haemoglobin is below 12.0 g/dl, giving 10–20 ml/kg over 3 hours. A plasma infusion should be given if the peripheral perfusion and pulse volume are poor. Circulatory and renal function are assessed by the urine output. Apart from routine care, the blood sugar level must be monitored with Dextrostix®. Antibiotics are indicated in conditions such as hyaline membrane disease, meconium aspiration, and congenital pneumonia.

Principles of and indications for oxygen therapy

Oxygen administered indiscriminately, particularly to the pre-term infant, may lead to retinopathy and blindness *(see Chapter 25, Disorders of the Eye)*. However, too little oxygen leads to hypoxic brain damage.

The main indication for oxygen therapy is cyanosis or a change in colour, such as pale extremities and a central duskiness. Oxygen should not be given for respiratory distress *per se*.

If the baby is obviously cyanosed or has had a cardiac arrest, 100% oxygen must be given. This must be reduced once a clinical response occurs, which may be delayed for up to 20 minutes. A baby with poor colour should be given 30 – 40% oxygen, which is again reduced with clinical improvement. This concentration of oxygen can be achieved by running 2–3 l/min into a headbox or incubator. Even at these low concentrations the arterial level may exceed 100 mm Hg. Oxygen therapy without additional ventilatory support is sufficient if the respiratory effort is good and there is reasonable tone and cry. Blood gas analysis should show no carbon dioxide retention and PaO_2 of 50 –100 mm Hg in an ambient oxygen concentration of up to 60%.

Ideally all newborns who are at risk of developing respiratory problems are delivered at centres with special care facilities. Transfer of selected infants to such centres is warranted where there is moderate to severe respiratory distress, or if there is deterioration (suggested by a need for increasing amounts of oxygen, a steady increase in the heart and respiratory rate, or repeated apnoeic or cyanotic attacks). Often seriously ill neonates may benefit from respiratory support, such as in haemorrhagic or septic shock. Babies with severe asphyxia, convulsions, hypothermia, or hypoglycaemia should not be transferred, but corrective management must be instituted in consultation with the referral unit.

Immediate respiratory difficulties

Failure of the baby to breathe at birth suggests asphyxia or respiratory depression, and is managed as outlined under *Resuscitation, above*.

Acute respiratory distress soon after birth requires careful clinical assessment to determine whether it is due to parenchymal lung disease, extra-pulmonary conditions, or congenital abnormalities. Early diagnosis of congenital abnormalities in particular reduces mortality and morbidity, as surgical intervention is often required.

Upper airway conditions which may present at the time of birth are choanal atresia and Pierre Robin syndrome.

The features of nasal obstruction are cyanosis and suprasternal recession during feeding or when the mouth is closed. The cyanosis is relieved by crying.

These are the classical signs of choanal atresia. The diagnosis is confirmed when it is not possible to pass a fine tube through the nasopharynx. A thick plug of mucus in the nostrils may have a similar clinical presentation, but the obstruction is immediately relieved by nasal suction.

Episodic dyspnoea and cyanosis are indicative of the tongue falling back, impacting into a cleft palate and occluding the airway. These features together with micrognathia make up the Pierre Robin syndrome, i.e., respiratory obstruction occurs in the supine position and is relieved immediately on turning the baby.

Stridor may follow resuscitation either as a result of vigorous suctioning or intubation. Vocal cord paralysis may also cause stridor. On direct laryngoscopy the traumatized larynx or asymmetrical movement of the cords can be seen. Congenital abnormalities of the larynx such as webs, cysts, and malacia may also be diagnosed by direct laryngoscopy. Babies with webs and cysts must be referred for management, but an urgent tracheostomy may be called for. Laryngomalacia can be diagnosed when the larynx appears to collapse with inspiration due to inadequate cartilage support. The condition is self-limiting, but often lasts for many months.

Persistent extension of the neck may follow an abnormal presentation *in utero*. This normally settles in a few days. Careful examination of the neck must exclude goitre. Neck extension and the presence of stridor suggests a vascular ring, which can be confirmed by an X-ray with a contrast swallow.

The baby who has increased secretions from the time of birth, chokes, coughs, or becomes cyanosed with feeding must be regarded as having oesophageal atresia. This is easily confirmed by failure to pass a nasogastric tube into the stomach *(see Chapter 28, Surgical Problems).* A chest radiograph with the tube *in situ* will confirm the presence of the pouch, with the coiled tube visible.

Respiratory distress with diminished breath sounds, either on one side of the chest or over the upper lobes, suggests a pneumothorax, which is readily confirmed radiologically. Other signs include increasing respiratory difficulty, cyanosis, restlessness, and apparent dextrocardia.

Apnoeic and cyanotic episodes

Apnoeic episodes and periodic breathing in the premature infant are considered to be one end of a spectrum of disturbed respiratory regulation. Periodic breathing is a manifestation of incomplete development of the modulating system of respiration. Apnoeic spells result when this delicate system is disturbed by a number of factors. Bradycardia and cyanosis may occur in premature babies after 20 seconds of apnoea. Should this persist, hypotonia and unresponsiveness may develop.

The following conditions may be associated with apnoeic episodes:
- immaturity
- respiratory distress, particularly when due to obstructed airways
- hyaline membrane disease
- congenital pneumonia
- central nervous system pathology, e.g., convulsions, intracranial haemorrhage, cerebral anoxia or oedema, and meningitis
- septicaemia
- metabolic abnormalities, including hypoglycaemia, hypocalcaemia, hyponatraemia, acidosis, hyperbilirubinaemia
- marked temperature fluctuations.

Drugs given to the mother, particularly diazepam and magnesium sulphate, may cause profound respiratory depression, resulting in failure to establish respiration, or apnoeic spells.

Convulsions as the possible cause of apnoea need special emphasis, as the typical features characterizing a seizure in the older infant are rarely seen in a neonate.

Management

The respiration of patients who are 'at risk' of apnoeic episodes must be monitored carefully. This includes the immature baby, those with respiratory distress of any cause, the asphyxiated infant, the cold baby, and those likely to develop metabolic abnormalities.

The basic management of an apnoeic or cyanotic episode is firstly gentle pharyngeal suction. Oxygen is given per mask and the baby is stimulated by flicking the foot. Intermittent positive pressure ventilation has to be commenced if bradycardia occurs. If the pulse rate increases but remains of poor quality, then plasma 10 ml/kg may be infused over 20 minutes, and respiratory support should be considered if a ventilator is available.

Further management depends on the specific cause. For example, if apnoea is a manifestation of convulsions, anticonvulsant therapy, lumbar puncture, and careful neurological assessment are important. Hypoglycaemia and electrolyte imbalance require specific therapy. Infection must be excluded. Intravenous furosemide 0.5 mg/kg/dose is given if pulmonary oedema is the cause. When apnoea of immaturity is diagnosed by exclusion, oral theophyilline 5 mg/kg is given, followed by 2 mg/kg 8-hourly.

Idiopathic respiratory distress syndrome (IRDS) (hyaline membrane disease)

This problem is the clinical manifestation of lung immaturity. The lipoprotein surfactant which is necessary for initiating and maintaining the physico-chemical characteristics of alveoli is deficient, either because of lack of production or failure of release from alveolar Type II cells. The air sacs collapse, the pulmonary capillary permeability is increased, and protein-containing fluid and red cells ooze into the sacs. The protein (fibrin) coagulates to form a membrane which lines the alveolar sac; the sac itself contains oedema fluid and blood. Within a few days, the alveolar macrophages gradually remove the membranes and, as surfactant is produced, the normal physico-chemical properties of the gas-liquid interface in the air sacs are restored and the alveoli are able to maintain a spherical shape in expiration.

The assessment of lung maturity and of alveolar Type II cells is possible by measuring the ratio of lecithin to sphingomyelin (L–S ratio) in the amniotic fluid. The more mature the fetus, the closer the L–S ratio approaches 2:1.

The **bubble test** is a simple bedside means of assessing lung maturity:

1 ml of amniotic fluid and 1 ml of absolute alcohol are shaken vigorously for 30 seconds in a clean 10 ml glass tube. After 15 seconds the bubble score is read. The higher the score, the more mature the lungs.

0 = no bubbles
1+ = a single ring of bubbles
2+ = 2 rings of stable bubbles
3+ = more than 2 rings of bubbles and a clear centre
4+ = all of the miniscus covered in bubbles

A score of 2+ can be considered 'safe' with regard to lung maturity.

The pathophysiological effects of IRDS on pulmonary function are as follows:

◆ reduced lung compliance
◆ ventilation perfusion imbalance
◆ pulmonary vasoconstriction resulting in a large right-to-left shunt of blood
◆ alveolar ventilation and functional residual capacity are reduced
◆ minute ventilation and work of breathing are increased.

These changes result in hypoxaemia, hypercapnia, and eventually metabolic acidosis.

The classical radiological findings are a ground-glass appearance, air-bronchogram, and reticular granular pattern. However, this characteristic picture does not exclude infection.

Management is as for respiratory distress.

Surfactant is commercially available as a bovine extract or a synthetic preparation. The bovine extract has been shown to be of value in babies weighing even less than 1 kg, and it has to be administered with ventilatory support. However, the cost of one vial is enormous, and this has to be weighed against the cost of intensive care. The complications of intraventricular haemorrhage and bronchopulmonary dysplasia still occur, but seem to be less severe. Surfactant should only be given to a baby with a definite hyaline membrane disease requiring ventilation.

Table 5.10   Lesions of the central nervous system

A   Developmental defects

1   Neural tube defects
Encephalocele, myelomeningocele, spina bifida occulta, anencephaly

2   Defects in growth and differentiation
Chromosomal defects, porencephaly, hydrancephaly, megalencephaly, holoprosencephaly

3   Defects in cerebrospinal fluid circulation
Hydrocephalus, Dandy–Walker malformation, aqueduct stenosis

B   Perinatally acquired conditions

1   Hypoxic ischaemic encephalopathy

2   Intracranial haemorrhage
Subdural, subarachnoid, intraventricular, intracerebral, intracerebellar

3   Metabolic encephalopathies
Hypoglycaemia, kernicterus, hypothyroidism

4   Infections

Massive pulmonary haemorrhage

This catastrophic situation most commonly arises in the low-birth-weight infant during the acute or recovery phase of an illness such as asphyxia, infection, hypothermia, or coagulation defects. It occurs most commonly between the second and fourteenth day.

The treatment with transfusion and ventilation is unsatisfactory, as the mortality rate is near 100%. Probably of greater importance is the prevention of predisposing factors.

Meconium aspiration

This condition usually occurs in SGA infants. The passing of meconium *in utero* does not mean inevitable aspiration or intrauterine hypoxia. However, significant morbidity and mortality may be decreased by gentle suction of the mouth and nose at delivery of the head, followed by direct pharyngeal and/or tracheal suction immediately after delivery. The aspiration of meconium may have a number of effects on the lungs and heart:

◆ small airways obstruction with areas of atelectasis and air trapping

◆ complete tracheobronchial obstruction, with sudden development of cor pulmonale and death

◆ acute pneumonitis presenting with various degrees of severity, shock, and acute pulmonary oedema, or respiratory distress within an hour

◆ pneumothorax.

If there has been severe asphyxia and hypotension, cerebral oedema and renal problems with fluid overload may readily occur.

The natural history is one of full clinical and pulmonary recovery within 3–5 days, unless severe asphyxia or pneumonitis cause death.

Management is as for respiratory distress.

Persistent pulmonary hypertension of the newborn (PPHN)

In this condition right-to-left shunting through the foramen ovale and ductus arteriosus occurs as a result of high pulmonary vascular resistence. Profound hypoxia resulting in cyanosis occurs soon after birth. The heart is structurally normal, the chest X-ray may show pulmonary oligaemia, and the ECG is most often normal.

PPHN may present as a primary disorder (lungs appear normal or oligaemic on chest X-ray) or with RDS, meconium aspiration, polycythaemia, and diaphragmatic hernia.

Mechanical ventilation with a high FiO_2 has little effect on the severe hypoxia. Correction of the acidosis and systemic hypotension may be followed by improving hypoxia as pulmonary vascular resistence improves. Where available, tolazoline (1 mg/kg/IV) as a slow bolus dose, followed by an infusion at 0.1–1 mg/kg/hr may assist in pulmonary vasodilation. However, this drug is a general vasodilator, and may cause systemic hypotension, which can be corrected by the administration of plasma.

Recently magnesium sulphate has been shown to be of possible benefit at a dose of 200 mg/kg body weight IVI over 20–30 minutes, followed by a continuous infusion of magnesium sulphate at a rate of 20–50 mg/kg per hour.

Transient tachypnoea of the newborn (TTN)

This brief, self-limiting, relatively benign condition follows a normal full-term pregnancy. The infant usually has mild respiratory distress which settles within a few days. Some may require oxygen. Radiological changes are those of perihilar streaking, fluid in the lung fissures, and a slightly enlarged cardiac silhouette.

Chronic lung disease

Chronic lung disease is diagnosed if a baby is ventilated and/or oxygen-dependent for 28 days or more. The chronic lung conditions are bronchopulmonary dysplasia, Wilson Mikity syndrome, chronic pulmonary insufficiency of prematurity, and pulmonary interstitial emphysema. Chronic lung disorder may also be associated with patent ductus arteriosus, pulmonary haemorrhage, infection, and milk aspiration.

The principles of **management** include adequate nutrition, treatment of cardiac failure if present, maintaining the haemoglobin above 12 g/l, and the oxygen saturation between 85 and 92%. The chest X-ray and electrocardiograph should be checked regularly for the development of right-heart involvement. Two drugs which may be of use are theophylline and dexamethasone. Theophylline may help to wean the baby from oxygen therapy or the ventilator, and in addition may improve lung compliance. Dexamethasone may bring about an improvement in some babies.

Disorders of the central nervous system

The common disorders of the central nervous system in the neonate fall into two major categories: developmental defects and perinatally acquired conditions (*see Table 5.10*).

Only the commonly encountered conditions and those requiring urgent treatment will be discussed.

Meningomyelocele

Meningomyelocele is the most common neonatal central nervous system disorder referred to neurosurgeons. This midline defect of the skin and vertebral arch containing both meninges and neural tissue occurs most commonly in the lumbosacral region. The aetiology is poorly understood. The prevalence is 0.2– 0.4 per 1 000 births, with variation in different population groups, and minor epidemics possibly related to maternal viral infections acquired in the first trimester. There is evidence that adequate folate supplementation preconceptually and during the first trimester will prevent this condition. The risk of recurrence is increased in subsequent pregnancies. Associated congenital abnormalities are most commonly the Arnold-Chiari malformation and aqueduct forking.

The diagnosis is usually quite obvious at birth, with motor and sensory impairment and bladder and bowel incontinence. Cranial ultrasound is used to demonstrate the initial ventricular size and to monitor subsequent distension. Associated abnormalities can be excluded by CT scan. Careful neurological assessment of the lower limbs and of bladder and bowel function is important for prognostic purposes.

Management

(See Chapter 28, Surgical Problems.)
Postoperatively the orthopaedic, renal, and general problems must be evaluated. The head circumference must be closely monitored, as **hydrocephalus** is a common sequela, requiring ventricular shunting. Prenatal diagnosis of neural tube defects by means of serum alpha-fetoprotein determination must be offered to the mother for her future pregnancies.

Spina bifida occulta

In this condition, which occurs most commonly at L5 and S1, there is a defect of the vertebral arch with failure of posterior fusion of the vertebral laminae, and frequently absent spinous processes. Associated vertebral body anomalies such as hemivertebrae may occur. The overlying skin may be quite normal, or there may be a tuft of hair, telangiectasia, or subcutaneous lipoma. It is often an incidental finding. Less commonly there are neurological signs, including those associated with meningomyelocele, e.g., unilateral leg and foot lesions or bladder dysfunction. Diagnosis is by X-ray of the spine, and further investigation is indicated only if there is progression of neurological signs. Associated tumours may be removed without neural tissue damage.

Anencephaly

Anencephaly is obvious at birth, with absence of the vault of the skull and cerebral hemispheres. The brain stem and basal nuclei may be seen at the base of the skull. These infants are stillborn or die within hours or days of birth.

Microcephaly

True microcephaly is not associated with destructive disease and is a disorder of cell proliferation, so that brain growth as a whole is defective and the resultant head size is below the 3rd centile. Developmental abnormalities affecting the fetus or the young infant may also lead to poor brain growth. Pathologically there is a decrease in total brain weight, and a decrease in the number, size, and complexity of the gyri. The frontal lobes are usually more severely affected; following perinatal insults there may be associated gliosis and neuronal loss in the cerebral cortex. Often the cerebellum is relatively spared and appears disproportionately large. Clinically the head is small compared to the body, and the circumference well below the 3rd centile. The forehead tends to recede, and may appear relatively large. Initially motor development appears reasonable, but as the head fails to grow, motor and mental retardation become more apparent. The outcome is better if the baby with a small head demonstrates head growth along a particular centile without fall-off. Skull X-rays, serological tests, and a lumbar puncture assist in the diagnosis of microcephaly due to intrauterine infection. Periventricular calcifications occur in congenital cytomegalic infection; diffuse cerebral calcifications occur in congenital toxoplasmosis.

The **fetal alcohol syndrome** is a very important cause of microcephaly and growth retardation. This condition *(see Fig. 5.8)* must be suspected in the baby with the following features:
◆ small palpebral fissures
◆ absent philtrum
◆ abnormal palmar creases.

Microcephaly must be distinguished from cranial synostosis affecting the sagittal and coronal sutures, which results in a small head. The prematurely closed suture can usually be palpated clinically, and raised intracranial pressure is evident as papilloedema and on a skull radiograph. This condition calls for surgical intervention.

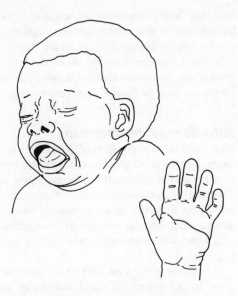

Fig. 5.8 Clinical features of fetal alcohol syndrome

Hydrocephalus

This term refers to an abnormally large head with raised intracranial pressure. Where the flow of CSF out of the ventricular system is obstructed, the pressure effect is from within the brain. In the communicating variety, on the other hand, there is interference with CSF flow or absorption outside the brain.

Aetiology is unknown in the majority of congenital varieties of hydrocephalus, where there is a range of malfunctions. In a small proportion, congenital infections and genetic factors play a roll. Meningitis, trauma, and intracranial haemorrhage are the common causes of acquired hydrocephalus.

Clinical features may be obvious at birth, or even diagnosed antenatally. At times the head enlargement develops gradually with very few symptoms early on, but subsequently anorexia, vomiting, irritability, and lethargy are seen. A bulging fontanelle and separation of the sutures are invariably present. Superficial venous engorgement is variable, and the classical sign of the 'setting sun' eyes appears late.

Benign enlargement of the head (or constitutional macrocephaly) must be differentiated from hydrocephalus. Once soft tissue swelling of the

scalp has been excluded, serial head circumference measurements will demonstrate proportional growth. There will also be no evidence of raised intracranial pressure.

Subdural fluid accumulation must also be considered in the differential diagnosis *(see following section)*. Very rarely intracranial cysts or tumours present a similar clinical picture.

Intervention is generally advisable, as the prolonged pressure effect causes atrophy of white matter. In the first instance it is important to record and plot serial head circumference measurements. Early referral for shunting is necessary as soon as excessive head enlargement is demonstrated. If cranial ultrasonography is available and demonstrates progressive enlargement of the lateral ventricles along with the development of a full fontanelle, referral for shunting is indicated.

The prognosis depends on the severity of associated malformations and the extent of subsequent brain damage.

Complications are not uncommon, and often necessitate reinsertion of the shunt. Patients with arrested hydrocephalus require prolonged observation for low-grade pressure buildup.

Subdural fluid collections

This is the second most common cause of abnormal head enlargement. The three main pathological types are haematoma, hygroma, and effusion, and all are managed along similar lines.

Bleeding in the subdural space is due to disruption of bridging veins from the cerebral surface to the major venous sinuses *(see Fig. 5.6)*. Birth trauma accounts for the majority of cases. Less commonly, bleeding disorders and dehydration cause subdural bleeds. Hygromas result from laceration of the pia-arachnoid, and effusions as the result of infections. In an acute subdural bleed the lysing blood clot creates an osmotic gradient which draws fluid into the space, enlarging the lesion and thus promoting further bleeding.

Hygromas do not expand, because the pia is less vascular and the effusions are absorbed with resolution of the infection.

Diagnosis

This is based on the history of either trauma, infection, or persistent fever. Transillumination is positive unless there is frank pus or blood. In acute subdural bleeds subhyaloid haemorrhage may be seen on fundoscopy. CT scan is the investigation of choice.

Treatment

Subdural clotted blood may be difficult to drain by needling, and require a burrhole. However, the chronic subdural collection is easily tapped *(see Chapter 31, Procedures)*. Chronic collections may be tapped repeatedly over 3–4 weeks, and if they do not subside, surgical intervention is indicated, possibly with a temporary subdural peritoneal shunt. In the acute variety the blood must be evacuated as discussed previously.

Prognosis

This depends on the nature of the underlying cause, size, onset, duration, and location of the lesion, and the response to treatment. Acute subdurals in the neonatal period generally have a poor prognosis.

Intracranial haemorrhage

Intracranial haemorrhage contributes significantly to neurological morbidity in both term and pre-term babies. Where primary health care facilities are good, generally only the pre-term (and particularily the very-low-birth-weight) baby is affected. However, where facilities are deficient, a large number of term babies are affected, and should receive preferential care. The extent of the injury and the outcome depend on the underlying pathogenic factors. There are four major categories of haemorrhage in the newborn: subdural, primary subarachnoid, periventricular-intra-ventricular haemorrhage, and intracerebellar *(see Fig. 5.6)*.

Subdural haemorrhage

Major factors involved in the traumatic process resulting in subdural bleeds are cephalopelvic disproportion, the duration of labour, and the method of delivery.

Massive infratentorial haemorrhage manifests from the time of birth. The signs are due to brain stem compression, viz., deviation of the eyes, unequal pupils, rapid respiration, and opisthotonus. If haemorrhage progresses, coma ensues, the pupils become fixed and dilated, ocular bob-

bing, and finally respiratory arrest occur. If the haemorrhage is less catastrophic the infant may survive, with hydrocephalus developing later.

Subdural haemorrhage over the cerebral convexities may be asymptomatic if minor. Seizures are usually focal, with other focal cerebral signs.

Subarachnoid haemorrhage

This common haemorrhage is related to asphyxial injury, and the development of the haemorrhage probably occurs as a result of vascular injury, as discussed in intraventricular haemorrhage *(see below)*. Small bleeds occur, commonly without clinical manifestations. Very few will have a structural lesion such as an aneurysm or vascular malformation.

The clinical features are difficult to outline because of the associated manifestations of asphyxia. Convulsions may occur on the second day of life. Between seizures these babies appear very well, and the prognosis is excellent. A massive haemorrrhage runs a fatal course and is often associated with trauma. The cerebrospinal fluid is bloody, and later xanthochromic, with a high protein and an increased cell count.

Intraventricular haemorrhage (IVH)

This classical intracranial haemorrhage of the pre-term infant occurs within the first 72 hours of life, often in association with respiratory distress. It commences as a haemorrhagic infarct of the periventricular white matter, and then bursts into the ventricles. The delicate vessels of the periventricular white matter form a large, unsupported network of capillaries which ruptures easily. In 20–40% of lesions the haemorrhage is confined to the brain tissue (germinal matrix) and does not rupture into the ventricles. As the fetus matures, the germinal matrix becomes less vascular, so this form of haemorrhage is rare in the term baby.

The **pathogenesis** has as yet not been fully clarified. However, hypoxia and ischaemia are major factors, in addition to raised cerebral venous pressure during resuscitation. Furthermore, there is marked fibrinolytic activity in the periventricular area of the newborn, which promotes spread of the haemorrhage.

The **clinical presentation** is variabale and depends on the size and rate of bleeding. Small

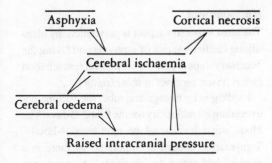

Fig. 5.9 The cerebral consequences of asphyxia

haemorrhages may produce no signs. With large haemorrhages, loss of consciousness, convulsions, a full fontanelle, and anaemia may occur. Altered muscle tone, behaviour disturbances, and progressive head enlargement may be the only signs.

IVH may present in one of two ways:
◆ sudden catastrophic neurological deterioration with convulsions on day 2 or 3
◆ gradual loss of consciousness with hypotonia.

The classical clinical features make the diagnosis easy. Ultrasonography is used for confirmation and in difficult cases a CT scan may be indicated.

Generally no definite guidelines for **treatment** have been established. Intervention is not indicated for those with severe haemorrhage, as the mortality is in the region of 90% and the remaining patients suffer severe morbidity. In those with smaller bleeds, repeated CSF drainage may reduce the pressure. Blood transfusions, anticonvulsants, and eventually shunting may be indicated. Aproximately 35% of babies with IVH develop posthaemorrhagic hydrocephalus.

Recent evidence indicates that the outcome in the milder degrees of haemorrhage depends on the initiating events and circumstances, rather than the extent. With steady improvement in the management of these small babies the incidence and complications of IVH are decreasing.

Periventricular leucomalacia

Periventricular leucomalacia (PVL) occurs when ischaemia is prolonged or dominant. This degenerative process results in multiple small cysts with varying clinical features which are determined by the site and extent of the injury.

Parasagittal cerebral injury

This classical cerebral lesion occurs in the term infant. There is necrosis of the cerebral cortex and subcortical white matter, with a characteristic bilateral symmetrical distribution involving the parasagittal and superomedial aspects of the cerebral hemispheres. The 'watershed' infarct emphasizes the ischaemic nature of the lesion which follows cerebral hypoperfusion. In severe cases necrosis extends to a large proportion of the lateral cerebral convexity. Clinically, spastic motor deficit, seizures, and intellectual impairment occur.

Focal ischaemic cerebral injury

Focal ischaemic lesions may also occur as a result of generalized cerebral hypoperfusion, with the middle cerebral arteries being involved most frequently. Infarction occurs, with subsequent cystic development which may or may not communicate with the lateral ventricles. Thromboembolic phenomena include disseminated intravascular coagulopathy and cerebral infarcts. Clinically the unilateral lesion results in hemiparesis, but multiple lesions may cause quadriparesis.

Hypoxic ischaemic encephalopathy (HIE)

This results from significant asphyxia of the fetus or newborn. Asphyxia is the failure of gas exchange at placental level in the fetus, and pulmonary level in the newborn. Perinatal asphyxia is predominantly an antenatal event, with no more than 10% occurring postpartum. In the author's opinion HIE is probably the major cause of cerebral palsy in the Third World. The pathogenesis of brain damage resulting from asphyxia is illustrated in *Fig. 5.9.*

As fetal respiration is controlled by placental circulation, asphyxia implies some degree of intrauterine ischaemia. The systematic response to hypoxia, hypercapnia, and mixed acidosis is to maintain cerebral blood flow at the expense of other organs. It follows that if an episode of hypoxia is sufficiently prolonged and severe, other organs such as the myocardium also function poorly. With subsequent decreased cardiac output,

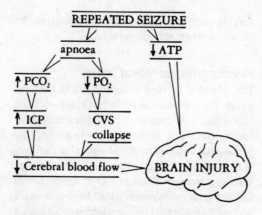

Fig. 5.10 The pathogenesis of brain damage in neonatal convulsions

hypotension occurs and perfusion of the brain, kidney, lung, and gut is compromised. The clinical effects are those of ischaemia of these organs.

Clinical features

These are caused by hypoxia and ischaemia occurring simultaneously or in sequence. With severe intrauterine asphyxia and/or ischaemia, the infant is in coma initially and has convulsions. Birth asphyxia is occasionally followed by a lucid interval of 12–18 hours.

The classical features of HIE are vomiting, an abnormal cry, and irritability, leading to unresponsiveness and eventually coma.

Convulsions at times are subtle and expressed as **apnoeic or cyanotic attacks** and usually occur within 12–18 hours. The respiration is often irregular, with a Cheyne-Stokes pattern suggesting diffuse bilateral hemisphere pathology. With a severe insult brain stem signs occur, such as fixed, dilated pupils, and abnormal or absent eye movements. Motor weakness is the main clinical manifestation of primary ischaemia. The fontanelle may become full as a result of cerebral oedema.

Subsequent evaluation is often confounded by the effects of therapy, such as phenobarbitone. An early improvement, however, suggests a good prognosis. Generally mild HIE is diagnosed when neurological signs such as feeding and tone disturbances last 24 – 48 hours. Moderate HIE includes convulsions and signs existing for 4–5 days. Severe HIE is diagnosed if the physical signs are severe and persist for 10 –14 days or more.

Management

The most important aspect is prevention, by identifying the fetus at risk of asphyxia and taking the necessary steps to prepare for prompt resuscitation (*see relevant sections in this chapter*).

Feeding is by nasogastric tube, the volume not exceeding 80 ml/kg/day for the first 2–3 days. The blood sugar level must be monitored 4-hourly. Temperature control is important, as there is a marked inclination to instability. A simple yet effective measure is to raise the head to 30° above the plane of the body. For established HIE with convulsions, the following medication is recommended:

- phenobarbitone 15 mg/kg IM stat.
- then 5–8 mg/kg/day orally (*see also Convulsions, below*).

Further management is largely determined by the level of consciousness and the severity and number of seizures. Anticonvulsant therapy is gradually reduced, guided by the cerebral state.

Complications such as pneumonia, hypoglycaemia, and inappropriate antidiuretic hormone secretion must be borne in mind constantly.

Long-term surveillance of the child is essential to detect complications and to prepare the parents accordingly. Appropriate rehabilitative measures must be introduced.

The **prognosis** depends on the duration and severity of the cerebral insult. A neonate with prolonged loss of consciousness and generalized hypotonia with severe convulsions very rarely makes a complete recovery. Cerebral palsy, microcephaly and lesser degrees of neurological impairment are the sequelae of survivors of profound cerebral hypoxia. Fortunately there is an appreciable proportion of those who make rapid and early progress who remain free of any deficit.

Convulsions

Neonatal seizures result from an insult to the brain. In themselves they are injurious to the neurones by rapid consumption of energy-producing metabolites. Furthermore, the concurrent respiratory disturbance causes hypoxia and hypercapnoea (*see Fig. 5.10*).

Clinical types

Subtle convulsions are very common. The physical signs include deviation of the eyes, repetitive blinking or fluttering of the eyelids, drooling, sucking, cycling movements of the lower limbs, rowing movements of the upper limbs, tonic posturing of a limb, apnoea, cyanotic episodes, an abnormal cry, and stertorous respiration.

Tonic seizures indicate severe encephalopathy. **Clonic convulsions** may be focal or multifocal. Lastly there are **myoclonic seizures,** which are single or multiple flexion jerks of groups of muscles.

Jitteriness is to be distinguished from convulsions: it is not accompanied by loss of consciousness or abnormal eye movements, and stops as soon as the limbs are held. However, it easily recommences with stimulation.

The **most common causes** of neonatal convulsions are HIE, birth trauma, metabolic disturbances such as hypoglycaemia and hypocalcaemia, hypothermia, intracranial infections, electrolyte disturbances (particularly sodium imbalance), and narcotic and alcohol withdrawal.

Management

Convulsions must be controlled as a matter of urgency. Anticonvulsant therapy is outlined in *Table 5.11.*

Table 5.11   Anticonvulsant drug dosage

Drug	Dosage
Seizure control	
Diazepam	0.5 mg/kg/dose PR
or	
Phenobarbitone	15 mg/kg/dose IM
or	
Phenytoin	5 mg/kg/dose IM
Maintenance therapy	
Phenobarbitone	3–5 mg/kg/day in 3 divided doses PO
Phenytoin	3–5 mg/kg/day in 3 divided doses PO

Supportive care must be provided as for any unconscious neonate. The airway must be kept clear with regular gentle naso- and oropharyngeal suction. The baby is nursed prone or on its side, with regular changing of position to facilitate the drainage of secretions. The frequency and duration of convulsions are noted. Oxygen is given for cyanosis.

The temperature must be monitored carefully, as sedated babies rapidly become cold. Blood sugar levels should be monitored 4-hourly, and the baby must be tube-fed, commencing with 80–100 ml/kg/day. When seizures have ceased for 24 – 48 hours, the anticonvulsant dosage may be reduced gradually over days.

Prognosis

The nature of the underlying neurological disease will determine the eventual outcome in the individual baby with seizures. Generally:

◆ convulsions due to HIE give a 50% chance of normal development

◆ associated hypoglycaemia has a similar outcome

◆ intracranial infection causes 20 –50% morbidity

◆ severe intraventricular haemorrhage causes 65–100% morbidity with a mortality of 50 – 65%.

Follow-up

It is essential that all babies who have experienced convulsions are assessed neurologically at regular intervals in order to detect deficits, which usually manifest at 9 –12 months. Minor problems are often not detected during the pre-school period. With expert counselling of the parents and correct management, many difficulties may be overcome within the home. Infants with significant neurological deficits may require the assistance of a physiotherapist, occupational therapist, and clinical psychologist. Hearing, vision, and speech assessments may be necessary.

Haematological problems

(See also Chapter 18, Blood Disorders.)

Acute anaemia

Pallor is an important physical sign which may indicate asphyxia or anaemia, usually due to acute blood loss before, during, or after delivery. Awareness of the significance and management of pallor is important, as rapid clinical decompensation and death may occur.

The causes of acute anaemia may be related to the placenta, such as abruptio, tearing of aberrant placental veins, and feto-maternal or twin-to-twin transfusion. Blood loss may occur during a traumatic delivery with intracranial or intra-abdominal haemorrhage. After birth blood loss may occur when the infant is held above the level of the placenta if the cord is unclamped. Cephalhaematoma, soft tissue bruising, and bleeding from the cord are further common causes. Rarely, coagulation defects or thrombocytopenia may cause bleeding.

Clinically the baby may be pale but warm, initially with normal heart rate and pulse volume. Some minutes or hours later peripheral vasoconstriction occurs, with tachycardia, a thready pulse, and low blood pressure. During the second phase the baby becomes restless and finally lethargic and quiet. Without intervention death will certainly ensue. When in doubt, serial haematocrit and haemoglobin (Hb) estimation at hourly intervals will indicate the need for transfusion.

Management

This depends on clinical assessment of severity, and is outlined in *Table 5.12*.

Severely anaemic infants will require oxygen and at times respiratory support. The blood sugar must be monitored while awaiting and during emergency transfusion. Besides a full blood count and smear, it is a wise precaution to check the prothrombin index to exclude haemorrhagic disease of the newborn.

Chronic anaemia

Chronic anaemia at birth is suggested by pallor and a well-compensated cardiovascular system, hepatosplenomegaly and sometimes jaundice. Oedema may be present if the anaemia is very severe, but pallor may be the only clinical sign of chronic anaemia. Blood group incompatibility, particularly Rh disease, must be excluded. Chronic intrauterine infections, mainly congenital syphilis, may present with anaemia.

Anaemia presenting late in the neonatal period may be due to frequent blood sampling, infection, or lack of iron or vitamin E. Anaemia in the pre-term at 4 – 6 weeks is usually due to the physiological anaemia of prematurity.

Ideally a record should be kept of blood volumes removed at each venipuncture. Elemental iron 2 mg/kg is given daily once the baby is well. The VLBW infant should also receive 25 IU of vitamin E daily. Appropriate investigations should be undertaken if blood group incompatibilities, acute infection, or chronic intrauterine infection are suspected.

Polycythaemia

Polycythaemia is diagnosed when the haematocrit is over 65%, and is associated with hyperviscosity which may have serious consequences, such as necrotizing enterocolitis. The infants at risk are those with hypervolaemia following twin-to-twin or materno-fetal transfusion, those who are small for gestational age, dysmature infants, and infants of diabetic mothers. In these conditions polycythaemia must be excluded by means of an Hb confirmation 4 –8 hours after birth.

Serious signs of hyperviscosity include central cyanosis, respiratory distress, apnoea, convulsions, abdominal distension, cardiac decompensation, and hypoglycaemia. Less ominous features include poor feeding, vomiting, irritability, lethargy, and hypotonia.

A partial exchange transfusion should be performed, using 20 –30 ml/kg of fresh frozen plasma, for any patient with a haematocrit over

Table 5.12   Management of blood loss according to severity

Colour	Pulse	BP	Hb	Haematocrit	Management
Good	Normal	Normal	> 15	65%	Observe, check Hb/HCT 2 hours later
Good	Normal	Normal		30–35%	Transfuse — not urgent
Pale*	Normal	Normal		Irrespective	Transfuse — urgent, cross-match
Pale*	Thready	Low		Irrespective	Transfuse immediately. Use a plasma expander while awaiting blood

* With no response to oxygen

70%. An infant with a haematocrit of 65% with any of the serious signs should be treated similarly. In view of the great risk of complications, such as cerebral infarcts, it is recommended that the plasma is infused rapidly into a peripheral vein, while blood is withdrawn in equal volumes from the umbilical vein.

Bleeding disorders

Bleeding disorders in the neonate may be classified as follows:

- haemorrhagic disease of the newborn
- consumption coagulopathy
- platelet disorders
- congenital deficiency of coagulation factors.

Haemorrhagic disease of the newborn

This disease is more common in Third World countries with poor socio-economic conditions. Bleeding due to vitamin K-dependent factors (II, VII, IX, X) classically occurs 48 hours after delivery, but may be seen within hours of birth. Bleeding commonly occurs from injection sites, cord stump, nose, and gastrointestinal tract, or there may be intraperitoneal and subaponeurotic haemorrhage. Multiple sites are commonly involved.

The diagnosis is confirmed by prolonged prothrombin time which improves within 2–4 hours following the administration of vitamin K 1–2 mg IV. Using Apt's test (see below) one can distinguish fetal from maternal blood if the baby has haematemesis and malaena. Similarly, if haematemesis persists after a stomach washout, it is almost certainly not maternal blood.

Pre-term infants respond with a slower rise in the prothrombin index and may require fresh plasma or fresh whole blood in order to control bleeding.

It is essential that all babies, including those of low birth weight, receive vitamin K 1 mg IM at delivery in order to prevent this disease.

Apt's test:

- 1 ml vomitus or meconium + 1 ml water; spin this mixture
- 5 parts supernatant + 1 part 0.25% NaOH
- a pink colour for more than 2 minutes = fetal Hb; yellow = adult Hb.

Consumption coagulopathy

Neonates who suffer infection or hypoxia are liable to develop this form of bleeding disorder, which tends to occur particularly in special care units. The coagulation cascade is probably induced by the release of thromboplastin following tissue damage mainly in the liver and brain. Widespread deposition of fibrin occurs in smaller vessels with the consumption of Factors V, VIII, and fibrinogen. Platelets tend to aggregate, resulting in thrombocytopenia. The red cells are distorted by the fibrin deposits in the smaller vessels, leading to the fragmented cells seen on the blood film.

Consumption coagulopathy may be associated with systemic infection, asphyxia, hypothermia, severe acidosis, and macerated twin. It usually presents in a seriously ill neonate with purpura, bruising, and bleeding from many sites, including haematuria and intraventricular haemorrhage in the pre-term.

Diagnosis: Clinical manifestations and associations as above are highly suggestive. The full blood count reveals anaemia and thrombocytopenia, and red cell fragmentation on a smear. If facilities are available the following tests must be done: prothrombin, partial thromboplastin, and thrombin times, all of which may be prolonged. A factor assay will reveal a classically low Factor V level. Fibrinogen levels are reduced in severe cases, and fibrin degradation products are elevated.

Management: The baby must be treated vigorously for underlying conditions, and the clotting defects corrected with fresh plasma 10 ml/kg, platelet concentrates, and fresh whole blood. Heparin therapy is only of value if instituted very early, and is potentially hazardous.

Thrombocytopenia

The clinical expression of thrombocytopenia in the neonate is very variable. The platelet count is usually below 50 000/mm^3. Common causes of thrombocytopenia are overwhelming bacterial infections, chronic intrauterine infections, consumption coagulopathy, maternal drugs, autoimmune disease, severe erythroblastosis fetalis, repeat exchange transfusions, and congenital leukaemia. Specific treatment for the underlying condition will reduce the bleeding tendency. Platelet transfusions may be considered if the count is less than 10 000/mm^3. An exchange transfusion with whole blood is also recommended.

Thrombasthenia

Bleeding disorder with the features of thrombocytopenia may occur in the presence of normal platelet count and coagulation factors, but platelet function is defective. Chronic ingestion of aspirin by the mother may give rise to this problem.

Congenital deficiency of coagulation factors

These are rare conditions. The usual presentation is one of prolonged bleeding from skin puncture sites. Classical haemophilia (Factor VIII) and Christmas disease (Factor IX) are the most common deficiencies (see Chapter 18, Blood Disorders).

The diagnosis rests on the family history and the demonstration of the relevant deficiency.

Gastrointestinal disorders

Gastrointestinal disturbances are common problems in the newborn. The major concern is to exclude surgical conditions, and therefore reference should be made to *Chapter 28, Surgical Problems*.

Vomiting

Vomiting is a very common symptom of the newborn in the first few hours of life. The most likely cause of vomiting in association with the first few feeds is irritation of the gastric mucosa by swallowed blood, meconium, or mucus. A gastric lavage will confirm this diagnosis and is therapeutic. Maternal sedation may also induce vomiting.

Vomiting may be the first sign of serious organic disease, which should always be suspected if vomiting is persistent, bile-stained, or associated with abdominal distension or constipation.

Causes

Infections, both enteral and parenteral, are commonly associated with vomiting, which is accompanied by temperature disturbances and other physical signs suggestive of infection. Besides meningitis, septicaemia, urinary tract infections, and necrotizing enterocolitis must also be considered.

Intestinal obstruction must be excluded *(see Chapter 28, Surgical Problems)*.

Intracranial injury, congenital abnormalities, and infection may cause persistent vomiting. Rarer causes include metabolic problems such as uraemia, congenital adrenal hyperplasia, and inherited enzyme disorders such as galactosaemia.

Abdominal distension

This is a fairly common physical sign in the newborn, and may be a sign of serious illness. It should be established whether the distension is due to gas, fluid, or organ enlargement, and whether associated physical signs such as constipation and vomiting are present.

Gaseous distension occurs as a result of the accumulation of air in the gut due to obstruction or paralytic ileus. The causes of obstruction are congenital abnormalities of the gut, hernias, volvulus, and malrotation. Necrotizing enterocolitis should always be considered in the ill LBW baby with abdominal distension.

Meconium ileus — an early expression of cystic fibrosis — is a condition which must be considered in babies of Caucasian origin who present with partial or complete obstruction. Perforation of the gut with meconium peritonitis may occur.

Paralytic ileus occurs as a result of asphyxia, shock, electrolyte imbalance, and infection, which may be generalized or confined to the gut.

Abdominal masses contributing to abdominal distension are most commonly due to organ enlargement such as hepatosplenomegaly, renal masses and hydronephrosis, dilated bladder, liver cysts, and tumours and ovarian masses. Other rare causes include gut duplication, mesenteric cysts, and retroperitoneal tumours. Urogenital causes are not uncommon, so abdominal ultrasound and urological investigations may be urgent to detect correctable abnormalities.

Ascites is a rare clinical finding in the newborn, and most commonly occurs in babies with generalized oedema. This is seen in severe anaemia (as in Rh disease), cardiac failure, hypoproteinanaemia as in nephrotic syndrome, and chronic intrauterine infections.

In the neonate the **basic investigations** for sepsis should always be carried out. For abdominal distension an erect abdominal radiograph will confirm the presence of a surgical condition. Ultrasound of the abdomen is important in evaluating a mass in the abdomen, and often an intravenous pyelogram is necessary to assist in making a diagnosis. A diagnostic laparotomy may be the only way to a final diagnosis.

Management

When a baby presents with persistent distension, the examination must aim at excluding surgical conditions. Specialized investigations may be necessary to confirm or exclude the various surgical conditions. A nasogastric tube is passed and gastric suction applied. An intravenous line is established to supply adequate fluid and calories, so that a normal blood sugar level and fluid and electrolyte balance are maintained. Careful monitoring of intravenous fluids and the urine output is essential. A paediatric surgical opinion should always be sought.

Diarrhoeal disease

As in the older child, diarrhoeal disease in the newborn is usually a short, self-limiting illness. Significant morbidity and mortality do occur, however, and the infant presents a risk of spreading the disease. Epidemics of diarrhoeal disease may occur in neonatal units, particularly if facilities are poor, with overcrowding, inadequate hand-washing, and ineffective disposal of soiled linen.

The most common cause of loose stools in a neonate is dietary in origin. In the fully breast-fed infant a loose stool with each feed is not uncommon, and is due to a mild lactose intolerance. This self-limiting condition clears within days or weeks. However, *E. coli,* salmonella, shigella, and the rotavirus may cause neonatal diarrhoeal disease.

It is extremely difficult to differentiate parenteral from enteral infection in the newborn. The clinical presentation may vary from mild disease to severe dehydrating disease with acidosis and electrolyte imbalance. Similarly, many babies are afebrile, while others become hypothermic, or pyrexial to 39 °C.

In the seriously ill baby basic investigations for septicaemia should be undertaken, and it is essential to determine the electrolyte and acid base status.

Treatment

Fluid replacement and electrolyte balance are critical in the newborn. For mild to moderate cases of dehydration, oral therapy with a sugar electrolyte solution including potassium is satisfactory. The severely dehydrated neonate requires a plasma infusion of 20 ml/kg for rapid correction. Fluid requirements must be determined accurately, and the intake and output carefully monitored. Antibiotics are usually given for very ill babies, commencing with a penicillin and an aminoglycoside. Supportive therapy, as discussed under septicaemia, must be provided for every baby.

Prevention

This is the most important aspect of management of neonatal diarrhoea. Environmental control and regular surveillance are essential. The patient with acute infective diarrhoea must be isolated, strict hand-washing techniques practised by the mother and all attendants, and soiled linen must be disposed of appropriately.

Necrotizing enterocolitis

The incidence varies in different centres, being rare in some and reaching epidemic proportions in others. It occurs more commonly in infants below 1 500 g.

The pathogenesis is poorly understood, but bowel ischaemia seems to be a critical factor. Perinatal asphyxia, prematurity, possibly sepsis, shock, and exchange transfusions are further contributing factors. Following the ischaemic insult, gas-producing organisms invade the bowel wall, proliferate, and produce classical pneumatosis intestinalis. Organisms associated with this disease include *E. coli,* klebsiella, aerobacter, pseudomonas and *Clostridium difficile.*

Clinical features

Abdominal distension is the earliest sign, usually occurring on the third to fifth day, but it may occur within a few hours of birth and as late as one month of age. A poor colour and shock may ensue. Stools are usually scanty, but blood-streaked in 20–25% of cases.

Investigations

A low white count may be present; thrombocytopenia, particularly a *falling* platelet count, is a poor prognostic sign, and disseminated intravascular coagulation may be present. The erect X-ray of the abdomen will show intestinal distension, intramural air, and possibly intrahepatic portal venous gas. Signs of pneumoperitoneum will be present if the gut has perforated.

Management

The general principles of septic infants must be observed. All feeds are stopped; intravenous alimentation (total parenteral nutrition, TPN) is mandatory. Antibiotics are commenced once appropriate cultures have been taken, and reviewed according to results. A nasogastric tube is passed and left open to drain, to prevent accumulation of air and gastric content. Consultation with a paediatric surgeon is essential, as immediate surgical intervention will be necessary in the event of perforation, and also weeks later when strictures may develop.

Prognosis

Prompt diagnosis, resting the gut, and intravenous alimentation have vastly improved the outlook in this disease. In the individual patient, however, the degree of prematurity and associated conditions will affect the prognosis. In some centres mortality rates have decreased from 75% to less than 20%.

Jaundice

In the sub-tropics and tropics neonatal jaundice is associated with conditions such as ABO incompatibility and G6PD deficiency, which occur more frequently than rhesus incompatibility.

The incidence of jaundice varies greatly within a particular unit and with ethnic groups. For instance, in China and Japan it is particularly prevalent. Clinical jaundice becomes apparent at 85–120 mmol/l (1 mg/dl of bilirubin = 17 mmol/l).

Bilirubin encephalopathy

Bilirubin encephalopathy occurs when the fat-soluble unconjugated free bilirubin rises to levels that result in altered membrane function. Bilirubin crosses the blood-brain barrier and areas of the brain with high blood flow and high metabolic rates are susceptible to bilirubin toxicity. Kernicterus is the term which refers to the yellow staining of the basal ganglia and hippocampus seen at autopsy in infants dying of bilirubin toxicity.

Factors interfering with albumin binding, allowing a higher level of free bilirubin in the circulation, are a low serum albumin (< 30 mg/l), certain drugs such as sulphonamides which compete with bilirubin for binding sites on albumin, non-esterified fatty acids (associated with TPN), and acidosis. The pre-term infant is at risk of encephalopathy at appreciably lower serum bilirubin levels than the term baby. Bilirubin encephalopathy is rarely seen in term infants with levels below 400 mmol/l unless there is underlying pathology or factors which enhance the deposition of free bilirubin.

Asphyxia, sepsis, acidosis, hypoglycaemia, and RDS predispose to kernicterus.

In general hyperbilirubinaemia originating from sources other than rhesus incompatibility does not commonly cause kernicterus.

The **clinical picture** of bilirubin toxicity may be transient or one of irreversible brain damage. The signs may not develop for several hours after toxic levels have occurred. Initially the signs are reluctance to take feeds, temperature instability, irritability, and cycling movements. An exchange transfusion at this stage may arrest the process. Progression of the disease manifests as generalized increase in extensor tone with opisthotonus and crossed extension of the legs. The cry is high-pitched, and paralysis of the extra-ocular muscles causes a 'setting sun' sign. Terminally, gastric and pulmonary haemorrhage may occur. In the surviving infant, hypotonia eventually occurs, with developmental delay. Long-term manifestations include choreoathetosis or spastic cerebral palsy, clumsiness, intellectual impairment, and high-tone deafness. Dental dysplasia may occur. In the pre-term infant the initial physical signs may be quite different, including fisting, an increase in tone, and apnoea.

Physiological jaundice

Up to 50% of normal newborns and considerably more pre-term infants become jaundiced in the first week of life. The normal newborn has a number of inadequacies in bilirubin metabolism and transport:

- increased red cell breakdown
- defective uptake, conjugation, and excretion of bilirubin
- inadequate hepatic perfusion
- increased enterohepatic circulation of bilirubin.

These result in raised unconjugated serum bilirubin levels in the first week of life. In physiological jaundice the bilirubin level does not exceed 220 mmol/l. In the term neonate it peaks at 102–119 mmol on the third day, and in the pre-term at 170–204 mmol on the fifth to seventh day. The diagnosis of physiological jaundice is largely by exclusion.

Hyperbilirubinaemia

Jaundice is pathological if it occurs within the first 24 hours of life, exceeds 220 mmol/l in the term infant or 204 mmol/l in the pre-term baby, rises by more than 85 mmol/l per day, or if the direct serum bilirubin exceeds 34 mmol/l. Similarly if jaundice persists for more than a week in the term baby and more than 2 weeks in the pre-term baby, it must be regarded as pathological.

The usual causes of jaundice in the first week of life are as follows:

- blood group incompatibility
- bleeding and bruising, e.g., cephalhaematoma
- infection, e.g., intrauterine or acquired
- immaturity
- maternal diabetes.

Causes of late-onset jaundice are:

- infections, e.g., Gram-negative sepsis
- neonatal hepatitis syndrome
- metabolic disturbances, e.g., galactosaemia
- storage disease, e.g., lipid, carbohydrate
- endocrine, e.g., hypothyroidism
- miscellaneous, e.g., Down's syndrome.

Rhesus haemolytic disease
Pathogenesis

There are three distinct rhesus antigens, Cc, Dd, and Ee. C, D, and E are dominant, and c, d, and e are recessive. About 85% of Caucasians have the D antigen. Rh negativity usually denotes absence of the D antigen. In that case when fetal cells leak across the placenta into the maternal circulation they stimulate antibody production in the mother to the specific fetal antigen. These antibodies, in turn, cross the placenta, causing the destruction of the circulating red cells of the fetus. Rh disease increases in incidence and severity with increasing blood, feto-maternal bleeding at abortion, amniocentesis, or external cephalic version. These factors may be responsible for the occasional case of Rh disease in the first pregnancy.

Severity of the disease is also related to parity and to the stage of pregnancy during which the antibody crosses the placenta. The earlier the antibody crosses the placenta, the more severe the disease. Haemolytic disease commencing in the second trimester may result in severe anaemia, hepatosplenomegaly, liver damage causing hypoproteinaemia, oedema (i.e., hydrops fetalis — *see below for further details*), cardiac failure, and ascites. When haemolysis occurs nearer to term, the infant is born less anaemic but rapidly develops jaundice which may be severe.

Prevention

Antenatal investigation of Rh-negative women for the presence of rhesus antibody will detect the affected fetuses. Amniocentesis with measurement of the bilirubin concentration and optical density has been the method of assessing severity. More recently, tertiary centres have been performing cordocentesis, measuring the haematocrit and analyzing the blood groups. Direct fetal transfusion is performed if indicated.

All Rh-negative women must be given human Rh hyperimmune gammaglobulin (100–200 mg IM) within 48 hours of any procedure which could result in sensitization. The gammaglobulin binds to the fetal cells, which are then rapidly removed from the maternal circulation. This procedure has resulted in the dramatic decline in incidence of Rh haemolytic disease.

101

Management of the infant

The jaundiced infant is managed as outlined below. Low-grade haemolysis may continue in the affected infant, resulting in anaemia at 2–4 weeks, and may require a transfusion at that time. The early administration of iron and folate supplementation may reduce the severity of the late anaemia.

ABO incompatibility

The frequency of ABO blood group incompatibility is similar in tropical and non-tropical areas. However, as Rh disease occurs very rarely in the tropics and sub-tropics, ABO incompatibility assumes greater importance. It is difficult to prove the latter, but it rarely presents with such severe manifestations as does Rh disease, e.g., hydrops fetalis, severe anaemia, and early onset of jaundice. Although the Coombs' test is often negative, sensitization may be suggested by the presence of immune anti-A or anti-B antibodies in the baby's serum or on the surface of the red cells. It has also been suggested that the primary effect of maternal antibodies directed against A and B blood group conceptions is widespread tissue necrosis rather than specific red cell destruction. ABO incompatibility therefore plays an important role in the pathogenesis of early abortion.

In an analysis of 1 237 jaundiced black neonates admitted to a large unit (King Edward VIII Hospital, Durban) over a 9-month period, 163 (13%) were found to have severe jaundice (i.e., serum bilirubin > 300 mmol/l). Of these, 68 showed ABO incompatibility and only 2 had Rh disease. Sixty-three patients required an exchange transfusion, 44% having ABO incompatibility, which therefore is a major cause of severe jaundice in African newborns.

The usual ABO incompatible combinations in this series were:

Mother	Infant
O	A
O	B
B	AB

Hyperbilirubinaemia in the group with ABO incompatibility was aggravated by low birth weight, haemorrhage, and infection. Anaemia and hepatosplenomegaly were unusual features.

Management of hyperbilirubinaemia

Figure 5.11 gives guidelines for the management of hyperbilirubinaemia. The aim of therapy is to prevent kernicterus. Careful observation of the baby is important to detect and correct any of the above-mentioned predisposing factors. The

Guidelines for the Management of Bilirubinaemia
(1mg/100ml = 17 mmol/L)

Serum Bilirubin mmol/L	< 24 hrs		24-48 hrs		49-72 hrs		< 72 hrs	
	< 2500g	> 2500g	< 2500g	2500g	< 2500g	> 2500g	< 2500g	> 2500g
< 85								
85-150	Phototherapy if haemolysis							
170-240	Exchange if haemolysis		< < < < < < < < < Phototherapy > > > > > > > >					
250-320	< < < < < Exchange > > > > >				< < < < < Phototherapy > > > > >			
>= 340	< < < < < < < < < < < < < < < < Exchange > > > > > > > > >> > > > > >							

Fig. 5.11   Guidelines for the management of hyperbilirubinaemia

Table 5.13   Serum bilirubin levels and exchange transfusion

Age	> 2.5 kg	1.8–2.5 kg	1.3–1.7 kg	< 1.3 kg
Day 1	204	170	153	136
Day 2	255	221	204	187
Day 3	289	255	238	221
Day 4	340	289	255	238
Day 5	340	289	255	238
Day 6	340	306	272	255
Day 7	340	306	289	272

specific forms of therapy are phenobarbitone, phototherapy, and exchange transfusion.

Phenobarbitone

When this is used prophylactically it reduces the serum bilirubin (SB) effectively by enhancing hepatic uptake, conjugation, and excretion. Although it may cause drowsiness and slow feeding, particularly in LBW infants, the advantages generally outweigh the disadvantages where phototherapy is not available.

Phototherapy

This should also be regarded as both prophylactic and curative. Optimal results are obtained with blue light, but daylight is adequate. Napkins must be left untied so that the maximum surface is exposed. Phototherapy should be given to all LBW infants as soon as jaundice is noticed, to all pre-term infants with extensive bruising, and to full-term infants with SB over 200 mmol/l or any haematoma.

Phototherapy should be discontinued as soon as there is a sustained fall in the unconjugated bilirubin level. Adequate hydration must be maintained throughout the therapy, with frequent breast-feeds or 50–100 ml/kg/day extra fluids (in addition to normal feeds). The eyes must be covered throughout the procedure.

Side-effects include hyperthermia, loose stools, and skin rashes.

Exchange transfusion

The SB levels at which an exchange transfusion must be considered are given in *Table 5.13*.

Although the SB level gives an indication of the potential risk of kernicterus, each baby has to be assessed individually. An exchange transfusion at a lower level may be required if risk factors are present *(see above)*.

The frequency of monitoring SB levels depends on the severity of the jaundice, clinical condition, and available facilities. Mild to moderate jaundice may require daily assessment, whereas severe jaundice requires 4- to 6-hourly determinations. If a bilirubinometer is being used the standards must be checked regularly.

Preparation for the procedure: The infant must be kept warm, adequately hydrated, and the stomach emptied prior to the exchange transfusion. Congestive cardiac failure and acidosis must be corrected where possible before commencing.

The procedure is carried out under sterile conditions, in a warm environment or in an incubator, particularly when dealing with premature or ill infants. It is advisable to use whole blood or packed cells less than 48 hours old, preserved with citrate and warmed to room temperature. Disadvantages of this blood are that it is more acid, and that it has a higher potassium and lower calcium content, thus predisposing the infant to acid-base and electrolyte disturbances. Heparinized blood, on the other hand, is fresh and has none of the above problems, but cannot be stored. Whole blood is most commonly used because the plasma albumin helps to bind the bilirubin, thus increasing the efficiency of the exchange transfusion. Packed cells are used more often in severely anaemic infants or those in cardiac failure.

Technique: The infant is immobilized by splinting loosely, to allow easy access to the umbilical area. The cord stump is trimmed to within 1.5 cm of the umbilicus, and an 8 FG (or 6 FG in LBW infants) catheter is inserted into the umbilical vein, until venous blood appears in the catheter. A 20 ml (10 ml for LBW) deficit is established at the onset and corrected at the completion of the exchange. Aliquots of 10–20 ml are exchanged at a time. Pre- and post-exchange blood samples are taken routinely for SB, blood cultures, FBC, and electrolyte estimation. The volume of blood exchanged is 150–180 ml/kg. The procedure should take about 90 minutes. The infant is carefully monitored throughout for colour and temperature change, restlessness, and rising or falling pulse and respiratory rates. Cardiac and apnoea monitors may be used.

Complications can be avoided by careful attention to detail. They relate to metabolic problems and haemodynamic alterations during the procedure. Chilling of the infant occurs readily if the blood is not warmed or the environmental temperature is too low. Heart failure from hyper- or hypovolaemia is avoided by slow, small-volume exchanges. Bradycardia, arrhythmias, and cardiac arrest may occur if the donor blood is old, acidaemic or hyperkalaemic, or if the catheter is situated in the heart. Hypocalcaemia is a risk with citrated blood. Fresh citrate-phosphate-dextrose blood, as opposed to acid-citrate-dextrose blood, will avoid most complications related to the blood itself.

Air or pulmonary embolism may occur. Necrotizing enterocolitis occurs rarely, possibly as the result of haemodynamic changes transmitted to the mesenteric vessels. Septicaemia may result from a septic cord or contaminated equipment.

Hydrops fetalis

(See also Miscellaneous section, below.)

Hydrops fetalis is the term used to describe a grossly oedematous fetus which may be anaemic, has hepatosplenomegaly with ascites, and pleural effusions. Besides Rh disease, congenital infections — most commonly syphilis, cytomegalovirus and toxoplasmosis — may cause hydrops fetalis. Cardiac failure, hypoproteinaemia due to hepatic and renal disease, twin-to-twin transfusion, thalassaemia, and a host of miscellaneous conditions may rarely be responsible for this condition.

The management involves respiratory support, removal of the ascitic and pleural fluid (if they contribute to respiratory embarrassment), and

slow correction of the anaemia by exchange transfusion, creating a deficit of 10–20 ml of fluid during the procedure. Furosemide may be of assistance in controlling the cardiac failure. Haemorrhage may be prevented by the administration of vitamin K after birth and exchange transfusion with fresh whole blood. Hypoglycaemia may also occur in these infants, so it is important to monitor the blood and correct hypoglycaemia as it develops.

Infection

The reported prevalence of infection in neonatal units varies greatly — from 7–30% — depending on how assiduously infection is sought and on the conditions prevailing in a particular nursery. For each death caused by infection, up to 100 non-fatal cases may occur.

The prevention of infection is very important, and prompt recognition is necessary for optimal management. It is equally important to stop antibiotic therapy when the investigations and subsequent clinical picture do not support the diagnosis of infection.

Antibiotic therapy is not only a discomfort for the patient and a considerable expense, but the development of resistant organisms is a constant hazard.

Predisposing factors

Certain conditions and functions increase the risk of infection in the neonate. Amniotic fluid infection syndrome is a common condition which is particularly prevalent in poor socio-economic conditions and is associated with pre-term labour.

Factors which predispose to infection of the neonate are:

- maternal infection
- low birth weight
- obstetric or resuscitative procedures
- anatomic: long cord stump, delicate or
- cracked skin
- immature host defense mechanisms
- nursery environment: crowding, under-
- staffing
- poor hand-washing facilities.

Common organisms

The common bacterial pathogens are the Gram-positive organisms such as Group B streptococcus, *Streptococcus faecalis, Staphylococcus aureus* and *Listeria monocytogenes*. Gram-negative organisms are *E. coli* and *Klebsiella pneumoniae* species. Infection due to herpes, enteroviruses, chlamydia and *Pneumocystis carinii* may present in the same manner.

Superficial infections

A constant vigilance for infection of the following sites is essential: skin, umbilicus, eye, mouth, and perineum.

Systemic antibiotics are rarely indicated. Any pustules and abscesses of the skin should be opened and the pus collected for a Gram stain and culture. The lesions are cleaned with alcohol and left exposed to air. Strict hand-washing should be observed, and the baby isolated if possible. For staphylococcal (coagulase-positive) infections, PhisoHex® may be used to clean the area.

Discharge from the eyes requires prompt treatment, preceded by a Gram stain and culture. The eyes must be cleaned with saline and broad spectrum antibiotic instilled 2- to 4-hourly. If the eyelids are red and swollen (blepharitis), parenteral penicillin is given for 3 days. Gonorrhoeal ophthalmia requires parenteral penicillin unless penicillin-resistant.

For oral thrush, nystatin suspension is instilled after each feed. Nystatin cream must be applied to the perineal area when this is involved. Monilial infection of the mother often calls for concomitant therapy.

An umbilical flare without induration may be regarded as a superficial infection. Shortening the stump and spraying the area frequently with alcohol is all that is required. Dressings should not be applied, but the area must be observed for spread of infection.

Septicaemia

The diagnosis of infection may be very difficult in the newborn because of subtle and non-specific presentation. Certain clinical features, however, are highly *suggestive* of infection, whilst others indicate *obvious* sepsis.

Septicaemia should be *suspected* when three or more of the following are present:

- any predisposing factors
- unstable temperature
- lethargy
- poor colour
- apnoea
- feeding difficulties
- vomiting
- abdominal distension
- sclerema
- superficial sepsis.

A combination of the following signs is *strongly indicative* of serious infection: purpura, anaemia, jaundice, hepatomegaly, splenomegaly, full fontanelle or a swollen joint.

Chronic intrauterine infection should be diagnosed in the presence of a combination of hepatosplenomegaly, jaundice, anaemia, and purpura. Of these infections the most common is syphilis, but others to be considered include toxoplasmosis, rubella, cytomegalovirus, herpes, TORCHES, and lysteriosis. In syphilis typical skin lesions and/or metaphysitis may occur in isolation or in addition to this constellation of signs *(see Chapter 8, Infectious Disorders, and Chapter 24, Dermatological Disorders)*.

Investigations

Once infection is suspected, a full blood count and smear must be done, as well as blood culture, urinalysis and culture, cerebrospinal fluid (CSF) examination and culture, and relevant skin, umbilical, or eye swabs. A C-reactive protein is very useful; in conjunction with the white cell count it gives support to a clinical diagnosis of sepsis. Both of these are also of value in assessing response to treatment. A chest radiograph should be considered even in the absence of signs of respiratory distress. A Gram stain on the gastric aspirate before the first feed is helpful if intrauterine sepsis is suspected: the presence of organisms and pus cells is indicative of infection.

Management

Antibiotics are usually commenced once infection is suspected. Penicillin and an aminoglycoside are given initally until culture reports are available, when antibiotics are either stopped or changed according to microbial sensitivity. The duration of antibiotic therapy depends on the nature of the organism and the clinical condition of the patient. As a general rule the neonate with proven septicaemia is treated for 7–10 days. Supportive care of the infected neonate is as important as the specific antibiotic. Hypothermia must be prevented. The blood sugar must be monitored carefully, and feeds given by nasogastric tube where indicated. Parenteral fluids may have to be omitted until the baby is over the acute phase, particularly where there is abdominal distension.

The regular monitoring of peripheral perfusion and pulses will indicate the need for blood pressure support, e.g., plasma 10–20 ml/kg over 1 hour. Supplementary oxygen and electrolyte and acid base balance are also important aspects of care. A blood transfusion may be necessary if the haemoglobin drops below the optimum.

Prevention

This is the single most important aspect of neonatal infection. All personnel handling neonates must be trained with regard to the prevention and dangers of infection. Overcrowding must be avoided. As contamination from the hands of attendants is the most important source of infection, hand-washing before and after handling an individual baby is recommended.

Antiseptic spray of the hands of all attendants before touching a baby is a more realistic objective.

Careful attention to the umbilical cord and meticulous cleaning of the skin before venipuncture are mandatory. Isolation facilities for highly infectious illnesses, such as acute infective diarrhoea, must be available in all units.

Pneumonia

Pneumonia in the neonatal period is an important cause of morbidity and contributes to mortality. Infection may be transmitted via the placenta, by aspiration, or acquired subsequently.

Transplacental lung infection may be part of a generalized infection. The clinical features will include those of respiratory distress and the specific disease. Occasionally septicaemic infections cross the placenta.

Aspiration pneumonia is acquired during birth by aspirating infected material, and can occur with intact membranes (amniotic fluid infection syndrome) or if ruptured for more than 12 hours. Sometimes aspiration of maternal faecal material at the time of delivery may result in pneumonia. Clinically the liquor may be offensive, and the onset of the illness occurs within minutes or hours of birth. Signs of respiratory distress may be mild or severe, and may be delayed for a day or two. The microbes involved are group B β-haemolytic streptococcus, pneumococcus, and coliform organisms.

In acquired pneumonia the signs and symptoms of respiratory distress usually appear after the first week of life. Common bacteria are coagulase-positive staphylococci, streptococci, and at times *E. coli* and *Klebsiella pneumoniae*. Respiratory syncytial virus, influenza A and B, adenovirus, and echoviruses have been associated with outbreaks of pneumonia in nurseries. Chlamydia and *Pneumocystis carinii* may occasionally be responsible for infection, particularly in premature babies.

Another form of nursery-acquired infection may occur in those babies supported by respirators. This disastrous, often low-grade, chronic pneumonia from organisms such as klebsiella and pseudomonas contributes to mortality and chronic pulmonary disability. These organisms are harboured in the equipment, such as humidifiers and suction apparatus. Once established, it is extremely difficult to eradicate the organism.

Investigations

These are as for septicaemia and must include the chest radiograph. Appropriate investigations for viruses should be considered according to available facilities. If intrapartum pneumonia is suspected, an examination of gastric aspirate, as discussed under septicaemia, is of great value.

Treatment

Antibiotic therapy is given along with supportive care as outlined for septicaemia. Respiratory support must be considered if facilities are available.

Meningitis

This is perhaps the most difficult diagnosis to make on clinical grounds, as the *classical signs occur very late* in the neonate. A full fontanelle and convulsions are always serious signs, but are frequently not due to meningitis. Should these signs occur in the presence of meningitis, however, the prognosis is poor.

Meningitis is therefore diagnosed on clinical suspicion, and any infant suspected of having sepsis must have a CSF examination. Ventriculitis is a characteristic feature of neonatal meningitis, and is very resistant to treatment.

Intrathecal and intraventricular therapy is no longer undertaken. Drugs such as penicillin, chloramphenicol, and co-trimoxazole cross the blood – brain barrier but do not eradicate the organisms. Particular difficulty is experienced with Gram-negative organisms which are often responsible for the ventriculitis. The beta lactam antibiotics, such as the third generation cephalosporins, and the new penicillin — piperacillin — are of great value in the management of these difficult cases. These antibiotics given intravenously not only cross the blood–brain barrier, but do clear the infection. There is still some controversy as to whether aminoglycoside or cephalosporin should be used for the septicaemic aspect of the illness.

Penicillin is still the drug of choice in group B streptococcal meningitis. Therapy must be given for a minimum of 14 days in all cases, and sometimes extended to 21 days, depending on the clinical and CSF response.

Osteitis and septic arthritis

Two anatomical reasons account for these two conditions occurring together so frequently. Firstly, the capsules of the hip and shoulder joint are attached below the metaphysis of the femur and humerus respectively. Infection of the epiphyseal cartilage will rupture into the joint space, causing purulent arthritis. Secondly, during the first year of life capillaries perforate the epiphyseal plate of the long bones and provide a communication between metaphysis and joint space, so that spread occurs readily.

The most common causative organism is *Staph. aureus*, followed by group B streptococcus and Gram-negative organisms. This disease may follow certain invasive procedures, such as femoral vein puncture and umbilical catheterization.

The most indicative physical sign is decreased movement of the affected limb; redness and swelling are late signs. Non-specific signs, as discussed under septicaemia, may also occur. Of all the serious infections, this is most often diagnosed late.

Investigations

Blood cultures, a full blood count, and a diagnostic tap of the joint should be carried out on all suspected cases. The Gram stain will indicate the choice of antibiotics. The earliest radiographic sign is widening of the joint space; elevation of the periosteum and joint destruction are not seen before the second week of the illness.

Treatment

Antistaphylococcal antibiotics should be commenced if Gram-positive cocci are demonstrated. An aminoglycoside is indicated for Gram-negative organisms. An antistaphylococcal agent and an aminoglycoside are indicated if no organisms are seen. The minimum period of therapy is 3 weeks. The joint should be splinted. Supportive therapy should be commenced as for septicaemia.

Prognosis

Resolution of the bony pathology lags behind clinical recovery. Patients rarely die, but the morbidity is high, particularly for the weight-bearing joints. Dislocation may occur, with resultant shortening of the limb, contractures, and muscle damage.

Acute infective diarrhoea
(See gastrointestinal section, above.)

Fluid and electrolytes

Maintaining fluid and electrolyte homeostasis has revolutionized the care of the neonate at risk. Not only has survival improved, but also the quality of life of the survivors. Inadequate fluid, calories, and electrolytes (such as in starvation) result in a number of hazardous biochemical derangements such as hypoglycaemia, pre-renal uraemia, acidosis, hypernatraemia, and hyperbilirubinaemia.

The following are situations in which parenteral fluids should be considered in place of oral feeds:

◆ at birth: severe birth asphyxia, weight less than 1.5 kg, major surgical conditions, severe respiratory distress

◆ later: respiratory distress, apnoea, cyanosis, intolerance of oral feeds.

Water, glucose, electrolytes

Basal fluid requirements are approximately 60 – 150 ml/kg/day, increasing with age. The less mature the baby, the greater are the losses, in particular with the use of the open incubator, radiant heaters, and phototherapy lamps. Osmotic diuresis due to glycosuria in the stressed infant receiving a 10% dextrose infusion, excess fluid losses from the gut as with vomiting and diarrhoea, and diuretic therapy are further examples of increased fluid requirements.

Fluid retention, overload, and oedema may occur as the result of excessive parenteral fluid or repeated clearing of arterial lines after blood-sampling. Bolus doses of dextrose, various drugs, and bicarbonate may similarly disturb the fluid balance. The result of fluid overload is congestive cardiac failure, pulmonary oedema, increased risk of patent ductus arteriosus, electrolyte imbalance (e.g., hyponatraemia), and oedema of various organs including the gut, predisposing to necrotizing enterocolitis and cerebral oedema. Fluid retention occurs in severely ill infants suffering asphyxia, poor renal function, and 'leaky' capillaries, with resultant hypotension and acidaemia. Further inappropriate ADH secretion may occur in those with neurological and pulmonary problems. Poor cardiac output and poor renal function may manifest as fluid retention due to severe RDS, asphyxia, sepsis, and the effects of IPPV and CPAP.

Infants therefore vary greatly in their water requirements, and need an assessment of fluid balance 6- to 12-hourly depending on the clinical state. The following are guidelines of normal urine values: urine volumes 50–100 ml/kg/day, osmolality 75–300 mOsmol/kg, and specific gravity 1 005–1 012.

The glucose requirement is adjusted to the blood sugar level. Most infants are commenced on a 10% glucose infusion, but hypoglycaemia or hyperglycaemia may develop. The blood sugar level should be determined with Dextrostix® 4-hourly initially, and then 8-hourly.

The initial intravenous infusion should contain 30–50 mmol/l of sodium and 20 mmol/l of potassium, with adjustments according to the electrolyte levels. Sodium, potassium, calcium, and the acid base status are monitored according to the clinical condition, which may be necessary daily, every 3 days, and then weekly once the infant has recovered.

Metabolic disturbances
(Also see Chapter 20, Endocrine and Metabolic Disorders.)

Hypoglycaemia
The prevalence of hypoglycaemia is generally quoted at approximately 70% in SGA babies, and 25% in the pre-term and LGA baby. The diagnosis of hypoglycaemia is based on a blood sugar level (BSL) below 1.7 mmol/l during the first 72 hours and below 2.2 mmol/l thereafter (1 mmol/l = approx. 18 mg per cent). In term and growth-retarded babies, 1.1 mmol/l is the critical level. It is a wise precaution to take a second sample to confirm the diagnosis before the commencement of treatment.

Hypoglycaemia occurs as a result of a decreased rate of delivery of glucose from inadequate or depleted glycogen and fat stores.

Hyperinsulism is responsible for the hypoglycaemia of babies born to diabetic mothers and those with severe erythroblastosis fetalis. An increased rate of consumption of blood glucose occurs in conditions such as hypothermia, asphyxia, respiratory distress, and infection. There is also a distinct possibility of rebound hypoglycaemia if a glucose infusion is interrupted for any reason.

Clinical features
As the brain relies on glucose as its only source of energy, cerebral signs predominate. However, many hypoglycaemic neonates, particularly those with diabetic mothers, are asymptomatic. The signs are related not only to the actual BSL, but also to the rate of fall. Symptomatic babies present with restlessness, irritability, jitteriness, sweating, eye-rolling, convulsions, coma, apnoeic episodes, cyanosis, lethargy, and poor feeding. As these features are non-specific and can be caused by a wide range of problems, it is important to ensure that they are reversed by the treatment.

Management

▶ The BSL must be monitored within 1 hour of birth in infants at risk of hypoglycaemia, i.e., SGA and pre-term neonates, those of diabetic mothers, and those who have been asphyxiated or hypothermic.

Thereafter it must be determined 2-hourly for the first 8 hours and then 6-hourly for the rest of the first 24 hours. Dextrostix® can be used for screening, but biochemical analysis is advisable for more accurate BSL determination.

Feeding must commence within 2 hours of birth in all these infants. If an infant is too ill to tolerate a gastric feed, a 10% glucose solution must be infused IV as soon as possible.

The hypoglycaemic patient is given 2 ml/kg of 50% glucose diluted to 20%, IV at a rate of 1 ml per minute. Then a 10% glucose solution is infused at 65 ml/kg per 24 hours (0.5 g/kg/hr). The blood sugar is monitored 4-hourly and small-volume milk feeds are commenced as soon as possible. When the patient is asymptomatic and the BSL has stabilized, the infusion is decreased slowly, while increasing the milk feeds.

If the blood sugar does not reach normal levels, a 15% glucose infusion should be considered. The maximum glucose concentration that may be infused is 20%. If control is not achieved after 48 hours, infection must be excluded. Drugs such as hydrocortisone 4 mg/kg IV or IM 12-hourly, or glucagon 0.1 mg/kg per dose IM may be infused repeatedly 6- to 12-hourly. However, appropriate biochemical investigations must be considered in prolonged hypoglycaemia.

Hyperglycaemia

Hyperglycaemia is defined as a BSL over 8 mmol/l with glycosuria. It may occur as a consequence of severe stress, asphyxia, and sepsis, especially in the very-low-birth-weight infant. This aggravates any existing lactic acidosis, which in turn will increase the risk of neuronal and myocardial injury.

Hyperosmolar solutions will induce an osmotic diuresis which can result in significant dehydration. Transient neonatal diabetes occurs very rarely in the SGA baby within the first six weeks of life. Usually there is failure to thrive with extreme hyperglycaemia and dehydration without acidosis. Insulin corrects the hyperglycaemia.

Management

The aim is to reduce the concentration of glucose in the infused fluid. The blood and urine sugar must be monitored carefully to detect the fall in the glucose levels. If these simple measures fail and the blood sugar remains above 20 mmol/l insulin is infused at a dosage of 0.05–0.1 unit/kg/hr, with very strict monitoring of the BSL to detect hypoglycaemia. The very ill infant can be very sensitive to insulin, and the BSL may fall within 15–20 minutes of the insulin injection.

Infant of the diabetic mother

Good diabetic control during pregnancy decreases the risk of the majority of the problems which the infant of the diabetic mother (IDM) is likely to suffer. Unfortunately control during pregnancy does not reduce the incidence of malformations. To achieve the latter it is critical to ensure preconceptual control.

The difficulties of the IDM are due to the large size of the baby in uncontrolled maternal diabetes, and relative immaturity for the gestational age.

The **problems** include:
♦ birth injuries because of the large size: brachial plexus injury and fractures of the humerus following shoulder dystocia are the most common
♦ hypoglycaemia which may develop within the first 1–2 hours after birth and may recur within 24–48 hours. This complication implies poor maternal control during the 24 hours preceding delivery
♦ poor feeding and sucking
♦ jaundice
♦ hypocalcaemia
♦ respiratory distress syndrome
♦ polycythaemia
♦ cardiomyopathy which may lead to cardiac failure. The diagnosis is confirmed on electrocardiograph. Propranolol is the drug of choice
♦ small left colon syndrome presenting as transient obstruction which resolves spontaneously
♦ renal vein thrombosis which presents as macroscopic or microscopic haematuria. Transient renal damage occurs but permanent injury may also ensue
♦ congenital malformations, which vary from 5–13%. Anomalies include neural tube or vertebral defects, sacral agenesis, and cardiac

malformations such as ventricular septal defect, transposition, and coarctation *(see Chapter 17, Cardiac Disorders)*.

Management

This includes 3-hourly monitoring of the BSL from birth, and early feeding if there is no respiratory distress. The IDM requires careful scrutiny for the above-mentioned conditions, and appropriate intervention.

Hypocalcaemia

Approximately one-third of LBW babies and about 50% of the infants born to mothers with diabetes develop hypocalcaemia, which may occur within the first 3 days of life or later. The latter is usually seen in artificially-fed infants as a result of the high phosphate content of cows' milk.

In term infants a serum calcium level of less than 2 mmol/l is regarded as hypocalcaemia, and in pre-term infants 1.8 mmol/l. The normal serum calcium range in the full-term baby is 2.1–2.7 mmol/l, and in the pre-term 1.9–2.8 mmol/l.

Predisposing factors

The neonate suffers relative hypoparathyroidism caused by the suppression of the fetal parathyroid by transferred maternal parathyroid hormone. This function improves within a few days of birth. Pre-term infants are relatively calcium-deficient, and factors such as asphyxia, correction of acidosis, and exchange transfusions with citrated blood may precipitate hypocalcaemia.

Clinical features

Hypocalcaemia may be asymptomatic and detected in routine blood chemistry analysis. Common physical signs are twitching, jitteriness, frank seizures, and a high-pitched cry. The electrocardiogram will show prolonged Q–T segments.

Treatment

In babies with the predisposing factors, 3 ml of 10% calcium gluconate may be added prophylactically to each 100 ml of glucose infusion from the first day of life, and the calcium level monitored.

Asymptomatic infants may be given oral calcium gluconate or lactate 1–3 g daily in divided doses, and the blood level is then monitored.

Symptomatic infants should receive 2 ml/kg of 10% calcium gluconate diluted in 5% glucose and infused very slowly. Calcium may have to be given intravenously or orally over days or even weeks, and the dose gradually decreased and stopped.

Hypomagnesaemia

This disturbance is very infrequent, and is diagnosed when the serum magnesium level is below 0.62 mmol/l. The normal serum magnesium level in the term baby is 0.7– 0.9 mmol/l. Signs are indistinguishable from hypocalcaemia, and may occur in the SGA baby, the infant of the diabetic mother, or during exchange transfusion with citrated blood. Hypomagnesaemia is corrected by giving 0.1– 0.3 ml/kg of 50% magnesium sulphate IV or IM 12-hourly, with a maximum of 3 doses.

Hypermagnesaemia

This uncommon disturbance occurs when eclamptic mothers are treated with magnesium sulphate. Profound central nervous system depression with apnoea may occur, necessitating ventilation for a number of hours.

Hypernatraemia

Hypernatraemia by definition is a serum sodium level above 150 mmol/l. This electrolyte disturbance is serious, as it results in a shift of water from brain tissue, causing brain cell shrinkage and pressure differences which may result in dilatation and rupture of capillaries. Cerebral venous thrombosis or haemorrhage may occur.

Insufficient fluid administration, and dehydration from excessive insensible water loss are the main causes. Phototherapy lamps and radiant heaters tend to cause hyperthermia and diarrhoea. Excessive sodium bicarbonate administration during resuscitation is a further iatrogenic element to be borne in mind.

Clinical features are usually non-specific and occur at a late stage, with lethargy, irritability, and convulsions.

Treatment

The serum sodium level should be lowered gradually over 24 – 48 hours to avoid cerebral oedema. A solution containing sodium chloride must be used, as a plain glucose solution encourages cerebral oedema. Plasma is a safe substitute.

Prognosis

This depends on the underlying cause, and the duration and degree of the electrolyte imbalance. Death or permanent neurological sequelae may be caused by an episode of hypernatraemia, and are related to the complications as discussed earlier.

Hyponatraemia

Hyponatraemia is a serum sodium level below 125 mmol/l. Central nervous system injury occurs as water is drawn into the brain cells.

VLBW infants under 32 weeks' gestation are unable to conserve sodium, and may lose more than 3 mg/kg/day in their urine. Severe asphyxia or respiratory distress may cause inappropriate secretion of antidiuretic hormone (IADH), with loss of sodium in the urine, water intoxication, and diarrhoea resulting in hyponatraemia.

Clinical signs include lethargy, poor feeding, apnoeic attacks and shock.

Treatment

This depends on the cause of the hyponatraemia. In the case of water intoxication or IADH secretion, fluid restriction is very important before attempting correction with sodium itself. Hyponatraemia due to excessive losses in diarrhoea or urine is corrected by the use of a simple formula: mmol sodium required = (125 minus serum sodium level) x 0.6 x weight in kg. Ventilation may be indicated for the apnoeic attacks, and plasma 20 ml/kg is given to the shocked patient.

Hypokalaemia

Hypokalaemia is defined as a plasma potassium level below 3 mmol/l. The major causes of this complication are poor intake, alkalosis, diarrhoea, and diuretics.

Clinical manifestations are marked hypotonia, arrhythmia, and ileus. Prolonged hypokalaemia may lead to renal tubular changes with decreased concentrating ability and interstitial nephritis.

The correction is achieved by giving potassium chloride either IV or orally, 1–3 mmol/kg.

Hyperkalaemia

The definition of hyperkalaemia is a plasma potassium in excess of 7 mmol/l. The electrocardiograph is a guide to toxicity: peaked T waves, a prolonged PR interval, absent P waves, and arrhythmias may be evident.

The causes are severe catabolism, acute renal failure, hypoxia, shock, acidosis, and congenital adrenal hyperplasia.

The management includes electrocardiographic monitoring and IV calcium gluconate (10 %) 0.5–1 mg/kg over 2–4 minutes (which is effective in 30–60 minutes). Acidosis is corrected by giving 1–2 mmol/kg of sodium bicarbonate (effective within 1–2 hours). Salbutamol 4 mg/kg IV by bolus injection is much safer than the administration of glucose and insulin. Kayexalate® (cation exchange resin) 1 g/kg/day may be given orally or rectally. If these methods fail then an infusion of glucose and insulin may be administered. Glucose 0.5–1 g/kg is given, with 1 unit of insulin for every 4 g glucose. BSL must be monitored meticulously, as there is a danger of a precipitous drop. Finally, one may have to resort to peritoneal dialysis.

Miscellaneous

Temperature instability

As temperature regulation in the neonate is very delicately balanced, it is readily upset, with dire metabolic consequences. Both hypo- and hyperthermia increase the metabolic rate. If there is associated hypoxia or hypoglycaemia, metabolic acidosis will complicate the picture and possibly cause tissue damage. In the care of neonates a neutral thermal environment is essential — which will allow a normal temperature to be maintained at a minimum metabolic rate. There are marked individual variations depending on the size, maturity and state of health of the baby. It is important to achieve this environment, so that insensible water loss is kept to a minimum and energy can be utilized optimally for growth.

Energy for heat production is obtained from glucose stored in the liver and myocardium. In the absence of further intake these stores are depleted within 4–8 hours. Thereafter brown fat at special body sites will release free fatty acids in response to noradrenaline stimulation. Heat is lost mainly by evaporation and radiation, and to a lesser extent by conduction to clothing, sheets, etc., as well as by convection currents.

Hypothermia

In LBW babies hypothermia raises the mortality by at least 25%. The commonest cause of hypothermia is a low ambient temperature at birth. The asphyxiated, hypotonic, SGA baby requiring resuscitation is at greatest risk: hypoxia interferes with heat production, whilst hypotonia diminishes metabolisn in the muscles and increases exposure from extended limbs. Furthermore the LBW, SGA baby has no brown fat stores on which to draw. This is particularly likely to occur if there is a need for resuscitation and during transport. Associated sepsis further interferes with the metabolism and hence with heat production.

The metabolic rate and oxygen consumption increase rapidly with cooling. Clinically, vasoconstriction occurs and apnoea may ensue. The adverse effects of hypothermia include metabolic acidosis, hypoglycaemia, decreased surfactant production, and a rise in free fatty acids. The latter interfere with bilirubin binding and increase the risk of kernicterus. Slow or delayed weight gain may occur. The overall effects are reflected not only in an increased morbidity, but also in a striking mortality.

Management:

 Prevention of heat loss is essential; rewarming the neonate is difficult, time-consuming, and fraught with further complications.

Asphyxia in particular must be anticipated *(see High Risk Pregnancy and Neonate sections, above)* and precautionary measures introduced. At birth every baby must be dried and wrapped in a pre-warmed towel. The head must be included, as it is the site of appreciable heat loss. Skin-to-skin contact with the mother provides warmth and prevents heat loss. When this is not possible and additional risk factors are present, warmers, cotton wool, alumi-nium swaddlers, and incubators can be used.

Rewarming of the cold baby is critical when hypothermia has been prolonged, and must be carried out with as low a temperature gradient as possible. Again skin-to-skin contact with the mother is very effective, and can be carried out in

any situation. The BSL must be monitored and metabolic acidosis corrected. Complications such as infection, haemorrhage, and cerebral insults must be anticipated and treated appropriately.

Neonatal cold injury

Prolonged exposure to cold results in neonatal cold injury. Not infrequently the temperature is 32 °C or less. There is oedema, generalized redness, poor feeding, and lethargy. Sclerema, hypoglycaemia, shock, hypoxia, decreased surfactant production, convulsions, uraemia, and pulmonary haemorrhage may be encountered. There is an increased risk of sepsis and haemorrhage associated with cold injury. The mortality in this serious condition is very high. Treatment is as for hypothermia plus symptomatic management.

Overheating

When exposed to unnecessarily high environmental temperatures a baby becomes overheated. Term babies in incubators are particularly at risk. There is vasodilatation with increased insensible water loss, which results in dehydration and hypernatraemia. Apnoeic episodes may occur, and heat stroke and death may ensue.

Management is by lowering the environmental temperature, giving fluids either orally or by nasogastric tube, and correcting any serious metabolic disturbances.

Oedema

Oedema is a common clinical problem amongst neonates. Approximately 75% of the newborn weight is due to water (adult value 65%). Extracellular water in the skin and subcutaneous tissue accounts for 16% of the infant's total body water (compared to 8% in adults). Accumulation of oedema fluid can be brought about by decreased plasma oncotic pressure or decreased tissue hydrostatic pressure. Immediately after birth the extracellular fluid mass is greater than the intracellular fluid compartment. This early phase is referred to as physiological oedema. During the first few days, however, the situation is reversed, and weight loss occurs. Within a few days of birth the glomerular filtration rate rises, with improved urinary concentration and no change in serum proteins. The body water may also be influenced by the amount of blood infused from the placenta and the mode of delivery: elective Caesarean section babies have a higher water content. The term baby tends to retain salt and may show oedema if challenged with a salt load.

The pre-term infant may have persistent moderate oedema, probably due to increased capillary permeability rather than hypoalbuminaemia. Factors such as poor perfusion, acidosis, shock, sepsis, severe respiratory distress, and hypothermia aggravate this situation.

Common causes of severe neonatal oedema are Rh disease and severe haemolytic states, chronic intrauterine infection, and congenital nephrotic syndrome *(see Hydrops Fetalis, above)*. In the VLBW baby with respiratory distress, fluid retention causes fairly severe oedema. Inappropriate anti-diuretic hormone (IADH) secretion is commonly responsible for oedema in the presence of hypoxic ischaemic encephalopathy and severe parenchymal lung disease. This is characterized by hyponatraemia.

Careful assessment of salt and water intake is important in the oedematous baby. One needs to rule out excessive maintenance fluids and plasma or bicarbonate infusions. The weight, urine output, peripheral perfusion, blood pressure, and temperature must be carefully monitored. The known causes of oedema must be considered and appropriate treatment instituted.

Fluid restriction is the first step in controlling oedema. Should this fail, a volume expander such as plasma and salt-poor albumin may be infused, followed by a diuretic such as furosemide. Underlying metabolic and temperature disturbances need to be corrected. Oedema due to IADH secretion frequently clears with fluid restriction. Very rarely is salt replacement necessary.

Failure-to-thrive

Failure-to-thrive means that a baby fails to gain weight adequately. This must be distinguished from dwarfism, where length is the affected growth parameter. Following the initial weight loss in the first few days after birth, the healthy term baby should regain the birth weight by the tenth day, and the pre-term infant by the fourteenth day. Thereafter the expected weight gain is a minimum of 150 g per week, and a baby who does not gain weight at this rate must be regarded as failing to thrive.

The most common cause is infrequent feeding practices: firstly those related to breast-feeding, such as difficulty with sucking, poor technique, and inadequate frequency of feeding; secondly dilute or infrequent formula feeds may be the problem. In the pre-term infant careful calculation of volumes, calories, proteins, and water is essential. Often insensible water loss is underestimated, particularly in VLBW infants and those nursed in incubators, under phototherapy units, or radiant warmers.

Metabolic acidosis develops in some otherwise healthy pre-term babies, particularly during rapid growth, when hydrogen ions are produced which may not be excreted by the immature kidney. This build-up of acidosis will in turn result in poor weight gain, which is easily corrected by giving oral sodium bicarbonate 2–4 mmol/kg/24 hours.

Anaemia and occult infections, such as urinary tract and chronic intrauterine infections, are not uncommon causes. Subclinical cold stress occurs when babies nursed in temperatures below thermoneutrality use calories in an attempt to maintain body temperature and thus do not gain weight. Congenital heart defects with cardiac failure, urinary and gastrointestinal tract malformations, chronic chest conditions, metabolic diseases, endocrine disorders, and brain damage may all cause failure to thrive.

The common causes must be excluded by taking a careful history, particularly in respect of feeds, vomiting, and stools, and by doing a detailed, relevant, clinical examination. Special investigations must be selected with circumspection.

A very important aspect of thriving is the mother–child relationship. Some infants with growth failure and developmental lag have been shown to have suffered as a result of psychosocial disturbances, such as maternal depression. On correction of these problems the infants improved both physically and developmentally. This form of failure to thrive is at one end of the spectrum of child abuse and neglect. The pre-term baby and one of twins are particularly at risk for this problem.

M. Adhikari

6

Feeding of infants and toddlers

Introduction

The Alma-Ata declaration and many subsequent international health movements have pin-pointed improvement in nutrition as a major goal for improving health. In many developing countries, improved nutrition alone has resulted in significant positive changes in national health. In turn, these changes have served as motivation to tackle other health determinants.

Few, if any, of the factors directly affecting health are as intimately linked with society and the environment as is nutrition. Culture, religion, politics, societal hierarchy, economics, education, transport, urbanization, population growth, climate, agriculture, disasters such as drought, floods and war — to name but a few — all have an influence on the amount of food available to the individual on a daily basis. In developing countries and disadvantaged communities, the high mortality and morbidity rates of young children and women of child-bearing age are stark proof of this fact.

Improving nutrition and nutrition-related behaviour therefore necessitates a multi-disciplinary public health approach, which must extend beyond the traditional 'medical' team. It has to involve the community itself, with important inputs coming from agriculturists, sociologists, and educationists. Ultimately however, it has to be recognized by all health workers that although nutrition does imply nutrients, the bottom line is *food,* a highly emotive, controversial, personalized commodity. Changes in eating patterns cannot be imposed on people, they have to be accepted and put into practice. For the most vulnerable groups, endorsement must come from the community.

Adequate food is a basic human need. The physiological, psychological, and social implications of balanced nutrition are important determinants of an individual's growth and development throughout the life cycle. The new-born infant can only express the need for food by becoming restless and crying. The mother's response is to breast-feed her child, and at the same time to communicate affection and care as nature intended. Human milk remains the perfect food for the infant, and under normal conditions the child will thrive on this. Breast milk is a complex physiological secretory fluid which is specific for the nutritional needs of the infant and cannot be duplicated by an artificial feed.

As the child grows older and the nutritional requirements change, solid foods with a higher nutrient density need to be gradually introduced. This transition also creates the ideal opportunity to introduce the young child to the eating habits and culture of the family and community.

In the majority of urban and rural developing and deprived communities, a marked decline in breast-feeding has been documented. Substitute feeds are often accompanied by inadequate and inappropriate weaning diets, leading to malnutrition. The subsequent lowered nutritional status contributes directly to the high infant and childhood morbidity and mortality seen in developing communities. Successful infant and toddler feeding therefore remains a matter of great concern for health professionals and parents, and is a subject with which health professionals should be fully acquainted.

The importance of a well-nourished mother

When a healthy woman with a good nutritional status falls pregnant, and maintains an adequate food intake, the prospects are excellent for an uncomplicated pregnancy, a healthy infant, and the capacity to adequately breast-feed her baby. The possibility of a rapid return to optimal health following delivery is also enhanced.

Over and above the needs of the fetus, nutrients are also required for additional maternal tissues and stores, viz., the placenta, increased blood supply, and preparation for lactation. Initially these nutrient requirements are minimal, but as the pregnancy progresses, the requirements increase. Energy intake should be such that it provides for the additional requirements of pregnancy, but not in excess (resulting in rapid weight gain). The emphasis has to be placed on quality rather than quantity — quality protein sources. In addition, ensuring adequate supplies of vitamins A and C, calcium, and iron in the diet need special attention. A sufficient intake of water and the ingestion of complex carbohydrates — providing fibre — should also be stressed. Refined carbohydrate and fat consumption should not be excessive. Table salt is the most common source of sodium, and use should be limited.

In deprived communities the weight of women of child-bearing age is frequently significantly lower than that of women with an acceptable food intake. The chronically undernourished mother may be anaemic, stunted, and show signs of pelvic deformity. She is more susceptible to complications during pregnancy and labour, and the infant is more likely to have a low birth weight (LBW). These infants have poor survival rates, especially if they are further compromised by poor sanitation, infection, and inadequate care.

The undernourished mother can breast-feed, and the quantity and quality of her milk is maintained at the expense of her own reserves for relatively long periods. However, the demands of 'women's work' in rural settings — gathering fuel and water, caring for the family, agricultural tasks — may contribute to early weaning. As ovulation is no longer suppressed, this increases the likelihood of yet another pregnancy, which further taxes her health. In urban settings, the need to resume work shortly after the birth or after a limited period of maternity leave, in order to earn an income, presents a similar situation. Coupled with this are the inadequacies of child-care facilities. In many cases, this results in the infant being weaned shortly after birth and sent home to be cared for by the grandmother, and consequently not breast-fed. The vicious circle of undernutrition, LBW, stunting, poor nutrition, and pregnancy, LBW is repeated again and again.

Intervention programmes have shown that small daily supplements of food, which mainly increase energy intake, improve mothers' nutritional reserves. This also resulted in fewer LBW infants and enhanced periods of breast-feeding. However, unless the community understands and acknowledges the special requirements of the pregnant female, she and her unborn child may continue to be deprived of the nutritional attention they deserve.

Pregnancy in early adolescence is fraught with complications: the mother is not physiologically fully developed, is still growing, and her nutritional needs are higher than those of an adult woman. Many teenagers are poorly nourished due to a high consumption of 'junk' foods or because of an inadequate total intake of food. The additional burden of pregnancy therefore necessitates particular attention to the food intake of this group in urban and/or deprived communities.

Pica and compulsive eating because of 'cravings' can compromise the nutrient intake of the pregnant woman. Food or non-food items consumed may interfere with normal appetite and food intake and can contribute to poor nutritional status during pregnancy. It should be borne in mind that in many traditional communities, pica has cultural connotations.

Specific requirements of the infant

See Table 7.1 in Chapter 7, Nutritional Disorders, for a summary of the energy and protein requirements of infants as determined by expert committees of the WHO. It should be noted that these figures represent an energy requirement per kg which is two to three times that for adults. The protein requirements are between two and four times higher.

Figures of recommendations for other nutrients are also published by the WHO, as well as by the National Academy of Sciences in the form of Recommended Dietary Allowances (RDAs). It should be remembered that the figures are not intended to be strictly applied to individual infants, but merely as useful guidelines.

Breast milk and infant formulae supply adequate nutrients for the first 4–6 months of an infant's life. There are, however, two nutrients that need special consideration. Human and cows' milk are poor sources of vitamin D. The infant will manufacture adequate vitamin D as long as his skin is exposed to sunlight daily. Due to the fact

115

that infants are born with sterile gastrointestinal tracts, parenteral vitamin K is administered soon after birth.

Formats of infant feeding

The trends in infant feeding in industrialized countries since the late 1920s show an initial sharp decline in breast-feeding, followed by a gradual return only after the 1970s. The reasons for this have been well documented. One aspect of particular concern is the fact that women in poorer communities tend to follow the example of their educated and more well-to-do counterparts. Unfortunately this tendency is still apparent in many developing communities, both urban and rural. There are various scenarios which operate to perpetuate this unfortunate situation. Artificial feeding is regarded as a status symbol by many. Working mothers frequently have to leave their babies in the care of others, and institute weaning very early. This is often due to a lack of, or inadequate, facilities at their place of work, which were they available would enable them to continue breast-feeding. Many of these mothers are unaware of how to maintain lactation. Other complicating factors needing attention are the numerous unsubstantiated beliefs and attitudes about breast-feeding.

Although breast-feeding is still practised extensively in many developing communities, there are definite signs of decline. Early introduction of artificial feeds, or inadequate weaning foods go hand in hand with infant gastroenteritis and other infections.

Breast-feeding

Although apparently regarded as a *natural* instinctive reaction of all women, breast-feeding is a learned behaviour. Unless the new mother is given support and correct information, she may be tempted to wean her infant onto an artificial formula when she encounters problems.

Advantages

◆ Human milk is constituted to provide virtually all of the infant's nutrient requirements for a period of 4–6 months. The composition of the milk changes in line with the infant's requirements and growth pattern.

◆ Protection against certain infections, which is conferred by the presence of antibodies and macrophages in the colostrum and breast milk, is a major benefit of breast-feeding. Immunity against enteral, and to a lesser extent parenteral, infections is derived from the antibodies. As a result it is uncommon for a fully breast-fed infant to contract infective diarrhoea or necrotizing enterocolitis.

◆ Breast milk is hygienic, convenient, and readily available for the infant. It requires no preparation or sterilization. These factors need serious consideration when a breast-feeding mother is contemplating the use of artificial feeds on returning to work outside her home.

◆ Breast-feeding strengthens the psychological bonding process between mother and child. This is especially important in the later development of the child's personality and in the socialization of the child.

◆ Ovulation is suppressed by demand breast-feeding especially if the baby feeds at night. The duration of lactational amenorrhoea associated with regular continued breast-feeding varies, but may continue for 12 months or longer. However, this should not be considered a totally reliable method of contraception, as 3–7% of breast-feeding women do fall pregnant. The benefits of breast-feeding for child spacing have nevertheless been well established.

◆ It has been suggested, but not convincingly shown, that the incidence of allergies in infants exclusively breast-fed for the first 4–6 months of life is less frequent than for infants who have been fed cows' milk. Colic also appears to occur much less often in breast-fed babies.

◆ Breast-feeding is less expensive than any substitute, even if the mother has to eat slightly more. An additional factor to consider is that the breast-fed infant's ration does not have to be shared by other members of the family.

◆ Breast-fed babies are rarely overweight.

◆ The incidence of Sudden Infant Death syndrome is lower in breast-fed babies.

◆ Breast cancer occurs less frequently in women who have breast-fed.

Physiology of lactation

Several factors are involved in stimulating the formation and secretion of human milk. The two pituitary hormones, prolactin (lactogenic hormone) and oxytocin, exert the major effect. In addition, a combination of direct and indirect interactions between mother and infant such as physical contact, eye contact, odour, and the sound of the infant's crying, provide further stimulation.

Prolactin promotes the formation of milk in the alveolar cells of the breast. It is stimulated by nerve impulses following suckling and inhibited by breast engorgement, pain, and anxiety *(see Fig. 6.1)*. Oxytocin causes the myoepithelial cells of the alveoli to contract, forcing the milk into the larger ducts and sinuses towards the nipple (let-down reflex), from where it can readily be emptied by the infant *(see Fig. 6.2)*. Activation of this reflex by feeding is delayed for a few days, but subsequently secretion is immediately triggered even by the mere thought of feeding the baby.

During the first few days after birth, the breast secretes colostrum, which is light orange in colour and contains considerably more protein and minerals than 'mature' human milk. A high concentration of antimicrobial factors is also present, which provides protection to the infant against Gram-negative organisms. Colostrum is then supplanted by 'transitional milk', which contains more protein than mature breast milk. Mature breast milk follows gradually during the subsequent 3–4 weeks of breast-feeding.

On average, approximately 100 ml of milk is available daily at the start of lactation. During the second week the amount increases to roughly 500 ml daily. With well-established breast-feeding, the average daily volume of milk is about 700–800 ml. Some of the important factors affecting lactation are outlined in *Table 6.1*.

Basic requirements for breast-feeding

◆ A positive attitude to breast-feeding by the mother, and support from the father, family members, and the health team.

◆ An infant with a well-developed sucking reflex.

◆ Frequent suckling.

◆ Sufficient rest and sleep to stimulate prolactin secretion.

◆ A nutritionally adequate diet for the mother.

Table 6.1 Factors affecting lactation

	Favourable	Unfavourable
Environment	Calm, relaxed	Noisy, stressful
Frequency of feeds	Frequent	Infrequent
Breast contents	Empty	Engorged
Emotional state	Relaxed	Anxious
Physical state	Comfortable	Painful, tense
Drugs	Metoclopramide	Oestrogen
	Oxytocin	Testosterone
	(sub-lingual)	Bromocriptine
		Sedatives
		(large doses)

Practical aspects

First feeding: Much is to be gained by putting the infant to the breast as soon as possible after birth. The intimate contact promotes bonding which is beneficial for both mother and child. The secretion of prolactin and oxytocin is also stimulated; the latter hormone aiding uterine contraction, and so diminishing the possibility of post partum haemorrhage. The initial feeding is aimed at establishing proper suckling rather than supplying a large volume of milk.

Method of breast-feeding: The baby should be offered the breast whenever the need arises. Rooming in, or keeping the baby as close as possible to the mother during the first few days after delivery, promotes successful breast-feeding. Mother and child must be comfortable, the mother either lying down or in a sitting position. The infant should be held in a semi-sitting position, with the head supported against the mother's breast. When the nipple is stroked against the baby's cheek, the rooting reflex will become operative, causing the baby to open the mouth and move the head in search of the nipple. The nipple and an appreciable portion of the areola should fill the infant's mouth in order to prevent sore, cracked nipples due to excessive sucking, and to ensure gum pressure through chomping on the milk ducts immediately under the areola *(see Fig. 6.3)*. Some infants are able to suck strongly very soon, whereas others are weaker, easily tired, and lose interest quickly. Short, frequent feeds are preferable for both mother and child, and prevent engorgement.

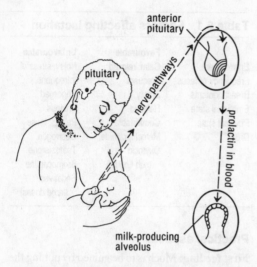

Fig. 6.1   The milk-producing (prolactin) reflex
Suckling stimulates nerve endings in the nipple and areola. The impulse is conducted to the hypothalamus via the vagus, causing the anterior pituitary gland to release prolactin. The hormone acts directly on the milk-secreting glands.

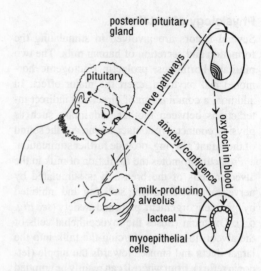

Fig. 6.2   The milk ejection (let-down) reflex
Suckling stimulates the posterior pituitary gland to release oxytocin, which causes ejection of the milk from the myoepithelial cells and ducts. Pleasurable sensation and confidence promote this process, whilst pain and anxiety inhibit the reflex.

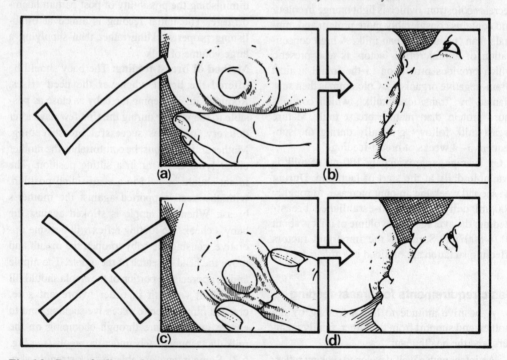

Fig. 6.3   Breast-feeding technique
a. The mother presents the whole areola to the baby.
b. The nipple and greater part of the areola are in the baby's mouth; this promotes efficient feeding as the gums can compress the milk ducts.

c. The nipple only is presented by the mother.
d. The baby sucks on the nipple, which is likely to cause pain and excoriation.

As the child drinks, the milk composition changes: the initial secretion (fore-milk) appears thin and watery, but contains a high proportion of protein, vitamins, and minerals. The milk secreted at a later stage (hind-milk) is whiter and creamier, and has a much higher fat content.

The baby should preferably drink from both breasts at every feed, and each feed should start from the alternate breast. Duration of feeds is variable, and determined by the infant and the feeding technique. After the feed, the infant should be held upright over the mother's shoulder to facilitate bringing up any swallowed air. The time it takes for the milk to leave the stomach varies from one child to another and from one feed to another. Demand feeding has replaced the rigid routine of the past, dictated by the clock. As the volume of milk that the infant can handle at one feed increases and stabilizes, a regular routine of five or more feeds per 24 hours may be established, i.e., every 3–4 hours.

Babies should not be fed to placate them when they are wet, uncomfortable, or restless. An infant should be fed to provide nourishment, and not as a substitute for attention.

After the age of 4–6 months, the child's requirements cannot be obtained solely from breast milk. Suitable supplementary weaning foods need to be introduced gradually to ensure an adequate nutrient intake. Assessment of whether the child is receiving an adequate intake can be made by measuring weight and development against established norms such as growth charts, e.g., Road-to-Health Charts (*see Chapter 4, Fig. 4.2*).

Inexperienced mothers need continued sympathetic support with regard to feeding the new infant after returning home. Influences of various kinds (such as difficulty in establishing a breast-feeding regime, feelings of inadequacy, the need to return to work to earn money, and prejudice against breast-feeding from family and friends) may induce her to stop breast-feeding. Firm but diplomatic counselling of decision-makers at home is required if the mother is to succeed. Once she has breast-fed successfully and is convinced of the benefits, she will be confident about assisting other mothers.

Problems: real and imaginary

Lack of time, and in many cases inadequate understanding of the principles and implications of breast-feeding by many health professionals, may be negative factors in the promotion of breast-feeding. Numbers of patients, the actual hospital or clinic routine, and limited staff are all counter-productive in establishing a situation favouring breast-feeding. Particular problems may include:
♦ separation of the mother and child at birth and for protracted periods afterwards
♦ maintaining rigid schedules of 3- to 4-hourly feeds
♦ nipple confusion in the infant, following offers of bottle feeds during the first few days
♦ inadequate time available for individual attention to help the mother establish breast-feeding, and impatience with the hesitant new mother.

The mother's fear that the milk is insufficient and/or of poor quality: This can be linked to the appearance of the fore-milk, which is thin and watery, and that of the admixture of fore-milk and hind-milk (pus-like). The mother needs to understand that changes in milk composition occur with suckling. It must also be explained to the mother that the relatively small stools of the breast-fed infant are due to the minimal amount of indigestible material present in the milk. The mother should be reassured and encouraged to continue breast-feeding provided the infant is growing according to accepted norms, appears satisfied, and passes a normal amount of urine (approximately 6–8 wet nappies per day, or a wet nappy after each feed, provided the infant does not get any other fluid besides breast milk).

In many developing communities **traditional beliefs** are firmly entrenched. Colostrum may be regarded as poisonous, or it may be felt that affliction or bewitchment can occur through breast milk. Such traditional beliefs have to be handled tactfully and with discretion.

A crying baby immediately after feeding may be associated with insufficient milk. This is, however, more likely to be due to gastric discomfort and distension from swallowing air during feeding. Occasionally this may be the result of an imbalance between fore-milk and hind-milk in favour of the less satisfactory former. This may be obviated by allowing the infant to feed entirely from one breast at a time, thus ensuring an adequate fat intake.

Nipple excoriation or sore and cracked nipples result commonly from faulty feeding techniques. Prolonged and/or vigorous sucking is the underlying cause, rather than chomping *(see above)*. A non-absorbent, tight bra may also contribute to maceration of the nipples. If nursing the infant is too painful, a nipple shield may provide relief. Alternatively, the milk can be expressed by hand or hand pump and fed to the baby by spoon.

Engorged breasts interfere with proper drinking and further compromise draining of the breast. More frequent feeding (if practical) can overcome this problem, or expressing the milk manually and then feeding it to the infant by spoon.

Abscess formation and mastitis can ensue from a damaged nipple and engorgement. As the abscess is sealed off, continued breast-feeding is recommended, as this promotes drainage of the breast. Suitable antibiotics should be prescribed.

Emotional stress and fatigue may result in decreased lactation. A primary deficiency of prolactin is extremely rare. *True* inadequate lactation may manifest itself in unsatisfactory weight gain if the deficiency is slight. If the deficit is severe, the infant cries frequently and feeds greedily. This may contribute to the swallowing of air, and even vomiting. The baby may also have a tendency to be constipated and pass greenish 'starvation' stools. The diagnosis can be confirmed by giving complementary feeds *after* breast-feeding and noting the volume consumed. More frequent breastfeeding to stimulate milk production through prolactin secretion remains the accepted method of treatment. At the same time one should ensure that the mother drinks enough fluid and that she is reassured and supported. Supplementary feeding is seldom required, and should only be introduced as a last resort.

'Aesthetic perceptions' may prejudice mothers against breast-feeding. Leaking or sagging breasts, breasts regarded merely as sex symbols, and breast-feeding viewed as an obstacle to a satisfactory sex life, are all cited as reasons not to breast-feed. In all these cases sympathetic counselling, regular drainage of the breasts, and a suitable supporting bra will alleviate the perceived problems. Furthermore, it must be stressed that it is repeated pregnancies, and not breast-feeding,

which are the cause of the breasts sagging eventually.

The mother who has to **return to regular employment shortly after the birth** of her infant is faced with many problems. These include the lack of day-care facilities at work, and leaving the baby with a child-minder. Bottle-feeding would then appear to be the solution to her problems. The mother needs to be convinced that it is possible for her to continue breast-feeding. She has to be provided with acceptable and practical alternatives, such as feeding before leaving for work and on return, as well as during the night. The stimulation of a hungry baby drinking will encourage lactation. Breast engorgement can be prevented by expressing milk, which should be kept cool and given to the infant by spoon (or at a later stage in a cup), when the mother is at work.

The mother should also understand that the introduction of bottle-feeding may preclude the continuation of breast-feeding.

Less exertion is required by a child drinking from a bottle, and she may rapidly lose interest in feeding from the breast.

Many employers now provide facilities at the work site, and the mother may well be able to continue the child's normal breast-feeding routine. Appropriate support and effective antenatal health care and education will enable the mother to find solutions for problems associated with leaving the child when she has to work.

Contra-indications to breast-feeding

While breast-feeding remains the best for the infant — physiologically, psychologically and socially — there are some legitimate reasons for a mother not to breast-feed her baby. If one of these does occur, the health professional has a responsibility to help the mother not to feel inferior or a poor quality mother *(see Table 6.2)*.

Artificial feeding

It is well documented that artificial feeding is associated with numerous problems. Artificially fed infants have higher mortality and morbidity rates than breast-fed babies, and the incidence of hospitalization among artificially fed infants is more frequent. In addition, the early introduction of foreign protein macromolecules through feeds,

Table 6.2   Contra-indications to breast-feeding

Absolute	Relative
Mother: Psychosis	**Mother:** Pregnancy
HIV in developed	Infections** e.g.,
countries	typhoid
Serious systemic	AIDS
disease	herpes
Carcinoma of the breast	septicaemia
	pneumonia
Drugs*:	
Radioactive iodine	
Cytotoxins	
Thiouracil	
Infant: Galactosaemia	**Infant:** Abnormalities[+]:
Phenylketonuria	mouth or swallowing
	mechanism
	Low birth weight[++]
	Lactose intolerance

Notes: * *Alternative drugs should be considered before introducing artificial feeds.*
** *The severity of the illness will determine whether breast-feeding should be terminated or continued.*
[+] *If suckling is totally impossible, expressed breast-milk should be fed to the child by tube or spoon.*
[++] *Every effort should be made to establish breast-feeding, as this will contribute greatly to an LBW baby's survival and catch-up.*

as well as the problems arising from the preparation of artificial feeds, predispose such infants to problems which are rare in the breast-fed infant. Before the final decision is made to substitute artificial feeding for breast-feeding, the situation should be assessed in its totality. A second opinion should be considered, as the consequences, especially in the case of disadvantaged families, are far-reaching. If the indications for terminating breast-feeding are relative rather than absolute, the mother may simply require advice and support with regard to some of the common problems encountered *(see above)*.

Specific problems associated with artificial feeds

Cost: The total cost involved in artificial feeding goes beyond that of just the purchase price of the feeds themselves. The bottles, teats, cleaning materials, disinfectants, fuel, and medication required, cause the total expenditure to escalate. Added to this is the fact that an adequate intake by the infant and the nutritional status of the family as a whole may be put in jeopardy.

Malnutrition: Misunderstanding, illiteracy, and limited funds can all lead to overdilution in order to make the product 'last longer', and result in undernutrition. This is of particular importance when the highly modified feeds with a low protein content are used. Undernutrition further compromises the infant's immune system against infections.

In contrast, in more well-to-do families, the chances of overfeeding the infant are increased. This is likely to result in an obese child who is also at risk, particularly for respiratory infections.

Infection: Artificial feeds do not contain antibodies and macrophages, which provide the breast-fed infant with protection against infections. Artificial feeds provide an ideal culture medium for micro-organisms, due to inadequately cleaned and sterilized containers, inadequate and contaminated water supplies, poor sanitation, and limited fuel. Added to these factors, the mother is often uninformed or does not understand the need for care in the preparation of artificial feeds. Gastrointestinal and other infections are far more common in infants fed on artificial feeds.

Allergy: The gastrointestinal mucosa of the young infant is permeable to large protein molecules. Allergic disorders are said to be more common and severe in infants fed on artificial feeds.

Types of artificial feeds

If a mother is not in a position to breast-feed her baby, she must be provided with alternatives. The most obvious choice is cows' milk, or products which are based on cows' milk and modified to more closely resemble human milk. The composition of cows' milk reflects the needs of a calf much more closely than those of a human infant. Undiluted cows' milk has a higher protein and ash content than human milk, resulting in a high solute load. Due to the high casein content of cows' milk, tough, hard-to-digest curds are formed in the infant's stomach. In contrast, breast-milk contains a higher proportion of lactalbumin, a protein that forms soft, flocculent, easy-to-digest curds. Studies have indicated that even if cows' milk is pasteurized, it may cause intestinal blood loss which could contribute to iron deficiency anaemia. The vitamin and mineral content of cows' milk is far from optimal for an infant. In many cases the levels are very high, especially of minerals, or nutrients are supplied in a form which is unavailable to the human infant.

Commercial formulae have been developed in an attempt to overcome the limitations of cows' milk. (*See Table 6.3* for types of formulae available in South Africa.) In the case of an infant who has to be artificially fed, it is preferable to use a modified milk for at least the first 4 – 6 months.

The Recommended Dietary Allowances (RDAs) for infants tend to be based on the intake of normal, thriving infants, and only a few nutrient recommendations are based on balance studies. Nutrients are present in commercial formulae in amounts which meet the RDA's. Consequently there are significant differences between the nutrient content of breast milk and comparative amounts of the formula milks. Alterations are made to the ratios of the macronutrients, predominant types of protein, and the solute load. Iron is supplied in much larger quantities in formula milks due to its lower availability in formulae compared to breast milk (*see Table 6.3*).

Types of cows' milk

Due to the high solute load and increased risk of hypertonic dehydration related to cows' milk, it is not advisable for an infant under the age of 4 – 6 months to receive unmodified cows' milk in any form. In cases where financial constraints do not allow for the purchase of infant formulae, *diluted* cows' milk may be given for the first 4 months of feeding. This necessitates supplementation with 35 mg of vitamin C and 400 IU of vitamin D. The former can be obtained from vitamin C-rich fruit juices (such as orange or guava), which should initially be diluted.

Types of full cream milk

Fresh milk: Pasteurized milk should be boiled before use. UHT or sterilized milk may be diluted from the container. A ratio of 2 parts milk to 1 part boiled, cooled water is an appropriate dilution, 5 ml sugar should be added for every 100 ml diluted milk.

Evaporated milk (Ideal®, Carnation®): The volume of evaporated milk has been reduced to half that of fresh cows' milk by means of heat treatment. It should be appropriately diluted (1 part water : 1 part milk) before it can be used similarly to fresh milk, as above.

Milk powders (Nespray®, Klim®, Farmer's Pride®): This is cows' milk from which practically all the water has been removed. To reconstitute the milk, 1 part powder is mixed with 3 parts boiled, cooled water (volume for volume). The reconstituted milk is then used as specified for fresh cows' milk, above.

Types of reduced fat and skim milk

These are available as fresh, evaporated, or powdered milks. These milks have a high protein and mineral content and the essential fatty acid levels are low. They should therefore not be used as a milk feed for children under the age of 12 months.

Formulations which are unsuitable for infants and children

A number of products are available which are *totally* unsuitable for infant feeding. Mothers *must* be made aware of these, and of the potential dangers of giving them to their children. The products can be categorized as follows:

Primary dairy blends (Numel®): Although these are manufactured solely from milk, their energy, vitamin, and mineral content make them unsuitable as substitutes for breast milk. These products should not be confused with imitation milk blends.

Imitation milk blends (Carnation®, Make-a-litre®, Sungold®, and others): These blends are composed of milk solids and creamers. They contain approximately half the protein and calcium found in cows' milk. The vitamin, mineral, and energy content of these products are unsuitable for young children.

Creamers (Coffee-mate®, Cremora®, Ellis Brown®, Gold Cross®, and others): These are primarily composed of corn syrup and vegetable fat, and contain *no* milk solids. They should therefore *never* be used for drinking or as a supplement, particularly for children.

Condensed milk (Gold Cross®, Gold Medal®, and Nestlé®): This is cows' milk which has been heat treated to remove much of the moisture. Large amounts of sugar are then added to the milk, making it unsuitable for infant feeding.

Primary dairy blends, imitation milk blends, and condensed milk are unsuitable substitutes for breast milk. Creamers should never be used for drinking as a substitute for milk.

South African Code of Ethics for the Marketing of Breast Milk Substitutes

South Africa endorses the Code of Ethics accepted by the WHO Assembly in 1981 which applies to developed and developing countries. The aim of the South African Code is to control the promotion of artificial feeds, not to ban the sale or use of infant feeds. Its essence is to protect children from the abuse or misuse of such products. All health personnel, especially those involved with infant nutrition, should be familiar with the Code.

The aim of the Code is to contribute to the provision of safe and adequate nutrition for infants by the protection and promotion of breast-feeding, and to ensure the proper use of artificial feeds.

The scope of the Code applies to infant formulae; other milk products, foods, and beverages; feeding bottles and teats.

Principles of the Code:
◆ There should be no advertising or other form of promotion to the general public of products within the scope of the Code.
◆ Manufacturers and distributors should not provide free samples or gifts of products to the public.
◆ There should not be any contact between the marketing personnel and mothers.
◆ There should be no promotion to induce sales directly to the consumer at retail level, such as special displays, discount coupons, premiums, special sales, loss-leaders, or tie-in sales for the products.

◆ Neither the container nor the label should have pictures of infants or text which may idealize the use of infant formulae.
◆ No health care facility should be used for the promotion or advertisement of infant formulae or other products within the Code.
◆ No financial or material inducement should be offered to health workers or marketing personnel for the promotion of the products.

Specialized requirements for certain infants

Allergic infants seldom develop an allergy to breast milk. Allergic reactions to certain artificial feeds are, however, more common. If the child is diagnosed as being truly allergic and breast milk is unsuitable, a substitute feed has to be found. A number of **hypoallergenic foods** are available. These are Nutramigen®, and soya protein-based feeds (Infasoy®, Isomil®). Goats' milk feeds, suitable for certain infants, can also be obtained.

Inborn digestive or metabolic errors

Infants suffering from congenital or acquired deficiency of digestive or cellular enzymes require modified feeds from which the offending substrate has been removed. This is because these substances hinder normal catabolic processes; and therefore the particular substrate, and frequently its precursors, accumulate to toxic levels. High concentrations of these metabolites may result in osmotic/fermentative diarrhoea in the case of defective digestive enzymes. Intracellularly, the high levels of metabolic precursors interfere with other cellular metabolic processes, retarding growth. Minor alternative pathways may begin to operate, resulting in the formation of potentially lethal metabolites. These may also interfere with normal maturation of certain tissues or result in pathological tissue changes.

Absolute or relative lactase deficiency

Lactase deficiency is by far the most common enzyme deficiency. Congenital lactase deficiency of the neonate is extremely rare. However, a lack of lactase is frequently encountered when there is damage to the intestinal brush border, such as in protein-energy malnutrition (PEM). Improvement of nutritional status and substrate challenge

Table 6.3 Nutrient composition of breast milk, compared with infant formulae and other milks available in South Africa

Content per 100 ml	Breast milk	Pre Nan	S26 Preemie	Alfaré	Nan	S26	Similac PM60/40	Isomil	SMA	Infasoy	Pelargon	AL 110
Energy kJ	280	293	340	273	281	281	280	280	274	281	285	281
Cal	67	70	81	65	67	67	67	67	65	67	68	67
Protein g	1.2	2.0	2.0	2.2	1.5	1.5	1.5	1.8	1.5	2.5	2.0	1.9
CHO g	7.4	7.9	8.6	7.0	7.6	7.2	7.3	6.9	7.2	8.0	8.1	7.4
Fat g	3.6	3.4	4.4	3.3	3.4	3.6	3.8	3.6	3.5	2.8	3.1	3.3
Ca mg	35.0	70.0	80.0	54.0	42.0	42.0	40.0	70.0	46.0	115.0	70.5	60.0
P mg	15.0	45.0	45.0	34.0	21.0	28.0	20.0	50.0	36.0	65.0	55.0	40.0
Mg mg	2.8	8.0	7.0	8.0	4.5	4.5	4.2	5.0	4.0	9.4	6.3	6.7
K mg	60.0	75.0	75.0	82.00	66.0	56.0	58.0	77.0	62.0	100.0	88.8	80.0
Na mg	15.0	26.0	32.0	39.0	16.0	15.0	16.0	32.0	18.0	32.0	29.6	23.0
Cl mg	43.0	40.0	53.0	68.0	46.0	40.0	40.0	59.0	42.0	80.0	66.3	49.0
Fe mg	0.08	1.1	0.07	0.04	0.04	0.05	1.0	1.2	1.2	1.2	0.8	0.8
Cu mg	0.04	0.06	0.07	0.04	0.04	0.05	0.06	0.05	0.047	0.058	0.04	0.04
I µg	7.0	7.0	8.3	3.3	3.4	6.0	4.1	10.0	3.4	6.9	3.4	3.4
Mn µg	1.5	4.8	6.0	4.6	4.8	10.0	3.4	20.0	15.0	10.0	4.8	4.7
Zn mg	0.3	0.53	0.8	0.5	0.5	0.5	0.5	0.05	0.5	0.5	0.5	0.5
Renal SL (mOsms/l)	82	22	128	145	96	92	93	126	95	162	134	123
Ca:P	2.3	1.6	2.0	1.6	2.0	1.5	2.0	1.4	1.28	1.77	1.28	1.4
Vit.A IU	200	10	240	195	201	200	200	200	200	230	205	200
Vit.D IU	32.4	70	48	39	40	40	40	40	40	48	41	40
Vit.E IU	0.52	1.4	1.5	0.8	0.8	0.95	1.7	1.7	0.95	1.08	0.8	0.8
Vit.K IU	1.5	8.4	7.0	5.0	5.5	5.5	5.5	10.0	5.5	6.6	5.6	5.5
Vit.C mg	3.8	11.0	7.0	5.0	5.4	5.5	5.5	5.5	5.5	6.6	5.5	5.4
Thiamin mg	0.01	0.04	0.08	0.04	0.04	0.07	0.065	0.04	0.067	0.04	0.04	0.04
Ribofl. mg	0.03	0.1	0.13	0.09	0.1	0.1	0.1	0.06	0.1	0.12	0.1	0.09
Niacin mg	0.23	0.7	1.2	0.5	0.5	0.5	0.7	0.9	0.5	0.61	0.5	0.5
Biotin µg	0.76	1.6	1.8	1.4	1.5	1.5	3.0	0.03	1.5	1.7	1.6	1.5
Folacin µg	5.2	42.0	48.0	6.0	6.0	5.0	10.0	10.0	5.0	6.0	6.2	6.0
Pantothenic acid µg	0.26	0.31	0.36	0.3	0.3	0.21	0.3	0.5	0.21	0.24	0.3	0.3
Vit.B6 mg	0.00	0.06	0.05	0.05	0.05	0.04	0.04	0.04	0.042	0.48	0.06	0.05
Vit.B12 µg	0.01	0.16	0.2	0.1	0.15	0.13	0.15	0.3	0.13	0.12	0.16	0.15
Choline mg	8.9	5.3	12.7	5.0	3.0		8.0	0.01	≥ 39.0	4.7	5.1	5.0
Inositol mg	17.5	3.1	3.2	3.0		3.0	16.5				3.1	3.0

Table 6.3 Nutrient composition of breast milk, compared with infant formulae and other milks available in South Africa (continued)

Content per 100 ml		Breast milk	Cows' milk	Nespray	Nutramigen	Portagen	Lactogen 1	Lactogen 2	S26 Infagro
Energy	kJ	280	276	275	281	281	281	280	281
	Cal	67	66	66	67	67	67	67	67
Protein	g	1.2	3.5	3.36	1.9	2.4	1.69	3.1	2.5
CHO	g	7.4	4.9	4.9	8.8	7.8	7.4	7.5	8.0
Fat	g	3.6	3.7	3.64	2.6	3.2	3.4	2.8	2.8
Ca	mg	35.0	117.0	121.0	82.5	63.4	61.0	112.0	115.0
P	mg	15.0	98.0	98.0	48.9	47.6	49.0	90.0	65.0
Mg	mg	2.8	11.0	11.0	7.3	13.7	5.5	10.0	9.4
K	mg	60.0	137.0	156.0	68.0	84.5	77.0	141.0	100.0
Na	mg	15.0	51.0	46.0	31.3	31.7	27.0	46.0	32.0
Cl	mg	43.0	103.0	103.0	46.9	58.1	59.0	106.0	80.0
Fe	mg	0.08	0.05	0.8	1.3	1.3	0.8	1.2	1.2
Cu	mg	0.04	0.03	0.03	0.06	0.0967	0.04	0.04	0.058
I	µg	7.0	4.7	4.7	4.7	4.8	3.5	3.3	6.9
Mn	µg	1.5	4.0	4.0	104.1	200.0	4.7	4.6	10.0
Zn	µg	0.3	0.35	0.35	0.4	0.08	0.5	0.5	0.5
Renal SL	(mOsms/l)	82	209	223	133	145	116	210	162
Ca:P		2.3	1.3	1.23	1.3	1.3	1.2	1.2	1.77
Vit A	IU	200	103	195	167	528	200	200	230
Vit D	IU	32.4	1.4	52.0	42	53	40	41	48
Vit E	IU	0.52	0.06	0.06	1.1	2.1	0.8	0.8	1.08
Vit K	IU	1.5	6.0	6.0			5.5	5.5	6.6
Vit C	mg	3.8	1.1	1.1	5.4	5.5	5.4	5.4	6.6
Thiamin	mg	0.016	0.04	0.028	0.052	0.1	0.04	0.04	0.081
Riboff.	mg	0.031	0.18	0.18	0.062	0.13	0.09	0.09	0.12
Niacin	mg	0.23	0.09	0.09	0.833	1.4	0.5	0.5	0.61
Biotin	µg	0.76	2.0	2.0	5.36	5.1	1.5	1.4	1.7
Folacin	µg	5.2	4.0	4.0	10.4	10.6	6.0	5.9	6.0
Pantothenic acid	µg	0.26	0.35	0.28	0.312	0.68	0.3	0.3	0.24
Vit B6	mg	0.006	0.064	0.064	0.042	0.138	0.05	0.4	0.048
Vit B12	µg	0.01	0.4	0.24	0.2	0.2	0.15	0.18	0.12
Choline	mg	8.9	13.0	13.0	8.9	8.7	5.1	5.1	4.7
Inositol	mg	17.5	13.0	13.0	3.149	trace	3.1	3.0	-

stimulate the synthesis of lactase. A disaccharide-free feed (AL 110®) is available for cases of severe fermentative diarrhoea where lactase is absent or deficient. Soya-based products are also suitable, as they do not contain lactose.

Lipase deficiency

In cases of fat malabsorption due to lipase deficiency, e.g., cystic fibrosis, Portagen® — which contains mainly medium chain triglycerides — is available. These do not require intestinal hydrolysis and micelle formation for absorption.

Rarer matabolic abnormalities

Special feeds for the rarer types of metabolic abnormalities such as phenylketonuria, galactosaemia, and hypercalcaemia are not freely available in South Africa. They are, however, obtainable at relatively short notice from overseas, where the incidence of these conditions is significantly higher. These diseases require highly specialized dietary modification, and the cost of the special feeds is exorbitant.

Weaning

The first year of life is characterized by a significant growth and development spurt. The infant has normally trebled its birth weight at the age of 12 months. The energy requirements of infants per kilogram of body weight are approximately two to three times those of adults. After about 6 months of age, the nutrient density of milk becomes insufficient to meet the infant's requirements. Additional nutrient sources are therefore necessary *(see Fig. 6.4)*. The reason is that the relatively small stomach of the infant cannot contain the amount of milk required for normal growth and development. At this stage the infant is also interested in new experiences, oral muscles have developed, and teeth are erupting. Weaning therefore provides the ideal situation in which to introduce the child to new textures, tastes, and flavours. Delaying the introduction of new foods may result in difficulties, as the child becomes too used to the consistency and texture of a liquid feed. This could also cause a lag in growth and development, as the child may not receive its full nutrient requirements. The introduction of solid foods before 4 months is unnecessary and may create problems,

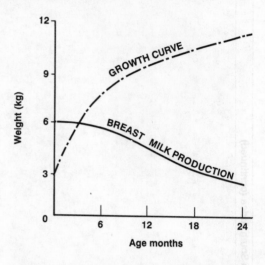

Fig. 6.4   Breast milk production cannot meet the demands of the rapidly growing infant during the second half of the first year.

such as supplanting the extremely important milk feed and increasing the possibility of food-linked allergies.

Custom and fashion also play an important role in a mother's decision as to when weaning should be commenced. In many traditional societies there are relatively strict norms which dictate when a new phase in the child's rearing may be initiated. Child health services need to dovetail the advice and general health education given to the mother with the child's own phase of growth and development and with cultural norms for the society concerned. Weight – height charts provide the best monitoring guide.

Weaning does not mean the sudden complete substitution of breast milk with solid foods. Weaning entails maintenance of breast-feeding along with the gradual introduction of suitable solid foods which form part of the daily diet of the family. Breast milk still makes up a major part of the infant's diet. The composition of breast milk does not change substantially, and one third of the infant's protein needs can still be obtained from breast milk during the second year of life. Underprivileged mothers should be encouraged to breast-feed their babies for as long as possible, for 2 years or more. Supplementation of the child's diet with suitable weaning foods is, however, imperative. This will lower the chances of the child developing potentially lethal conditions such as gastroenteritis and malnutrition.

Special, sophisticated, commercially prepared infant foods are expensive and unnecessary. All communities are exposed to clever advertising, and the mother should be made aware that these foods are not essential for her infant. The child may develop a preference for these items, and may later refuse the normal family fare. Such foods may be convenient and ready for use, but in under-privileged communities their consumption may compromise the infant's food intake and nutri-tional status. Furthermore, the use of commer-cially prepared foods may create dependence at the cost of self-reliance, and can therefore be harmful.

The infant should be introduced to the new foods slowly, and a regular routine instituted. In-itially very small amounts (5 ml) should be of-fered. The solids are mixed with milk to a consistency between that of a semi-fluid and a purée. The infant has to learn to use the tongue to move the food to the back of the mouth, and to accept new tastes and textures. The amount is gradually increased to approximately 125 ml within 2 months. Once the baby starts chewing, at 6 or 7 months of age, foods need only be mashed, and later finely chopped. When the child begins to handle food, small pieces (finger foods) should be offered, such as strips of bread, fruit, and vegeta-bles.

Cereals contribute carbohydrate and other nu-trients to the diet. They are usually the first solid foods introduced to the infant, as they can be mixed with milk, and the child slowly becomes accustomed to the different texture of more solid food. The normal cereal staple used by the family, such as maize porridge, is quite suitable. It is of the utmost importance that the mother understands that the child needs *more* than just cereal, and that breast-feeding should continue.

To increase the protein quantity and quality of the cereal feed, skim milk powder can be mixed into the porridge — 25 ml of powder per 250 ml is an acceptable proportion. Other good protein sources include: dried beans (cooked and mashed); peanuts, lentils, dried peas or dhal (soaked and the skins removed before cooking).

Cooked vegetables (pumpkin, potatoes, sweet potatoes, *amadumbe*, the various spinach types,

imfino, and carrots) can be fed to the child, initially as a strained purée. Later these can be given mashed, either mixed with the cereal or separately. Beetroot is also suitable, but to avoid anxiety the mother must be told that it will change the colour of the child's stools. Strongly flavoured vegeta-bles (cabbage, turnips, onions) are best introduced later. Locally-available fresh, ripe, fruit (banana, pawpaw, guava, orange segments, apple, pear, peach) *raw*, peeled, and mashed or grated, will provide important sources of vitamins, especially vitamin C. Fruit or vegetables in which the edible part is bright green, orange, or yellow are excellent sources of carotene, the precursor of vitamin A. Sugar and salt should preferably not be added, in order to allow the child to become familiar with the natural taste of the food.

Other foods which follow in the infant's diet are eggs, meat, fish and cheese. Fat in one or other form provides a concentrated source of energy, and some also contribute fat-soluble vitamins and essential fatty acids. Fat should be incorporated as a spread on bread, or stirred into the staple cereal porridge.

Margarine, oil, butter, or animal fat added to a meal substantially increases the energy value: two teaspoons (10 g) added to a 65 ml meal for a 2-year-old will increase the energy value by ap-proximately 33%.

Fried foods are difficult to digest and are not suitable for the small child. Too much fat will delay the emptying time of the stomach and so interfere with normal appetite. An excessive in-take of fat and too much refined carbohydrate such as sugar and very sweet foods could be the direct cause of obesity. Highly spiced foods may lead to gastric discomfort and indigestion. These should only be introduced when the child has been ex-posed to the simply prepared foods familiar to the family. Eventually the child will be accustomed to eating the full range of dishes which comprise the regular family diet.

One of the important causes of protein-energy malnutrition is the fact that a small child cannot consume enough of the traditional staple cereal diet to provide his energy, protein, and other nu-trient requirements. This problem can be over-come to an extent by increasing the frequency of feeds and the addition of fat.

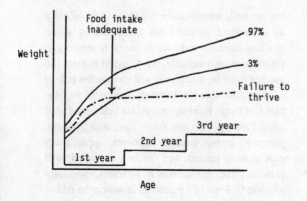

Fig 6.5   Inadequate food and failure to thrive

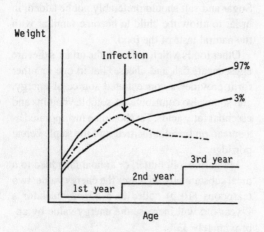

Fig 6.6   Infection and failure to thrive associated with inadequate food intake

After iron stores are depleted (within 4–6 months of birth), it will be necessary to add a source of iron to the child's diet. Mothers should be encouraged to include adequate quantities of iron-rich foods in the weaning diet. These include such items as liver, meat, egg yolks, dried beans and peas, as well as green leafy vegetables.

Assessment: Road-to-Health Chart

Regular monitoring of the child's weight plays an important role in ensuring optimal health and nutritional status. The weight is plotted on a Road-to-Health Chart *(see Chapter 4, Fig. 4.2)*. The exact position of the child's weight on the graph is less important than whether the line plotted follows the same general direction as the curves

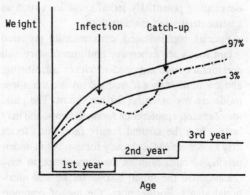

Fig 6.7   Infection and adequate food intake associated with catch-up growth

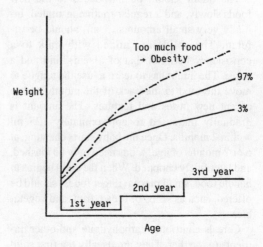

Fig 6.8   Too much food, resulting in obesity

on the growth chart. Some examples of possible abnormal growth responses are illustrated in *Figs 6.5–6.8*.

If the infant has been solely breast-fed, it is likely that growth and development will be within the normal range. An infant who has been given artificial feeds is at a much higher risk of becoming malnourished and/or sick, due to reasons already discussed. This will be easily detected from the growth chart. The weaning period may be a particularly hazardous one for the infant if milk feeds are not continued. Again, potential problems may be elucidated by plotting the weight regularly.

The growth chart should not be seen as a tool to be used solely by health personnel. It is important that the mother understands what the lines on the card represent. It can become a valuable teaching aid during health and nutrition education.

Feeding the toddler

At the age of one year the child's first growth spurt is tapering off. In line with this, the total amount of food required per kilogram of body weight is less than that for an infant or school child. This is demonstrated by a smaller appetite in the well-nourished child whose weight–height development pattern stays within the accepted norms. Regular weight and height assessment remains an important aspect of the child's health care routine.

The eating behaviour of healthy toddlers shows certain specific tendencies. They begin to act independently and may show distinctive food preferences or dislikes. Occasional fluctuations in appetite or a sudden dislike for a previously favourite food is not unusual. Toddlers are easily distracted from a meal, or may be so involved in a game that a mealtime is of no consequence. They are also well aware that food and food-related behaviour can be used to manipulate others to their own advantage.

In most societies toddlers participate in the family meal. They may be expected to begin to handle utensils such as a spoon, drink from a cup, and start to behave in accordance with societal norms for eating. In the ideal family situation where the toddler is in the care of a parent, grandparent, or other responsible member of the extended family, these behaviour changes are handled without much trauma. However, where the mother has returned to work and is away from home for a long period each day, the child may be left with a relative, neighbour, older sibling, or in a day-care centre. There is then a particular danger that nutritional adequacy will not be maintained. In underprivileged communities this may well be the beginning of serious malnutrition problems, as lack of finances and limited knowledge of nutrition can aggravate the situation. Once the child's nutritional status is compromised, the immune mechanisms are negatively affected and a subsequent infection may precipitate severe states of malnutrition.

The toddler still cannot handle large quantities of food. So although the appetite is significantly reduced, between-meal feeds are extremely important. Even though the total amount of food required has decreased, the proportional amount of quality protein, calcium, and other vitamins and minerals needed by the toddler remain a priority. If breast-feeding can be maintained well into the second year of life, the need for these nutrients is partly met. A judicious selection of supplementary foods must be made from those consumed by the family to ensure nutritional adequacy. If breast-feeding cannot be maintained, *real* milk (fresh, powdered, soured, evaporated, UHT, or sterilized) remains the supplement of choice for the toddler.

Imitation milk blends and creamers should under *no* circumstances be used for children.

This is particularly important if the normal family diet is primarily a cereal one. The addition of relatively small amounts of legumes, peanuts or peanut butter, meat, poultry, fish, eggs, or soya protein products (TVP), to the staple cereal will significantly improve the protein quality of the diet.

In many Asian and African countries the use of traditional foods in the diet of young children — which in the past has been out of favour — has recently received much attention. Slightly fermented foods such as soured milk, yoghurt, and soured cereal porridges have a lower pH, which reduces the chances of bacterial growth and subsequent contamination. The lower pH also serves to accelerate hydrolysis of starches and disaccharides, and in the case of milk-based foods results in a finer protein coagulate which is easier to digest.

A major difficulty in maintaining adequate nutrition in the toddler is the problem of the low nutrient density of the bulky cereal staple. In order to make the starch granules available for enzymatic hydrolysis, the milled cereal has to absorb water. Cooking accelerates the fluid absorption process and makes the end product palatable. Cereals contribute carbohydrate and considerable amounts of protein to the diet. The latter can be supplemented by relatively small amounts of milk or legumes, to provide quality protein for growth. However, the viscous porridge or cooked granular dish is bulky. A young child cannot physically cope with the amount required to maintain adequate nutritional status and promote growth.

Traditional food preparation methods such as germination of seeds, wherein amylases are produced which hydrolyse polysaccharides into shorter dextrin chains, are being used in India, Latin-America, and Africa. During the rapid hydrolysis, the water in the viscous cooked cereal is released, and the cooked cereal liquifies rapidly without increasing in original volume. Thick cooked cereal mixtures have to have water added to make them into a gruel suitable for young children, which at the same time dilutes the nutrient density. In contrast, the addition of ground germinated seeds to cooked cereal results in a liquid consistency without additional fluid. In southern Africa the traditional use of germinated sorghum, millet, and wheat needs to be investigated.

Goal achievement

The WHO definition of health — 'a state of complete physical, mental, and social health, and not merely the absence of disease' — is particularly pertinent in relation to optimal nutrition. Nutrition has a direct bearing on physical growth and development, on mental ability, and on the child's socialization and functioning in society. A child who is undernourished does not have the interest or the energy to interact with the environment or her parents in a manner which would promote optimal socialization or development.

Growth must still be monitored regularly, using a Road-to-Health Chart. Growth may be seen as an indirect means of assessing mental and social health. However, it is imperative that other signs of development also be used. The child must be seen in entirety and treated as a 'small person' in his own right.

Priorities in the feeding of infants and toddlers

The emphasis on primary health care and expansion of the community-centred, hospital-based health scheme in South Africa puts a number of nutrition-related topics which affect developing communities into the spotlight. These need to be addressed, irrespective of the size of the community, at the national as well as the local level.

♦ Development of a co-ordinated, responsible approach to nutrition education between the public and the private sectors. Too many different and confusing messages are being received by consumers.

Applicable global research data must be incorporated. Planning should be done in co-operation with local communities. The emphasis must be placed on addressing local needs in the light of local food practices, production, and potential.

♦ Developing a programme to create an awareness of the importance of adequate nutrition for vulnerable groups. This must address leaders and decision-makers in all communities, at all levels of society.

♦ Involvement of the media to communicate nutrition information in a responsible manner. Programmes must be based on research data and not on information supplied by self-proclaimed nutrition experts.

♦ Development of a training programme for 'grass roots' nutrition educators nominated by communities.

♦ Development and scientific evaluation of suitable 'weaning mixtures' and foods acceptable to local communities.

♦ A central data bank to evaluate and communicate information on local foods, eating patterns, and food preparation practices.

♦ Inclusion of a compulsory basic nutrition module in the training programme of all medical students, nurses, supplementary health professionals, teachers, social workers, and agricultural officers. This should create an awareness of the basic principles, and of the diversity and complexity involved in establishing and maintaining optimal nutrition in communities.

N. Nel
F.M. Ross

7

Nutritional disorders

Protein-energy malnutrition (PEM)

Historical background

Mention of starvation and nutritional disorders dates back as far as the sixteenth century. Wasted, emaciated, or marasmic infants had various clinical names attached to them — such as 'hypothrepsie' or 'dystrophy', according to the severity of the wasting of their body tissues. *Oedematous* forms were referred to as nutritional dystrophy, infantile pellagra, nutritional oedema, Mehlnährschaden, wet marasmus, and more recently kwashiorkor. The contradictions in terminology were rooted in regional differences, age of weaning, local foods, and the prevalence of infection.

In 1959 the various syndromes were brought together by Jelliffe under the all-embracing term of protein-calorie (energy) malnutrition (PEM), with the realization that protein and/or energy deficiency played a central role in their aetiology.

The wasted, non-oedematous forms of PEM, now generally referred to as marasmus, received extensive paediatric literature coverage in Europe and North America during the last century and first half of this century. By 1950 this type of PEM had disappeared from these regions, and had become a major problem in the Developing World. In the early 1900s paediatricians in Germany described Mehlnährschaden — an oedematous form of PEM that they were seeing — and in 1933 Cicely Williams drew attention to this form in Ghana, and named it kwashiorkor. The term means literally 'first-second' and refers to the sickness the older child develops when the next baby is born, or when the mother becomes pregnant again.

The children Williams described all had a history of an abnormal diet: they had been weaned onto maize porridge, low in protein content, and within 3–4 months began to sicken. This indicates well the circumstances in which PEM most commonly develops: poverty, or inability — for one reason or another — to give adequate protein and/or energy to children during the weaning period, from 6 months to 2 years.

After the Second World War, heightened interest in PEM followed a report by Brock and Autret (1952), who described kwashiorkor as 'the most serious and widespread nutritional disorder known to medical and nutritional science'. A classic monograph by Trowell *et al* (1954) dealt with all aspects of kwashiorkor. At that time it was known that high-protein foods (of both animal and plant origin), as opposed to low-protein cereal, prevented and cured kwashiorkor. There was, however, speculation as to whether it was the deficiency of protein itself, or the associated vitamins, minerals, or unknown factors within the protein food, that was responsible for the syndrome.

All sorts of treatment were recommended at that time, including 'hog's stomach' and vitamin B_1, although milk was the mainstay of dietary therapy. By 1956, research led to the finding that a vitamin-free formula of synthetic amino acids, glucose, and minerals could initiate recovery from kwashiorkor. These and other studies took the nutritional mystique out of the syndrome. We now know that deficiency of protein (as a source of amino acids), together with varying degrees of deficiency of energy, are responsible for the broad spectrum of syndromes now described as PEM (marasmus, kwashiorkor, marasmic-kwashiorkor, and nutritional dwarfism). Although there has been some controversy in the literature about the relative importance of protein and energy in the pathogenesis of PEM, both are obviously important, as is the quality of the protein.

Epidemiology

PEM characteristically occurs amongst pre-school children aged 6 months to 5 years. However, no age is immune, and juvenile and adult cases of PEM can occur as a result of certain environmental and nutritional circumstances, or disease (e.g.,

Table 7.1   Summary of energy and protein requirements

	Energy per day		Energy per kg/day		Proteins g/kg/day
	k cals	kJ	k cals	kJ	
0–3 months			120	500	2.4
3–5 months			115	480	1.9
6–8 months			110	460	1.6
9–11 months			105	440	1.4
1–3 years	1 360	5 700	101	424	1.2
4–6 years	1 830	7 600	91	382	1.0
7–9 years	2 190	9 200	78	326	0.9
Adult man	3 000	12 600	46	192	0.6
Adult woman	2 300	9 200	40	167	0.6

Note: k cals = kilocalories   kJ = kilojoules

intestinal malabsorption). Manifestations in older individuals are less frequent and clinically less obvious, because protein and energy requirements per kilogram mass are not as great as in childhood.

Important factors in the epidemiology of PEM: Poverty, Third World, developing communities, unemployment, societies in transition, migration, squatter communities, natural disasters (drought, famine, flood), war, infection, family breakdown, working mothers, and alcoholism.

PEM is found where food is scarce, and is particularly prevalent in the so-called developing countries or Third World. There is a high prevalence in all African countries, in India, South-East Asia, the Middle East, the Caribbean, and South and Central America.

In urban areas, PEM occurs largely in families of low socio-economic status and in broken homes. Here poverty, large numbers of children, and lack of education preclude the purchase of sufficient food — particularly the relatively expensive, high-protein foods. Cheap or refined carbohydrate foods tend to form the basis of the diet. The world-wide migration of people from rural to urban areas is aggravating the PEM problem enormously, and it affects large numbers of children in city squatter communities.

In rural areas in poor countries PEM is endemic. It increases in prevalence during periods of drought, famine, or other disaster, when cereal staples are often the only foods available. Lack or contamination of water promotes intestinal and other infection, and this in turn worsens nutritional status.

In both urban and rural areas, but particularly the former, the sociological phenomenon of the working mother has dietary implications for pre-school and primary school children. Many of them have only two meals a day, which prevents adequate growth and is a likely cause of PEM. Childcare facilities are often unavailable, inadequate, or spasmodic.

The prevalence of the individual syndromes of malnutrition varies in different communities and parts of the world. In a poor community, severe forms may affect 2–3% of the child population, with 10–60% suffering from milder forms. Age of weaning, availability of food, local or individual prejudices and customs, environmental and economic circumstances, and family stress are some of the more common factors which will collectively or individually determine prevalence and clinical picture. When the dietary intake of apparently healthy children is only marginally adequate, infection or other stress factors may precipitate PEM in epidemic proportions. Thus in well-nourished communities, morbidity and mortality from gastroenteritis, measles, or tuberculosis is negligible, but may be 20–50 times higher in poor communities.

Individual cases of PEM may occur whenever disease, surgery, or trauma interferes with the intake, absorption, or utilization of nutrients.

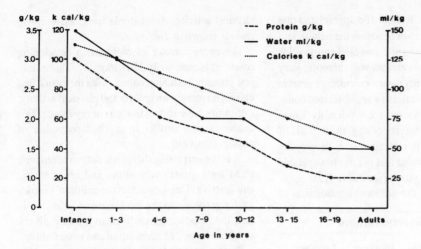

Fig. 7.1   Protein, calorie, and fluid requirements

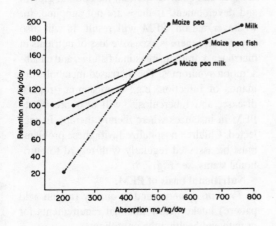

Fig. 7.2   Relationship of source of protein to nitrogen retention. At low levels of absorption (intake), nitrogen from a vegetable mixture is not as well retained as it is from a mixture which contains a small amount of animal protein. At higher levels of absorption, nitrogen retention of a vegetable mixture equals that of milk. Therefore when appetite is poor, animal protein or milk should be included in the diet

Causes of PEM

Intake of protein and/or energy below minimal requirements for growth and health is the basic cause of PEM. Infection plays a central role: in children with borderline nutrition, infection precipitates PEM. The high world-wide prevalence is likely to be aggravated by the current inflation of food prices. This is brought about by food produc-

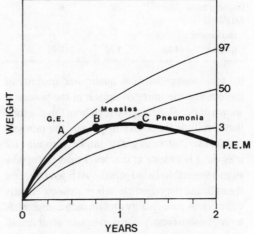

Fig. 7.3   Common infections in the development of protein-energy malnutrition (PEM)

tion and distribution failing to keep pace with population growth, and has forced a scientific appraisal and determination of the minimal requirements of protein, energy, and other nutrients for health. A summary of energy and protein requirements, as determined by expert committees of the WHO, is given in *Table 7.1*, and the relationship to water requirement in *Fig. 7.1*.

The requirements for children, particularly in the pre-school age group, are relatively greater per kg mass than those for adults. This is because of the demands for growth, and the younger a child, the faster his growth. It should be appreciated that the quality of a protein depends on the pattern and quantity of essential and non-essential amino acids that it contains. Requirements will therefore vary immensely with quality: when calculating protein requirements for a toddler in a sophisticated country, the doctor works on a considerably lower figure (e.g., 1–1.5 g/kg/day of egg, meat, milk, or fish protein) than his colleague in a developing country, where the basic diet is largely vegetable protein (1.5–2.0 g/kg/day) *(see Table 7.2).*

An illustration of the practical implications of

Table 7.2   Protein requirement

	Milk or egg protein	Mixed veg. protein	Single veg. protein
Chemical score	100	70	60
FAO/WHO requirement g/kg/day	1.19	1.70	2.08

the relationships between quality and quantity of protein and the nitrogen uptake in the tissues is shown in *Fig. 7.2.* It can be seen from this diagram that if milk is the source of protein, the nitrogen uptake at 200 mg/kg/day intake (protein 1.2 g/kg/day) is greater at that level than the uptake from a vegetable-based protein. At higher intakes, the milk and the vegetable-mix protein are equally effective. A poor-quality protein such as maize has a very unsatisfactory nitrogen uptake at all levels. It can therefore never meet growth and health requirements if used without supplementation.

All food contains energy, or calories, so there is no difference in energy requirement between vegetarian or animal protein diets. However, an adequate energy intake is essential for proper utilization of protein. Energy requirement is made up of three components: maintenance, growth, and

Table 7.3   Energy requirements

		kJ/kg/day
Maintenance	1.5 x BMR (220 kJ/kg)	330
Growth		20
Physical activity		80
Total		430

physical activity. An example for a one-year-old child is shown in *Table 7.3.*

The energy intake of children in developing countries is commonly 320 kJ/kg/day. This is only just enough for maintenance, with the result that there is no margin for growth and physical activity.

Studies have shown that an energy intake 30% below normal results in marked reduction of physical activity.

It is not surprising therefore, that children with PEM have growth retardation and are apathetic and inactive. This may affect the children's capacity for response to the environment, affecting in turn the response given to them by care-givers, resulting in lack of stimulation and educability.

Protein quality, total protein, and energy intake are thus all equally important for optimal growth and development. If these are not supplied, for whatever reason, PEM will result. It will also occur where there is excessive loss of nutrients in diarrhoea, vomiting, intestinal fistulae, and malabsorption syndromes. The increased metabolic demands of infection, e.g., septicaemia, tropical disease, and tuberculosis, will also precipitate PEM in instances where dietary therapy is neglected. Children hospitalized with these problems must be assessed regularly with regard to nutritional status *(see Fig. 7.3).*

Nutritional basis of PEM:

1. *Protein* quantity and/or quality (amino acid pattern) intake below minimal requirements for growth and health, with or without

Energy intake less than energy expenditure on muscle activity, heat production, growth, and other energy requirements.

2. Excessive loss of protein and energy in diarrhoea and acute and chronic disease.

Pathogenesis

Growth failure (nutritional dwarfing)

The first effect of PEM is on growth, as manifest by:

♦ a slowing or cessation in linear growth

♦ slowing or cessation in weight increase, or loss of weight (mass)

♦ decrease in mid-upper-arm circumference

♦ delayed bone maturation (age)

♦ normal or diminished weight/height ratio

♦ normal or diminished skinfold thickness.

The most useful indices are weight and height. International rather than local reference levels should be used in assessment of growth performance, because the former are stable, whereas in developing areas, secular increase or decrease in weight and height occurs with changing environmental circumstances.

Patterns of growth failure vary considerably. There may be *acute loss* due to sudden restriction of energy, or to acute infection or diarrhoea. Here there will be diminished weight/height ratio. At the other extreme, *chronic shortage* of protein and/or energy leads to failure of weight and height gain, with little or no change in weight to height ratio. Other parameters such as mid-upper-arm circumference (MUAC), skinfold thickness, and bone age maturation are useful in assessment of growth when age is not known. Eruption of deciduous teeth may be delayed slightly in PEM, but there is much less effect than that occurring in height, weight, and bone age.

Body composition

There is a profound change in body composition. This involves the amount and distribution of body water, body fat, minerals, trace elements, and total body protein, particularly muscle wasting.

Total body water (TBW): With cessation or slowing of growth, there is a gradual increase of TBW as a percentage of body weight *(see Fig 7.4)*. This is mainly due to the disappearance of fat stores, and wasting of muscle and other tissues. There is an inverse relationship between being underweight and total body water content. Thus children with marasmus who exhibit the most tissue wasting have the highest TBW. The high body water content of children with PEM resembles that of newborn infants. The children are therefore not only small for their age, but have the body water composition of much younger children. Associated with an increase of TBW is a proportionate rise in extra-cellular fluid (ECF). Children with oedema have more water in the extracellular space than those without oedema. On recovery, some of the excess ECF is taken up into the cells, and some is lost by diuresis, causing an initial loss of weight.

Potassium: Total body potassium is severely reduced in PEM. In kwashiorkor it is approxi-

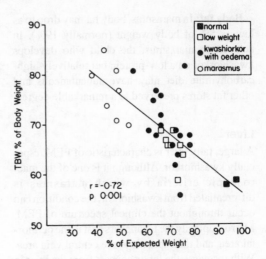

Fig. 7.4 Total body water (TBW) has a direct relationship to expected weight. If weight is below 80% expected weight (approximately 3rd percentile) it is highly likely that body composition will be abnormal

mately 31 mEq/kg and in marasmus 39 mEq/kg (normal = 45–55 mEq/kg). The loss is due to wasting of lean tissue and loss in diarrhoeal stools. The metabolic effects are: promotion of oedema because of reciprocal sodium retention, hypotonia of muscles, diminished insulin secretion, and renal function disturbance. Serum potassium concentration may or may not reflect the overall potassium deficiency.

Other minerals: There is some evidence of a magnesium deficiency in PEM, and autopsy studies have shown diminished total body calcium and phosphorus. Iron deficiency can occur as in any other condition.

Trace elements: There is limited evidence that zinc deficiency occurs in PEM, and aggravates ulcerative skin lesions. Zinc supplementation improves these, and leads to better retention of nitrogen during recovery. New information is appearing on vanadium, deficiency of which may stimulate the sodium pump and so promote oedema.

Total body protein: This is severely reduced in PEM. In particular, non-collagen protein is affected. Collagen protein is affected to a very limited extent. Muscle mass is greatly diminished, and may be only 30% of normal mass for age.

Body fat: In marasmus, body fat may drop to as low as 5% of body weight (normally 19%). In contrast to marasmus, the child who develops kwashiorkor on a low-protein but relatively high-carbohydrate diet may have subcutaneous and other fat stores preserved to a remarkable degree.

Liver

A large, fatty liver is characteristic of PEM, especially kwashiorkor. Although it is one of the macroscopic criteria by which marasmus is differentiated from kwashiorkor, the condition can occur throughout the clinical spectrum of PEM. Microscopically the fat appears first in the periportal area, and then spreads to the central vein area. With recovery, the fat disappears from the liver in about three weeks, and follow-up biopsies have failed to reveal any damage. The lipid that accumulates is triglyceride, and it has a similar fatty acid pattern to adipose tissue. Plasma lipids — particularly cholesterol, triglycerides, and phospholipids — are usually low in kwashiorkor and low to normal in marasmus. Free fatty acids (FFA) are raised in both conditions.

It seems likely that the fatty liver results from a combination of increased flux of fatty acids from adipose tissue, with decreased hepatic synthesis of beta-lipoproteins, which normally transport triglycerides from the liver. On treatment, plasma triglycerides and cholesterol rise dramatically.

Pancreas

Macroscopically, there is no striking abnormality; histologically, there is atrophy of the acinar cells, but not of the islet tissue. Exocrine secretion is depressed, but recovers within the first few days of treatment.

From the endocrine point of view, various patterns of immunoreactive insulin (IRI) have been noted in marasmus and kwashiorkor. After oral glucose, IRI is abnormally low in every patient with kwashiorkor, and in most with marasmus. After intravenous glucose, normal insulin responses are sometimes seen, presumably associated with the greater glycaemic stimulus. In both groups there is a great improvement after 3–6 weeks of therapy, and 2–10 months later insulin levels are within normal limits. A high potassium intake has a stimulating effect on early insulin

release in kwashiorkor, and chromium may also be important in this respect.

Glucose tolerance is impaired in kwashiorkor, and is normal or impaired in marasmus due to the above. Poor utilization of glucose by peripheral tissues may be another factor accounting for impaired glucose tolerance. The occurrence of hypoglycaemia in some cases has a complex aetiology, possibly related to deficiency of glucagon or diminished lean tissue, e.g., muscle, which in turn means lessened stores of glycogen.

Gastrointestinal tract

Diarrhoea is a major problem in PEM, so it is not surprising that there are profound structural and functional changes. Macroscopically, the bowel is atrophic throughout its length, and microscopically particularly in the duodenal, jejunal, and colonic sections. The mucosal changes range from almost normal to severe villus atrophy, with only convolutions or ridges being seen. On light microscopy, the brush border of the mucosal cells may be abnormal, and there is a lymphocyte and plasma cell infiltrate in the mucosa and submucosa.

On electron microscopy, there are gross epithelial cell changes, with a sparse brush border and shortened microvilli. The nuclei are irregular, and there is disorganization of the mitochondria and cytoplasmic organelles. The disaccharide enzymes are frequently diminished, especially lactase, and this may be related to the mucosal atrophy. Marked improvement of the mucosal histology and of the enzyme levels occurs with dietary therapy, though in a few children, lactase deficiency may become permanent.

The functional effects of the above changes are manifest in lactose intolerance and, in some cases, sucrose and glucose intolerance. With regard to protein absorption, there is little effect, except in cases with severe diarrhoea. Fat malabsorption does occur however, and lasts for a short while after treatment has commenced. It is due to low pancreatic lipase levels, reduced transit time, impaired micellar solubilization of lipids, and decreased conjugated bile acids. Infection, e.g., with *Giardia lamblia*, may be important in producing malabsorption (*also see Chapter 11, Gastrointestinal Disorders*).

The pathogenesis of the diarrhoea of PEM has, therefore, several factors, of which the following seem important:

◆ Enteric infections with pathogens, e.g., salmonellae, shigellae, *E. coli, E. histolytica, Giardia lamblia,* and viruses, e.g., rotavirus, intestinal moniliasis, have all been identified to a greater or lesser degree in different geographical situations.

◆ Contamination of the upper small bowel with bacteria is also thought to contribute.

◆ The grossly atrophied bowel mucosa must play an important part in the pathogenesis of diarrhoea, as in many instances, symptoms will resolve as soon as improved nutrition brings about restoration of mucosal surface and enzyme activity.

Endocrine system

In PEM the standard pathological description of the endocrine glands is that of atrophy, affecting particularly the pituitary and adrenal glands. However, recent studies have shown that endocrine function bears little relationship to the macroscopic appearance of the glands.

Pituitary: Human growth hormone levels are normal or supranormal in both marasmus and kwashiorkor. This fits in well with the observation of intense metabolism and growth once protein and energy are supplied in the diet. Thyroid-stimulating hormone (TSH) is elevated, and TSH response to synthetic thyrotrophin-releasing hormone is prompt, exaggerated, and sustained with a normal reserve. There is no deficiency of the antidiuretic hormone.

Adrenals: Plasma cortisol levels in kwashiorkor and marasmus are elevated. There is good functional reserve, as shown by prompt response to corticotrophin. Because of hypoalbuminaemia, there is decreased binding of cortisol and a higher 'free' content in the plasma. This may contribute to the clinical features of the 'moon facies', abnormal glucose tolerance, and oedema. Aldosterone secretion rates and plasma levels are also normal or elevated in PEM.

Thyroid: No evidence of thyroid deficiency or abnormality has been described in PEM. Certainly 'catch up' growth is dramatic when food is supplied.

The mechanism of growth retardation in PEM is therefore not related to pituitary, adrenal, or thyroid dysfunction, but rather to the lack of energy and/or protein intake.

Protein metabolism

A striking feature of PEM is hypoalbuminaemia, which is more marked in kwashiorkor, but also present to a lesser degree in many cases of marasmus.

Extensive investigations into protein metabolism in PEM have, in summary, shown the following:

Plasma proteins: On a low-protein diet the catabolism of albumin is reduced to about half the normal rate. Total albumin mass is reduced by about 50%, the extravascular pool being more depleted than the intravascular pool. The albumin synthesis rate is reduced when dietary deficiency occurs, and rises immediately when the diet is corrected. It appears to be controlled by the rate of amino acid supply, particularly the branched-chain amino acids.

The metabolism of the gamma globulins and immunoglobulins is quite different. Synthesis and turnover are unaffected, and may even be increased in the presence of infection.

Total protein turnover: Synthesis and catabolism are greatly decreased in PEM, and there is increased re-utilization of ammonia from endogenous urea. The synthesis rate in muscle is decreased by 58%, but no decrease occurs in the liver. This supports the concept that muscle acts as a buffer in the adjustment of protein metabolism to deficiency in the diet. The skin may also act as a protein reserve, and re-utilization of amino acids in the liver is enhanced when protein supplies are short.

Nitrogen balance: Protein is adequately digested, even though pancreatic enzyme function is reduced. Absorption of nitrogen may be reduced from a normal rate of 90% to 70–80% of the intake. However, nitrogen retention is much more efficient in the child with PEM than in the well-nourished child, and again, full utilization is made of whatever protein is offered to a child with PEM.

Mechanism of oedema

The presence of oedema is a striking physical sign in kwashiorkor as opposed to marasmus *(see Classification, below)*. It is also a fact that a child with 'marasmus' can become oedematous overnight and thus change to having 'marasmic kwashiorkor', and vice versa.

The pathogenesis of the oedema is complex, but is closely related to total body potassium depletion (from diarrhoea) and reciprocal retention of sodium and water. It is aggravated by the low colloidal osmotic pressure of the plasma (hypoalbuminaemia), decreased cardiac output and glomerular filtration rate, infection, and anaemia. Deficiency of vanadium has recently been postulated as another possible cause of promotion of oedema. Hypersecretion of ADH and aldosterone has been put forward as a cause, but does not appear to be important in this respect. Certainly potassium supplements early in treatment, speed up resolution of oedema.

▶ **Summary of pathogenesis**

The current explanation of the characteristics of PEM is that energy intake, total nitrogen (protein) intake, and quality of protein (amino acid pattern) are all important in the pathogenesis of PEM. Severe energy shortage results in marasmus (wasting). A protein intake less than minimal requirements will result in hypoalbuminaemia and failure of growth, even in the presence of adequate energy intake. Where the protein from a sole source is lacking in an essential amino acid (N.B. all cereals lack lysine, and maize is deficient in lysine *and* tryptophan), failure of growth and hypoalbuminaemia will result. In the areas where PEM occurs, inevitably vitamin, mineral, and trace element deficiencies can complicate the basic syndromes to varying degrees, as does infection.

Golden and Rambath have recently hypothesized that all the serious features of kwashiorkor, e.g., oedema, fatty liver, infection, and mortality can be explained by excess free radicals. These act in a situation where protective factors are diminished, e.g., glutathione peroxidase, vitamins A and E, and zinc. While the theory is attractive as a possible mechanism of the pathological features of kwashiorkor, children still have to be short of protein and/or energy before their growth slows

and they become susceptible to the toxic effects of free radical excess.

Classification of PEM

There is a spectrum of clinical syndromes that fall under the umbrella term of protein-energy malnutrition, ranging from kwashiorkor to marasmus, and including pellagra. The criteria for distinguishing between them remain essentially clinical, and at the moment, the most widely-accepted classification is that sponsored by the Wellcome Trust in 1970 *(see Table 7.4)*. It is based on the presence or absence of oedema and the deficit of body weight.

Table 7.4   Protein-energy malnutrition Wellcome classification

Weight (percentage of standard*)	Oedema	
	Present	*Absent*
60–80	Kwashiorkor	Underweight
60	Marasmic kwashiorkor	Marasmus

* Standard — 50th percentile NCHS standards

It is recognized that there are exceptions, in that a child having all the clinical features of kwashiorkor (oedema, skin changes, etc.) may fall above the 80% standard weight; but the simplicity of this classification is its main merit. It also allows for international comparison. One disadvantage is that age must be known, and scales available. In the absence of these, the health worker must rely on clinical signs.

Pellagra, which has very similar clinical features to kwashiorkor, but which usually occurs above the age of six years, can also be regarded as a form of PEM. Although pellagra is specifically associated with deficiency of niacin, it must be appreciated that the precursor of niacin is the amino acid tryptophan, an essential amino acid.

Clinical features of PEM

Clinical presentation of PEM depends very much on the degree and duration of protein and/or energy deficiency, the age of the individual, previous nutritional status, and on modification produced by disease, and by possible associated vitamin, mineral, and trace element deficiencies.

Underweight (growth failure, nutritional dwarfing)

Of the four syndromes, the underweight child is the one that is the most common and important presentation of PEM, and the most frequently missed if the classification is not used.

It is inevitable that cessation or slowing of linear growth, failure to gain weight, or actual loss of weight are the first effects of a diet inadequate in protein and/or energy. In areas where marasmus and kwashiorkor are found, there are many children whose dietary deficiency has not been sufficiently severe to produce clinical disease or symptoms. These children are underweight and undersize, while at the same time they have relatively normal body proportions, e.g., weight/height ratios. Because of the latter, the diagnosis is frequently missed unless weight and height for age are charted. There are no specific physical stigmata, and the only biochemical abnormality may be a slightly reduced serum albumin concentration. Children with this type of mild PEM are very susceptible to the effects of infections such as gastroenteritis, respiratory disease, or infectious fevers, e.g., measles and tuberculosis.

It is essential that all health workers recognize these underweight or growth-retarded children: failure to appreciate the underlying presence of PEM in patients who present with a variety of ailments will lead to ineffective therapy, repeated hospital visits, and frequently a fatal outcome.

In the diagnosis of growth retardation due to PEM, any child who is below the 3rd percentile weight or height for age is suspect (80% expected weight or 90% expected height). Other causes of growth retardation should be excluded, e.g., chronic renal disease, malabsorption syndromes, endocrine abnormalities, metabolic disease, congenital abnormalities, and chronic infections. Of all the syndromes of PEM, the underweight child is the most important numerically, as well as from a medical and public health point of view. This fact can be best appreciated when it is recognized that the high morbidity and mortality rates of pre-school children in poor countries are invariably associated with a high prevalence of growth retardation. This can range from 10–60% or more of children 5 years and under in developing populations.

Kwashiorkor

This is a severe and characteristic form of PEM which occurs mainly after weaning from the breast or bottle. Its maximum prevalence is between 9 months and 2 years, but no age is immune. The diet is commonly devoid of milk or other high-protein food, and consists principally of refined carbohydrate, cereal, and/or vegetable foods. Presenting symptoms are mainly those of failure to thrive, oedema, anorexia, diarrhoea, skin and mucous membrane lesions, and misery or apathy.

On clinical examination the important features are:

Growth failure, as manifested by low body weight and decreased length for age. Oedema and excess subcutaneous fat from a high carbohydrate diet may give a deceptively chubby appearance.

Muscle wasting: This causes increasing weakness, resulting in an inability to run, walk, sit, or hold the head up.

Oedema appears first on the dorsum of the feet or over the lower tibia. It can be slight, or generalized and gross, depending on the state of hydration and the availability of salt and water in the diet. Ascites rarely occurs, and this is a distinguishing point in the differential diagnosis of renal, hepatic, and cardiac oedema.

Dermatoses: These are pellagroid in type, and characterized by pigmentation, desquamation, depigmentation, and ulceration. In gross cases their appearance is similar to a burn. The lesions are distributed in exposed and unexposed areas of skin, in contrast to pellagra, where lesions occur in exposed areas only. In toddlers the perineum and buttock areas are particularly affected. The mouth often shows reddening, with atrophied tongue papillae and fissuring at the corners (angular stomatitis). The hair is sparse, thin, easily pulled out, and in tropical regions changes its colour to red or grey. The eyes may reveal xerophthalmia, as there is frequently an associated vitamin A deficiency.

Mental and neurological changes: Apathy and irritability are always present. The children are constantly unhappy, and there is no play activity. A few children develop parkinsonian-like tremors ('kwashi shakes', Kahn's syndrome) which disappear after 2–3 weeks of treatment.

Other features frequently associated with kwashiorkor are a large, firm liver (due to fat infiltration); anaemia due to protein, iron, or folic acid deficiency; diarrhoea (stool weight 300 – 500 g/day); and infection of all kinds, particularly pneumonia, septicaemia and gastroenteritis. A less frequent finding is mild purpura due to low prothrombin and platelets. Diarrhoea is persistent and debilitating. Fluid levels are often seen on X-ray of the abdomen.

Atrophied bowel wall, invasion of small bowel by bacteria, and hypokalaemia may all contribute to small bowel dilatation and abdominal distension. Hypokalaemia may cause an ileus. Wasting of the thymolymphatic system is reflected in small tonsils, a depressed cell-mediated immunity (CMI), and an occasional inability to produce fresh antibody. Depression of CMI may encourage severe infection, in particular measles, tuberculosis, moniliasis, septicaemia (mostly Gram-negative), and herpes simplex. Herpes infection often disseminates, causing fits, hepatomegaly, purpura, pox-like herpes skin lesions, collapse, and death.

As the tuberculin test is often negative in the presence of active tuberculosis, a routine chest X-ray is indicated. The prognosis is poor, with likelihood severe infection, hypothermia, hypoglycaemia, jaundice, and collapse due to dehydration.

Course of the disease: Most deaths occur in the first 3 days from uncontrollable infection, diarrhoea, or electrolyte imbalance. The mortality rate with good treatment and care should not exceed 10%. Those who recover may gain weight (because of water retention) for the first 3–4 days, then have a massive diuresis, with loss of oedema and weight reduction from the 5th day. Thereafter there is a steady gain in weight. Persistent oedema suggests infection or other complications. A smiling child is a welcome sign of improvement, and hospitalization is rarely necessary for more than 2–3 weeks, depending on home conditions.

Marasmus

This is the childhood equivalent of starvation, and occurs when the diet is grossly deficient in energy. Such a diet also necessarily fails to meet protein requirements. Marasmus is most common during the first year of life. It may become manifest in wholly breast-fed infants when the milk is quantitatively insufficient, but more frequently it occurs after early weaning onto dilute or low-energy (low-density) bottle feeds or cereal paps. In the age group 1–5 years, marasmus occurs when food of any kind is unavailable, as in war, civil unrest or famine conditions, extreme poverty, or lack of care. Often it is produced by prolonged starvation during treatment of diarrhoea or other infections.

The presenting symptoms are: failure to thrive, irritable crying, or alternatively apathy. Diarrhoea is frequent, and vomiting is sometimes a complaint. The children are usually ravenously hungry, but some are anorexic.

On examination, the child has a shrunken, wizened, stark appearance, due to the absence of subcutaneous fat. The degree of underweight for age is extreme, the children being less than 60% of their weight for age. Watery diarrhoea or the passing of semi-solid, bulky stools with a low pH is usual. Voluntary muscles are weak and atrophic. The dermatosis, hair changes, mucous membrane lesions, and oedema characteristic of kwashiorkor are not features of pure marasmus. A mixed picture often occurs, however (*see marasmic kwashiorkor, below*).

In the differential diagnosis, marasmus must always be distinguished from severe weight loss produced by chronic pyogenic disease, tuberculosis, syphilis, AIDS, and tropical infestations. Psychological factors, especially maternal deprivation, can be severe enough to bring about marasmus through depression of appetite or rumination.

Marasmic kwashiorkor

The pure syndromes of marasmus and kwashiorkor are probably not as common as the many borderline cases and intermediate conditions which have some clinical signs of both. This is due to the fact that, in practice, diets vary enormously — sometimes from season to season. Local

Table 7.5   Clinical features of PEM

	Underweight	Marasmus	Kwashiorkor	Marasmic kwashiorkor
Weight	↓	↓↓	↓	↓↓
Height	↓	↓	↓	↓
Dermatosis	O	O	+	+
Oedema	O	O	++	+
Apathy, irritability	O	+	++	++
Muscle wasting	+	++	++	++
Enlarged liver	+/-	+/-	++	+
Anaemia	+/-	+	++	+
Infections	+/-	+	++	++

Key :   ↓ = Decrease
    ↓↓ = Marked decrease
    O = No manifestation
    + = Mild
    ++ = Severe
    +/- = Presence variable

conditions determine the availability and intake of carbohydrates, water, minerals, and vitamins.

In addition, infection and diarrhoea modify presenting symptoms and signs. The term marasmic kwashiorkor is used to describe the wasted, intermediate forms of PEM which have a variety of clinical dematoses and/or oedema characteristic of kwashiorkor. Similarly, a child on a high carbohydrate/low protein diet may look plump and have no oedema or dermatosis, yet is growth-retarded, apathetic, and weak (so-called pre-kwashiorkor). Confusion sometimes arises when a child who appears to be marasmic is admitted to hospital and becomes, by definition, a case of kwashiorkor overnight because oedema and skin lesions are more apparent when hydration has improved.

Immunodeficiency in malnutrition

Malnutrition and infection, which are both problems of disadvantaged children, are very closely interlinked. The child who is malnourished is often infected, while infection in the sub-optimally nourished child may precipitate frank marasmus or kwashiorkor. There is a considerable body of data arising out of clinical observations and epidemiological studies which shows that infections are more common in poorly-nourished

than in well-nourished patients. Infections in such children tend to be more severe, are more frequently associated with complications, and account for a higher mortality. Measles, which is often severe in African children, can be positively dangerous when it occurs in combination with malnutrition. Severe infection in any child with PEM denotes a poor prognosis.

Malnourished children exposed to poor environmental conditions are particularly susceptible to respiratory and gastrointestinal infections, and to septicaemia. The infecting agents responsible for these diseases range from viruses to helminths. *Herpes simplex* infection of the oral cavity is frequent, and causes much distress. Malnutrition is one of a few conditions (the others being the neonate, malignancy, and measles) in which the herpes virus tends to disseminate and cause life-threatening illness. The hepatitis viruses (A and B) and varicella may also be more damaging in malnutrition. Tuberculosis is common and debilitating, while Gram-negative septicaemia is serious enough to warrant aggressive therapy. Staphylococcal infections and shigella dysentery occur frequently. Mucocutaneous candidiasis poses feeding problems, and the fungus disseminates occasionally. Infection with the protozoan

E. histolytica can cause fulminating dysentery and liver abscess, while *Pneumocystis carinii* may cause a progressive pneumonia which is difficult to diagnose. *Giardia lamblia* infestation of the bowel is common, and aggravates the nutritional deficiencies. The presence of parasites such as roundworms and hookworms is almost invariable in these children. Deficiencies of vitamins such as A and D, nutrients such as iron and folates, and trace elements such as zinc, may also cause a predisposition to infection.

The frequency and severity of infections in PEM suggest defects in protective mechanisms of the immune response. This is supported by the clinical findings of an anergic response to infection. Even serious infection can be silent and unaccompanied by fever, while microbial invasion terminates in gangrene rather than suppuration. Hidden infections must always be suspected in any child presenting with malnutrition, and excluded by thorough investigation.

Immunity to infection is complex, and involves the interaction of a number of different components of the normal immune response. PEM affects many of these components *(see Table 7.6)*, and possibly protection from free radical damage.

Deficiencies of vitamins, iron, folate, and zinc depress some of the factors listed in *Table 7.6*.

Long-term effects of malnutrition

Growth retardation

Follow-up of cases of kwashiorkor occurring within the first 2 years of life has revealed that growth retardation is reversible if social circumstances and food intake are adequate. In fact no difference can be detected in growth achievement between ex-kwashiorkor cases, their siblings, and the children of the community from which they come.

Malnutrition and intelligence

Malnutrition and poverty are so closely interwoven that the effects on development of one cannot be distinguished from the other. Therefore the consequences of malnutrition on intellectual function must be seen as being inseparable from those of a poor socio-economic environment. It follows that therapeutic interventions should include not only food, but improvements in other

Table 7.6 Immunodeficiency in malnutrition

Tissue integrity ↓
Thymo-lymphatic atrophy
Cell-mediated immunity ↓
    T cell number ↓
    T cell function ↓:   Delayed cutaneous hyper-sensitivity ↓
        Lymphocyte transformation by mitrogens and antigens ↓
        Lymphokine production +/-
Humoral immunity +/-
    B cell number N
    Serum immunoglobulins N or +
    Serum antibody response variable
    Secretory antibody (IgA) response ↓
Polymorphonuclear function ↓
    Metabolic abnormalities
    Chemotaxis N or ↓
    Phagocytosis N
    Intracellular killing ↓
Complement proteins ↓
Other factors
    Serum transferrin ↓
    Lysozyme ↓
    Interferon ↓
    Alteration of gut flora
Key: ↓ decrease
    + increase
    N normal
    +/- variable

essential components of life, such as the residential environment, employment, and education.

In general, studies show that the majority of malnourished children have mild and reversible deficits in tests of intelligence.

Where malnutrition is endemic, children who have had PEM in earlier years enrol late in school, drop out early, and have impaired aptitudes. Children with stunting (i.e., chronic PEM) do less well in school than their peers. Nutritional rehabilitation, and health and educational inputs can improve aptitude and school performance.

In a 15-year follow-up there was no difference in scholastic attainment or social adjustment between PEM survivors and the children of the socio-economic environment from which they came. With respect to intellectual development, the survivors could not be distinguished from their siblings at the age of 10 years, on intelligence testing.

Long-term effects of PEM

◆ Growth retardation, stunting. Reversible with nutritional intervention.

◆ Reduced intellectual potential. Reversible with stimulation and environmental improvement.

◆ Late school enrolment, early school drop-out, impaired aptitude, and poor school performance. Reversible with nutritional rehabilitation, health and educational inputs.

◆ Stunting, small adult stature, apathy, and lack of initiative where PEM and poor socio-economic environment prevail throughout childhood.

Nutritional intervention

Successful nutritional intervention in families where kwashiorkor has occurred (which ensures adequate growth in subsequent siblings in the first 2 years of life), results in a significant improvement of intelligence, as tested at the age of 10 years, even though family diet between the ages of 2 and 10 years results in impaired growth. This and other similar work has highlighted the problem of separating the effects of malnutrition on brain growth *per se* (the physical aspect), from the effects of poor stimulation. The two often go together: with malnutrition in the early years (pre-school), a child's capacity for exploring, learning, and gaining experience is reduced due to apathy, weakness, etc. It is probably through this mechanism, rather than biochemical or structural change to the brain, that malnutrition exerts its main effect. In support of this view, it has recently been shown that stimulation of children recovering from PEM in hospitals, brings their intelligence up to normal for their age.

In conclusion, it can be stated that the effects of PEM in children are reversible if adequate treatment, sustained improvement of dietary intake, stimulation, and social circumstances allow. However, extended deprivation of food throughout the growing period (18 years), is likely to lead to adult stunting and diminished intellectual potential. Environmental and nutritional enrichment in the first 2 years of life reduces the chance of intellectual impairment in the long term.

Laboratory findings

The classical biochemical finding in PEM is reduced serum albumin concentration. It may be relatively insensitive as an index compared with the earlier manifestation of PEM (growth failure or marasmus), but hypoalbuminaemia, if found, is characteristic of the condition. A useful interpretation of serum albumin concentration is as follows:

Concentration (g/l)
> 35   Normal
30–34   Subnormal
25–29   Low
< 25   Pathological.

Once serum albumin concentration drops below 30 g/l, it has been shown that there is a drop in serum insulin, a rise in human growth hormone, diminished serum valine and alanine, a drop in serum beta-lipoprotein and cholesterol, and a drop in serum colloid osmotic pressure.

Measurement of serum ablumin concentration must be done by an acceptable method, with a proper laboratory standard, if it is to be used as a biochemical index of PEM.

There has been a world-wide search for other biochemical tests for PEM. These have included measurements of transferrin, blood urea (which is always low), serum amino acid patterns, urinary hydroxyproline secretion, urinary creatinine-height index, 3-methylhistidine excretion, etc. None of these has proved useful in practice. Abnormalities of serum electrolyte concentrations such as hypokalaemia, hypocalcaemia, hypomagnesaemia and low plasma zinc are frequently found, but are not diagnostic of PEM *per se* — rather of its complications.

With regard to anaemia, the diets that lead to PEM are frequently lacking in iron, folic acid, and other vitamins. There is thus a moderate degree of anaemia in most cases of mild PEM. The part played by protein deficiency is not entirely clear, but it is likely to be a factor in its own right. Almost every morphological type has been described, and anaemia can be particularly severe in cases complicated by infection. In tropical areas malaria must be excluded.

The prothrombin index is commonly depressed, and responds to vitamin K. Leucopenia and thrombocytopenia may occur, but tend to recover with treatment.

Hypoglycaemia is sometimes a feature in the very severe case of PEM, calling for screening (using Dextrostix®) whenever there is any drowsiness, loss of consciousness, or other suspicious signs.

Infection and malnutrition often go together. Blood cultures, urine culture, and rectal swabs should be done in all cases of severe PEM, to detect treatable infections.

Tuberculin test: This is mandatory in all patients, as tuberculosis is a common precipitating cause of PEM. If the test is negative on admission, it should be repeated on discharge, as some cases will have become positive with improvement of nutritional status.

Treatment

Mild PEM

This refers to those children identified in clinics, school, crèches, and so on who have growth retardation or are underweight, but who are not ill enough to be admitted to hospital. The children in this group make up the greatest number of cases of PEM, and are most at risk from the effects of gastroenteritis, and infections in general.

Health services in developing areas should be specially orientated towards detecting and managing the child with mild PEM. These children will present to the primary health care worker with a variety of complaints, and their state of nutrition must be detected clinically or by weighing.

The mainstay of treatment is the provision of adequate amounts of protein and energy. A protein intake of 2–3 g/kg/day with an energy intake of 100–150 k cal./kg/day (420–630 kJ/kg) should be prescribed.

The most important aspects regarding the provision of this kind of diet to an ambulatory patient are:

◆ As much of the diet as possible should consist of available staple foods. Advice on increasing the usual diet by introducing an extra one or two meals a day will frequently suffice (no child can grow on less than three meals a day). Increasing the energy density of weaning foods will also help to supply basic requirements.

◆ Specific supplements, whether of energy or protein, should be cheap and easily available.
◆ Changes in diet should be acceptable to the patient, the mother, the family, and the traditions of the community.

Many different forms of supplementation have been introduced in various parts of the world, making use of locally-produced foods. The aim of these is to improve the biological value of the protein, and the protein and energy content of the staple foods. In Africa, staples such as maize, bread, or rice can be supplemented with milk, egg, or fish, but these — if indeed they are available — are expensive. Vegetable protein supplements such as beans, peas, lentils, and nuts (peanuts) are excellent substitutes for animal protein, and often considerably cheaper.

If milk is available, it remains the best form of protein supplement for a basic cereal diet. There is 1 g of protein in each 30 ml of whole or skimmed milk. This means that 30–60 ml of milk/kg of body mass will supply 1–2 g protein/kg, which is sufficient, together with the basic diet, to cover any child's protein requirement. Even 15 ml of milk/kg/day added to a cereal diet will be sufficient to promote recovery and prevent malnutrition. From a practical point of view, 600 ml of milk added to the pot of porridge daily would be sufficient for four children.

Clinics usually have dried milk powder or other sources of high protein foods to issue to patients who need protein supplementation in treatment over the short term. Here it is important to appreciate that it takes much time and patience on the part of doctors, nurses, and nutritional advisors to obtain the understanding and co-operation of the mother.

Follow-up is essential for every case, and the best measure of efficacy of dietary treatment is weight gain, which should be monitored at least until the child has reached the normal centile range in the Road to Health Chart *(see Chapter 4, Community Paediatrics)*.

Any child presenting with mild PEM should be checked and treated for infection, the social and economic circumstances assessed, and advice and assistance given where possible.

▶ **Clinical features of severe kwashiorkor include:**

Drowsiness or stupor
Poor capillary filling
Temperature < 35 °C
Open skin lesions
Significant infection, (e.g., pneumonia)
Persistent diarrhoea
Obvious anaemia
Jaundice
Failure to respond to out-patient therapy.

Severe cases of PEM

(See above.)
These cases should be hospitalized due to the danger of death from dehydration, electrolyte disturbances, hypoglycaemia, and infection. Treatment can be divided into the following phases :

Resuscitation: Dehydration, severe anaemia (Hb less than 6 g %), hypoglycaemia, and electrolyte imbalances must be managed appropriately in the first instance. For the first 24 hours, routine maintenance administration of half-strength Darrow's solution or equivalent ORS (oral rehydration solution) should be given orally or intravenously, at a level of 100–150 ml/kg/day. Additional amounts (50 ml/kg for mild dehydration and 100 ml/kg for severe dehydration) should be prescribed where indicated *(also see Chapter 11, Gastrointestinal Disorders)*. In the presence of shock or severe anaemia, plasma or blood should be given initially at a dose of 20 ml/kg. This therapy will assist in correcting dehydration and acidosis. Mineral supplements in the form of potassium (to a total of 6 mEq/kg/day), calcium (to 3 g/day), and magnesium (to 2–3 mEq/kg/day) have been found helpful in correcting gross deficiencies and cardiac arrythmias that are frequently present. Zinc sulphate or acetate in a dose of 2 mg/kg/day assists in correcting possible deficiencies of this trace element.

During this 24-hour period of resuscitation, no food or milk should be given. This precaution lessens the complication of vomiting and gastric distension that frequently occurs if feeding is started too soon.

Hypoglycaemia: Mild, asymptomatic hypoglycaemia should be treated with 25% dextrose water orally. When severe (less than 1.1 mmol/l), often

with associated hypothermia, dextrose should be given intravenously in the form of 50% solution (0.5 g/kg) and maintained as a 10% dextrose electrolyte solution.

Infection: If the child has open skin lesions, overt infection, or is critically ill, antibiotics should be given immediately, preferably after blood cultures and other bacteriological specimens have been obtained. Initially antibiotics should be given intravenously where possible. Penicillin, ampicillin, and sulphonamides (sulphadiazine or co-trimoxazole) have proved very useful. If a stronger combination is needed, penicillin and kanamycin, gentamycin, or amikacin are valuable. Where parasitic infections such as malaria, amoebiasis, giardiasis, ancylostomiasis and ascariasis are endemic or present, these should be dealt with as soon as possible.

Underlying tuberculosis is a frequent concern, and must be treated immediately if there is any suspicion of this infection. The possibility of HIV infection or AIDS must be considered when there is failure of response to therapy.

Diet and supplements after resuscitation

After initial resuscitation measures, it is usually possible to commence feeds on the second day. Small, frequent, skim or full-cream milk feeds, orally or by nasogastric tube (60–90 ml/kg/day), should be started. This can be gradually increased by 20 ml/kg/day to a total of 150 ml/kg/day. Too rapid an increase in food intake can lead to gastric distension and vomiting.

Cereals and other foods are gradually introduced after 3 or 4 days, until the child is on a full diet by 7–10 days after admission to hospital. Supplements of potassium, zinc, and magnesium should be maintained for at least 5 days after admission.

If milk is not available, or is poorly tolerated because of lactose intolerance, milk substitutes such as soya milk or egg added to porridge or other lactose-free food or formula (usually expensive) may be given.

Vitamin supplementation: It is wise to add vitamin A, due to the danger of xerophthalmia, and because it has recently been claimed that vitamin A therapy decreases the morbidity and mortality of infections. All children should have a single intramuscular injection of 33 000 µg of water-miscible vitamin A on admission, and then 5 000 µg orally daily for 5 days. Most children respond rapidly to an adequate protein intake without the B group of vitamins, particularly if milk is used as a protein source. Vitamin D should be given if there is evidence of rickets, and as the prothrombin index is often low in kwashiorkor, vitamin K 2–5 mg is necessary.

Folic acid is important in anaemic patients. As yet there is no firm evidence of the value of vitamin E, but this may change if free radicals are shown to be important in the pathology of kwashiorkor. Iron supplements are commenced after 10–14 days' therapy, when transferrin levels can be assumed to have returned to normal.

Usually there is an obvious improvement in the child within the first 2–3 days of treatment. Appetite returns, and apathy and irritability lessen. Many children with marasmus may become temporarily oedematous, and oedema may increase in kwashiorkor. This is not a bad sign, and represents sodium retention while the child is still potassium-depleted. Diuresis and loss of oedema (and weight) will occur by the 8–10th day. In 2–3 weeks, the child is smiling once more, gaining weight, and is ready to go home.

Play therapy and tender loving care during the hospital stay will help to restore quickly the child's natural interest and learning abilities. No specific therapy is needed for skin lesions, apart from protecting ulcerated areas from moisture and contamination.

It is important to ensure that before the child's discharge from hospital, the parents understand the reasons for the child's illness and know what to do for follow-up care and prevention.

Follow-up

Every case of PEM should be followed up at regular monthly intervals after discharge to check on gain in weight. It is desirable that the child should catch up to at least the third percentile on the weight chart, or that growth rate should parallel the percentile lines. Mothers are particularly interested in this aspect, and if properly instructed will aid the doctor or clinic nurse in achieving this goal. There are relatively few cases that relapse, and usually these occur in exceptional instances.

Table 7.7 Treatment of PEM

Mild PEM	3–5 meals/day. Enrich basic diet with animal or vegetable protein, carbohydrate and/or fat.
Severe PEM	Hospital admission, resuscitation, antibiotics, mineral and vitamin supplements.

Nutrition education and explanation for mild and severe PEM.

Care must be taken to ensure that other members of the family, such as the father and grandmother, also understand the causes of and preventive measures for PEM. It is important that the relevant social services are mobilized to assist these families. There are various schemes — both governmental and voluntary — in most countries, whereby subsidized milk or food can be obtained at welfare clinics for children recovering, or at risk, from malnutrition. Full use should be made of these schemes by all health workers.

Prevention

PEM is essentially a problem of poverty, whether this is brought about by famine, social or family disorganization, unemployment, or migrant labour. The eradication of PEM is therefore an extremely complex challenge, and one that faces two-thirds of the world population. The World Bank and numerous international agencies have struggled with variable success for the last 30 years to improve the lot of the world's poor. The following macro-economic measures have been found to be effective in alleviating malnutrition in developing countries:

♦ Economic growth which includes participation of the poor; this is an investment for future well-being.

♦ Social security for the poor; this includes easy access to food ('food security'). Such intervention meets the immediate needs for food consumption.

South Korea and Singapore have emphasized the first option, while Costa Rica, Jamaica, Sri Lanka and China have taken the second route to improving nutrition. It has been shown that even countries with a low per capita GNP can successfully provide social security. When dealing with malnourished children, the health team should be aware of what help can be obtained from locally-available services and resources, to promote

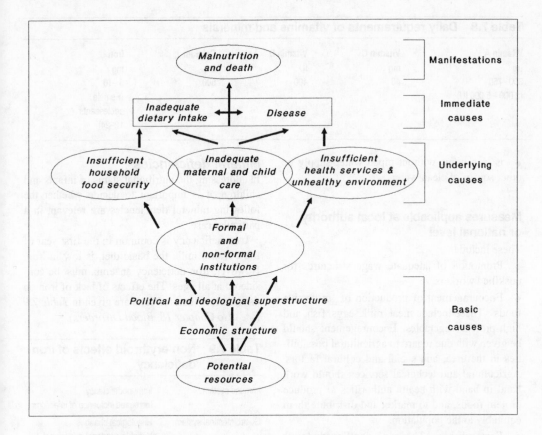

Fig. 7.5   *Causes of malnutrition, indicating levels of intervention (Source: 'UNICEF Strategy for improved nutrition of children and women in developing countries'. UNICEF Policy Review 1990–91.)*

recovery and assist prevention. Some of the complexities in the aetiology of PEM and the levels of intervention required are given in *Fig. 7.5.*

Preventive measures applicable at a clinic or community level

Doctors, nurses, and all members of the health team working in infant welfare clinics, health centres, hospital outpatient departments, or the wider community should include nutritional assessment in the clinical examination of every child. This applies in particular to children who present with gastroenteritis, pneumonia, or other infections. Attention to dietary needs is an essential part of treatment of these children, to avoid poor results, relapse, and constant re-attendance for minor and major illnesses.

Points of particular importance in preventive care have been summed up conveniently in a now

widely-used UNICEF mnemonic: GOBI FFF and Facts for Life *(see Chapter 4, Community Paediatrics).*

The child at risk

◆ is in poor social circumstances and is not being, or has not been, breast-fed

◆ is a twin

◆ has diarrhoea, pneumonia, tuberculosis, or another infectious disease

◆ has a mother who is in poor social circumstances, in poor health, incompetent, or who already has many children

◆ has a father who is alcoholic or out of work

◆ has lost one or other parent by death or desertion

◆ has a working mother and there is inadequate child-minding

Table 7.8   Daily requirements of vitamins and minerals

Vitamin A	Vitamin C	Vitamin D	Calcium	Iron
µg	mg	IU	mg	mg
300–750	40	400	500	5–10
(2 000 – 5 000 IU)				(Female adolescents 12–24)

♦   is in a home without piped water supply or other source of clean water.

Measures applicable at local authority or national level

These include:

♦   Promotion of adequate wage structures for unskilled workers.

♦   Encouragement of production of 'protective foods'. These include meat, milk, eggs, fish, and high-protein vegetables. Encouragement should be given with due regard to agricultural possibilities in the area, and social and cultural factors. Agricultural and technical services should work hand in hand with health authorities to produce protein foods, and to market and distribute them equitably to the population.

♦   Food subsidies: These can significantly lower the price of basic and essential protective food for the poor.

♦   Health education: The mass media should be widely employed for propagation of sound advice on nutrition.

♦   Notification of nutritional diseases: This helps to identify families at risk so that assistance in one form or another can be given.

Vitamins and minerals

Deficiencies and toxicities

In contrast to protein and energy, requirements for vitamins do not differ significantly with age. Some requirements are listed in *Table 7.8*.

Vitamins and minerals are present in most mixed diets, but under certain circumstances pure deficiencies do occur. In children in South Africa, vitamin D deficiency is common in the first year of life; pellagra occurs in maize-eating populations, but scurvy is uncommon; and overt vitamin A deficiency is particularly associated with PEM.

Mineral deficiencies

In addressing the nutritional status of infants and children, it is important to decide whether the following mineral deficiencies are relevant in a particular case.

Iron deficiency is common in the first year of life because milk, the basic diet, is low in iron. However, iron deficiency anaemia must be considered at all ages. The effects of lack of iron on tissues other than red cells are given in *Table 7.9* (*see also Chapter 18, Blood Disorders*).

Table 7.9   Non-erythroid effects of iron deficiency

Immune system:	Immunodeficiency
	Increased incidence of infections
Gastrointestinal system:	Histological changes
	Variable duodenal and jejunal atrophy
	Hypochlorhydria
	Impaired absorption of food, D-xylose, vitamins
Thermoregulation:	Impaired homeostatic response to hypothermia
Physical work:	Reduced efficiency
Cognition and behaviour:	Impaired or abnormal

Sodium, potassium and magnesium: (*see Chapter 20, Endocrine and Metabolic Disorders*). Diarrhoea, vomiting, or loss of fluid from the gastrointestinal tract from suction, fistulae, ileostomy, and colostomy may give rise to acute or chronic deficiencies of these minerals. They form part of most therapeutic supplements in treatment of these conditions, and must never be omitted in serious cases.

Calcium deficiency occurs in some areas where milk is in short supply (*see Chapter 21, Metabolic*

Bone Disorders). Infants, school-age children, and the elderly may be affected.

Trace element deficiencies

Fluoride: The chief source of fluoride is drinking water, which, if it contains 1 part per million (ppm) or 1 mg/l, supplies 1–2 mg per day. Soft water contains less, and deficiency leading to dental caries may occur *(see Chapter 29, Oral and Dental Problems).*

Iodine deficiency occurs in some areas and gives rise to goitre and hypothyroidism *(see Chapter 20, Endocrine Disorders).*

Zinc: There is currently much interest in this trace element, but a reliable clinical measure of zinc deficiency is lacking. It has been proved unequivocally that deficiency of zinc is a feature of the rare disease acrodermatitis enteropathica. Zinc supplements improve the lesions dramatically.

Claims are made that zinc deficiency causes stunting of growth in certain populations, such as in the Middle East. It has also been shown that serum zinc levels can be very low in cases of kwashiorkor with ulcerative skin lesions, and in small-for-date infants. In all instances, other factors and deficiencies bedevil the assumption that zinc deficiency *per se* is the cause of the lesions, and therapeutic uses of zinc supplements are as yet controversial.

Vitamin deficiencies and toxicities

Vitamin A (retinol)

This fat-soluble vitamin is found in full-cream milk, butter, egg-yolk, and fish oils, among other things. Its provitamin, β-carotene, is responsible for the yellow/red colour of vegetables and some fruits. Dark green leaves are a good source of β-carotene, and carrots are an excellent source. Where animal foods are seldom eaten, all vitamin A intake comes from such sources. β-carotene is transformed by intestinal mucosa to retinol, which along with dietary vitamin A is absorbed by chylomicrons, transported to the liver, and stored as retinyl palmitate. Thence it is released into the circulation as retinol bound to retinol-binding protein (RBP). The old-fashioned international unit of vitamin A is equivalent to 0.3 µg of retinol.

Retinol is essential for vision in dim light, and for integrity of tissues, particularly the epithelial tissue of the eye and the skin. Daily requirement of Vitamin A ranges from 300 µg in infants to 750 µg in adolescents.

Pathogenesis of deficiency: The human infant is dependent on milk for her supply of the vitamin. Later, carotene-containing vegetables and fruit are an additional source, but in many rural districts the supply is inadequate, especially in the dry season, and these foods may be too expensive for poorer urban dwellers. The diets of children with vitamin A deficiency are almost invariably deficient in other nutrients, especially in protein and energy content. In Africa, vitamin A deficiency tends to occur with PEM, particularly in severe kwashiorkor and marasmus, whereas in the East, where the staple diet is rice, it may occur in a more specific and endemic form. In the development of eye lesions associated with vitamin A deficiency, precipitating factors such as gastroenteritis, measles, and tuberculosis are important, in addition to a hot, dusty climate.

Epidemiology: Night blindness and xerophthalmia are found in the Middle East, Africa, India, South and East Asia, and Latin America. The peak incidence is between 2 and 5 years. The exact incidence is unknown, but one estimate is that keratomalacia causes 20 000 children per annum to become permanently blind.

The reported frequency in severe PEM varies from 74% in Indonesia, to 1–2% in Lebanon, Uganda, and South Africa. These differences are explicable on the basis of the vitamin A content of the basic diet.

Another less dramatic but no less devastating aspect of vitamin A deficiency is susceptibility to infection. Studies in developing countries have shown a strong association between vitamin A deficiency and increased incidence of respiratory and diarrhoeal infections. In addition, infections have been shown to reduce serum concentrations of vitamin A. This vicious circle can be broken by vitamin A supplementation, as has been shown in trials in Indonesia, India, and Nepal, where vitamin A supplementation resulted in significant reduction in morbidity and mortality from common childhood infections. There is now adequate evidence that vitamin A supplementation during complicated measles shortens the duration of complications, lowers the incidence of new infections, and reduces the mortality rate It should therefore be included as part of the primary health care routine. One of the ways in which vitamin A is thought to have its effect in reducing the severity and incidence of infections is by repairing and maintaining the integrity of the epithelial tissue of the respiratory and gastrointestinal tract, thus providing an effective barrier against infectious agents.

Clinical features

Eye: Although night blindness is the typical clinical feature of vitamin A deficiency in older children or adults, xerophthalmia is characteristic of the deficiency in infants and younger children. The earliest sign is dryness of the conjunctivae (xerosis conjunctivae). There is a loss of transparency, and thickened vertical folds of conjuctivae appear. Often a small plaque of silvery-grey hue, Bitot's spot, is raised above the surface of the conjunctiva *(see Fig. 7.6).*

The next stage is corneal xerosis, characterized by unwettability and loss of transparency, which leads to haziness of the cornea. This is reversible, but irreversible corneal ulceration can be the next stage. Perforation and iris prolapse may occur.

Keratomalacia, a passive softening of the cornea, is another manifestation that can occur suddenly, even during therapy. Again there may be perforation and panophthalmitis as a complication.

Xerophthalmia is seen particularly in association with severe PEM, and should always be looked for in these children. A retinol plasma

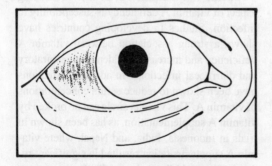

Fig. 7.6 Bitots' spots resulting from vitamin A deficiency

concentration of less than 15–20 μg/100 m*l* (normal 20–50 ug/100 ml) is suggestive of deficiency. The plasma RBP is also low.

Skin: Perifollicular keratosis (phrynoderma, 'toad skin') is thought to be due to vitamin A deficiency. It has also been associated with exposure to dry, cold atmosphere, and with deficiency of fatty acids and the vitamin B complex group. It is therefore difficult to ascribe the condition solely to vitamin A deficiency.

Sunbathing enthusiasts believe that vitamin A oil protects or relieves the skin from sunburn, but the scientific evidence for such claims is uncertain. Acne in adolescents is currently being treated with concentrated vitamin A preparations, with variable results.

Differential diagnosis: Xerophthalmia may also be due to disease of the lacrimal glands, e.g., pemphigus or trachoma, or it may result from overexposure of the conjuctiva or cornea.

Treatment: Vitamin A in a dose of 30 mg (100 000 IU) of retinol daily for 3 days should be started as soon as the diagnosis is suspected. Half of the dose should be given orally and half intramuscularly as a water-miscible retinyl palmitate. All cases of PEM should receive vitamin A prophylactically in the form of fish-liver oil or a vitamin supplement containing vitamin A. Antibiotics help in prevention and treatment of secondary infection. Local treatment of the eye will only be required if disorganization is already present, in which case an ophthalmologist should be consulted. Children with complicated measles should be given 60 mg of retinol (in the form of retinyl palmitate) daily for 2 days.

Cancer: Much research is currently in progress into the possible role of vitamin A deficiency in the aetiology of various types of cancer.

Prevention of vitamin A deficiency: Green leafy vegetables, squash, pumpkin, carrots, and yellow and orange fruits are good sources of ß carotene. In areas where xerophthalmia is endemic, encourage diets including whichever sources are locally available and/or cheap.

Where blindness from keratomalacia is a major public health problem, single, large prophylactic doses of 60 mg (200 000 IU) of retinol in oily solution should be given orally at 4- to 6-monthly intervals to all children, if personnel and facilities are available. Other means of fortification of local food such as sugar are being investigated.

Vitamin A toxicity: Acute poisoning has occurred following overdose of sunburn tablets or vitamin preparations, or excessive ingestion of fish- or shark-liver. The symptoms are restlessness, headache, and vomiting, sometimes with signs of raised intracranial pressure. Recovery with no residual damage occurs on removal of the vitamin A source.

Chronic poisoning from extended excessive dosing occurs occasionally. In its mildest form, carotenaemia (or yellow staining of skin) occurs, particularly in children who have had over-enthusiastic dosing with carrots or vitamin preparations. In more severe forms, the clinical picture can include coarse, sparse hair, cracking of lips, and dry skin. Arthralgia, headache, and weakness can occur, and in the long bones, thickening of shafts and widened metaphyses have been reported.

A fasting serum retinol value of more than 250 µg/100 ml is diagnostic. Recovery occurs with withdrawal of the vitamin.

Vitamin E

The actions of vitamin E (tocopherol) are mainly antioxidant, and effects of its deficiency in humans are still controversial. It is present in human tissues and widely distributed in foods, so primary deficiency of the vitamin is unlikely. In paediatrics at present, it is accepted that deficiency in premature and small for date infants results in haemolytic anaemia. Prophylactic vitamin E to prevent or treat this is given routinely in some neonatal units. Apart from small infants, vitamin E deficiency is sometimes considered in cystic fibrosis patients with severe malabsorption. Claims that it is of value in habitual abortion, sterility, muscular dystrophies, diabetes, coronary heart disease, and skin disorders have no scientific basis of proof. Its value as a counter to free radical excess situations is under investigation.

Vitamin B complex

Thiamine (vitamin B_1): Thiamine is the least labile portion of the B complex, and deficiency leads to beriberi. In children in Africa, clinical beriberi is very rare, as the basic diet of maize or wheat contains vitamin B_1. It does occur in the Far East in those populations that exist solely on polished rice or highly refined wheat flour. Infants breast-fed from a mother on such a diet may develop beriberi at 2–5 months. In southern Africa, infants with recurrent attacks of diarrhoea have been found to have biochemical evidence of B_1 deficiency, but no clinical features were noted. Beriberi occurs in adult alcoholics in most countries.

The clinical features of beriberi in infants are those of acute cardiac failure, occurring suddenly with cyanosis and/or oedema, aphonia because of laryngeal paralysis, and pseudomeningeal signs, with drowsiness and head retraction.

Lowered erythrocyte transketolase activity is suggestive of beriberi.

Treatment: Emergency administration of 50–100 mg of thiamine hydrochloride, IM or IV, should be followed by oral maintenance of 5–10 mg daily for several days. Recovery is rapid.

Nicotinic acid deficiency (pellagra): Nicotinic acid is biosynthesized from the essential amino acid tryptophan. Diets low in nicotinic acid or tryptophan lead to the deficiency disease pellagra. Africa appears to be the only continent where pellagra is an important public health problem. In parts of southern Africa it remains endemic, with outbreaks in the spring and summer months. The reason for this is that the basic diet of a great proportion of the population is maize. Maize protein is deficient in tryptophan, and although maize contains nicotinic acid, it is present in a bound form unavailable to the consumer. Unsupplemented maize porridge diets are thus pellagra-producing. Pellagra, because of its association with nicotinic acid and its precursor tryptophan, can be regarded both as a vitamin deficiency disease or as one of the syndromes of PEM.

Clinical features: Traditionally pellagra has been known as the disease of the three D's: dermatitis, diarrhoea, and dementia. In children, dementia is rare, and pellagra is characterized by the skin lesions and features akin to protein deficiency.

The disease affects children from the age of 5 years. The skin lesions of pellagra are almost identical to those of kwashiorkor. In fact, before kwashiorkor became established as a term for severe protein malnutrition, it used to be labelled 'infantile pellagra'.

The lesions consist of erythema or pigmentation over areas exposed to sunlight or other irritants. Thus in infants with kwashiorkor, the perineum and buttock areas are affected, but in older children with pellagra, the lesions are on the neck (Casal's necklace), forehead, face, back of hands, wrists, forearms, and legs; covered areas are spared.

A red, beefy tongue, angular stomatitis, and cheilosis are frequently present. The more severe features of kwashiorkor, e.g., gross oedema, diarrhoea, apathy, or infection are not as prominent in pellagra, because in older children protein requirement is not as critical as in the rapidly-growing infant or toddler. It is advantageous to regard pellagra in children as a manifestation of kwashiorkor in an older child. In affected families, children under 3 years will have kwashiorkor, and the older children pellagra.

Diagnosis is made on clinical appearance and history. A reduced N-methylnicotinamide excretion in the urine is helpful academic confirmation. Fasting plasma tryptophan ranges from 1.0 to 4.5 mg/l in pellagra, and from 6.5 to 8.8 mg/l in healthy adults.

As in PEM, there may be a degree of hypoalbuminaemia.

Treatment: Nicotinamide or nicotinic acid (100 mg orally every 4 hours) will give relief, but it is more important to improve the diet with sources of animal protein, e.g., milk, meat, cheese, fish, eggs, or with legumes such as beans, peas, and lentils. Recovery is complete and rapid.

Prevention: A mixed diet, or maize enrichment with nicotinic acid, will assist in preventing pellagra. Commercial maize enrichment is now becoming more universal in southern Africa and pellagra is less common than it used to be.

Riboflavin (vitamin B_2): Deficiency of this vitamin rarely occurs alone, and is usually associated with kwashiorkor or pellagra. The skin lesions of riboflavin deficiency cannot be distinguished from these conditions.

Pyridoxine (vitamin B_6): Most foodstuffs contain this, and isolated deficiency is very rare. Convulsions have been described in established deficiency due to heat-processing of commercial milks, malabsorption, or drug antagonism (isoniazid).

Folic acid and B_{12} deficiency: Megaloblastic anaemia is associated with these deficiencies *(see Chapter 18, Blood Disorders)*. Where there is a poor diet, or malabsorption associated with anaemia, deficiency of folic acid should be considered. Folic acid deficiency in pregnancy may result in neural tube defects in the newborn, e.g., myelomeningocele.

Vitamin B_{12} deficiency tends to occur in vegans (those who are true vegetarians and who eat no animal protein at all, as compared to the lacto-ovo vegetarians who do allow eggs and milk in the diet). Dietary B_{12} deficiency from a pure vegetable diet may take months or even years to develop, and is thus hardly ever seen in children.

Vitamin C (ascorbic-acid) deficiency (scurvy)

The minimum requirement of vitamin C is 40 mg/day for all age groups. It is found in fresh vegetables and fruit.

In infancy, requirements are met by breast milk, which is rich in vitamin C, or by fruit juices or artificial supplements when feeding is by bottle. It is important to appreciate that cows' milk is low in Vitamin C, and that boiling or processing destroys the vitamin. Infants fed solely on unsupplemented processed milks are thus prone to develop scurvy at 4 – 6 months of age.

Vitamin C promotes the release of free folic acid from conjugates in food and, most important, facilitates the absorption of iron. In the tissues, vitamin C deficiency results in defective function of intercellular ground substance. In skin, bone, and blood vessels, the deficiency leads to defective collagen, resulting in poor wound healing, rupture of capillaries, and haemorrhage.

Clinical features: Scurvy in paediatrics is a disease of infancy, usually at the age of 4–10 months. The presenting symptom is irritability, made worse by picking up or by moving limbs. This is due to the tenderness and swelling of subperiosteal and other haemorrhages. For this reason, patients are often referred to surgeons with a provisional diagnosis of osteitis. The pseudoparalysis induced by pain leads to a characteristic frog-like position of the legs.

Haemorrhage may occur in any tissue. Gum bleeding is rare in infants before tooth eruption. There is beading of the ribs at the costochondral junction. X-ray changes of long bones are diagnostic. Periosteal elevation because of haemorrhage is a striking feature, and is especially well seen in recovery, when it becomes calcified. There is a ground glass appearance in the shaft, thinning of the cortex, and broadening of the zone of provisional calcification.

In the epiphyses, the ground glass appearance within the centre of ossification, and the surrounding dense epiphyseal line, give the appearance known as 'ringing' of the epiphyses.

On recovery there is a return to normality without deformity.

Scurvy must be differentiated from other bleeding disorders and causes of purpura. Herpesvirus stomatitis is occasionally mistaken for scurvy.

Osteitis, septic arthritis, and non-accidental injuries *(see Chapter 4)* have to be excluded, and because of skeletal abnormalities, rickets and congenital syphilis must be distinguished.

Treatment must be immediate because of the danger of further bleeding.

Ascorbic acid (250 mg 4 times a day) causes prompt improvement and initiates healing.

Prevention: Scurvy tends to occur only in the first year of life. A source of vitamin C (fruit juice or vitamin preparation with 40 mg vitamin C) must be given daily from birth to infants on artificial (bottle) feeding.

Summary of vitamin deficiencies

Vitamin A: Xerophthalmia, increased morbidity and mortality

Vitamin B
complex: Pellagra, macrocytic anaemia

Vitamin C: Scurvy, anaemia, poor iron absorption

Vitamin D: Rickets

Vitamin E: Haemolytic anaemia (newborns), neuropathy, ataxia

Vitamin K: Haemorrhagic disease (newborns)

Vitamin K (phytomenadione)

This fat-soluble vitamin occurs in plants, and is also produced by bacteria in the gut. Vitamin K is a co-factor for the synthesis in the liver of prothrombin. Primary deficiency of this vitamin in the neonate occurs because the gut is sterile and there is very little vitamin K in breast and cows' milk. Infants in the first week of life therefore have low prothrombin in their blood. There is spontaneous improvement in a few days, but haemorrhagic disease of the newborn may supervene in the interim. Bleeding from the second to fifth day of life can occur from any internal or external site, and may be fatal. The condition can be completely avoided by administration of 1 mg of vitamin K_1 IM at birth. This should be a routine at every delivery.

Vitamin K deficiency after the newborn period tends to occur with hyperalimentation regimes, liver disease, biliary obstruction and fistulae, intestinal malabsorption syndromes, and as a result of long-continued antibiotic therapy. Prophylactic administration of vitamin K_1 by mouth or by injection will prevent bleeding in these circumstances.

Diseases of overnutrition
Obesity
Definition

Obesity is overweight due to excess fat. In childhood, obesity may be defined as the infant or child who is too heavy for his length or height. An obese child is obvious on inspection, but to determine obesity objectively, weight and length must be charted on standard growth reference curves. If the weight is 10% over the desirable weight for length, overweight should be suspected unless there is another cause for this discrepancy; 20% or more over the desirable weight for length is definite obesity. In practice, this means a child who is 10–20 percentiles more in weight than his percentile length or height is obese. Skinfold measurements can be used as additional evidence, and charts are now available for these in childhood. In adults, men should be considered obese if the triceps skin exceeds 15 mm, and women if it exceeds 25 mm.

Prevalence

Between 3 and 13% of children and teenagers suffer from obesity. It is more common in girls than boys, particularly during adolescence.

Pathogenesis

The immediate cause of obesity is a positive energy balance. Excess fat is laid down if energy intake exceeds energy expenditure. Whether there is a metabolism in obese children that predisposes to obesity is a matter of debate. It is suggested, for example, that some individuals have an abnormality of brown adipose tissue that prevents their responding to a low environmental temperature by a rise in metabolic rate. According to this theory, overfeeding causes the lean person to expend more energy because of increased non-shivering thermogenesis induced by brown adipose tissue, and to lose the excess energy as heat. The person prone to obesity does not do this to the same extent, and her only alternative is to store the excess energy as fat.

Whether there is an abnormality of metabolism or not, obesity in infants tends to occur with artificial feeding as opposed to breast-feeding in the first year of life. This is because many infant formulas are supplemented with refined carbohydrate in the form of glucose, sucrose, or lactose.

Mothers tend to encourage infants to finish the bottle — the baby is unable to control milk intake as is possible on the breast. In pre-school and school years, obesity is propagated by the eating habits of families that favour the excess consumption of refined foods (sugar, cold drinks, white bread, cakes, sweets) as opposed to unrefined carbohydrate sources (fruit, potatoes, brown bread, vegetables). Also, an excess of fat, e.g., butter, fried foods, fatty meat, will promote obesity. Genetic factors predisposing to obesity appear to be less important. Although obesity is more common in the children of fat parents, pseudo-hereditary influences such as family eating patterns and environment appear to be the operative factors. Lack of exercise, and psychological causes of overeating, e.g., boredom, insecurity, poor family relationships, or mental and physical handicaps, are important factors affecting obesity in modern-day society. It is unlikely that there is anything particularly bad in the prognosis of early-onset obesity, *provided that it is not allowed to progress unchecked.*

Clinical assessment

Obesity as defined above should be recorded at all ages at infant welfare clinics, at pre-school assessments, at school, and during adolescence. The doctor or primary health care worker should include the presence of obesity in the diagnostic assessment, so that appropriate advice can be given before the condition becomes chronic and complications occur.

Complications

Infancy and pre-school: Fat infants and children are prone to repeated respiratory infections. In diarrhoea and vomiting, dehydration is more difficult to assess in a fat child, and this may result in inadequate fluid therapy. Impaired glucose tolerance is a problem which may eventually lead to diabetes.

School age and adolescence: The psychological effects of obesity in this age group may be profound, leading to feelings of rejection and poor self-image which in themselves propagate the overeating habit or, alternatively, could precipitate anorexia nervosa.

Long term: Complications include increased mortality and morbidity from hypertension, diabetes, heart disease, or joint problems.

Differential diagnosis

Large infants: During the first year of life large infants are frequently confused with obese infants. During the first 6–12 months, an infant tends to put on more fat than muscle, and looks chubby. The distinction between the two is made clear by charting weight and length *(see Fig. 7.7)*. The large, as opposed to obese, infant will have a length corresponding to the weight on the percentile lines.

Endocrine disorders: Hypothyroidism, Cushing's syndrome, and Fröhlich's syndrome (craniopharyngioma) may present with apparent obesity, and weight for height will be increased. However, the height in these cases is usually below the third percentile, whereas in true obesity height is within normal limits.

Rehabilitation from malnutrition: During recovery from severe PEM (marasmus or kwashiorkor) catch-up weight gain precedes catch-up length. Convalescent cases, therefore, may go

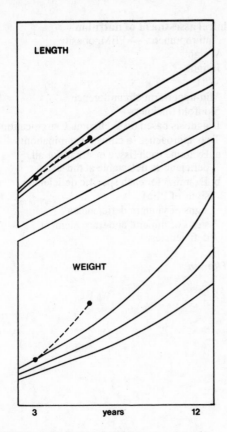

Fig. 7.7 Weight/height discrepancy reveals obesity

through a period of apparent obesity. In these instances, measurement of length at monthly intervals will reveal the growth spurt, and weight/height discrepancy will disappear with time.

Rare congenital disorders associated with mental deficiency and dwarfism, e.g., Prader–Willi syndrome, have to be considered in cases where the clinical picture does not fit with simple obesity.

Treatment

A well-motivated parent and patient are essential if treatment is to be attempted. Obesity runs in families, and it is usually impossible to distinguish what is genetic and what is environmental. However, the paediatrician should watch the weight gain of children so that parents can be advised at the earliest sign of obesity. A dietician can be of great assistance for all age groups.

In infancy: Excessive gain of weight compared to height can be detected on weight charts. Here,

simple advice should be given to cut down feeds to requirements, e.g., after the age of 6 months 500 ml of milk per day is enough on a weaning diet. Avoiding adding sugar to feeds, and using it sparingly on porridge, will cut energy intake. In practice, using skim milk in place of whole milk effectively cuts energy intake without need for further dieting. The aim should always be to keep weight static rather than to promote loss of weight. This will enable the infant to continue growing and so 'grow into her weight'.

In children: The best time for treatment is at primary school entry, since a modest reduction in the normal rate of fat storage between the ages of 5 and 12 will convert the obese 5-year-old into a normal-weight child at entry to secondary school.

In adolescence: This is a more complicated age for treatment, but emphasis should be on:

◆ Increased activity: many obese adolescents are extremely inactive.

◆ Sensible dieting: concentration on foods with high fibre and low fat, e.g., salads. Avoidance of refined carbohydrates (cold drinks, cakes, sweets, white bread). Porridge, brown bread, potatoes, and rice can be eaten in moderation. Diet should be adapted as closely as possible to family and cultural eating habits.

◆ Psychological support: frequent counselling and follow-up visits assist self-discipline.

Group therapy is often helpful. Organizations such as Weighless are very effective, but are expensive.

Prevention

The detection and treatment of obesity in infancy and childhood will prevent multiple complications in later life. Health education — during and after pregnancy, at infant welfare centres, and via the school medical service — is therefore mandatory if prevention is to be effective. Proper use of growth and weight charts will detect early predisposition to obesity, and should be emphasized in all doctors' rooms and clinics.

Overnutrition and malnutrition in children related to cardiovascular disease

Recently it has been suggested that childhood poverty and malnutrition followed by later affluence may be a leading determinant of degenerative arterial disease in adulthood. Speculation aside, an elevated serum cholesterol is now an established cardiovascular risk factor, and intervention is indicated when it is above 4.2 mmol/l in children and adolescents. This intervention takes the form of appropriate advice on lifestyle, e.g., a 'prudent' diet (fat intake limited to 20–30% of total energy intake), daily exercise, and control of stress. This is particularly so when there is a family history of cardiovascular disease, diabetes, or familial hyperlipidaemia. In the latter instance, screening of children above the age of 2 years is indicated.

Nutritional assessment

The clinical assessment of nutritional status should form part of every clinical examination.

Clinical assessment of nutrition

1 Anthropometry — PEM, obesity
   Weight
   Height
   W/H
   Mid-upper-arm circumference
   Skinfold thickness
2 Diagnosis based on Wellcome Classification
3 Two approaches to clinical examination:
   a. Examine each tissue or organ for all deficiencies detectable at the site.
   b. Examine for each specific deficiency:
   signs of PEM
   signs of vitamin deficiencies
   signs of mineral and trace element deficiencies.

J. Hansen

8

Infectious diseases

The advent of acquired immune defiency syndrome (AIDS) has had a considerable impact on the spectrum and character of infectious diseases. A separate chapter deals with this disease specifically (see Chapter 10), but it must be stressed that AIDS victims are particularly susceptible to several of the diseases described in this chapter, especially viral, fungal, and other opportunistic infections.

Fever and septicaemia

Fever is a common presenting symptom, and may be the sole reason for a consultation in about 20% of cases attending a hospital out-patients department. High temperatures (in excess of 41 °C) are more often due to bacterial infections than are lower temperatures. In infancy, bacterial infections are accompanied by fever in the majority of cases. However, newborns and malnourished children often do not manifest a high temperature, despite severe underlying infection. About 97% of premature babies with bacterial infections do not have fever. The reason for this paradoxical situation is the presence of anergy in these babies. It is important to know the mechanisms maintaining normal temperature in order to understand fever.

Control of body temperature

In healthy individuals body temperature is strictly maintained within a narrow range (±3 °C). The body requires 3 levels of control to achieve such fine temperature regulation:

◆ receptors to detect thermal changes in the skin, spinal cord, and hypothalamus

◆ a reference mechanism situated in the hypothalamus which maintains temperature at a set point (cf., thermostat)

◆ effector channels to retain or release heat in order to keep temperature at the set point. This is achieved by regulating the metabolic rate (heat production), vasoconstriction or vasodilatation, sweating, and behavioural responses (e.g., putting on warm clothing).

Changes in environmental temperature

In cold weather heat is retained in the body by vasoconstriction, increased heat production (by brown fat in neonates, by means of shivering in children), and lack of sweating. In hot weather there is increased loss of heat from the body through vasodilatation (by radiation and convection), and sweating (by evaporation). These responses to changes in environmental conditions keep internal body temperature at the set point.

Changes to the set point in the hypothalamus

At the onset of sleep the set point is reduced, thereby lowering the internal body temperature through the appropriate thermoregulatory mechanisms. The opposite happens in febrile states: the hypothalamic set-point is displaced upward, and therefore the internal body temperature is higher than normal. This higher temperature is maintained by decreasing heat loss (through vasoconstriction) and increasing heat production (by increasing metabolism and shivering). The threshold for the set point is raised in infections by the following process: bacterial products (e.g., endotoxins) stimulate mononuclear phagocytes to release a pyrogen, interleukin I, which increases synthesis of prostaglandins in the hypothalamus. It is not known how prostaglandins reset the hypothalamic thermostat. Acetylsalicylic acid acts by reducing synthesis of prostaglandins. Thermoregularity mechanisms are not fully developed in neonates, especially pre-term babies, and hence they do not adjust adequately to changes in ambient temperatures and do not produce fever in response to infection.

Clinical considerations

Certain signs which relate to the appearance and behaviour of the child suggest a potentially serious infection. These observations include changes in the cry, reactions to stimuli (smiling, anxiety, crying), level of consciousness, skin colour, and hydration.

The aetiology of fever varies according to circumstance.

Neonates are often afebrile despite being infected, but if they have fever one should suspect severe bacterial disease and treat accordingly. Malnourished children are equally anergic, although some infections such as herpes regularly produce a high temperature.

The common causes of mild to moderate fever in well-nourished children are benign fevers probably due to viral disease, upper respiratory tract infections, pneumonia, and some of the common exanthems.

Pyrexia of unknown origin

Pyrexia of unknown origin (PUO), especially when prolonged, presents special problems of diagnosis and management. The clinical examination of the child has to be systematic and thorough before a provisional diagnosis of PUO is made, i.e., there are no significant physical signs except fever. The cause in such cases will depend on the type of infections prevalent in the local environment. The most frequent underlying infections in many developing communities outside the malarial belt are tuberculosis, typhoid, and amoebiasis.

If features of any of these infectious diseases are found, the diagnosis is not difficult. In the absence of any pointers, a number of clues should be specifically sought.

Lymphadenopathy, a doughy abdomen, wasting, positive tuberculin test, chest radiograph, a history of contact and of gradual onset of ill health suggest tuberculosis. Miliary TB is especially difficult to pin-point; the only positive findings may be tachypnoea and fever.

A swinging temperature, 'toxic' appearance, splenomegaly, a tumid abdomen, leucopenia, and a background of unsanitary living conditions indicate typhoid.

High fever, leucocytosis, anaemia, tenderness in the right hypochondrium, rectal ulcers, bloody stools, and positive serology usually mean amoebic dysentery or liver abscess. It will be noted that a detailed history, careful abdominal palpation, and a few well-targeted investigations will aid in the diagnosis of these conditions.

Urinary tract infection in children may present insidiously with pyrexia alone. It is of the utmost importance to exclude infection at this site, as the implications of this are serious. A clean-catch specimen of urine or suprapubic aspiration confirms the diagnosis. White cells seen on microscopy of the urine are suggestive of urinary tract infection.

In endemic regions, or for visitors to such areas, malaria must be at the top of the list of differential diagnoses; a blood smear establishes the diagnosis.

Extreme toxicity, encephalopathic features, and a focus of tenderness in bones or joints should alert the clinician to the likelihood of staphylococcal osteitis, arthritis, and septicaemia. Occult abscesses cause loin tenderness, and pelvic abscesses can be detected on rectal examination.

The likelihood of pertussis should be entertained in any infant with moderate pyrexia, an anxious look, slight periorbital oedema and a spasmodic cough. A chest radiograph and white cell count are useful.

Infective endocarditis occurs infrequently in children, but because of the grave outcome if the disease remains undiagnosed, special attention must be paid to excluding it. Among Third World children, fever, changing murmurs, and anaemia are the common features of presentation. Blood cultures, white cell counts, urine examinations, chest X-rays, and an echocardiograph (if available) assist in diagnosis. To exclude rheumatic fever one should carefully palpate for nodules, examine for arthritis, and listen for murmurs.

The consequences of an unsuspected meningitis are very serious, so even in the absence of any clues, a cerebrospinal fluid examination must be undertaken. This investigation may also suggest the possibility of encephalitis or of a brain abscess. Hypothalamic lesions (e.g., tumours) may cause PUO.

In well-off communities where health care facilities are appropriately utilized, an apparently benign fever may reflect the early stage of severe infections such as meningitis, pneumonia, arthritis, and septicaemia, due to organisms such as *H. influenzae* or *pneumococcus* in infants and children, and to Gram-negative organisms or *Streptococcus B* in neonates.

Enteroviral infections occasionally cause prolonged fevers, and a macular skin rash should raise the examiner's suspicion of these organisms being responsible for the PUO.

Where there is multisystem involvement and the above causes have been addressed, collagen diseases must always be considered. Each of these diseases has certain characteristic features which aid in establishing the diagnosis. For example, fever, musculoskeletal features, rash, and glomerulonephritis suggest systemic lupus erythematosus. Rarely, the signs do not fall within a recognized pattern of a single syndrome, but reveal overlapping features of several autoimmune disorders. Auto-antibodies, especially anti-nuclear factor, are helpful. However, antibodies to body constituents may be present in healthy black children.

Dehydration, hyperthyroidism, and high environmental temperatures are some metabolic causes of fever. Malignancies such as lymphoma may also produce fever, and therefore bone tenderness, lymphadenopathy, anaemia, and splenomegaly should be specifically sought.

Features suggesting specific organisms are given in *Table 8.1*. *Table 8.2* lists the probable infections which occur in association with some specific disease states.

Investigations

There can be no uniform rules governing the type and number of investigations to be done in cases of fever; the approach is determined by the epidemiology of local diseases, the presence of underlying disorders, the age of the patient, and physical signs detected. At primary care level investigations should be done only if there is suspicion of a specific disease, or if the fever does not settle within 3–4 days. The following investigations are frequently undertaken if it is necessary to probe the cause of pyrexia: urine, full bood count (including malaria), chest radiograph, tuberculin test, blood culture, lumbar puncture, stools, and serological tests such as a Widal.

Treatment

Therapy should obviously be directed to the cause of the fever. However, in many cases the aetilogy is not immediately clear, and the clinician has to treat on the basis of probability. In our experience, for example, a child with PUO would be put on treatment for tuberculosis and typhoid, and occasionally for amoebiasis, until a firm diagnosis has been made. If there is a suspicion of tuberculosis it is far better to start specific therapy immediately, and to discontinue treatment if investigations do

Table 8.1 Features suggesting specific organisms

Meningococcus	Petechiae, meningitis, arthritis, Waterhouse-Friedrichsen syndrome
Chronic meningococcaemia	Pyrexia of unknown origin, erythema nodosum
Streptococcus pneumoniae	Lobar pneumonia, meningitis
E. coli	Jaundice pyelonephritis
S. typhi	Headache, confusion, intestinal disturbance
Staphylococcus aureus	Skin infection, bullous lesions, osteitis, lung abscess, pericarditis, subacute pyomyositis
Haemolytic streptococcus	Anaemia
Streptococcus viridans	Low-grade infective endocarditis
Brucella	Undulant fever, arthritis
Listeria monocytogenes	Meningitis, miliary granulomata
Yersinia	Convulsions, painful joints
Y. pestis	Gross purpura, bubonic glandular enlargement, pneumonia
Clostridium welchii	Gas gangrene
Psuedomonas	Necrotic, septic, purplish skin lesions
Avirulent organisms	e.g., *Staphylococcus albus* and *epidermidis, Streptococcus faecalis* in state of depressed immunity such as kwashiorkor, leukaemia

not support the diagnosis. Basic side-room techniques (urine, CSF, stools, white cell count) must be done immediately in order to facilitate a rational choice of antibiotics.

Should antipyretics be given? There is no agreement on this, although in practice most clinicians would answer in the affirmative. Children tolerate temperatures of 38–40 °C fairly well, but above 41 °C problems arise. These include anorexia, irritability, discomfort, and the likelihood of convulsions in those who are susceptible. The disadvantages of reducing the temperature are the risks of side-effects of the drugs, and masking the underlying cause. Fever also appears to benefit immune responsiveness by its effect on increased phagocytosis, enhanced leucocyte mobilty, lymphocytic activation, interferon production, and decreased iron mobilization. The final decision to treat rests on an assessment of risks and benefits — not only to the child, but also to anxious parents and attendants.

Symptomatic treatment of a child with fever is as follows:

Physical methods: Tepid baths, sponging, removal of excess clothing, maintaining hydration.
Drugs: Paracetamol 5–10 mg/kg 6-hourly; Ibuprofen 2–5 mg/kg 6-hourly.

Dysentery

The word dysentery is derived form the Greek *dys* = bad, and *entera* = bowels. Traditionally it implies the passage of blood and mucus in the stools as the result of the infection of the large bowel by bacteria (shigella), or amoebae *(Entamoeba histolytica)*. A number of other bacteria and parasites may cause dysentery when they invade the colonic mucosa.

Bacteria

- shigella
- salmonella, including *S. typhi*
- entero-invasive *E. coli*
- campylobacter
- yersinia
- *Clostridium difficile.*

Parasites

- *E. histolytica*
- *Balantidium coli*
- malaria
- *Trichuris trichiura*
- *Schistosoma mansoni*
- ankylostoma.

Although in the vast majority dysentery is infective in orgin, non-specific ulcerative colitis is occasionally encountered in childhood.

When blood and mucus are passed without any faecal matter, intussusception must be considered. This may occur *de novo,* or as a complication of acute infective diarrhoea or dysentery of any cause.

Dysentery may present with frank blood where the haemorrhage from an eroded vessel obscures the presence of mucus. In these cases other causes of bleeding must be considered, e.g., Schönlein-Henoch purpura, Meckel's diverticulum, and

Table 8.2   Fever in children with underlying disease

Underlying disease	Likely organisms
Protein-energy malnutrition	Respiratory and gastrointestinal infections, septicaemia, herpes (disseminated), adenovirus, fungi
Post-measles	Herpes (disseminated), adenovirus, Gram-negative or Gram-positive organisms, TB, candida
Schistosomiasis	Typhoid, hepatitis B
Sickle-cell anaemia	Pneumococcus, *H. influenzae,* salmonella
Rheumatic fever	Infective endocarditis, brain abscess
Malignancies	Septicaemia, Gram-negative organisms, fungi, protozoa
Neprotic syndrome	Pneumococcus, other bacteria
Hydrocephalus (with shunt)	Ventriculitis, septicaemia
Renal tract anomalies	Gram-negative infections
Congenital heart disease	Infective endocarditis, brain abscess

polyps. Blood on the surface of the stool is likely to be caused by ano-rectal pathology, e.g., fissure-in-ano. In the newborn, necrotizing enterocolitis rarely presents as bleeding per rectum.

Bacillary dysentery (shigellosis)
Shigellae are Gram-negative, non-motile, aerobic, slender rods. Their natural habitat is limited to the intestinal tract of man and other primates. Four strains or sub-groups are responsible for bacillary dysentery: *Shigella dysenteriae, Shigella flexneri, Shigella boydii*, and *Shigella sonnei*.

Epidemiology
Shigella organisms occur in all parts of the world, remaining endemic even in developed countries, where *S. sonnei* accounts for most cases. In tropical areas both epidemic and endemic forms occur. The infecting dose is small, and spread from person to person is particularly likely to occur in overcrowded home conditions or in institutions. Children with diarrhoea are more likely to spread infection than asymptomatic carriers. In the tropics, infection may be spread by flies or by contaminated food.

Clinical picture
The incubation period is short, from 1–4 days. The onset is abrupt, with fever, abdominal pain, and watery stools (often, but not invariably, containing blood and mucus). In young infants, vomiting may be the presenting symptom. The illness may be mild and self-limiting, especially in *S. sonnei* infections in developed countries, but may be severe, with marked dehydration leading to circulatory collapse. Encephalopathy, meningism, and convulsions may occur. Disseminated intravascular coagulation and haemolytic-uraemic syndrome may complicate the clinical picture. A reactive arthritis is a well-recognized association in genetically predisposed individuals. Rarely, the organisms may be isolated from the bloodstream.

Management
Mild cases require no specific therapy, and chemotherapy in particular is unnecessary because it does not influence the course of the disease or the carrier state. In severe cases, replacement of fluid and electrolytes is necessary, and antibiotics such as co-trimoxazole or ampicillin may be given, depending on the sensitivity of locally prevalent strains.

Salmonellae
These are Gram-negative, motile, non-lactose-fermenting, aerobic rods. The majority of the more than 1 700 serotypes known are primarily parasites in animals, but may cause gastroenteritis or septicaemia in humans. The enteric fever organisms, *S. typhi* and *S. paratyphi A, B,* and *C,* are exclusively human parasites and will not be considered further here *(see Typhoid, below)*. Transmission is by ingestion of dairy products, undercooked or cold meat, or contaminated food and water. Human carriers play a role in spreading the bacteria. Formerly regarded as being primarily enteropathic in action, it is now recognized that an invasive colitis (i.e., entero-invasive) can occur and produce ulceration of the colon.

Clinical manifestations
An incubation period of 12–24 hours is followed by abrupt onset of diarrhoea, vomiting, abdominal pain, and fever. Stools are usually watery, but may contain blood and mucus.

The severity of the illness varies from a mild, self-limiting attack of diarrhoea and vomiting which lasts a few days, to that in which the child is acutely ill with high fever and severe dehydration. Abdominal distension due to colonic dilatation may occur. Marked irritability, meningism, encephalopathy, and convulsions may occur. Temporary improvement is often followed by frequent relapses of diarrhoea, but persistence beyond 4 weeks is uncommon. Continued fever in a severely ill patient usually indicates septicaemia or, in the very young, localization of the infection in the meninges, bone, spleen, lung, or some other site. Salmonella infections of the bone commonly occur in sickle-cell anaemia.

Treatment
Antibodies are not indicated in infections localized to the bowel. They do not influence the clinical illness and may prolong the carrier state. Many salmonellae show multi-resistance to chemotherapeutic agents. Septicaemia or metastatic foci are

161

indications for antibiotic therapy. The drug of choice will depend on the sensitivity of the organisms. Response to therapy may be slow.

E. coli infections
Certain strains of O serogroups of *E. coli* have been incriminated in outbreaks of dysentery in many parts of the world. These produce invasive inflammatory changes in the colon, unlike the enteropathogenic and enterotoxigenic strains which affect the small intestine and cause gastroenteritis *(see Chapter 11, Gastrointestinal Disorders)*.

Campylobacter infections
Infections occur world-wide, more commonly in older children and young adults. Infection is frequently from animals: cows, sheep, dogs, and cats have been implicated. After an incubation period of 3–5 days, fever, nausea, vomiting, and abdominal pain precede the onset of diarrhoea with watery stools which may contain blood and mucus. Colitis may be indistinguishable from other causes of inflammatory bowel disease, and occasionally it may mimic an acute abdomen. A reactive arthritis has been a complication.

Management
As it is usually a self-limiting disease, antibiotics are not indicated, but erythromycin may be beneficial in certain severe forms.

Yersinia enterocolitica
This organism is a recognized cause of diarrhoea in children, and commonly invades the terminal ileum, but may cause dysentery. Animals are probably the reservoir for the infection.

Pseudomembranous colitis
Diarrhoea in association with antibiotic therapy is common but usually mild. Rarely, a severe form of diarrhoea of sudden onset and accompanied by abdominal pain and blood in the stools occurs about one week after the commencement of antibiotics. Dehydration, electrolyte disturbances, and shock soon develop, and the mortality rate is high in the absence of treatment. Patchy, confluent, white or yellow-green plaques consisting of mucus, fibrin, inflammatory cells, and necrotic epithelium which may slough and leave shallow ulcers of the bowel, are pathological findings. Clindamycin and lincomycin are the antibiotics most commonly implicated, but many antibiotics — including penicillin, ampicillin, tetracycline, and chloramphenicol — have been associated with pseudomembranous colitis.

It was previously believed to be caused by the overgrowth of bowel organisms such as staphylococci, which were resistant to the antiobiotic being employed. Now there is ample proof that a toxin produced by *Clostridium dificile* is the cause of pseudomembranous colitis. Vancomycin is the treatment of choice, but is not effective in every case, and is expensive and toxic. Metronidazole may be of use, but has itself been incriminated in producing pseudomembranous colitis. Recognized in the pre-antibiotic era in association with surgical procedures and severely debilitating conditions, it is possible that ischaemia may play a role in the development of this serious state.

Pseudomembranous colitis is rare in childhood.

Entamoeba histolytica
Amoebiasis is the state of harbouring the parasite *E. histolytica*.

Incidence and epidemiology
It has been estimated that 10% of the world's population is infected, but in the majority of infections *E. histolytica* is a harmless commensal. The incidence of infection and disease is highest in subtropical and tropical areas, but lack of sanitation and personal hygiene are more important factors than are climatic conditions. The parasite is harboured in the large intestine and is spread by faecal contamination of food and water. No age group is exempt from infection. Dysentery and hepatic amoebiasis may occur in infants as young as 3 weeks of age, when the source of infection may be from the mother's perineum. Mothers of infants with amoebiasis are commonly found to be harbouring *E. histolytica* cysts.

Aetiology and pathology
(See Fig. 8.1.)
Infection is acquired by swallowing cysts, which are $10-20\,\mu$ in size and contain up to four nuclei.

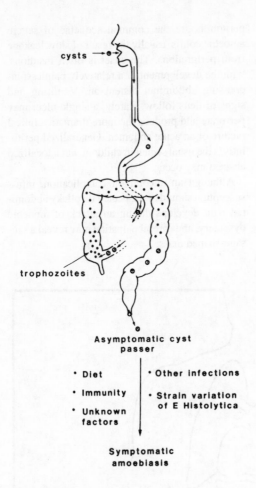

cysts

trophozoites

Asymptomatic cyst passer

* Diet
* Immunity
* Unknown factors

* Other Infections
* Strain variation of E Histolytica

Symptomatic amoebiasis

Fig. 8.1 **E. histolytica**

Motile trophozoites emerge from the cysts and travel to the caecum, where they colonize. They are also continuously carried further down the large bowel, the largest number tending to collect in areas of greatest faecal stasis such as the caecum, lower ascending colon, sigmoid colon, and rectum. Trophozoites ingest bacteria and particles of faecal matter, grow, and multiply by binary fission, but usually cause no harm to their host. When they reach the lower bowel where faeces are more solid, they encyst, the single nucleus divides by four, and these mature infective cysts are passed in the stool. Trophozoites are usually passed in the stool, but any cause of diarrhoea may lead to their more rapid passage down the colon. The finding of trophozoites in a diarrhoeic stool does not necessarily indicate that the amoebae are

causing the diarrhoea. It is a matter of conjecture as to why invasion of the bowel wall occurs in some individuals and not in others. Diet, immune status, and other bowel infections may all play a role. There is some evidence that certain strains of *E. histolytica* may be more pathogenic than others. Invasion is accomplished by lytic enzymes secreted by trophozoites, which damage the bowel wall and capillaries. Trophozoites ingest red cells and produce ulcers varying in extent from the pinhead-sized lesions confined to the caecum, to extensive, deep, confluent ulceration throughout the bowel. Studies have shown that in severe cases, trophozoites invade colonic blood vessels and cause well-demarcated areas of infarction. Extension through the bowel wall leads to peritonitis. Rarely, the extension occurs to the skin of the perineum. Access to the liver is via the portal vein. Here tissue necrosis leads to abscess formation. Rupture of the abscess may involve adjacent spaces or tissue. Blood-borne embolic spread to remote sites such as the lung or brain is encountered occasionally.

Clinical manifestations

Intestinal amoebiasis may be asymptomatic. Non-invasive parasites produce no symptoms, and even mild colonic invasion evidenced by the passage of haematophagous trophozoites may not produce symptoms.

Symptomatic intestinal amoebiasis varies in severity from mild intermittent diarrhoea which may last for weeks or months, to severe fulminating dysentery, with the passage of many blood-stained, mucoid stools which contain little or no faecal matter. The onset tends to be insidious, but may be abrupt in children.

Abdominal discomfort and colonic tenderness may be found, and liver tenderness elicited in the absence of hepatitis. Fever is usually absent or slight, and the appetite unaffected. Proctoscopy or sigmoidoscopy frequently reveals ulcers, varying in size and covered with a yellow exudate. The intervening bowel is normal.

In severe cases, dehydration and symptoms and signs of electrolyte imbalance develop rapidly. Generalized abdominal tenderness and distension suggest impending peritonitis, even in the presence of bowel sounds *(see Table 8.3)*.

Local complications
(See Fig. 8.2.)
Table 8.4 lists the complications of invasive amoebiasis as seen in Durban. Perforation and

Table 8.3 Helpful features in the diagnosis of transmural spread of amoebiasis and impending perforation

Malnutrition
Toxicity
Abdominal distension
Straight X-ray abdomen:
   'Crenated' colon with loss of haustrations
   'Fixing' of colon in left iliac fossa with surrounding mottling
Failure to respond within 24 hours to metronidazole

peritonitis are the common sequelae of severe amoebic colitis, usually the result of slow leakage from perforations. The onset is often insidious, with the development of a relatively painless, increasing abdominal distension. Vomiting and signs of ileus follow. Rarely, a single ulcer may perforate and produce the more dramatic clinical picture of an acute abdomen. Generalized peritonitis is the usual sequel in children, but a localized abscess may occur.

Although an uncommon complication, intussusception should be suspected if colicky abdominal pain develops during an attack of amoebic dysentery, and careful palpation may reveal a sausage-shaped mass.

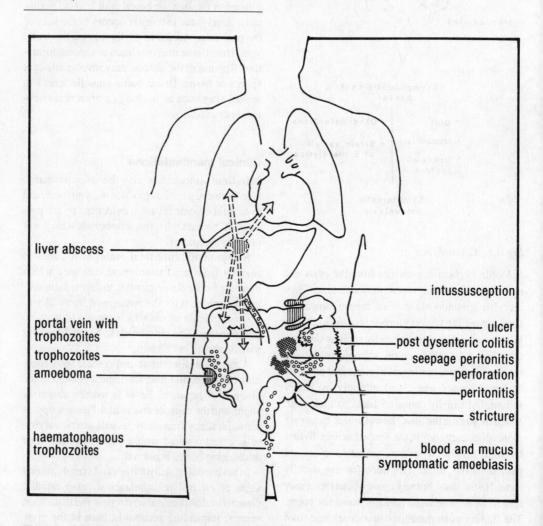

liver abscess

intussusception

portal vein with
trophozoites

ulcer
post dysenteric colitis

trophozoites

seepage peritonitis

amoeboma

perforation

peritonitis

stricture

haematophagous
trophozoites

blood and mucus
symptomatic amoebiasis

Fig. 8.2 Complications caused by **E. histolytica** *infection*

Strictures at sites of severe ulceration tend to be more common in the descending colon and rectum. They present as palpable masses of faeces in the left iliac fossa, and not usually as intestinal obstruction.

Amoeboma, a granuloma of the bowel, presents as a tender mass, most commonly in the right iliac fossa.

Haemorrhage as a result of erosion of a blood vessel in the bowel wall may be profuse and lead to shock and collapse.

Post-dysenteric colitis is a sequel of severe colitis, and may be seen in children who have survived a seepage peritonitis. Continued diarrhoea or dysentery leads to severe debility and emaciation, requiring weeks or months of supportive therapy. Repeated stool examination should be made to exclude a relapse of amoebic dysentery.

Table 8.4   Complications of invasive amoebiasis — King Edward VIII Hospital, Durban, 1960 – 82

Frequent complications	No.	Mortality%
Dysentery, peritonitis and ALA*	18	100
Dysentery and peritonitis	90	89
Dysentery and ALA*	163	50
Dysentery	1176	22
ALA*	273	17
Total	1720	28

Rare complications	No.	Mortality (No.)
Pericarditis	7	5
Intussusception	7	4
Amoeba	5	1
Apendicitis	3	3
Brain abscess	2	2
Colonic stricture	2	-
Volvulus	1	1
Total	27	16

* ALA = Amoebic liver abscess

Systemic complications

Hepatic amoebiasis is the most common extra-intestinal complication. Amoebic liver abscess is the only pathologically proven form.

In childhood, the majority of liver abscesses present in the first 3 years of life, with no gender preference. A history of previous or concomitant dysentery is found in more than 50% of cases, and swelling of the abdomen is a common complaint. Fever, tender hepatomegaly, and anaemia are almost invariable findings.

Hepatic amoebiasis should be considered in the differential diagnosis whenever there is unexplained fever, and in all instances of liver enlargement, especially when associated with anaemia.

Palpation often reveals a mass in the liver, which may be visible. A single abscess most often involves the right lobe, resulting in elevation of the diaphragm and signs at the right lung base. Multiple abscesses are more common in infancy and early childhood, but jaundice is rare. Extension or rupture of a liver abscess is a serious complication. In children, rupture into the peritoneal cavity occurs more commonly than into the pleural space. Because amoebic liver abscesses are usually bacteriologically sterile, extension into the peritoneal cavity is accompanied by less severe illness than that produced when amoebic colitis is complicated by peritonitis. A left lobe abscess may cause an effusion in, or rupture into, the pericardium, resulting in sudden, severe distress and signs of cardiac tamponade. An effusion of the adjacent pleural space may complicate abscesses situated near the superior surface of the right lobe of the liver, whilst rupture of the abscess through the diaphragm leads to an amoebic empyema.

Bacterial contamination of the liver abscess may cause persistent fever and failure of the abscess to resolve, despite adequate anti-amoebic therapy.

Other very rare extra-intestinal complications are cutaneous amoebiasis involving the perianal area and perineum, or blood-borne amoebic abscesses of the brain or lungs.

Diagnosis

Identification of haematophagous *E. histolytica* trophozoites in bowel contents or liver pus establishes the diagnosis of invasive amoebiasis. These motile trophozoites are most readily seen in freshly passed specimens or scrapings obtained from ulcers at sigmoidoscopy, or in freshly aspirated pus. Repeated stool examinations may be needed before the parasite is identified. Amoebic cysts are less fragile, and retain their characteristic features for hours after being passed, but as the number of cysts fluctuates, a single negative finding does not exclude the diagnosis.

Aspiration of bacteriologically sterile pus is strongly suggestive of amoebic liver abscess. The pink or reddish-brown colour ('anchovy pus') may not be seen; the pus is often yellowish-grey on first aspiration.

A full blood count very commonly reveals anaemia and neutrophil leucocytosis in amoebic liver abscess, whilst a chest radiograph may show elevation of the right diaphragm. Ultrasound examination of the liver is helpful in diagnosing the presence and number of abscesses. Radioactive liver scanning provides similar information.

Serology: The gel diffusion test is an invaluable clinical tool, and is positive in almost all children with invasive disease. Repeat tests in those who are negative will show seroconversion. A number of other serological tests are available, but the advantage of a fluorescent antibody test based on whole amoeba is that it can be used to monitor IgG and IgM response.

Treatment

(Also see Chapter 28, Surgical Problems.)
Imidazole derivates — metronidazole (Flagyl®) 50 mg/kg/day for 5–7 days, or tinidazole (Fasigyn®) for 3 days, are highly effective in the vast majority of cases. In uncomplicated amoebic dysentery these preparations are given by mouth, and symptoms subside rapidly. If they persist after 48 hours, the diagnosis should be questioned.

In severe amoebic colitis with impending or established peritonitis, metronidazole should be given intravenously until such time as oral therapy becomes possible. Fluid and electrolyte losses should be corrected, and gastric suction employed until signs of ileus subside. Profound anaemia indicates the need for blood transfusion. Gram-negative septicaemia and chest infection, which are often present, are indications for broad spectrum antibiotic therapy. Steroid therapy is contra-indicated.

Amoebic liver abscesses may respond to metronidazole alone, but large abscesses — those present as palpable masses and producing marked elevation of the diaphragm or causing persistent localized tenderness — should be aspirated with a wide-bore needle. Persistence of symptoms despite adequate amoebicidal therapy is also an indication for aspiration. Repeated aspirations may be necessary. On rare occasions, posteriorly situated abscesses may require aspiration under direct vision at laparotomy.

Until more experience is gained, the role of surgery in the management of seepage peritonitis, complicating severe amoebic colitis, remains in doubt. The value of surgical repair is obvious in those rare instances where a single ulcer perforates to produce an acute peritonitis. Surgery is not indicated in the management of strictures and amoebomas.

Asymptomatic individuals with amoebic cysts or trophozoites in the stool should be treated, because they are exposed to potential pathogens which may lead to disease at a later date. Diloxanide furoate, 25 mg/kg/day for 10 days, or metronidazole should be given by mouth.

Balantidiasis

The large ciliate protozoan, *Balantidium coli*, is usually a harmless commensal in the large bowel of humans, but under rare circumstances may invade the terminal ileum and colon to cause ulcers or abscesses of the mucosa and submucosa. Chronic recurrent diarrhoea alternating with constipation may be a complaint, and occasionally severe dysentery with bloody, mucoid stools, tenesmus, and colic may develop. Fatal cases have been described. Metronidazole is the treatment of choice.

Malaria

P. falciparum infections occasionally present with passage of bloody, mucoid stools.

Dysentery caused by helminths

See Parasitic Helminths, below.

Bacterial infections

Pertussis (whooping cough)

Epidemiology

Pertussis is caused by the organism *Bordetella pertussis*. It shares minor antigenic components with *Bordetella parapertussis* and *Bordetella bronchiseptica*, both of which give rise to respiratory infections resembling pertussis.

Pertussis occurs world-wide, but the mortality is higher in poor communities. It is spread by droplet, and since attack rates are highest following household exposure, it is likely that prolonged exposure is important in the spread of the disease.

About 65% of cases occur under the age of 7 years. Morbidity is the same in urban and rural communities, and whether epidemic or endemic conditions prevail. Morbidity and mortality are highest in infants. A patient is infectious from 7 days after exposure to 3 weeks after the onset of paroxysms.

Immunity

No transplacental immunity is conferred to newborns. Acquired immunity is always lifelong. Acellular vaccines containing selected and detoxified antigens are in use in some countries. These have greater protective efficiency and markedly reduced side-effects compared with the original whole-cell vaccine still in use in most countries. Whole-cell vaccine may not prevent disease, but does decrease the severity and duration in those who develop it *(see below for vaccination details)*.

Pathogenesis

The organism does not invade tissues or blood, but it does cause necrosis of ciliate epithelium in the respiratory tract. Sticky mucus and sloughed cells which accumulate in bronchi result in obstruction, leading to patchy atelectasis and emphysema.

The neurological and haematological effects probably result from haemagglutinins present in the organism.

Clinical features

The incubation period is 7 days, and the course of the disease is divided into stages:

The catarrhal stage lasts for 1–2 weeks. The symptoms are of an upper respiratory infection with a short, dry, nocturnal cough.

The paroxysmal stage lasts for 2–4 weeks. The cough becomes paroxysmal; it is followed by a forceful inspiration usually associated with a whoop. At the end of a paroxysm the child often vomits mucus or feeds. Haemoptysis may occur.

The cough is most common at night, and is precipitated by eating, drinking, or crying.

In the young infant the cough is often atypical: the whoop may be absent and paroxysms may be less frequent.

The convalescent phase lasts 2–4 weeks, and is marked by a decrease in the severity and frequency of paroxysmal coughing, which finally ceases. Symptoms often recur for up to a year after the disease, whenever the child contracts an upper respiratory infection.

Diagnosis

The diagnosis is usually made on the distinctive clinical features of the cough. A leucocytosis in excess of 10 000/mm^3 (sometimes rising to 100 000/mm^3), with a relative lymphocytosis, occurs from the second to fifth weeks of disease.

Special techniques of nasopharyngeal culture or serology using the ELISA method are not usually needed to confirm the diagnosis.

Differential diagnosis of the cough:

◆ A cough suggestive of pertussis may occur in infants with bronchiolitis, chlamydial pneumonitis, or cystic fibrosis. In older children a similar cough may accompany interstitial pneumonia, inhalation of a foreign body, or pressure on the trachea by enlarged tracheobronchial glands.

◆ Infections with *B. parapertussis* and *B. bronchiseptica* produce a clinical picture indistinguishable from pertussis.

Treatment

Isolation from susceptible children is required during the infectious period. Severe cases, especially infants, are best managed in hospital, where close nursing supervision is available. Factors which provoke coughing should be avoided.

Frequent vomiting may affect nutrition. Small feeds, if necessary by nasogastric tube, may reduce frequency of vomiting. Bland rather than crumbly food is better in older children.

Antibiotics effective against *B. pertussis* (erythromycin, co-trimoxazole, chloramphenicol), if given within the *first week* of illness, before paroxysms develop, may shorten the course of the disease. If given later, the nasopharynx is cleared of organisms in 2–4 days and so the period of infectivity is shortened. A neonate who has been exposed to the infection should receive a prophylactic antibiotic.

Antitussives, sedation with phenobarbitone or promethazine hydrochloride, bronchodilators, and mucolytics have all been prescribed, but have not been shown to be more than marginally beneficial.

There is evidence that steroids are effective in reducing the paroxysms and shortening the course of the disease (prednisone 5–10 mg/kg/day for 1 week). This should be reserved for severe cases, especially in infants less than 9 months old.

Complications
Otitis media is common.
Respiratory tract: Pneumonia is responsible for most deaths under 3 years of age, and is due to bacterial or viral superinfection.

Atelectasis may only be detected by chest radiograph. Re-expansion of lobar or segmental collapse may not be achieved by chest physiotherapy, and bronchoscopy will be needed to aspirate the blocked bronchus. Bronchiectasis will occur in persistent atelectatic segments, a complication now rarely seen in the First World, but still a problem in poor communities.

Infrequently subcutaneous and interstitial emphysema or pneumothorax follow rupture of alveoli during violent coughing.

Encephalopathy with irritability, fits, or coma supervenes in 0.1– 4% of cases. This is due either to toxic or asphyxial brain damage, or to intracranial haemorrhage.

Treatment is supportive: meticulous nursing care, sedation, and oxygen.

Congestive cardiac *failure* may occur in a few cases with severe pneumonia. Myocarditis due to the exotoxin of the bacterium may also be a factor.

Treatment consists of oxygen, digitalis, and diuretics.

Increased venous pressure during coughing may lead to epistaxis, subconjunctival haemorrhage, skin petechiae, or intracranial haemorrhage. The frenum of the tongue may be traumatized on the lower incisors during coughing. Increased abdominal pressure during paroxysms may cause hernias or prolapsed rectum.

Prognosis
The case fatality rate has declined with reduction in severity of disease due to immunization and improved control of secondary pulmonary infection.

Complications worsen the prognosis, and these occur most frequently in infancy. About 10% of all cases and 70% of all deaths occur in the first year of life.

Typhoid
Typhoid fever is endemic in Africa, the Middle and Far East, south-eastern Europe, and Central and South America. Sporadic cases have a world-wide distribution, and occasional epidemics occur even in countries which, under normal circumstances, have a very low incidence of the disease. In Britain up to 400 cases, and one or two deaths, occur each year. In the majority of instances the infection is acquired while holidaying in countries where typhoid is endemic. In South Africa, annual notifications have remained remarkably constant, at about 4 000, for over 50 years.

Salmonella typhi and *paratyphi* differ from other salmonellae in that they are primarily human pathogens. Inadequate sanitation, and faecal contamination of water supplies are obvious modes of spread. Areas in southern Africa with the highest incidence have summer rains, with the peak incidence in the hottest months, i.e., January to March. However, cases occur throughout the year, and drought also leads to an increased number of cases. No age is exempt, but schoolchildren and young adults have the highest incidence. In Durban, 11% of children with typhoid are less than 2 years old. Transplacental infection may lead to neonatal typhoid. Both sexes are equally affected.

Pathogenesis
Swallowed organisms multiply in the reticuloendothelial tissues of the small intestine and, after an incubation period of 10–20 days, invade the bloodstream, resulting in symptoms and signs. Dissemination of organisms may lead to focal involvement of many organs. Focal necrosis of the liver and inflammation of the biliary passages and gall bladder are usually present. Re-invasion of the small intestine via the biliary tract leads to the characteristic hyperplasia, necrosis, and ulceration of Peyer's patches, which may progress to perforation or haemorrhage.

Lipopolysaccharide endotoxins in the cell wall of the bacteria may also affect many organs and give rise to symptoms, signs, and complications.

Clinical features

(See Tables 8.5 and 8.6.)
As typhoid is both a septicaemia and a toxaemia, practically any organ or tissue in the body may be involved. A wide variety of symptoms and signs occur, and their severity and duration vary greatly from patient to patient. Children admitted to hospital are frequently severely ill.

Fever is the most constant of all clinical manifestations, is commonly high (39– 40 °C) and may be sustained or intermittent. Severely anaemic children and those presenting in congestive cardiac failure may become pyrexial only when the anaemia has been corrected or the cardiac failure controlled. The temperature response to successful antibiotic therapy varies, but often takes as long as 7–8 days. Rigors may be seen at the height of fever. Relative bradycardia is rare in children.

Anorexia and abdominal pain are common in children old enough to complain, and constipation may be an early feature in the older child. In those under 5 years of age, diarrhoea and vomiting often dominate the clinical picture and mask the diagnosis, which may be missed unless the accompanying high fever alerts the clinician to the possibility of typhoid.

A tender, tumid abdomen together with hepatosplenomegaly in a febrile child in an endemic

Table 8.5 Symptoms in 1 400 children with typhoid fever

Symptom	%
Fever	75
Headache	56
Cough	47
Abdominal pain	43
Diarrhoea	40
Vomiting	27
Generalized pains	14
Joint pains	9
Constipation	9
Epistaxis	3

(From the *South African Journal of Hospital Medicine*, Vol. 2, No. 10, 1976.)

Table 8.6 Signs in 1 400 children with typhoid fever

Signs	%
Pyrexia	98
Tender/tumid abdomen	49
Hepatomegaly	49
Splenomegaly	36
Anaemia	40
Bronchitis	33
Thrombocytopenia	22
Leucopenia	17
Bradycardia	1
Rose spots	0

CNS signs	
Meningism	15
Delirium	15
Stupor	3

(From the *South African Journal of Hospital Medicine*, Vol. 2, No. 10, 1976.)

area is highly suggestive of typhoid. The incidence of splenomegaly varies in different childhood series, from a little over 30% in the Durban experience to almost 100% elsewhere.

Symptoms and signs of respiratory tract involvement are present in many patients, cough being a complaint in almost half, and signs of bronchitis in one-third. Headache is a frequent presenting complaint in the older child. Delirium and signs of meningeal irritation due to meningism are common. Myalgia, arthralgia, and sore throat sometimes head the list of complaints, but epistaxis is uncommon in children. Rose spots, regarded as a diagnostic sign, are invisible or absent in pigmented skins. In the Aberdeen (Scotland) endemic, rose spots were present in less than half of the affected children. Anaemia is present in up to 40% of patients on admission. When present, leucopenia helps in establishing the diagnosis, but is relatively uncommon. A moderate leucocytosis is often found when focal involvement gives rise to complications. Thrombocytopenia, unrelated to drug therapy, may be present in one-fifth of patients, but is seldom severe.

Complications

(See Table 8.7.)
Respiratory complications in typhoid are well-documented. Pneumonia, confirmed radiologi-

Table 8.7 Complications in 1 400 children with typhoid fever

Complications	%
Respiratory:	34
Bronchopneumonia (radiological)	2
Lobar pneumonia (radiological)	16
Neurological	5
Hepatitis	4
Nephritis	4
Cardiovascular	
Gastro-intestinal:	2
Intestinal haemorrhage	2
Perforation	1
Haemolytic anaemia	

From the *South African Journal of Hospital Medicine*, Vol. 2, No. 10, 1976.

cally, was present in one-third of patients, and in over half the number of fatal cases at necropsy in Durban. Very rarely, lung abscesses and pleural effusion or empyema are seen.

The incidence of **neurological** complications is higher in children than in adults. Convulsions are common in infants and pre-school children with typhoid, but are rare in the older child. Disturbances in consciousness, aphasia, ataxia, tremor, chorea, athetosis, hemiplegia, cranial nerve palsies, and peripheral neuropathy are some of the many varied manifestations encountered. Meningeal involvement, commonly seen as meningism, occasionally gives rise to a moderate pleocytosis, and very rarely to a frankly purulent cerebrospinal fluid which yields *S. typhi*.

Hepatic: Jaundice, with disturbances of liver function suggestive of hepatitis, occurs in 5% of patients. In Durban hepatitis was found in one-quarter of necropsy cases. Less commonly, mild jaundice may result from excessive haemolysis.

Renal: Albuminuria with pyrexia is often seen in uncomplicated typhoid. Glomerulonephritis, complicating typhoid, occurs in 4% of patients in Durban. Patients with typhoid glomerulonephritis differ from those with the post-streptococcal variety in that they have longer histories of oedema in the presence of fever before admission, and a less marked reduction in the third component of complement. Renal failure in typhoid may complicate

either glomerulonephritis or acute tubular necrosis. The latter may result from dehydration. Typhoid may precipitate the haemolytic uraemic syndrome. Pyelonephritis is also described as a complication, and was seen in two children at necropsy in Durban.

Cardiovascular: Over half of the children presenting with congestive cardiac failure in typhoid may be shown to have acute glomerulonephritis or profound anaemia. The rest have clinical and electrocardiographic evidence of myocarditis. This complication, regarded as a toxic manifestation, is often present in the most severely ill patients.

Haematological: In Durban, anaemia is sufficiently common to be regarded as a clinical finding rather than a complication. It is most severe in patients with long histories of typhoid, and is presumed to be the consequence of toxic marrow depression, together with some degree of blood loss.

Haemolytic anaemia due to typhoid is well-recognized, although rare. The incidence in Durban is less than 1%. Acute haemolysis with haemoglobinuria is very rare in Durban, having been seen on only two occasions among over 2 000 patients.

Thrombocytopenia in typhoid may be the consequence of marrow depression or disseminated intravascular coagulation. Rarely, purpura may be the presenting complaint.

Gastrointestinal

Intestinal perforation: (Also see Chapter 28, Surgical Problems.) This serious complication has occurred in 2 – 3% of cases seen in Durban. The mortality rate has dropped from 61 to 25% over the past 15 years. It may complicate typhoid at any age, even in infancy.

Intestinal perforation may occur at any time after the onset of symptoms, but is most common in the second or third week of illness. Apparent clinical response to appropriate antibiotic therapy does not prevent the occurrence of intestinal perforation. The symptoms and signs present abruptly, with classical features of an acute abdomen, but in the severely ill child the onset may be insidious and the diagnosis missed. The finding of air under the diaphragm on abdominal radiographs confirms the diagnosis of perforation.

A non-obstructive ileus without perforation and presenting with vomiting, increasing abdominal distension, and decreased or absent bowel sounds may also complicate typhoid. Distended loops of bowel and air-fluid levels will be seen on X-rays. The absence of air in the peritoneal cavity distinguishes ileus from perforation.

Intestinal haemorrhage has a similar incidence to that of perforation. Sudden collapse and peripheral circulatory failure precede the passage of blood per rectum. Milder rectal bleeding without shock also occurs in typhoid. This may be the presenting complaint, but more commonly blood loss is microscopic.

Skeletal: Arthritis usually involves large joints, and is uncommon. Involvement of an intervertebral disc, which may mimic spinal tuberculosis, has been detected occasionally. Osteitis is a rare late complication.

Other rare complications include parotitis, acute cholecystitis, splenic infarcts and abscesses, peripheral thromboses, orchitis, and alopecia.

Diagnosis

The diagnosis is most often missed or delayed in the very young or when children present with symptoms and signs of focal complications. Confirmation of diagnosis is by culture of blood, stool, or urine. Rarely, *S. typhi* may be isolated from cerebrospinal fluid or pus. Blood cultures are positive in the majority at presentation. Samples should be collected at the height of fever, and repeated whenever fever remains unexplained or occurs inappropriately in such clinical conditions as acute glomerulonephritis, hepatitis, cardiac failure, or profound anaemia.

Less commonly, cultures of stool and urine yield *S. typhi*, particularly in the first week of illness.

The Widal test is of limited value in diagnosis. At least 25% of children with proven typhoid fail to show a significant titre, and false positive results may be misleading in older children in endemic areas. A rising titre is supportive evidence for the diagnosis when the clinical picture suggests typhoid.

Newer serological tests, using counter-immuno-electrophoresis, may prove superior to Widal testing, and have the additional advantage of producing results within hours.

Treatment

Chloramphenicol, 50–100 mg/kg/day, remains a valuable form of therapy. Drug resistance, failure to respond, increased relapse rate, and convalescent carrier state, together with the rare but serious complication of bone marrow depression, have created the need for alternative forms of chemotherapy.

Amoxycillin, 100 mg/kg/day, has proved effective in treatment, and has the advantage of causing less serious toxic effects. Skin reactions and drug fever may be troublesome side-effects, but the former respond to antihistamines, and both to cessation of therapy. Antibiotic therapy should continue for 21 days as shorter courses lead to a significant increase in the relapse rate.

Recently it has been shown that a short course (5 days) of ceftriaxone (80 mg/kg IM or IV once a day) is as effective as 3 weeks of chloramphenicol. Ceftriaxone therapy is cost-effective since it greatly reduces the length of hospital stay.

Correction and maintenance of fluid and electrolytes and the provision of a nutritious diet are essential components of the treatment. Haemorrhage and shock require immediate and often life-saving blood transfusions.

Corticosteroids are believed to be the antitoxigenic, and have been recommended in severely ill patients. They apparently cause no increase in the incidence of perforation or haemorrhage. Perforation requires prompt surgical intervention if recognized reasonably early. Intravenous fluid therapy is recommended in advanced peritonitis and in the presence of ileus without perforation.

Relapses

Clinical relapse may occur within days or weeks of completion of therapy. In Aberdeen, Scotland, 21% of children relapsed after 14 days of antibiotic therapy. In Durban, experience with amoxycillin and chloramphenicol therapy over many years has shown that 21 days of therapy reduces the rate to 1% in amoxycillin-treated patients and 5% in chloramphenicol-treated patients. Relapse rate with ceftriaxone is similar to that with chloramphenicol.

Carriers

Convalescent carriage is relatively common. Most cases clear spontaneously without treatment. In Durban, convalescent carriers occur more commonly after chloramphenicol (6%) than after amoxycillin (less than 1%).

Permanent carriers are said to occur in 2–5% of all patients, but are very rare in children.

Prevention

Two new vaccines are licensed for prevention:
1. Ty21a attenuated live *S. typhi* oral vaccine in an enteric-coated formulation is given on alternate days for three doses. This gives 70–90% protection for 3 years, and does not cause adverse reactions.
2. Vi capsular polysaccharide vaccine given in a single parenteral dose results in 70–80% protection for 2 years. Trials for longer efficacy are in progress.

At present both these vaccines are given to schoolchildren. Information on the efficacy of Ty21a in infants is not available. Vi capsular polysaccharide vaccine is not effective in the very young, but trials of conjugates with proteins (e.g., tetanus toxoid) are underway to determine whether this improves immunological response in those under 2 years old.

The provision of a water supply free of contamination should be the aim in all endemic areas.

Syphilis

Humans are the natural host of the spirochaete *Treponema pallidum* and serve as the vector for spread of the disease which, in adults, is usually by sexual contact. In children, syphilis is most commonly acquired transplacentally, the fetus being infected by an infected mother. Rarely, infection may occur from contact with infectious lesions during passage through the birth canal. This constitutes congenital syphilis.

Sexual abuse or direct contact in a non-venereal manner may lead to syphilis in the older child.

The spectrum of syphilis in childhood is outlined in *Table 8.8*.

Congenital syphilis

Incidence: The incidence is not known, but the number of cases of congenital syphilis correlates with the incidence of primary and secondary syphilis in women and the adequacy of antenatal care. There appears to be a world-wide resurgence.

Pathogenesis: It was believed that spirochaetes were unable to penetrate the Langhans cells of the early placenta, and that infection of the fetus occurred only after the first 16 weeks, when these cells atrophied. However, it has been shown that infection may occur as early as the first trimester, even though histological evidence of syphilis is rarely seen until the second trimester. Clinico-pathological effects in syphilis are determined by host immune responses, and therefore a possible explanation is that the fetus is able to exhibit an inflammatory response only in the second trimester. Syphilis is not a common cause for early abortion, and adequate therapy of the mother during the first trimester prevents congenital

Table 8.8   Spectrum of syphilis in childhood

| | Congenital | | Acquired | |
	Early	Late	Endemic	Acquired
1. Transmission	Transplacental	Transplacental	Non-venereal (contact)	Sexual abuse
2. Pathogenesis	Host response to (T. pallidum)	Stigmata	Host response	Host response
3. Age	Newborn Infancy Early childhood (< 2 years)	> 2 years	Childhood 2 – 10 years	Any age
4. Manifestations	Extensive resembles 2° syphilis	Restricted, stigmata	Usually 2° and 3° stages	May go through 1°, 2° and 3° stages

syphilis in the fetus. Haematological spread from an infected mother involves the placenta, and may lead to pathology in many organs in the fetus.

The placenta in congential syphilis is large, pale, and greasy. Vasculitis may lead to infarction and intrauterine death, premature delivery, or intrauterine growth retardation.

Clinical manifestations: *(See Table 8.9.)* Prenatal infection may be obvious at birth, or signs and symptoms may be delayed for weeks or months. The lesions correspond roughly to those seen in the secondary stage of syphilis. Those occurring during the first 2 years of life are referred to as early congenital syphilis, and those manifesting after this time, late congenital syphilis. Overlapping may occur.

Early congenital syphilis: *(Also see Chapter 24, Dermatological Disorders.)* The *skin and mucous membranes* are commonly involved. The earliest sign is often a transient bullous eruption containing many spirochaetes (syphilitic pemphigus). Characteristically involving the palms and soles, the bullae rapidly rupture, leading to desquamation and a glazed pink appearance to the palms and soles. Reddish maculo-papules, not confined to the soles and palms, which darken with age but which may also desquamate, appear later.

Condylomata lata — flat, wart-like, moist structures near the anal margin — are occasionally seen and are highly infectious. Mucous patches in the mouth may lead to fissuring and scarring at the angles of the mouth.

Rhinitis frequently occurs after the first week or two. The mucous discharge from the nose (snuffles) may become tinged with blood, and is teeming with spirochaetes.

Hepatosplenomegaly is present in a very high percentage of cases. Jaundice may occur, but is less common.

Haematological involvement manifesting with anaemia is very common. Erythroblastosis, with many nucleated red cells on a peripheral smear, together with hydrops fetalis and haemolytic anaemia may produce a picture which has to be differentiated from isoimmunization. A leuco-erythroblastic picture with immature white and red cells may be seen on a peripheral blood smear. At autopsy, extramedullary haemopoiesis involving the liver and spleen is a common finding. Thrombocytopenia and disseminated intravascular coagulation may lead to purpura or bleeding from other sites.

Congenital syphilis is a rare cause of a leukaemoid reaction.

Table 8.9 Manifestations of congenital syphilis

	Early	Late
Skin	Bullae	
	Desquamation	
	Red maculo-papules	
	Condylomata	
Mucous membranes	Fissures	Scars at corners of
	Scars	mouth (rhagades)
	Rhinitis	Flat nasal bridge ('saddle nose')
Liver/ spleen	Hepatosplenomegaly	
	Jaundice	
	Hepatitis	
Haematological	Anaemia	
	Haemolytic	
	Leuco-erythroblastic	
	Normocytic, normochronic	
	Leukaemoid reaction	
	Thrombocytopenia	
	DIC	
Bones	Metaphysitis	Sabre tibia
	Diaphysitis	Bossing
	Periostitis	Deformities of maxilla
	Meningo-encephalitis	Chronic meningo-vascular disease
CNS	Convulsions	Hydrocephalus
	Hydrocephalus	Mental retardation
		Cranial nerve palsies
		Hemiplegia
		Paresis and tabes
Renal	Nephrotic syndrome	
Other	SGA	Malnutrition
	Pseudoparalysis	Hutchinson's teeth
	Oedema	Mulberry molars
	Pancreatitis	Caries
	Gastrointestinal disease	Nerve deafness
	Pneumonia alba	Painless synovitis
	Susceptibility to other infections	Interstitial keratitis
	Chorio-retinitis	Argyll Robertson pupil
		Optic atrophy

Bone involvement should be sought on radiographs of the long bones *(see Fig. 8.3)* in any infant suspected of being syphilitic. The long bones are most commonly involved, but, rarely, the phalanges (syphilitic dactylitis) and metacarpals may also be affected. Involvement of the maxilla may lead to facial deformities, and involvement of the skull to bossing.

Characteristically, multiple bones are involved, usually symmetrically, and the lower limbs tend to be more affected than the upper. The metaphysis, diaphysis, and periosteum may be involved; the epiphysis is spared.

Translucent bands in the juxta-epiphyseal areas are the earliest manifestations of syphilitic bone disease. Frank bone destruction at the metaphysis, appearing as 'rat bitten' or 'nibbled out' areas, tends to occur after the neonatal period. Wimberger's sign is this type of involvement of the upper medical aspects of the tibiae. Patchy, irregular, 'moth-eaten' lesions of the diaphysis, together with cortical thickening, are evidence of more extensive bone involvement, and fractures may occur. Periostitis, appearing as an elevation of the periosteum, is a common finding. Although a periosteal reaction may be a simple growth phenomenon or be caused by many other pathological states, when it involves many bones, syphilis periostitis may persist long after resolution of metaphyseal and diaphyseal lesions and lead to chronic

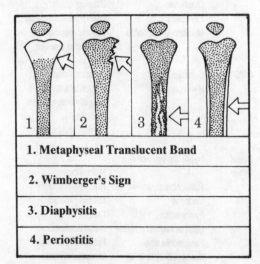

| 1. Metaphyseal Translucent Band |
| 2. Wimberger's Sign |
| 3. Diaphysitis |
| 4. Periostitis |

Fig. 8.3 Bone changes in syphilis

thickening. Involvement of the tibiae leads to the 'sabre' deformity of late congenital syphilis. Bone involvement causes pain, which is responsible for the irritability commonly found in infants suffering from congenital syphilis. In some instances, pseudoparalysis of a limb occurs (Parrot's pseudoparalysis). The exact cause of this is not defined, but may in part be due to bone disease.

CNS involvement, when present, leads to convulsions and, if untreated, can cause mental retardation and hydrocephalus. Routine examination of the cerebrospinal fluid will reveal abnormalities in more than one-third of patients.

Renal involvement should always be sought in the presence of oedema. The nephrotic syndrome is a well-recognized complication of syphilis. The onset is usually within the first 6 months, but may occur later without other clinical evidence of congenital syphilis. Immune complex deposition leads to a membranous nephropathy. Adequate antisyphilitic therapy results in complete resolution of the condition. Pretibial oedema is a frequent finding in early infancy, and may occur as a result of hypoproteinaemia unrelated to renal involvement.

Miscellaneous: Babies with congenital syphilis are not infrequently small for gestational age, and many fail to thrive as a result of gastrointestinal involvement. The pancreas and intestines frequently reveal spirochaetes at autopsy, a fibrous pancreatitis being a common finding.

A pericellular fibrosis of the lungs may also be found at autopsy (pneumonia alba). Pneumonia complicating congenital syphilis is usually of intercurrent bacterial orgin.

Patients with congenital syphilis have impaired cell-mediated immunity, and secondary bacterial infections, including septicaemia, occur frequently.

Late congenital syphilis: Scars of early syphilitic lesions and subsequent developmental changes give rise to stigmata. These include rhagades (scarring at corners of the mouth), sabre tibiae, bossing of the skull, 'saddle nose' and other deformities of the maxilla, together with characteristic deformities involving permanent teeth. The upper central incisors tend to be peg- or barrel-shaped, with convergent lateral borders and thickened bodies. The cutting edge becomes notched with usage (Hutchinson's teeth). Moon's mulberry molars have multiple small cusps instead of the normal four. These deformities cause a predisposition to caries.

A wide variety of neurological sequelae may result from chronic meningovascular syphilis, including hydrocephalus, cranial nerve palsies, hemiplegia, juvenile paresis, and tabes.

Late hypersensitivity reactions include interstitial keratitis, nerve deafness, and painless synovitis (Clutton's joints) commonly involving the knees.

Diagnosis: Symptomatic congenital syphilis may be mimicked by any of the causes of intrauterine infection and by bacterial infections acquired after birth.

The only way to make a definitive diagnosis of syphilis is through microscopic identification of the *Treponema pallidum* in secretions, by dark ground illumination, or by examination of the pathological tissues. However, although not foolproof, serological tests are of great practical value in establishing the diagnosis. Treponemal infection leads to production of both non-specific antibodies known as reagins, and specific antitreponemal antibodies. Examples of the non-specific serum antibody tests are the Wasserman, Kahn, and Venereal Disease Research Laboratory (VDRL). The last-mentioned is one of the most commonly employed as a screening test for syphilis, and as a quantitative serological method to assess the efficacy of treatment or activity of disease. A disadvantage is false positive reactions, which may be technical or due to other infections or connective tissue disorders.

Specific antibody tests have been devised in an attempt to overcome false positive reactions. Of these, the fluorescent treponemal antibody (absorbed) test (FTA Abs) has proved reliable in most instances. The FTA test detects both IgG and IgM antibodies. A baby born to a syphilitic mother may show a positive FTA IgG test merely as a result of passive transplacental transfer of maternal IgG, but a positive IgM test usually indicates infection of the infant. Biological false positive FTA tests may occur occasionally, but for practical purposes a positive FTA IgM test in young infants is indicative of congenital syphilis infection which requires treatment. Unfortunately, when syphilis is acquired by a mother late in pregnancy, her baby may not produce IgM FTA antibody until 3 months of age. A cerebrospinal fluid examination should always be done to exclude meningeal involvement.

Treatment: *(See Table 8.10.)* A symptomatic infant without meningeal involvement requires benzathine penicillin 50 000 units/kg/IM in a single dose. For a symptomatic infant without meningeal involvement, procaine pencillin G, 300 000 units IM daily for 10 days is essential. A symptomatic infant with meningeal involvement is given aqueous penicillin G, 50 000 units/kg/IV in two divided doses daily for 10 days.

Table 8.10 Treatment of congenital syphilis

1. Asymptomatic	50 000 u/kg benzathine penicillin IM single dose
2. Symptomatic without meningeal involvement	300 000 u daily procaine penicillin G IM x 10 days
3. Symptomatic with menigeal involvement	50 000 u/kg aqueous penicillin G IV x 10 days

Follow-up: Ideally all infants with congenital syphilis should be seen at 3-monthly intervals after completion of treatment, for quantitative VDRL tests and clinical examination to assess efficacy of treatment. Treatment should be repeated if the VDRL remains positive 12 months after therapy.

The mother and father of the infant should be investigated, and treated if necessary.

Prevention: Adequate antenatal care of the mother should include serological testing, and treatment where necessary, during the second and third trimesters of pregnancy.

Acquired syphilis

Transmission is either sexual or non-sexual. Acquired syphilis is usually transmitted sexually, the older child or adolescent being affected most commonly. Sexual abuse must always be ruled out, as syphilis is rarely the result of direct physical contact between an older child with an infected lesion and another child. Syphilis acquired in this way follows the usual pattern of primary, secondary, and tertiary stages, as seen in adults.

Endemic syphilis

This is found in small isolated areas of the Third World, including certain areas in southern Africa. It is transmitted by direct contact, and occurs predominantly in children between the ages of 2 and 10 years. Unlike venereally acquired syphilis, the primary lesion or chancre is rarely seen. Extensive involvement of the skin and mucous membranes is a characteristic feature in the secondary stage. In the tertiary stage, which usually manifests during adolescence or adulthood, granulomata of skin and bone produce disfigurement and pain. Cardiovascular and neurological involvement is rare, and tends to be mild.

Diptheria

Aetiology

Corynebacterium diphtheriae produces an exotoxin which is responsible for the disease process.

Epidemiology, pathogenesis, immunity

Diphtheria occurs throughout the world. In well-immunized communities the disease is rare, and tends to occur in adults, but where immunization is deficient, children of the poorer sector are most affected.

Virulent diphtheria bacilli lodge in the nasopharynx following droplet spread from a case or carrier. The toxin produced by the multiplying organisms causes local tissue necrosis which, along with the inflammatory and exudative reaction, combines to form a membrane. Toxin is then absorbed into the bloodstream and can affect all tissues, but has a predilection for myocardium and nerve tissue. Once fixed in cells the toxin cannot be neutralized; antitoxin is only effective against circulating toxin.

Occasionally disease may result from diphtheritic infection of skin lesions, e.g., a leg ulcer.

Immunity after an attack of diphtheria may not be permanent, and active immunization with toxoid should be started in convalescence. Immunity may be acquired by inapparent infection or with mild symptoms, and immune persons may become nasopharyngeal carriers.

Clinical features

The patient develops a sore throat, which may be followed by stridor. A white to grey membrane is seen in the nose or oropharynx, ranging in size from a small patch to massive involvement of tonsils, palate, pharynx, and glottis. Attempts to remove the membrane result in bleeding.

Clinical clues to the aetiology of the membrane are a serosanguinous nasal discharge, cervical adenopathy with periadenitis ('bullneck'), and toxaemia.

There are several significant facets of the disease:

◆ Upper airway obstruction by the membrane.

◆ Myocarditis may occur early in the disease (first or second week), especially when antitoxin therapy has been delayed.

◆ Neuritis may supervene 3–8 weeks after the onset, with a characteristic sequence of events. Initially, soft palate paresis occurs, then bulbar palsy, after which the muscles of accommodation are affected. Symmetrical areflexic motor paresis of the limbs, and diaphragmatic and intercostal paralysis may cease at any stage, and complete recovery follows. Recovery from paralysis usually takes place in reverse order to the onset progression.

◆ Thrombocytopenia and disseminated intravascular coagulation are seen in severe cases.

◆ Renal failure occurs from direct toxic effect on the kidneys and from disseminated intravascular coagulation, or is pre-renal following the low-output cardiac failure of myocarditis.

Management

The patient must be isolated. Culture of nose and throat swab is essential.

Antidiphtheritic toxin (ADS) is given if the diagnosis is strongly suspected clinically, as it is unwise to delay therapy until laboratory confirmation is received. Where there has been delay in the patient seeking medical care, a simplified dosage scheme for ADS is recommended. For nasal diphtheria or a small tonsillar patch of membrane, a dose of 40 000 IU is given; for a larger membrane, 80 000 IU. One half is given intravenously, diluted 1:20 in saline, and the other half is administered undiluted intramuscularly.

ADS is a horse serum, thus anaphylaxis may follow its administration.

An intradermal sensitivity test is performed initially, and if positive, precautions are taken to give the serum in a very dilute form over 24 hours.

Antibacterial therapy with penicillin or erythromycin is given for 10 days. Nose and throat cultures are redone at the end of treatment, as in some cases the organism is not eradicated and repeat therapy is indicated.

Myocarditis: Strict bed-rest is vital, and sedation may be necessary. The use of digoxin has been controversial, but current thinking is that it should be given in low dosage if cardiac decompensation occurs.

Upper airway obstruction by the membrane: Endotracheal intubation should be undertaken early. Extubation is usually possible in 4–5 days.

Neuritis: Aspiration is likely with palatal and pharyngeal paresis: such cases should be given thickened feeds through a nasogastric tube.

Endotracheal intubation will facilitate removal of secretions in those with a weak cough. Respiratory muscle paresis requires mechanical ventilation, which is seldom necessary for more than 10 days.

Contacts should be isolated until the results of their nose and throat cultures are known. Those with negative cultures can be released from isolation. Those with positive cultures require antibiotic treatment for 10 days, followed by a repeat culture.

Active immunization is recommended for contacts who have previously received a course of diphtheria toxoid or who are uncertain of their past immunization history.

Prevention

Diphtheria is readily preventable by means of vaccination *(see below)*.

Prognosis

Prognosis is affected by several factors:
◆ the virulence of the organism
◆ the larger the membrane, the greater the amount of toxin produced
◆ delay in receiving ADS therapy. These all increase the likelihood of myocarditis, neuritis, and renal failure occurring.

If an immunized child contracts the disease, it is usually mild. In those who are not immunized or who develop large membranes and receive specific treatment late or not at all, mortality rates go up to 50%.

Tetanus

Pathogenesis

Tetanus is caused by an exotoxin released by the anaerobe *Clostridium tetani* from a focus of infection. In the newborn the umbilicus is the common site of infection. In older children infection can be introduced at any site, contaminated wounds or retained foreign bodies being particularly dangerous. The toxin is released into the bloodstream, is picked up by the motor nerve endings, and travels in the perineural spaces to reach the anterior horn cells, where it accentuates the reflex arc markedly. This results in muscular hypertonia and usually intermittent muscle spasms. It is also transmitted along the neurones from the site of infection, aided by muscular contraction. The short VIIth cranial nerve and the powerful contraction of the masseter make trismus an early and constant sign. Muscles in the region of infection are also likely to be more severely affected, and the last to lose their hypertonicity.

The incubation period is seldom less than 5 days. The disease is more likely to be severe if the incubation is shorter than 8 days and the onset period from the first symptom to the first generalized spasm is less than 48 hours.

Clinical features

Mild forms may show only increased muscle tone, with extension of the neck and spine, walking on toes, and a characteristic risus sardonicus.

Usually generalized spasms are provoked by any slight sensory stimulus, but can occur spontaneously. Shock-like spasms of all muscles occur, with dominance of the more powerful muscles arching the back, extending the neck, and clamping the jaw — hence 'lockjaw'.

Pharyngospasm prevents swallowing of saliva, which may bubble from the mouth; laryngospasm and spasm of the chest muscles and diaphragm impair or stop breathing, causing apnoea, cyanosis, and sweating. Relaxation of the vocal cords following a spasm is at times associated with a stridulous cry. Saliva inhaled into the lungs, may predispose the patient to bronchopneumonia.

Muscles may be torn from their attachments, and bones may fracture, most commonly causing a compression fracture of a vertebral body.

The dominant problem is respiratory, with inadequate ventilation from spasm of the intercostal muscles and diaphragm, or apnoea from laryngospasm, causing death. Inhalation bronchopneumonia worsens the prognosis.

Consciousness is not disturbed, except as a result of severe anoxia. Terminal hyperpyrexia occurs.

So-called 'cephalic' tetanus occurs when the site of infection is the head. Sometimes the locus is otitis media, in which case a paralysis of the facial nerve on the side of the infection is associated with a risus sardonicus on the opposite half of the face.

Focal tetanus is limited to the muscles in the region of the site of infection. Most often it occurs if antitetanus serum neutralizes the circulating toxin, but not the spread of toxin along the regional neurones.

Neonatal tetanus may present as refusal to feed because of 'lockjaw'. Muscular spasms may be mistaken for convulsions. Marked rigidity of the abdominal muscles and the risus sardonicus give the diagnosis.

Untreated severe cases survive only 2–3 days. Survival beyond 10 days usually results in recovery. With modern methods of treatment the death rate can be reduced to about 10%. Previously it was about 50% for older children and over 90% for neonates.

Differential diagnosis

Trismus occurs in some children with dental abscesses, peritonsillar infections, and/or submaxillary lymphadenitis. Trismus, neck stiffness, and generalized spasms may be mistaken for encephalitis, meningitis, or intracranial haemorrhage. They are distinguished by the risus sardonicus, the normal state of consciousness, and normal CSF in tetanus. Dysphagia and spasms of the oropharyngeal muscles may simulate rabies (hydrophobic tetanus). A history of an animal bite may occur in either tetanus or rabies. However, hyperexcitability, maniacal behaviour, and paralysis suggest rabies.

Spasm of abdominal muscles in tetanus may simulate peritonitis, and that of the back muscles, spinal injury. Tetany is distinguished by carpopedal spasms and a positive Chvostek's sign. Strychnine poisoning does not produce a risus sardonicus, and the muscles relax between spasms.

Prevention:

◆ Immunization of pregnant women with toxoid protects their infants for the first 4–6 months.

◆ Triple vaccine in infancy with a booster a year later, and tetanus toxoid every 10 years thereafter.

◆ Wound care: cleansing and debridement if necessary. Toxoid is also given if the child is fully immunized but with previous booster more than 5 years previously. If the patient is unimmunized or the status unknown, a complete course of toxoid is given. If the wound is penetrating, contains a foreign body or soil, and/or is more than 6 hours old, human antitetanus immunoglobulin 250 IU is given IM (in opposite limb to toxoid). An antibiotic (penicillin, erythromycin, cephalosporin) is given for 5 days, or until the wound is healed.

Treatment

Treatment of non-neonates

Mild to moderate severity (i.e., incubation period ≥ 8 days and onset > 48 hours; trismus, hypertonia, reflex spasms ± 12 per 24 hours):

◆ Human antitetanus immunoglobulin 500 units IM.

◆ Sedation *(see below)*.

◆ Intrathecal human antitetanus immunoglobulin *(see below)*.

◆ Fluids are given intravenously unless there are no spasms, or spasms have been well-controlled for 4 days with sedation. Nasogastric tube can be passed 1 hour after sedation. As this may provoke laryngospasm, an Ambubag, oxygen, and chlorpromazine IV must be to hand.

◆ Mouth suction: 30 minutes after each sedation.

◆ Tracheostomy must be performed if laryngeal spasm occurs or there is retention of laryngeal secretions, which may occur with tight trismus or after some days of sedation.

Severe (i.e., incubation period ≤ 7 days, onset < 48 hours and reflex spasms > 12 per 24 hours):

◆ Human antitetanus immunoglobulin 500 units IM.

◆ Sedation *(see below)*.

◆ Fluids are given intravenously.

◆ Tracheostomy and intermittent positive pressure respiration (IPPR).

Treatment of neonates: The vast majority have severe tetanus and therefore require IPPR.

◆ Human antitetanus immunoglobulin is given 500 units IM.

◆ Sedation *(see below)*.

◆ Nasogastric tube is passed 30 minutes after sedation; laryngospasm (if provoked) can be overcome by positive pressure ventilation with well-fitting face mask and O_2.

◆ Fluids: expressed breast milk — small feeds are given to lessen danger of regurgitation and aspiration. Fluid intake may need augmentation by IV fluids .

◆ Mouth suction and turning of infant 30 minutes after each dose of sedative if IPPR is not available. Penicillin is given for pneumonia, and antiseptic measures are applied to the umbilicus.

◆ Monitor and maintain body temperature.

Sedation

Neonate

◆ Chlorpromazine, 12.5 mg IM 4- to 6-hourly, and phenobarbitone 5 mg/kg/dose IM 1–2/day prn,

or

◆ diazepam, 15–30 mg/day, IV or by nasogastric infusion.

Child

◆ Chlorpromazine, 25 mg IM or by nasogastric tube 4- to 6-hourly, and phenobarbitone, 5 mg/kg/dose IM 1–2/day,

or

◆ diazepam, 5–10 mg 4- to 6-hourly IV or by nasogastric tube.

Phenobarbitone may be added to the chlorpromazine regimen if required, to gain extra control of spasms. Diazepam may be given alone in the dosage recommended above, or combined with chlorpromazine, when the lower dosage range is suggested. If spontaneous spasms are still frequent or prolonged despite very heavy sedation, IPPR is indicated. If facilities for IPPR are not available and heavy sedation must be persisted with,

tracheostomy to facilitate suction and to prevent laryngeal spasm is necessary.

In neonates, however, tracheostomy without IPPR is of no value.

Intrathecal human immunoglobulin can influence outcome. It is the timing and not the dosage that is important.

If intrathecal human antitetanus immunoglobulin is given to the non-neonatal case before the onset of spasms or when spasms are still infrequent, the progress of the disease is altered and mortality reduced.

Since few neonates are seen before the onset of reflex spasms, intrathecal therapy is less effective. The dose is 250 IU given as a single dose.

Management of tetanus at various levels of health care

Primary level	Sedate
	TIG
	Clean wound
	Tetanus toxoid
	Refer to secondary facility
	any neonate or child
	with incubation ≥ 9 days
	and onset ≥ 48 hours
	Refer to tertiary facility
	any neonate or child
	with shorter incubation
	and onset
Secondary level	Regular sedation
	Fluid intake
	Nursing care
Tertiary level	Tracheostomy or intubation
	IPPR

Cholera

Vibrio cholerae, classical and *El Tor* biotypes, are motile, rod-shaped, curved Gram-negative bacteria, which can cause severe dehydrating diarrhoea and vomiting.

Epidemiology and transmission

Vibrios are spread by the oro-faecal route, and therefore cause disease in impoverished communities with poor sanitation. Cholera is endemic in the Middle and Far East, and has spread along the routes of human migration to Africa, Europe, and the Gulf States of North America. Human carriers and mild cases spread the disease (there are no animal hosts). Vibrios can survive free-living in reservoir water and in saline estuaries, and can spread to humans via fish in certain circumstances.

Classical *Vibrio cholerae* causes relatively few mild cases and carriers, but *El Tor*, which is the biotype found in the south-eastern areas of Africa, causes many asymptomatic or mild infections and chronic carriers.

Pathogenesis

When swallowed, most of the vibrios are destroyed in the stomach acid, but some pass into the upper small bowel, where alkaline conditions favour survival and multiplication. Vibrios are confined to the bowel lumen, but liberate an enterotoxin which enters the cells lining the intestine and stimulates adenyl cyclase, which in turn increases the concentration of adenosine 3.5 monophosphate. This inhibits sodium absorption and causes secretion of chloride and water. The faecal fluid so formed is isotonic with plasma; this characteristic dictates the replacement of similar fluid in therapy.

Clinical features

An incubation period of 1–5 days is followed by:
◆ profuse diarrhoea: stools quickly lose faecal characteristics and become colourless with mucus ('rice water')
◆ vomiting without nausea
◆ dehydration with thready pulse, hypotension, anuria
◆ muscle cramps of limbs and abdomen due to effect of hypocalcaemia and hypochloraemia on neuromuscular junctions
◆ normal body temperature.

The condition usually resolves within 3 days, but in exceptional circumstances lasts up to 10 days.

Cholera can be differentiated from food poisoning, where vomiting with nausea precedes diarrhoea associated with severe abdominal pain, fever, and green offensive stools.

Complications are those of fluid and electrolyte deficits.

Diagnosis

The clinical picture is almost pathognomonic, but can be confirmed by dark ground stool microscopy and culture. Agglutinating or toxin-neutralizing antibodies can be detected in the serum.

Management

◆ Isolation of patients with barrier nursing.
◆ Rapid fluid replacement *(see Table 8.11)*. Intravenous rehydration is required in those children with circulatory collapse or continued vomiting. The fluid administered to older children (and adults) should be isotonic with plasma and contain potassium, dextrose, and alkali. Infants and young children lose less sodium in stools, and half-strength Darrow's solution with 5% dextrose is satisfactory. Oral rehydration fluid and solids are introduced as soon as the patient can tolerate them.

Some patients may be rehydrated orally using a solution of NaCl 3.5g, $NaHCO_3$ 2.5g, KCl 1.5 g, glucose 20 g or sucrose 40 g in each litre of water.
◆ Antibiotics are given, as they curtail the duration of diarrhoea and reduce incidence of the carrier state. Any of the following can be used:
— tetracycline 50 mg/kg/day in 4 divided doses for 2 days
— chloramphenicol 75 mg/kg/day in 4 divided doses for 3 days
— furazolidine (Furoxone®)

over 12 years	2 tabs (taken as 1 dose)
6–12 years	1 tab
1–5 years	1 tab or 10 ml syrup
under 5 years	5 ml syrup.

◆ Strict input/output charting, frequent blood pressure readings, and serum urea and electrolyte measurements are necessary.

Prognosis

With rapid replacement of fluid and electrolytes, mortality rate is 1–2%. Mortality can exceed 50% when fluid replacement is inadequate.

Prevention

Clean water supply and safe sanitation are the ultimate aims. Chlorination of water using bleaching powder or solution kills vibrios quickly.

Drinking water and milk should be boiled. Strict personal hygiene must be observed. Adequate hand-washing and drying facilities are a priority,

Table 8.11   IV fluids for cholera

Preparation	Na+ mmol/l	K+ mmol/l	Mg⁺⁺ mmol/l	Cl⁻ mmol/l	Lactate mmol/l	Dextrose g/l
½ strength Darrow's	61	17	–	51	27	55
Ringer's lactate with 5 % glucose*	131	5	1.8	112	29	55
Plasmolyte L® with 5% glucose	131	5	–	108	29	55

* Add 10 mmol KCL to every litre

especially at toilets and where patients are being nursed.

Chemoprophylaxis of household contacts is recommended, using antibiotics as above.

Killed vibrio vaccine is given as two subcutaneous injections of 0.5 ml 4 weeks apart, with boosters every 6 months while at risk, as protection is only 50– 60% for 3– 6 months. Vaccination is not very helpful in control of epidemics. However, it is indicated for travellers to endemic areas, or for those with high risk occupations.

Quarantine is never efficient, since carriers may be intermittent excretors.

Cholera must be suspected in the presence of
Profuse watery diarrhoea
+
Vomiting without nausea

Management
Rapid fluid and electrolyte replacement
Antibiotics

Prevention in contacts
Chlorinate or boil drinking water
Chemoprophylaxis

Leprosy
Leprosy is a chronic infectious disease caused by *Mycobacterium leprae*, which usually involves peripheral nerves and skin, and occasionally other tissues. It is a major cause of disability in some Third World countries. Transmission of infected tissue occurs between humans through inhalation or across abraded skin, and children usually acquire the disease from affected parents. As there is a prolonged incubation period of between 3 and 7 years, leprosy in paediatric practice is a disease of older children. *(See Table 8.12 for further details.)*

Clinical features
(See Fig. 8.4.)
The clinical features of the disease are influenced by two factors:
◆   The character of the immune response: a powerful cell-mediated immune reaction to *M. leprae* results in *tuberculoid* leprosy, while a deficient response is associated with a *lepromatous* picture.
◆   The preferred sites of the infection are nerves and skin. Presentation is therefore determined by nerve damage or skin lesions.

The earliest clinical evidence is an ill-defined, hypopigmented macule which usually retains sensation, has a diameter of about 5 cm, and occurs at any site. This lesion heals spontaneously in most instances and has been classified as **indeterminate leprosy**. A minority of children progress to the more serious manifestations of leprosy. A comparison is drawn between the **tuberculoid** and **lepromatous** patterns of leprosy in *Table 8.12. (See also Fig. 8.4.)*

Between these distinct types of leprosy, various intermediate forms occur, with accompanying shifts in immunological status. Of these the most common are **borderline tuberculoid** (commonest in Africans) and **borderline lepromatous** *(commonest in Asians and Europeans)*.

Diagnosis
◆   The clinical features of anaesthetic skin lesions and thickened nerves are pathognomonic
◆   Skin smears for acid-fast bacilli or biopsy of skin or nerve tissue will confirm the diagnosis.

Table 18.12 Leprosy

	Tuberculoid	Lepromatous
Frequency in childhood	Common	Uncommon
Skin lesions	Few	Numerous, bilateral, symmetrical
	Well-defined edge	Poorly-defined edge
	Macule, raised erythematous edge, hypopigemented, anaesthetic, hairless	Macule, erythematous or hypogigmented, no obvious progress to form plaques and nodules, and there is loss of eyelashes and eyebrows
Nerve lesions	Thickened cutaneous nerve at site of or away from skin lesions	Little nerve involvement in early stages. In late stages peripheral nerves thicken and cause anaesthesia and muscle weakness
Disseminated lesions	—	Rhinitis; conjunctivitis; keratitis; iritis; nodules in nose, palate, ear lobes; lymphoedema; lymphadenopathy; hepatosplenomegaly; testicular atrophy; deformities due to infection and injury
Complications	Rare	'Lepra' reactions occur spontaneously or during therapy, i.e., exacerbation of skin and nerve lesions. 'Erythema nodosum leprosum' (ENL) i.e., painful erythematous nodules
Cell-mediated immunity	Marked	Deficient
Lepromin test (delayed hypersensitivity to *M. leprae*)	+	–
Pathology	Non-caseating tuberculoid granuloma (epithelioid cells, giant cells, lymphocytes), nerves destroyed, few AFB	Macrophages containing many AFB, scanty lymphocytes, nerves intact during early stages

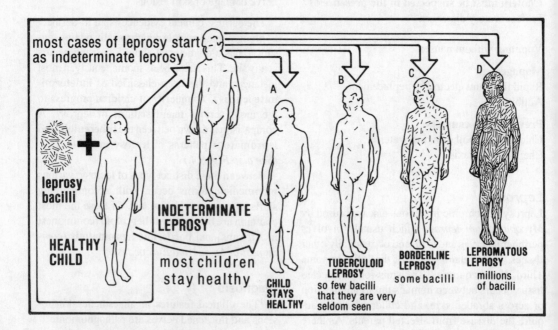

Fig. 8.4   Clinical varieties of leprosy

Management

Initial treatment for all varieties is dapsone (1 mg/kg/day), rifampicin (10 mg/kg/day), and clofazimine (adult dose 100 mg tds, paediatric dose not established) for 6 weeks.

Maintenance therapy:

◆ *Tuberculoid and borderline tuberculoid:* Dapsone daily until no signs of activity for 3 years.

◆ *Lepromatous and borderline lepromatous:* Continue dapsone, rifampicin, and clofazimine for 6 months; thereafter dapsone indefinitely.

◆ *Severe ENL and lepra reactions (see Table 8.12): Prednisone 2 mg/kg*

◆ *Education* to minimize complications, appropriate *physiotherapy,* and *surgery* where indicated.

◆ *Prevention:* BCG is used in some countries. Case-finding and prompt treatment limits spread.

Virus infections

Measles (rubeola)

Measles is an acute, highly contagious disease caused by an RNA paramyxovirus.

Epidemiology

The disease is distributed world-wide and is droplet-spread. It is communicable for about 7 days from the onset of the prodrome. In a Kenyan study, prolonged secretion of the virus, for up to 28 days in severe disease, was demonstrated in the more poorly nourished children. Infants up to the age of 3–4 months are protected by passively acquired maternal antibodies.

In developing countries, measles is common in infants under 2 years of age. Large families living in crowded conditions predispose to the disease being introduced into a household by an older sibling, and thus infants can acquire measles very early in life.

In disadvantaged communities measles is one of the most important causes of infant and childhood morbidity and mortality.

In developed countries, the disease occurs in pre-school age groups in towns and in older children in rural areas. Where vaccination is extensively practised, a marked reduction in the incidence of this disease has occurred.

Clinical features

After an incubation period of 10–11 days, a prodrome or catarrhal phase occurs, with fever, cough, coryza, and conjunctivitis. On the fourth day the rash appears. Koplik's spots appear 2 days before the rash and are usually present for 4 days. This **enanthema**, which is pathognomonic of measles, consists of small red spots on the buccal and labial mucous membrane, each with a minute white centre, not unlike salt grains.

The **exanthem** is an erythematous maculopapular (morbilliform) eruption, which spreads from the face to the trunk and arms and continues to the legs on the third day. It begins to fade by the third day, in order of appearance. Staining of the skin follows, and lasts for 1–2 months, while fine desquamation, sparing the hands and feet, may occur as the rash fades. After the second or third day of the rash, the temperature falls rapidly and convalescence ensues. If the child is feverish beyond the third day of rash, a complication should be suspected.

Complications

Pneumonia: Pulmonary complications are common, and are the main cause of death from measles.

Pneumonia following measles may be due to bacterial superinfection, often by a combination of Gram-positive and Gram-negative organisms. Just as frequently the cause is viral: the measles virus itself, or superinfection by adenovirus and herpesvirus, leads to bronchiolar and interstitial necrosis. Healing may be slow and incomplete, leading to obliterative bronchiolitis or bronchiectasis. Concomitant infection with measles and adenovirus produces the most severe symptoms, most prolonged course, and highest mortality rate.

Laryngotracheobronchitis (LTB): Mild laryngitis is a common feature of measles. More significant inflammation of the upper airway may occur, and obstruction of airflow results in stridor and retractions. LTB occurs during the period of the rash, but also in the post-measles state, when the cause is sometimes due to secondary infection by viruses such as adenovirus, para-influenza, or herpes simplex.

Encephalitis:

◆ *Acute:* This occurs in about 0.1% of cases, with onset usually during the rash, but it can occur before the rash appears or in the post-measles period. The CSF displays a typical viral picture, although in rare instances it may be normal. The course is variable, but in general 60% recover, 15% die, and the remainder have neurological sequelae.

◆ *Immunosuppressive measles encephalopathy:* Children with defective cellular immunity under cytotoxic therapy may have mild or atypical measles infection, followed by encephalitis 1–6 months later. The prognosis is poor, with survivors having severe neurological damage.

◆ *Subacute sclerosing panencephalitis (SSPE):* In about 1 in 100 000 cases of measles SSPE occurs some years after the initial disease (mean 6 years). This slowly progressive encephalitis almost always ends fatally. SSPE has followed most often where measles occurred in the very young. Despite this, the prevalence is no higher in communities where the disease is rife at an early age. In southern Africa there is clustering of cases in Zimbabwe and some provinces of South Africa, but it is almost unknown in Malawi.

Diarrhoea is a common complication, reducing food intake and contributing to a negative nitrogen balance. Florid malnutrition may be precipitated by measles in children with suboptimal nutrition. Cellular damage of the absorptive surface of the bowel leads to diarrhoea, protein-losing enteropathy, and lactose intolerance.

Otitis media, a common complication in measles, almost pales into insignificance in measles cases in developing communities, because of the high incidence of pneumonia, diarrhoea, and LTB. It should nevertheless be carefully watched for in all patients during convalescence, as it may not resolve, and can result in chronic infection and hearing loss.

Corneal ulceration following conjunctivitis is especially likely to occur in malnourished children.

Herpes simplex gingivostomatitis: There is an increased susceptibility to this condition in children with measles. Dissemination of the virus can occur, particularly in children with kwashiorkor.

Measles and the immune response: It has long been noted that a positive tuberculin test becomes negative after measles infection, and usually remains so for 2–6 weeks, except in malnourished children, in whom it may be negative for up to a year.

This fact prompted research into the immune status reaction during measles. It has been found that both B and T lymphocyte numbers are decreased, lymphocyte proliferation is inhibited, and the anti-bacterial function of polymorphonuclear leucocytes is defective. This is important, since it frequently allows the occurrence of secondary infection and the recrudescence of tuberculosis.

Prognosis

The prognosis for measles has improved as living conditions for children have improved. Worldwide, a high morbidity and mortality occur among the malnourished, in those under 1 year of age, and where an increased viral load occurs due to overcrowding of children in a home.

It has recently been shown that lymphopenia of less than 2 000/mm^3 in the first 2 days of the rash also indicates a poor prognosis and slow recovery from complications. This lymphopenia is due to a decrease in numbers of both B and T cells, and is significantly associated with the histocompatibility leucocyte antigen (HLA) AW32.

Treatment

Measles is usually an uncomplicated, self-limiting disease in well-nourished children, and requires supportive management consisting of an antipyretic and a cough mixture.

In less favoured communities, where the course is often complicated, more intensive therapy is required. Admission to hospital is warranted if a complication other than otitis media is present.

Pneumonia: Since it is not easy to differentiate between viral or bacterial pneumonia, antibiotics are used. Co-trimoxazole is frequently used, while penicillin with an aminoglycoside is recommended if the child is seriously ill.

Treatment of LTB: *See Chapter 13, Respiratory Disorders.*

Encephalitis: Management is supportive. Convulsions are controlled by barbiturates or diazepam. Nursing care is necessary for the child in a coma, with attention to nutrition and the prevention of intercurrent infections.

Diarrhoea: Continuation of milk feeds is recommended, along with oral or intravenous rehydration fluids if required. A low-lactose or semi-elemental feed may need to be substituted for cows' milk if diarrhoea becomes prolonged.

Otitis media: *See Chapter 14, Ear, Nose, and Throat Disorders.*

Conjunctivitis: Cleansing of the eyes with warm saline prevents infection of the viral conjunctivitis. Antibiotic eye ointment may also be necessary.

Vitamin A in measles: Vitamin A supplementation orally at the onset of the rash has been shown in controlled trials to halve the mortality rate and significantly reduce morbidity from pneumonia, diarrhoea, and conjunctival ulceration. The WHO recommends a dosage of 100 000 IU daily for 2 days.

Measles

Severe disease occurs in:
- infants < 1 year old
- malnourished children
- patients from crowded homes.

The disease must be considered to be serious when complicated by:
- pneumonia
- encephalitis
- diarrhoea
- LTB.

Measles commonly causes:
- malnutrition
- chronic pulmonary symptoms
- immune depression
- recurrent infections.

Measles can be prevented by vaccination.

Mumps (epidemic parotitis)

Epidemiology and immunity

Endemic in most urban communities, the mumps virus is spread by droplet infection and by infectious saliva from the human reservoir. Eighty-five per cent of infections occur under the age of 15 years. Infants are protected for about 6 months by passive placental transfer of antibodies. Immunity is lifelong after one attack.

The period of infectivity is from about 6 days before onset of symptoms to subsidence of salivary gland swelling: a period of 7–14 days in the average case. Inapparent infections occur in 30–40% of people; these remain infectious for a period similar to that of overt cases.

Clinical features

The incubation period is 17–21 days. Parotitis is unilateral in 30% of patients. Submandibular and, rarely, sublingual gland infection is encountered. There is tender swelling which reaches a maximum during the first day, but the opposite gland may be affected some days later. Opening the mouth may be difficult. There is oedema of the surrounding tissue, with the ear lobe displaced upwards and backwards. Stensen's duct may be inflamed. Sour food elicits pain along the duct and in the gland. Symptoms usually subside within a week.

Complications

Epididymo-orchitis occurs in about 25% of post-pubertal males.

Meningo-encephalitis: Clinical features are seen in about 10% of patients. The disease is usually benign, but high fever and marked meningeal signs do occur. The CSF shows a mildly raised protein content, with lymphocytes predominating.

Pancreatitis occurs in about 7% of patients, presenting with epigastric pain, fever, and vomiting.

Oophoritis, thyroiditis, and mastitis are rare complications.

All complications may precede or occur in absence of parotitis.

Deafness, post-infectious encephalomyelitis, facial nerve neuritis, myocarditis, arthritis, thrombocytopenia, and haemolytic anaemia are further rare complications which have been described.

Treatment

Treatment is entirely symptomatic.

Prevention

Mumps can be prevented by vaccination, usually in combination with measles and rubella vaccine (MMR), given at 15 months.

Chickenpox (varicella)

Chickenpox and herpes zoster are both due to herpes varicella-zoster virus (VZV), which is identical to *Herpesvirus hominis* on electronmicroscopy.

Varicella occurs at any age, with a peak age incidence at 5–10 years. It is spread by droplets or by direct contact with vesicular fluid. Infectiousness lasts from 24 hours before the rash until all lesions have scabbed; usually a period of 6–7 days.

Clinical features

After a 13–17 day incubation, a mild prodrome of 24 hours occurs, followed by a crop of red papules which develop rapidly into clear vesicles. Within 24 hours these become cloudy, then umbilicate and dry to scabs. Crops of vesicles erupt for 3–4 days, starting from the trunk and spreading to the face, scalp, conjunctivae, and mucous membranes. At the height of the disease the eruption consists of all stages of the rash. Systemic reaction is usually minor.

Complications

Complications are rare and consist of thrombocytopenia, pneumonia, myocarditis, hepatitis, glomerulonephritis, encephalitis, cerebellar ataxia, and Guillain-Barré syndrome. About 10% of Reye's syndrome cases are associated with chickenpox. Children on cytotoxic drugs and steroids are at risk of developing severe, disseminated, and fatal disease.

Differential diagnosis

Papular urticaria, bullous impetigo, scabies, and molluscum contagiosum.

Management

See Herpes Zoster, below.

Perinatal infection of infants

Infants born to mothers in whom varicella occurs within 7 days before or after delivery are at high risk of severe neonatal disease. Varicella develops in 33% of these neonates, often with a severe course, and has a 30–50% mortality rate.

Zoster immune globulin (ZIG) is recommended for these infants. However, since some infants who received ZIG developed chickenpox, prophylaxis with acyclovir given IV is preferred. This should also be given therapeutically if varicella has developed when the patient is first seen.

Fetal varicella syndrome can occur in 10–13% of fetuses whose mothers contract chickenpox in the first trimester of pregnancy, and in 5% after this period. The major features are skin lesions, cerebral atrophy, and eye abnormalities. Pregnant women in contact with varicella or who contract varicella should receive ZIG.

Herpes zoster (shingles)

See Varicella, above, for the causative organisms.

Pathogenesis

Chickenpox is thought to be the primary infection with VZV, and zoster to be a reactivation of the latent virus. There is an increased incidence of zoster in those immunodepressed by malignancy, drugs, or in AIDS victims.

The reactivated virus spreads from sensory ganglia along nerves to the skin and produces a vesicular eruption. The virus may be shed from skin lesions, producing varicella in susceptible subjects.

Clinical features

Pain and paraesthesiae occur over a sensory dermatome (spinal or cranial), followed in 2–4 days by a localized vesicular eruption. The disease may be complicated by meningitis, encephalitis, hepatitis, and post-herpetic neuralgia (uncommon in children).

Therapy of VZV infections

Prophylaxis:

♦ Varicella is prevented in susceptible contacts if zoster immune globulin (ZIG) is given within 72 hours of exposure. Prevention of disease is less effective in immunodepressed contacts.

♦ Zoster immune plasma (ZIP) is derived from convalescent zoster cases; 10 ml/kg intravenously is also effective in protecting susceptible contacts.

Management:
◆ Drying lotions and antipruritics can be prescribed for the rash.
◆ In complicated cases and in immunodepressed subjects, ZIP or acyclovir IV is often effective.
◆ Radiotherapy or cytotoxic drugs must be stopped, but steroids should be continued.

Herpesvirus type 1 (HVH1)
Infants are usually protected for a few months by maternal antibody to HVH1. Primary infection usually occurs between 1 and 5 years of age, but in an affluent society may be delayed to adulthood.

The virus spreads by close personal contact or by contamination with infected saliva. Primary infection is usually subclinical in childhood, with about 10% developing clinical disease. Lesions in the form of vesicles are localized in skin or mucous membrane. Viraemia and dissemination of the infection may occur in the immunodepressed (measles, malnutrition, malignancy). High-risk or very ill patients should receive acyclovir IV.

Clinical syndrome
Gingivostomatitis HVH1 is the common cause of stomatitis in children under 5 years. The onset is abrupt or insidious, with fever, salivation, and refusal to eat. Vesicles develop in the mouth, and rapidly rupture to leave ulcers covered with a yellow-grey membrane. The acute phase, which is self-limiting, lasts 4–9 days. Primary infection of fingers and abrasions occur in adults at risk, e.g., health workers. In stomatitis, oral hygiene is most easily achieved by giving small, frequent, fluid feeds. Local application of analgesic cream is useful, and in severe cases admission to hospital for tube-feeding may be necessary.

Eczema herpeticum: Widespread primary infection of eczematous skin can occur with HVH1. The vesicles develop in crops for 7–10 days, after which scabs form and healing occurs. Systemic reaction with high fever is common.

Meningoencephalitis is seen in all ages. HVH2 is the usual cause in neonates, and HVH1 in older patients. It can occur during primary or recurrent infection, carries a high mortality rate, and frequently produces permanent neurological sequelae in survivors. There is some evidence of improved prognosis with acyclovir.

Conjunctivitis and kerato-conjunctivitis are also manifestations of primary or recurrent infections. The diagnosis is suggested by herpetic vesicles of the eyelids (*see Chapter 25, Disorders of the Eye*).

Recurrent disease: The virus becomes latent in sensory ganglia. Recurrent attacks occur in 30% of cases, despite adequate serum antibody levels. The virus spreads to the skin along cutaneous nerves, and vesicles occur in mucocutaneous areas such as the lips. Recurrences are associated with pneumonia, meningitis, malaria, exposure to cold or sun, menstruation, viral respiratory infections, and emotional stress.

Disseminated herpes: In children with secondary immunodeficiency (usually measles or malnutrition) who have localized herpes simplex, dissemination of virus is to be suspected in the presence of neurological signs, increasing hepatomegaly, worsening pneumonia, pyrexia, and occasional bleeding. These patients are usually anaemic and septicaemic, and require vigorous therapy.

Herpesvirus type 2 (HVH2)
Infections are usually post-pubertal and transmitted venereally. The usual clinical expression is genital herpes, although cervical involvement is often subclinical. Sixty per cent of adults have antibodies to HVH2 in lower socio-economic groups, and 10% in higher groups. Five to ten per cent of cases are due to HVH1.

Neonates may contract HVH2 from maternal genital herpes. The resultant disease is usually disseminated and often fatal.

Infectious mononucleosis (IM)
Aetiology and pathogenesis
The disease is caused by the Epstein-Barr virus (EBV), which is a member of the herpes virus group. It infects B lymphocytes of humans and primates, and is transferred in saliva, from whence it can be isolated for at least 3 months after the acute infection, and for much longer in 30% of cases.

Epidemiology

EBV infection occurs early in life in underdeveloped communities, where 70–90% of the population becomes serologically positive by 6 years of age. In children, infectious mononucleosis (IM) is seldom recognized as a clinical entity; seroconversion tends to follow subclinical or non-specific illness.

In developed communities over 50% remain uninfected during childhood, and classical IM occurs in adolescents and young adults. But even in this population, subclinical infections are two to three times more common than manifest disease.

Clinical features

♦ Classical IM syndrome, seen mainly in young adults, has an insidious onset of malaise, headache, and nausea. After about 2 weeks, fever and pharyngitis occur, with or without tonsillar exudates and petechiae on the soft palate. In the majority there is also lymphadenopathy (mainly posterior cervical and epitrochlear) and hepatosplenomegaly. Occasionally there is oedema of the eyelids and a maculopapular rash.

♦ IM manifestations in infants and young children are rarely classical. The majority of seroconversions are subclinical or follow mild upper respiratory symptoms. Occasionally EBV infection is associated with hepatitis, Guillain-Barré syndrome, thrombocytopenia, and haemolytic anaemia.

Diagnosis

♦ Leucocytosis with 20–40% atypical lymphocytes is characteristic of IM.

♦ Heterophile antibody (Paul–Bunnell and 'spot' test). In all but 10–15% of cases of classical IM, the titre reaches a diagnostic level in 1 week and peaks at 3 weeks. Children, however, do not usually produce significant amounts of heterophile antibody.

♦ EBV-specific tests. These immunofluorescent techniques using different antigens detect specific viral antibodies.

♦ IgG antibody to viral capsid antigen (VCA): Titre peaks at 2–3 weeks, then declines, but persists for life.

♦ IgM antibody to VCA: This titre also rises early, but disappears within 2–3 months.

♦ IgG antibody to early antigen appears shortly after VCA appears, and disappears within 6 months of illness.

♦ Antibodies to EBV nuclear antigen: Titre rises late, but persists for life.

Using a combination of these tests, diagnosis of recent or past infection can be made in all cases of EBV infection.

Differential diagnosis

Fifteen per cent of classical cases of IM are Paul–Bunnell-negative.

Infections with cytomegalovirus, toxoplasmosis, and hepatitis virus must be considered.

Streptococcal sore throat and diphtheria must be excluded when the pharyngeal signs are prominent.

The rash and lymphadenopathy may be confused with those of rubella.

Treatment

Management is supportive and antibiotics should be avoided. Ampicillin in particular has been shown to cause a skin eruption.

Prognosis

Prognosis is good. Very rarely death has occurred from splenic rupture, Guillain-Barré syndrome, or haemolytic anaemia.

Cytomegalovirus infections

Cytomegalovirus (CMV) has the characteristics of herpes virus.

Epidemiology

When world-wide distribution is considered, congenital and acquired infection is generally higher in those with a low standard of living. Virus is excreted in the urine, faeces, milk, saliva, and upper respiratory tract, and there is cervical shedding in pregnant women. The virus may be transmitted from any of these sources.

Congenital CMV infections

Infection of the fetus occurs *in utero* and the majority are asymptomatic. In those with disease, hepatosplenomegaly, jaundice, purpura, microcephaly, cerebral calcifications, and chorioretinitis may occur together or singly. Neurological involvement may not be evident for some time (deafness, visual loss, cerebral palsy). Extraneural disease is usually reversible.

Confirmation of diagnosis is by detection of large, inclusion-bearing cells in urine, specific IgM antibody in cord serum, and by virus isolation. The differential diagnosis includes congenital toxoplasmosis, rubella, and *herpes simplex* infection, as well as bacterial sepsis.

Acquired CMV infections
These are usually inapparent, but can be associated in infants with pneumonia, paroxysmal cough, petechial rash, hepatosplenomegaly, and polyneuritis. Older children exhibit an infectious mononucleosis-like syndrome. The prognosis is usually good, except in those with increased susceptibility to infections, e.g., lymphoma, AIDS. Diagnosis is by virus isolation. Antibody titres are less reliable, as cross-reactions with other herpesviruses occur. CMV infections need to be differentiated from infectious mononucleosis and hepatitis due to A or B viruses.

Treatment
Supportive. No role for antiviral agents has been established.

Rubella (German measles)
Rubella is a world-wide endemic disease, with irregular epidemics, and is usually seen in older children and young adults. The disease is preventable by means of vaccination (*see below*).

It is droplet-spread, with an incubation period of 14–21 days.

There is a prodrome of malaise, coryza, conjunctivitis, and tender lymphadenopathy — usually of suboccipital, post-auricular, and cervical nodes. The pink-red, maculopapular rash appears on the face, spreads rapidly to the trunk and limbs, and lasts 3 days. Disease without the exanthem occurs, and the rash is difficult to see on pigmented skin.

Serological diagnosis: Haemagglutination-inhibition antibody level rises within 24–48 hours of the rash, peaks at 12 days, and persists. Complications, which are rare in childhood, are arthralgia, encephalitis, and purpura. The disease

is generally benign in children, and lifelong immunity is usual.

Congenital rubella
The main importance of the disease is the transplacental transfer of the virus to the fetus when a pregnant woman contracts rubella. The virus may spread widely in the fetus, damaging differentiating cells in many organs, and leading to abortion, stillbirth, or a malformed child. The risk of embryopathy is higher the earlier in pregnancy the mother is infected: in the first month 50% of fetuses exhibit embryopathy; by the fourth month the risk is 5%. Despite these observations and the prevalence of rubella, affected infants in black neonatal practice are very rare.

Embryopathy consists of one or several of the following:
◆ **Temporary damage**: Thrombocytopenia, hepatitis, skeletal change, pneumonia, haemolysis, and small size for gestational age.
◆ **Permanent damage:** Congenital heart disease, cataracts, microphthalmia, deafness, psychomotor retardation, microcephaly, and spastic quadriparesis.

Infants with embryopathy excrete virus for many months. Serological diagnosis is by IgM-specific antibody.

Respiratory syncytial virus infections
Respiratory syncytial virus (RSV) is the most important cause of respiratory tract infection in infants in the first few months of life, and transplacental antibodies are not protective.

In developed countries annual epidemics occur in winter. In the tropics the epidemiology is less clear, but outbreaks have coincided with the rainy season, or with festivals when large numbers of people congregate. About 50% of susceptible infants contract their primary infection in each epidemic. Reinfection can occur.

Infections are rarely asymptomatic, and the infant exhibits coryza, otitis, croup, bronchitis, bronchiolitis, or pneumonia. The latter two conditions carry a high morbidity, and are more common in infants living in crowded conditions.

It is suggested that the interaction of serum antibody and viral antigen in the lungs plays an important role in the pathogenesis of RSV disease, especially bronchiolitis.

Influenza infections

Influenza A and B

Influenza A virus is subject to major and minor antigenic changes which lead to regular pandemics. Influenza B virus undergoes only minor antigenic changes, with resultant major outbreaks at more variable intervals. In such epidemics, the attack rates with the new subtype are higher in children than in adults. The manifestation of infection in older children is fairly typical of influenza, but in younger children, coryza, croup, bronchitis, bronchiolitis, and pneumonia are caused. Bacterial superinfection is a common complication.

Parainfluenza infections

Parainfluenza types 1 and 2 infections occur in autumn epidemics, while type 3 is endemic. By the age of 5 years the majority of children have been infected by all three types.

Infections are usually symptomatic, and manifest as upper and lower respiratory disease. Parainfluenza type 1 most frequently causes laryngotracheobronchitis, and type 3 most frequently causes pneumonia.

Anterior poliomyelitis

Epidemiology

Poliovirus types 1, 2, and 3 are usually spread by oro-faecal contamination, but also by droplet in epidemics. Humans are the sole natural reservoir. The incubation period is about 10 days, and the latter part of the incubation period and first week of disease are the most infectious.

Poliomyelitis has been eradicated in communities where all children are vaccinated and living conditions are satisfactory.

Pathogenesis

The virus multiplies in the intestinal tract and its lymph nodes, with production of antibody. If the antibody response is rapid the virus is neutralized, but sometimes the virus proliferates and becomes invasive. Access to the central nervous system occurs either across blood vessels into the cerebellum or by spreading along the nerve pathways from the gut.

The virus affects the anterior horn cells of the cord and several areas of the brain. Damage may be reversible, with recovery; but may go on to irreversible nuclear destruction, when muscle paralysis results.

Clinical features

(See Figs 8.5 and 8.6.)

Inapparent infection: Approximately 95% of infections are subclinical, but give lasting immunity.

Abortive disease: A minor illness of a few days occurs, with fever, sore throat, headache, abdominal pain, nausea, and vomiting. Lumbar puncture at this stage shows a normal CSF.

Non-paralytic poliomyelitis resembles the abortive disease, with meningism and pain in the back and legs. However the CSF usually shows pleocytosis and a slightly raised protein level.

Paralytic disease: Weakness of skeletal or cranial muscle groups may follow closely upon the non-paralytic form or occur after a symptom-free period of some days.

◆ *Spinal form:* Involvement of muscles of neck, trunk, abdomen, thorax, diaphragm, and limbs.

◆ *Bulbar form:* Motor weakness of cranial nerves and/or dysfunction of medullary vital centres of respiration and circulation.

◆ *Bulbospinal form:* The above two forms frequently occur together.

◆ *Encephalitic form:* Irritability, disorientation, drowsiness, and tremors may be present.

The muscle paralysis is flaccid, with reduced or absent superficial and deep tendon jerks, and intact sensation. Improvement of muscle power following paralysis occurs up to 12 weeks after the onset. Muscle wasting is due to denervation of muscle, as well as disuse.

Diagnosis

The diagnosis is made on the clinical picture. The CSF is abnormal for about 10 days after onset of meningism. A rising serum antibody titre and culture of the virus from stool and urine is confirmatory evidence.

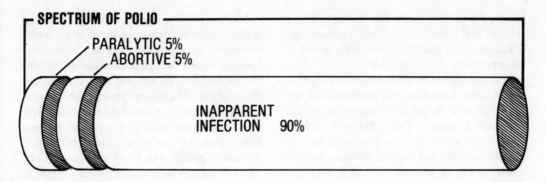

Fig. 8.5 Spectrum of poliomyelitis

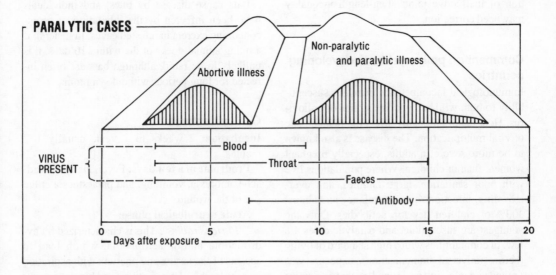

Fig. 8.6 Pathogenesis of the poliovirus

Complications

Superficial gut erosions with haemorrhage, hypertension, myocarditis, and transitory bladder paralysis are encountered at times. In the severely incapacitated, hypercalciuria may occur later, with urinary calculi.

Management

Acute phase of paralytic disease:

◆ The limbs are kept in the neutral position with cushions; warm packs are applied to the affected limbs, and analgesics prescribed until the pain has disappeared. Subsequently a programme of active and passive movements is commenced by a physiotherapist.

◆ In bulbar and bulbospinal disease care is taken to avoid aspiration, whilst respiratory muscle paralysis requires a period of assisted ventilation.

◆ Attendants should create a calm and confident atmosphere. Both patient and relatives need to be prepared for the prolonged treatment required and for permanent disability, should this occur.

◆ Isolation is essential during the acute phase.

Recovery phase: If trunk muscles are paralysed the patient should be kept recumbent, but otherwise should be encouraged to get up as soon as possible. Most recovery of muscle power will occur in the first three months. Active physiotherapy continues, aimed at strengthening residual muscle power. Deformity should be prevented by putting the affected limb through a full range of passive movements every day, and by fitting a splint to hold joints in their optimal position. Mobilization of the patient follows. with the aid of calipers to support flailing limbs.

Residual phase: Regular out-patient supervision is called for with regard to the physical and emotional state. Social and economic support is frequently necessary. The orthopaedic surgeon will advise on the adjustment of appliances to prevent deformity and improve function. Surgical treatment may be needed to overcome soft tissue contractures, and to improve function and/or prevent deformity by tendon transfer, or by stabilization of ineffective joints. Leg-length inequality may need correction.

Comment on poliomyelitis in developing countries

Immunological incompetence increases susceptibility to both wild and vaccine strains of poliovirus. Host factors probably affect the rate and site of viral multiplication. The disease is also known to be more severe in adults, especially pregnant women, than in children. Where populations live with poor sanitation, large families, and overcrowding, infections occur in infancy and almost 100% of children develop antibodies. Only the youngest are susceptible, and paralytic cases are few. In communities with a high standard of living (before universal immunization), exposure was limited and infection postponed, so that epidemics affected older children and young adults, many of whom became paralysed. As living standards improve in developing countries, the pattern of poliomyelitis is evolving from an endemic, low-paralysis-rate disease to one of epidemics involving older children.

Rabies (hydrophobia)

Rabies is a viral infection of the CNS, usually transmitted by contamination of a wound with saliva from a rabid animal.

Epidemiology and pathogenesis

Rabies is widespread in warm-blooded animals. The principal vectors vary in different countries. In Africa, meerkats, fruit bats, and stray dogs are the main transmitters of the disease to humans.

After entry through the skin, the virus possibly multiplies first in striated muscle, where antibody, interferon, and other host factors may retard nerve invasion. Ascent through sensory nerves follows, and once in the CNS, neuronal destruction occurs maximally in the brain stem, pyramid cells, cranial nerves, and posterior horns of the spinal cord. The virus then moves out along nerves to mucus-secreting and salivary glands, where the amount of virus is variable, which may explain why only 50% of bites by proven rabid dogs result in rabies.

Since animals lick their claws, scratches by rabid animals can transmit disease.

Bats cause disease by bites, and individuals have been infected by the inhalation of virus-containing excreta in infested caves. In general, if a biting animal does not die within 10 days, it is unlikely to be rabid, although bats are often infected for long periods without symptoms.

Clinical features

Incubation: 2 weeks to 1 year; usually 1–2 months.

Prodrome of a few days: Fever, malaise, headache, anorexia, vomiting, and paraesthesia at the site of the wound.

Acute neurological phase:
- *'Furious rabies':* This is characterized by hydrophobia and/or aerophobia, which lead to spasms of the larynx and pharynx with aspiration into the trachea. Hyperactivity and bizarre aggressive behaviour alternate with periods of lucidity. This is followed by ascending symmetrical paralysis, areflexia, and coma. Respiratory muscle paralysis or arrythmias are the usual cause of death.
- *'Dumb rabies':* In about 20% of cases there is an ascending symmetrical paralysis without a 'furious' phase. The CSF may show pleocytosis and elevated protein, or be normal. No survivors have been reported among unimmunized cases.

Laboratory confirmation

Fluorescent antibody test on brain and a rise in serum antibody titre are diagnostic.

Control of disease in endemic areas

- Domestic animals must be kept immunized with live attenuated virus vaccine.

◆ Measures against growth of vector population, e.g., meerkat, are a parallel approach.

Measures during an epidemic

◆ Revaccinate domestic animals, and keep them fenced in or tied up.
◆ Restrict movement of domestic animals between rabies and non-rabies areas.
◆ Eliminate stray animals.
◆ Vaccinate high-risk humans: veterinarians, health inspectors, etc.
◆ **Following exposure:** Prompt cleansing of wound with soap and water, then application of a viricidal solution, e.g., 10% povidone iodine. Vaccination must proceed according to the schedule below.

Vaccination schedule

Biting animals	Condition of animal at time of attack	Treatment of human
Wild	Regard as rabid	RIG* + V**
Domestic	Healthy***	None
	Unknown/escaped	RIG* + V**
	Suspected rabid	RIG* + V**

* RIG: Rabies immune globulin
** V: Human diploid cell vaccine
*** Isolate for 10 days if bite was apparently unprovoked

Management of patient when bitten by 'suspect' animal
◆ clean wound
◆ give RIG
◆ give human diploid cell vaccine.

'Suspect' animal is:
◆ wild animal
◆ domestic animal if unknown (escaped), or if the attack was unprovoked.

Confirmation of rabies is possible by autopsy on biting animal. Do not wait for this before giving RIG.

Viral haemorrhagic disease

This group of diseases occurs in Africa, Asia, and North America. Only those which have occurred in southern Africa will be outlined here.

Dengue fever

Aetiology: Four antigenic types of dengue virus and three other arthropod-borne viruses (Chikun-gunya, O'nyong-nyong, and West Nile fever) cause similar or identical disease.

Epidemiology: The dengue viruses are transmitted by mosquitoes of the stegomyia family, and the reservoirs are monkeys, birds, and other wild animals. Because of the limited flying range of mosquitoes, spread of an urban epidemic is mainly through movement of viraemic humans. Where dengue viruses are endemic, children and susceptible foreigners acquire overt disease, indigenous adults having become immune.

Epidemics of dengue fever have not occurred in southern Africa for 50 years. Chikungunya fever is prevalent in the Limpopo Valley and adjacent areas.

Clinical features: After an incubation period of 2–7 days a biphasic feverish illness develops, with headache, vomiting, myalgia, a transient macular, generalized rash, and lymphadenopathy. A secondary rise in temperature is accompanied by a generalized morbilliform, maculopapular rash, which spares the palms and soles. This lasts 1–5 days. Prolonged malaise and bradycardia during convalescence are seen in adults, but seldom in children. The platelet count and coagulation factors are normal. Diagnosis is confirmed by serology and virus isolation. Treatment is supportive, and the outcome is usually favourable.

Control of disease depends on measures against mosquito bites and mosquito breeding sites in stagnant water.

Dengue haemorrhagic fever (DHF)

DHF occurs where the different types of dengue virus are sequentially transmitted and second infections with heterologous types are common. DHF is a disease almost exclusively of children, and usually due to secondary infections. If it occurs during primary dengue infections, it affects infants whose mothers are immune. DHF is a biphasic illness similar to dengue fever, but hepatomegaly and a haemorrhagic diathesis occur, sometimes with circulatory shock. Thrombocytopenia, disseminated intravascular coagulation (DIC), and a rapid secondary-type rise in antibodies are the laboratory findings.

Treatment: Correction of shock and DIC.

Prognosis: Mortality rates vary from 5–40% depending on the effectiveness of management.

Rift valley fever (RVF)

Epizoötics of RVF, affecting sheep and cattle, have occurred in southern Africa since 1951. The disease is acquired by humans when handling carcasses and tissues of affected animals, and possibly from mosquito bites. RVF is spread among animals by mosquitoes. Person-to-person spread has not been noted.

After an incubation period of 4–6 days, a biphasic illness occurs, with fever, painful eyes, myalgia, diarrhoea and vomiting. During recrudescence of fever, encephalitis, hepatitis, and haemorrhagic diathesis are the main features. Management is supportive and fatalities do occur.

Marburg-Ebola fever

Marburg and Ebola viruses, while immunologically distinct, cause a similar disease. Epidemics have occurred in Uganda, Kenya, Sudan, and Zaire, and a small outbreak has occurred in South Africa, the primary case being a tourist who was probably infected in Zimbabwe. The viruses also cause infection in monkeys *(C. aethiops)*. The natural reservoir is unknown, as is the vector. Mosquitoes can be infected experimentally, but it is uncertain whether they transmit the disease.

The incubation period is 7–14 days, after which sudden fever, headache, malaise, arthralgia, diarrhoea, vomiting, and conjunctivitis develop. On the fifth to the seventh day an erythematous macular rash occurs, most marked on the upper arms and legs, followed by hepatic and renal damage and DIC.

Management: Since secondary person-to-person infection has occurred, strict isolation of the patient is necessary. Attendants must take meticulous care with barrier nursing. Treatment is symptomatic. The mortality rate is considerable.

Lassa fever

The reservoir for this virus, the rodent *Mastomys nataliensis,* is widespread in Africa, but the disease in humans has so far been limited to West Africa. Subclinical disease can occur, but high mortality rates of 35–65% among hospitalized cases have been reported. The modes of spread between people and from rodents to people have not been established, but virus has been isolated from the pharynx and urine. Rodents may contaminate the air, food, or water through their urine and saliva.

The incubation period is 3–16 days, followed by fever, chills, headache, pharyngitis, and myalgia. The febrile stage lasts 7–21 days. Hepatic and renal damage may occur, with haemorrhage into the bowel and lungs.

Crimean-Congo haemorrhagic fever (CCHF)

Hyalomma ticks, which are the vectors of the disease, occur widely in Africa, eastern Europe, and Asia. Antibodies to CCHF are found in cattle all over South Africa, suggesting the virus has occurred widely for years. Ticks are infected when feeding on viraemic small mammals (e.g., hares), and transmit the infection to livestock. While cattle and sheep do not become ill, they are briefly viraemic and can be a source of infection for people. Humans are infected from tick bites, from squashing ticks, or from contact with livestock tissue or with patients. Such nosocomial infection involves direct contact with infective blood. Mild and inapparent infections occur. Case fatalities occur in 15–70%, the latter being in nosocomial outbreaks.

The incubation is about one week, followed by sudden onset of severe headache, fever, and chills. Frequently dizziness, amnesia, confusion, and changed behaviour supervene, accompanied by myalgia, diarrhoea, nausea, anorexia, and vomiting. Fever is often biphasic, and hyperaemia of the face and chest occurs, with conjunctivitis, pharyngitis, bradycardia, and hypotension. Haemorrhagic diathesis appears in severe cases on the third to sixth day.

Special investigations may show anaemia, leucopenia, thrombocytopenia, abnormal coagulation factors, and raised liver enzymes. Management is supportive.

Differential diagnosis of acute haemorrhagic fever

Meningococcaemia, staphylococcal and streptococcal septicaemia, malaria, and trypanosomiasis are conditions to be considered.

The approach to a case of suspected acute haemorrhagic fever is to assume the worst: isolate and barrier nurse the patient, and take every precaution to prevent nosocomial spread; keep all contacts under close surveillance.

► Viral haemorrhagic disease

Suspect in the presence of the combination of: Chills, headaches, vomiting, diarrhoea, myalgia, arthralgia, fever (often biphasic), rash, conjunctivitis, hepatitis and/or encephalopathy and/or haemorrhagic diathesis.

Differential diagnosis: Septicaemia, malaria, trypanosomiasis.

Management: Barrier nursing, protect attendants supportive close observation of contacts.

Immunization

Schedule

Some of the infectious diseases can be prevented by immunization. An example of a schedule is given in *Table 8.13*.

Notes and comments

BCG: *(Also see Chapter 9, Tuberculosis.)* Adverse reactions are rare, and consist of ulceration at vaccination site, lymphadenopathy, and osteomyelitis. In children who fail to get BCG at birth, it is given at the first visit to the immunization clinic. BCG can be given again at school entry and school leaving if tuberculin testing is negative.

DTP: Common adverse reactions within 48 hours of vaccination are pyrexia (38.5 °C) and local induration and tenderness.

► Reactions which constitute absolute contraindications to continuing DTP are convulsions, encephalitis, focal neurological signs, and collapse with shock.

Probable contraindications to continuing DTP are excessive somnolence, screaming attacks of more than 3 hours' duration, and a fever above 40 °C.

DTP is not embarked upon if the infant has progressive neurological disease, a history of fits, or has a significant febrile illness. Babies with a mild upper respiratory infection, low-grade fever or diarrhoea can receive DTP.

The side-effects are largely due to the pertussis component of the triple vaccine. Thus children who have any contraindications to continuing or starting DTP, as well as those commencing the

Table 8.13   Vaccination schedule

Age	Vaccine
Birth	BCG (Bacillus Calmette-Guérin vaccine)
	OPV (oral live attenuated poliovirus vaccine) monovalent
3 months	DTP (Diptheria and tetanus toxoids, killed *Bordetella pertussis vaccine; 'triple vaccine'*)
	OPV (trivalent)
	BCG if there is no visbible evidence of previous BCG vaccination
4½ months	DTP, OPV (trivalent)
6 months	DTP. OPV (trivalent)
	Measles vaccine for high-risk infants*
9 months	Measles vaccine*
	OPV (trivalent)
15 months	Measles vaccine for low-risk infants
	Mumps vaccine
	Rubella vaccine
18 months	DTP: first booster
School entry	DT: second booster
	BCG repeat
9–10 years	DT: third booster
	Rubella vaccine for girls not previously immunized
School leaving	BCG if tuberculin test negative

* See text

programme after the age of 3 years, are given DT and not DTP.

A booster of DT at school entry is needed to ensure a protective level of diphtheria antibody into adulthood, but tetanus antibody levels are usually adequate without this. Tetanus toxoid boosters are recommended every 10 years.

New acellular pertussis vaccine: An acellular pertussis vaccine containing only one or two purified and detoxified antigens has been shown to be protective against whooping cough, and to cause fewer adverse reactions than the whole-cell vaccine. This new vaccine will take the place of the whole-cell vaccine in the DTP triple vaccine.

Poliomyelitis vaccine: OPV (Sabin) vaccine has the advantage of ease of administration and the induction of local gut immunity which prevents wild polio virus survival. Recipients also shed vaccine virus, which can spread to and protect the unvaccinated.

The risk of paralytic poliomyelitis was found in the USA to be 1 in 11.5 million doses. The major disadvantage of OPV in developing communities is that serological failures are sometimes unacceptably high after three or four OPV feedings. Many are due to widespread interference in the gut by other enteroviruses. To counter this, an extra (fifth) dose in the first year is suggested.

Breaks in the 'cold chain' from supplier of OPV to the field-worker may lead to inactivation of the vaccine and cause vaccination failures. A return to the inactivated Salk vaccine has been advocated. This vaccine, given by injection with boosters, gives a high seroconversion rate and has no complications.

Measles attenuated live virus vaccine: This vaccine may cause a fever or a mild measles-like illness 7–10 days after administration. The incidence of reactions is higher in the poorly nourished, but even those with kwashiorkor show seroconversion, although this is delayed. Because vaccine virus, like the wild virus, causes temporary immunoparesis, use of the vaccine in the malnourished should be restricted to those at home (as opposed to those at increased risk for superinfection, e.g., in a hospital), or to those whose nutritional rehabilitation has been initiated. Interim protection, if needed, is achieved by giving human measles immunoglobulin or pooled gammaglobulin, followed in 6 weeks by active immunization. Failures of seroconversion may be due to improper handling and storage of the vaccine, but also to the presence of maternal antibody in those under 1 year of age.

In developing communities the risk of measles in the first year is high, and carries increased mortality and morbidity. Therefore the younger the child is vaccinated the better. The Schwarz strain of vaccine virus (grown on chick embryo fibroblasts) is recommended at 9 months of age, but the new vaccine strain, grown on human diploid cells (Edmonston-Zagreb), when given in high titre at 6 months, achieves high seroconversion and protective rates. Field trials are in progress to determine whether a second dose is required at 9 months of age.

In low-risk communities with satisfactory socio-economic conditions, measles vaccine (Schwartz) is given at 15 months, when it can be administered with rubella and mumps vaccines.

In countries where measles occurs in older children and young adults:
◆ continue currently used schedules
◆ immunize groups with low coverage.

The occurence of measles in older children has arisen even where there has been moderately high coverage (90%) with vaccine, and is due to:
◆ coverage less than 100% in those < 2 years of age
◆ vaccine failures caused by:
— primary vaccine failures, amounting to 2–5% of vaccinated children
— vaccinating very young children with Schwartz vaccine
— waning immunity (in a small proportion of cases).

Measles vaccine can be given at the same time as the first DTP and OPV if the primary immunizing course is started after 1 year of age.

Rubella: The live attenuated vaccine RA 27/3 has a high seroconversion rate (95%) and virtually no untoward reactions when given to children. As with other live virus vaccines, it should not be given to pregnant women or to those who may become pregnant within 3 months of receiving vaccine. The teratogenic effect of rubella virus is well-known, but it is not yet established whether or not the vaccine is associated with embryopathy. Reinfections with rubella can occur: in epidemics there is a much higher incidence of reinfection in vaccinated people (80%) than in those with natural immunity (40%).

Mumps attenuated virus vaccine: This has no untoward reactions and produces antibody titres which are protective in 95% of cases, but are lower than titres following natural disease. While the use of this vaccine should not take priority over more essential community health needs, some complications of mumps are serious enough to warrant the use of a safe vaccine.

It is not yet known if vaccine-induced immunity in infancy against mumps and rubella will be lifelong.

Varicella vaccine: A vaccine is required for use in immunocompromised patients in whom varicella may cause severe and disseminated disease. A live attenuated varicella vaccine which is safe has been developed, with a high protective efficacy in healthy children. When given to leukaemic children, seroconversion and protection are slightly reduced, and reactions more frequent.

Hepatitis B vaccine: Vaccine is derived from formalin-inactivated HBS Ag particles obtained from plasma of carriers. A course of three doses given at monthly intervals produces no ill-effects in neonates, and immunogenicity is not reduced by pre-existing maternal antibodies. This vaccine is given with HB immune globulin to prevent transmission to the at-risk neonate. In children over 1 year, the second and third doses are given at 1 and 6 months after the first dose.

It is a safe vaccine with mild and occasional side-effects: sore arm, fever, fatigue, or nausea.

Vaccine is indicated in high-risk populations, e.g., selected health and laboratory workers, infants of HBS Ag-positive mothers (especially those who are also HBe positive), renal dialysis patients, institutionalized patients and their attendants, patients receiving repeated blood transfusions, illicit drug users, accidental needle stick injuries, and household contacts of hepatitis B subjects. Screening for immunity should be done before commencing vaccination.

Bacterial polysaccharide vaccines

Meningococcus: A bivalent meningococcal A/C vaccine is available. The infection in Africa is mainly due to Group A, although some cases of Group B have occurred.

Immune response to Group A antigen is satisfactory from the age of 3 months. A protective titre of antibodies develops in one week and last for 1–3 years. The other groups of antigens are poor immunogens under 2 years of age. Improved protein-conjugate vaccines have been developed, which are protective in the very young. The vaccine is indicated to control outbreaks of meningococcal disease, for travellers to epidemic areas, and for household contacts of a patient. The conjugate vaccine is undergoing trials in infants shortly after birth.

Pneumococcus: The vaccine is a polyvalent preparation of pneumococcal capsular polysaccharides. In recipients older than 2 years, protective antibody levels are achieved in 2 weeks and last for 5–8 years. The vaccine is indicated in high-risk patients, e.g., post-splenectomy, sickle-cell anaemia, nephrotic syndrome, Hodgkin's lymphoma.

The vaccine is poorly immunogenic in children less than 2 years. A conjugate vaccine of pneumococcus polysaccharides and a carrier protein could become available soon for use in children younger than 2 years.

Haemophilus influenzae B: Vaccine made from highly purified capsular polysaccharides is not protective in those under 2 years of age, who have the highest attack rate. The use of diphtheria or tetanus toxoid as the carrier protein for polysaccharide antigens rendered them more immunogenic in infants. Field trials are under way testing the conjugate vaccine in those under 6 months of age.

Typhoid vaccine: Vaccine containing killed organisms of typhoid and paratyphoid A & B (TAB) has been used for some years. It offers some, but not complete, protection, and is not very effective against large numbers of swallowed organisms, as may occur in developing countries. Thus where typhoid is endemic TAB vaccine has little place. It is not given under the age of 2 years or over 45 years. More recently new vaccines have been developed which are described above *(see section on Typhoid)*.

Cholera vaccine: Subcutaneously administered vaccine of killed *Vibrio cholerae* protects about 50% for about 6 months, and so a reinforcing dose is required every 6 months. Furthermore, the immune vaccinee can become a carrier and thus spread the organism.

Antitoxic activity can be induced by the oral route. Stable, nontoxigenic mutants of *V. cholerae* are available and being tested.

Contraindications to vaccination

Inactivated vaccines: *see under DTP.*
Live attenuated virus vaccines: pregnancy and immunodeficiency.

Those children allergic to eggs or egg products should not be given:

◆ duck embryo-grown rabies virus vaccine
◆ yellow fever vaccine
◆ inactivated influenza vaccine.

However, **these children can be given** human diploid cell rabies vaccine and vaccines grown in chick embryos, i.e.,

- measles vaccine
- mumps vaccine.

Immunization of HIV-infected children: WHO recommendations advise against BCG vaccination in symptomatic patients. Where the risk of tuberculosis contact is low it can also be omitted in asymptomatic children. There are no restrictions with regard to DPT, OPV, and measles vaccines.

Note: While every effort is made to complete an immunization schedule in the optimum time, in developing countries this is often not possible. However, perseverance is necessary. Every contact with a child by a health professional must be seen as an opportunity to bring the immunization schedule up to date.

Immunization programmes have failed because of:
- lack of political commitment by national decision-makers
- inadequate funding, staff, supplies, and equipment
- failure to implement comprehensive primary health care.

Use every contact with a child to bring vaccination schedules up to date.

Contra-indications to DTP are confined to:
- progressive neurological disease
- history of fits
- significant febrile illness.

Rickettsial infections

Rickettsiae have biological characteristics of both bacteria and viruses. They appear as pleomorphic cocco-bacilli on light microscopy, with a diameter of 0.3–0.5 microns..

The organism is transmitted to man from an animal reservoir by arthropod vectors such as the tick, louse, and mite. Small vessel endothelium is invaded, and subsequent proliferation of cells may result in thrombosis and/or plasma leakage. These changes occur principally in skin, meninges, brain, myocardium, kidneys, and lungs, and are responsible for the characteristic symptomatology.

Rickettsial infections in childhood can be grouped according to a number of different criteria into the following:
- typhus
- scrub typhus
- spotted fevers, e.g., tick-bite fever, Rocky Mountain spotted fever
- Q fever.

The main epidemiological and clinical features of these are summarized in *Table 8.14*.

Q fever, which rarely affects children, differs markedly from the others in that the mode of spread is by inhalation of infected animal material, with subsequent pulmonary symptomatology and varying degrees of systemic illness.

Clinical features

Generally rickettsial infections are mild in children and often escape diagnosis.

Tickbite fever (tick typhus) is seen predominantly in Caucasian children. Early exposure causing mild illness and producing long-lasting immunity might account for the infrequent occurrence of this disease in other groups.

The dominant features are pyrexia and headache, which rapidly reach peak intensity and respond poorly to symptomatic treatment. A small eschar at the site of the bite is found in most patients, with regional lymphadenopathy. The typical maculopapular, non-blanching rash appears on the second or third day in less than 50% of patients. A moderate splenomegaly is sometimes encountered. Significant cardio-

Table 8.14   Rickettsial infections: Summary of pertinent information

Disease group	Causative agent	Vector	Animal host	Incubation period (days)	Rash (day of onset)	Proteus strain (Weil-Felix reaction)
Typhus	*R. prowazeki*	Louse	Humans	14	4–7	OX19 +++
Scrub typhus	*R. tsutsugamushi*	Mite	Rodents	6–11	5–8	OXK +++
Tick-bite fever	*R. conorii, australis*, etc.	Tick	Mammals, rodents	5–8	2–3	Variable

vascular, respiratory, or neurological features are absent.

The disease is self-limiting, with symptoms settling after a week.

Epidemic typhus occurs at times of war and during population shifts when facilities for hygiene are inadequate and there is general dislocation. It is the most severe of the rickettsioses in children, although not as serious as it is in adults. The disease is spread by contaminated faeces of an infected body louse. The faeces gain entry through abraded skin or the upper respiratory tract. After an incubation period of up to 14 days, there is a sudden onset of severe pyrexia, headache, and malaise. The rash which appears 4–7 days after onset blanches on pressure initially but in severe cases is haemorrhagic.

In some cases the rash may be transient or not appear at all.

Stupor, delirium, circulatory collapse, and renal insufficiency suggest severe pathology, and these features may be accompanied by pneumonia. The untreated patient improves during the third week and recovers completely thereafter.

Diagnosis

Rickettsiosis must be considered in any patient with pyrexia of unknown origin. Meningococcaemia, typhoid, measles, meningitis, and encephalitis must be considered in the differential diagnosis. Typical features, i.e., rash and/or eschar, facilitate an early diagnosis.

Laboratory confirmation is not always possible. Although the proteus OX antigens are non-specific, rising antibody titres to these are helpful in diagnosis. Specific antigens for complement fixation tests and immunofluorescence are reliable but not readily available.

Treatment

Chloramphenicol and tetracyclines both suppress but do not kill rickettsiae. Nevertheless they have made a considerable difference to the severity of this disease complex.

Dosage (of either drug): 50–100 mg/kg/24 hours by mouth in 4 divided doses, or 30–40 mg/kg/24 hours IV in 8-hourly doses.

Drug treatment should be continued until the child has been apyrexial for 48 hours.

Supportive measures such as maintenance of hydration and nutrition are of utmost importance. Plasma or plasma expanders are used for circulatory collapse.

Prevention

Appropriate control measures must be instituted where conditions are conducive to epidemics. Rickettsiosis spread by ticks can usually be prevented by early search for and removal of ticks, as 2–3 days elapse before inoculation occurs.

Protozoal infections
Malaria

Although largely confined to tropical and subtropical regions of Africa, Asia, and America, increasing numbers of sporadic cases of malaria occur in non-malarious areas, as for example in individuals returning from visits to endemic areas. Freak transmission may also occur when an infected mosquito is conveyed to a non-malarious area by car or aeroplane.

In southern Africa, malaria is endemic in Malawi, Mozambique, northern Namibia, the lowveld of Zimbabwe, and northern Botswana. Epidemic outbreaks occur in the northern and eastern Transvaal and Zimbabwe, northern Natal and Swaziland, and in pockets in the northern Cape.

Aetiology and pathogenesis
(See Fig. 8.7.)

A vector-borne parasitic infection, malaria is caused by parasites of the genus plasmodium. Four species — *P. falciparum, P. vivax, P. ovale* and *P. malariae* — infect man and cause malignant tertian, tertian, ovale, and quartan malaria respectively. All four species occur in southern Africa. *P. falciparum* is the most prevalent and causes the most severe infection.

The life cycle is passed in two hosts: the asexual phase (schizogony) in man, and the sexual (sporogony) in the anopheles mosquito. After the female anopheles mosquito injects sporozoites into a human's bloodstream, development of the parasite occurs in the parenchymal cells of the liver (pre-erythrocytic phase). Invasion of the bloodstream and red cells by the parasite follows. Multiplication and maturation in the red cell leads

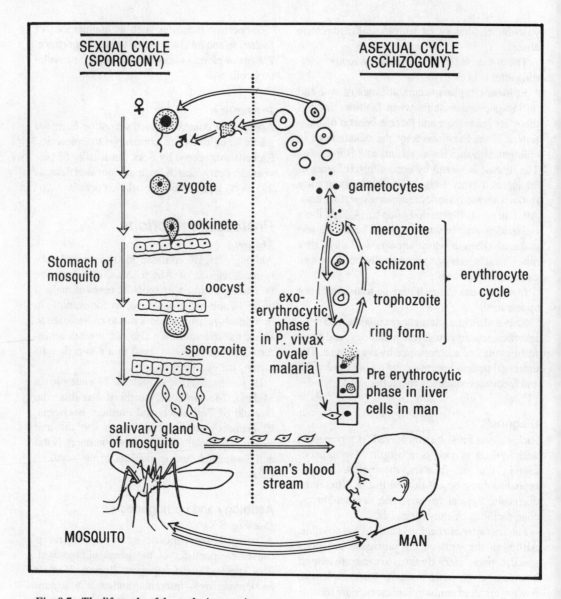

Fig. 8.7 The life-cycle of the malaria parasite

to red cell rupture. Reinvasion of red cells occurs and the cycle is repeated many times (erythrocytic phase). Attacks of fever are believed to correspond with the end of each erythrocytic cycle, occurring at 48-hour intervals in *P. falciparum*, *P. vivax*, and *P. ovale* infections, and at 72-hour intervals in *P. malariae* infection.

After schizogony has been repeated many times, sexual forms (gametocytes) appear and are sucked up by the mosquito to start the sexual cycle in the insect host.

In *P. vivax*, *P. ovale*, and *P. malariae* infections, parasites may re-enter liver cells, where they continue to multiply long after the initial bloodstream invasion has ceased (exo-erythrocytic cycles). Later reinvasion of the bloodstream results in a relapse of malaria. This may occur many years after the initial attack, especially in *P. malariae* infections, which have been known to relapse as long as 40 years after the initial infection. *P. falciparum* does not have an exo-erythrocytic cycle.

Although the bite of a mosquito is the usual mode of transmission, man may acquire the infection by means of a blood transfusion from an asymptomatic infected donor. Rarely, an infected mother may transmit the parasite to her fetus.

The ability of the malarial parasites to proliferate and produce clinical manifestations depends on their virulence, the size of the infecting dose, and the immune status of the host.

An attack of malaria is followed by a rise in immunoglobulin levels. Initially the IgM fraction rises steeply, but in chronic malaria the increase is predominantly in the IgG fraction. Transplacental passive immunity from mother to fetus probably explains the rarity of congenital malaria and the relative freedom from infection in young infants in endemic areas. As passive immunity wanes, clinical manifestations occur, but repeated exposures to infection lead to a tolerance between the host and the parasite. Clinical manifestations thereafter no longer occur provided the host continues to be exposed to infection. This state is known as *premunity*, and it is lost after a few years if the host leaves a malarious area. Re-exposure after this time results in a return of symptoms, but some degree of protection persists because fatalities rarely occur, unlike in a primary attack in a fully susceptible individual.

In certain hyperendemic areas an innate immunity to malaria may be present in addition to acquired immunity. G6PD deficiency and the sickle-cell trait appear to protect against *P. falciparum* infection, and the absence of the Duffy antigen in red cells in certain inhabitants of tropical Africa is believed to protect them against *P. vivax* infections.

An attack of malaria results in marked activity and hypertrophy of the reticulo-endothelial system, giving rise to enlargement of the liver and spleen.

Malarial pigment, released when parasitized red cells rupture, is phagocytosed by cells of the reticulo-endothelial system, giving rise to pigmentation of the skin and internal organs.

Destruction of red cells leads to anaemia with reticulocytosis and to jaundice.

In *P. falciparum* disease, infected red cells tend to adhere to each other and to the vascular endothelium. Interference with circulation and resulting tissue damage may affect many organs in the body, leading to a variety of complications.

Clinical manifestations

The incubation period is shortest in *P. falciparum* infections. Symptoms usually develop within 7–12 days of exposure, while in *P. vivax, P. ovale,* and *P. malariae* infections, 10–30 days may elapse after infection before clinical manifestations occur. Incomplete prophylaxis or partial immunity may suppress symptoms and signs for longer periods after infection has occurred. The onset is usually abrupt and often occurs in the morning.

Fever is the most common presenting sign, and initially tends to be remittent, but after some days typical periodicity is established.

In a classical attack, headache and muscle and joint pains rapidly progress to shivering and rigors. This is followed by flushing and complaints of feeling hot. Nausea and vomiting may occur, and severe headache and delirium may be present. Finally there is profuse sweating with relief of symptoms.

Cold, hot, and sweating stages are unusual in infants and children. Convulsions may occur during the height of the fever in the very young.

The spleen tends to be enlarged, and some degree of anaemia, together with a mild leucopenia, is usually present.

Infections due to *P. vivax, P. ovale,* and *P. malariae* commonly present in this manner, but *falciparum* malaria frequently presents atypically. The periods of fever may be irregular, and an undramatic picture of fever and constitutional symptoms may suddenly deteriorate when complications occur. These are usually the result of delay in diagnosis which allows for several cycles of replication of the parasite. Heavy parasitaemia is always a feature of complicated *falciparum* malaria.

Complications

Depending on which organ bears the brunt of infection, the following complications may be seen:

Cerebral malaria is the most dangerous complication, and is commonly present in fatal cases. Cerebral oedema and hypoxia produce symptoms varying from apathy to coma, disorientation to psychotic behaviour, focal, or sometimes even extra-pyramidal signs and, on occasion, convulsions. Rarely, frank malarial meningitis may be found.

Confusion is a warning sign that cerebral malaria is imminent.

Gastrointestinal involvement leads to severe vomiting, abdominal pain and distension with profuse watery diarrhoea or even dysentery, with the passage of blood-stained stools. Occasionally an acute abdomen may be simulated.

Hepatic necrosis with marked jaundice and disturbed liver function tests may dominate the clinical picture.

Acute renal failure with oliguria or anuria as a consequence of dehydration, hypotension, or intravascular coagulopathy may necessitate dialysis.

Massive intravascular haemolysis leading to haemoglobinuria and oliguria constitutes **blackwater fever.** This complication is believed to result from a hypersensitivity reaction of the host to his or her red cells, made autoantigenic by repeated quinine therapy and malarial infection. Pamaquine or primaquine therapy in the presence of G6PD deficiency may also cause *blackwater fever*. Rarely, it may be seen in a first attack of malaria before treatment is given.

Haematological involvement as shown by the presence of anaemia is invariable. Anaemia, if severe, may lead to cardiac failure. Even unparasitized cells have an increased osmotic fragility. Rarely, a positive Coombs' test suggests autosensitization. Purpura and bleeding from mucosal surfaces are consequences of disseminated intravascular coagulation.

Pulmonary complications are common in cerebral malaria. Oedema, congested capillaries, haemorrhages, and hyaline membrane formation may be found at autopsy, and present clinically with severe refractory hypoxaemia. Bacterial pneumonia may also occur.

'Algid' malaria is a term given to a syndrome which resembles Gram-negative shock. Severe complications are unusual in *P. vivax* or *P. ovale* malaria. Even in *falciparum* infections in the par-

tially immune, mild fever with general malaise lasting for a few days may be the only manifestation, and symptomless parasitaemia is not uncommon. Exceptions occur in pregnant women, who are liable to develop very severe attacks, as are splenectomized and immunosuppressed individuals.

Chronic malaria is seen in patients who have had inadequate or no treatment. As immunity develops, acute attacks gradually lessen. *P. falciparum* infections usually disappear within a year, and *P. vivax* infections within 2 years. Splenic enlargement, which may be massive and lead to hypersplenism, or rupture in response to trauma, is a feature of chronic *P. malariae* infections. Malarial nephrosis is a further important complication of quartan malaria. It is a common cause of death from renal failure in children in West Africa, unless the condition is diagnosed and treatment is instituted early.

Diagnosis

The symptoms and signs are rarely sufficiently specific to make a clinical diagnosis, and the only certain proof of malaria infection is the finding of the parasites in the peripheral blood.

A single negative finding does not exclude malaria. Repeated blood films may be required, and those taken during the height of fever are most likely to reveal parasites.

These may be more easily seen in thick films, but thin films may be necessary to identify the species of the infecting plasmodium. Small doses of antimalarial drugs or other drugs such as sulphonamides may result in negative films. The finding of malarial pigment in neutrophils or monocytes is strongly suggestive of malaria, even in the absence of parasites.

Bone marrow examination for detection of parasites may be of value, particularly in chronic malaria. Serological tests such as immunofluorescence for detecting antibodies may also be of help in the diagnosis of chronic malaria. When the diagnosis is strongly suspected but not proven, antimalarial therapy may be prescribed. Provided drug resistance can be excluded, failure of response to therapy makes the diagnosis unlikely.

Treatment

Uncomplicated attack: *Chloroquine* is the drug of choice for rapid elimination of the asexual forms in all four species. Dose: 10 mg base/kg orally immediately, followed by 5 mg base/kg 6–8 hours later, and 5 mg base/kg daily for 3 days. (Commercial names of chloroquine are Aralan® (not yet available in South Africa) and Nivaquine®. Standard tablet = 150 mg base.)

Primaquine should be given in addition to chloroquine in *P. vivax, P. ovale,* and *P. malariae* infections, for the hepatic or exo-erythrocytic phase of the parasite. Dose: 0.3 mg/kg orally, daily for 14 days. Primaquine is also effective against gametocytes of all four species.

Complicated malaria: *Supportive therapy* is as important as chemotherapy in severely ill patients, and includes maintenance of fluid and electrolyte balance. Accurate diagnosis of the cause of oliguria and uraemia and careful monitoring are necessary to prevent iatrogenic pulmonary oedema. Blood transfusion may be necessary.

In cerebral malaria *convulsions* are managed with diazepam and phenobarbitone or paraldehyde. *Hyperpyrexia* must be controlled. If *coma* persists for more than 24 hours, mannitol IV may reduce cerebral oedema; dexamethasone is no longer advocated for this purpose. Anticoagulant therapy has not been shown to improve prognosis.

Intravenous antimalaria therapy is started immediately: quinine 10 mg/kg in 5% dextrose or saline should be given over 4 hours and repeated after 12 hours until the patient is able to take by mouth and is not vomiting or shocked. Alternatively chloroquine 5 mg/kg is infused over 4 hours and repeated in 12–24 hours (maximum daily dose 10 mg/kg). The loading dose is omitted when oral therapy is substituted for parenteral drugs.

Hypoglycaemia is common in severe malaria and must be excluded in children with neurological signs before the diagnosis of cerebral malaria is made.

Hypotension may result from parenteral chloroquine. In the presence of liver and renal failures, the dose of antimalarials should be reduced.

Prophylaxis

A combination of chloroquine and pyrimethamine (Daraclor®) is recommended, and is available in tablets or syrup. The dosage is as follows:

Over 12 years	2 tabs (taken as 1 dose)
6–12 years	1 tab
1–5 years	½ tab or 10 ml syrup
6 weeks–12 months	5 ml syrup.

The first dose should be taken prior to entry into a malarious area, continued weekly on the same day each week for as long as the individual remains in the malarious area, and for 4 weeks after leaving the affected area.

Drug-resistant malaria

Chloroquine-resistant *P. falciparum* infections are largely confined to Asia and South America, but isolated cases have been described in East Africa. Visitors to these areas may acquire a drug-resistant infection. Quinine is the drug of choice in these instances: 25 mg/kg/day divided into three doses and given for 7–10 days.

Giardiasis

Aetiology and epidemiology

The flagellated protozoan *Giardia lamblia* has a world-wide distribution but is more prevalent in tropical and subtropical areas, and particularly in economically depressed communities. Children are infected more commonly than adults.

Infection is acquired by transmission from person to person due to swallowing of cysts, which may also contaminate food or water. The parasite lives in the duodenum and upper jejunum.

The oval cysts measuring 8–12 by 7–10 μm contain four nuclei when mature. The feeding stage of the parasite (trophozoite) is pear-shaped and contains two symmetrically placed nuclei, a pointed posterior, and a rounded antenna. The ventral surface has a sucking disc for attachment to the intestinal mucosa. The parasites do not appear to enter mucosal cells, nor have they been convincingly shown to cause any morphological change in these cells. The majority of infections are asymptomatic, and may persist for years or disappear spontaneously. The pathogenicity is unpredictable, and the severity of symptoms is not related to the density of infection. Under certain circumstances diarrhoea occurs.

Clinical manifestations

Giardiasis is a common cause of traveller's diarrhoea, and in such instances there is usually an explosive onset with foul-smelling stools accompanied by abdominal distension and flatulence. This diarrhoea characteristically has a longer incubation period and persists for longer than traveller's diarrhoea from other causes.

Giardiasis is also a well-recognized cause of outbreaks of diarrhoea in young children's nurseries. The diarrhoea is associated with loose, green stools and varies in severity. In some children, vomiting and dehydration are early complications. In others the diarrhoea is less severe but persists or relapses intermittently. Abdominal pain and tenderness may be features. Certain children become anorexic and fail to thrive.

Chronic diarrhoea may be associated with evidence of malabsorption *(see Chapter 11, Gastrointestinal Disorders)*. Whether giardiasis is the sole cause of malabsorption or whether it is always associated with some other cause of faulty intestinal absorption is unclear. No consistent or characteristic mucosal bowel pattern has been shown to be associated with giardiasis. Normal jejunal mucosa is present in some, whilst in others, changes may be found that are indistinguishable from coeliac disease or other causes of malabsorption.

Giardiasis often co-exists with protein-energy malnutrition and may compound intestinal malabsorption. In such cases it must be actively excluded and treated.

Although giardiasis is common in congenital hypogammaglobulinaemia, other causes of malabsorption must be considered in the presence of the latter.

Diagnosis

Stools tend to be greasy and contain no blood or mucus. Trophozoites may be seen in the stool, but are often extraordinarily difficult to detect. Cysts usually appear only when symptoms have been present for a week or more. Repeated stool examination may be necessary to verify the diagnosis. As examination of duodenal aspirates may be needed to identify trophozoites, empirical treatment is justified when clinical suspicion is strong.

Treatment

Metronidazole given as a single dose for 3 days eradicates the infection in 90% of cases. Children under 4 years require 50 mg daily, and those between 4 and 8 years 100 mg daily. Tinidazole in a similar dose is equally effective, and may be better tolerated by some children.

Prevention

Travellers to endemic areas should drink boiled water and even refrain from using tap water to clean their teeth. Fresh salads are also best avoided when travelling. In endemic regions improved sanitation and water supply are clearly necessary.

Toxoplasmosis

The protozoal parasite, *Toxoplasma gondii* has a world-wide distribution and infects a wide range of animals, including domestic cats and birds. Infection is acquired by swallowing oocysts which contaminate soil, by close association with cats, or by eating undercooked meat. Humans are relatively resistant to infection, and in the majority of cases infection is asymptomatic. *T. gondii* is an intracellular parasite and may cause depression of cell-mediated and humoral immunity. Latent infections may become active during immunosuppression, or primary infections may occur in immunocompromised individuals, especially those with lymphatic or haematological cancer. Toxoplasmosis acquired during pregnancy is often symptomless in the mother, or may cause only mild fever and malaise. Parasites form local lesions in the placenta and are released into the fetal bloodstream. It is generally believed that the earlier the infection occurs in pregnancy, the more severe the damage to the fetus. Abortion, stillbirth, or premature birth may result. The baby may show obvious neurological and visceral involvement at birth, or be apparently normal and develop clinical manifestations after a latent period of months or longer. More than 50% of babies born to mothers who acquire toxoplasmosis during pregnancy are uninfected.

Clinical manifestations

Congenital toxoplasmosis: Severely infected infants show features common to most intrauterine infections, such as jaundice, hepatosplenomegaly, anaemia, and skin haemorrhages. Microphthalmia, retinitis, and hydrocephalus may occur.

Intracranial calcification, seen on skull radiographs, is usually not present at birth, but is a characteristic feature later. Microcephaly, mental retardation, and convulsions may be later manifestations.

Acquired toxoplasmosis: Most infections are asymptomatic. Lymphadenopathy, especially of the cervical nodes, is the most common manifestation, and there is a predominance of mononuclear cells in the peripheral blood. Infectious mononucleosis is a common misdiagnosis.

Fever, myalgia, a transient maculopapular rash, hepatomegaly, and rarely pneumonia, myocarditis, and glomerulonephritis have been described.

Meningoencephalitis is the usual manifestation in immunocompromised individuals. Eye involvement in the form of necrotizing retinitis may be seen.

Diagnosis

Demonstration of the parasite in CSF or in sections from fresh tissue may be possible in early symptomatic congenital toxoplasmosis, but serological tests are more commonly used to establish the diagnosis.

The indirect fluorescent antibody test is the most reliable. Both IgM and IgG antibodies may be measured. In infants suspected of having toxoplasmosis, failure to demonstrate IgM antibodies immediately after birth does not exclude the diagnosis. Repeat tests may be necessary to show a rising titre. Antibody levels may take months or years to decline after infection.

Treatment

A combination of pyrimethamine 1 mg/kg/day and sulfadiazine 100 mg/kg/day in divided doses for 21 days is recommended for treatment of congenital toxoplasmosis. This treatment will prevent further harm from the infection, but has little effect on damage already present. Even asymptomatic infants with serological evidence of infection should be treated to prevent possible intellectual impairment at a later stage.

Both pyrimethamine and sulfadiazine may produce haematological complications, and blood counts should be monitored during treatment.

Acquired toxoplasmosis is usually a self-limiting disease and does not require treatment.

Prevention

Women should avoid handling cat litter and eating undercooked meat during pregnancy. Those who have antibodies prior to pregnancy are safe from infecting their fetuses.

Trypanosomiasis

Trypanosomes are elongated, motile protozoa with tapering anterior and blunt posterior ends. African trypanosomiasis is transmitted by the tsetse fly (genus glossina), and American trypanosomiasis (Chagas' disease) by bugs.

African trypanosomiasis

This occurs between the latitudes 14 °N and 29 °S and has a focal distribution within this area. Two varieties are recognized: the East African form (due to *Trypanosoma rhodesiense*) is transmitted by *Glossina morsitans*, a tsetse fly which inhabits savannah country, whilst West African trypanosomiasis (caused by *T. gambiense*) is transmitted by *G. palpalis* flies, which prefer riverine areas. Geographical overlapping of the two forms may occur. *T. rhodesiense* and *T. gambiense* are morphologically identical, but show differences in biological behaviour.

East African trypanosomiasis: Animal hosts (usually ungulates) and the tsetse fly harbour the trypanosome, and people only become infected when they visit an affected area. Children are rarely infected.

The disease in those who live near endemic areas, and who are presumed to have some degree of immunity, differs from that which occurs in people from non-endemic areas, who lack any immunity. In the latter, symptoms usually start abruptly 8 – 10 days after being bitten by a tsetse fly, and features closely resemble those of malaria. Paroxysmal bouts of fever, headache, debility, dizziness, and anaemia are common symptoms. A trypanosomal chancre at the site of the bite is helpful in establishing the diagnosis, but is rarely present. Central nervous system signs such as tremor, dullness, gait changes, slurred speech, and coma are more important clues for the diagnosis of sleeping sickness, but are late manifestations.

The prognosis is bad if treatment is delayed until the onset of semi-coma. Lymphadenopathy and splenomegaly may be present. Myocarditis and oedema may occur.

The duration of illness is usually 4–9 months.

West African sleeping sickness tends to have a more acute onset in Caucasians than in Africans. Recurrent fever, blotchy erythematous rash, lymphadenopathy, and hepatosplenomegaly, together with the appearance of the trypanosomal chancre are helpful pointers to the diagnosis in Caucasians. Insomnia and personality changes may be noted early in the disease. Later, cardiac failure and central nervous symptoms dominate the clinical picture.

The course of the disease in Africans is more protracted. Children are more commonly infected than in *T. rhodesiense* sleeping sickness.

Diagnosis: Identification of the parasite in thick blood films, lymph node aspirations, or on bone marrow aspiration is necessary to establish the diagnosis. Repeated examinations may be necessary. Late in the disease trypanosomes may be seen in the CSF, which also shows a pleocytosis and elevated protein level.

Treatment: In early cases, suramin 20 mg/kg is given IV at 7-day intervals for 5 doses. Suramin is nephrotoxic and should not be given to anyone with renal disease. Urine examination should be performed after each injection, and therapy stopped if casts or haematuria are found.

Once CNS involvement is present, IV melarsoprol (not yet available in South Africa) is given: 0.4 mg/kg on 3 successive days at weekly intervals over 4 weeks. Anaemia should be corrected, and parasites should be eliminated from the blood and lymphatic system by giving suramin before commencing this therapy.

American trypanosomiasis (Chagas' disease)

Trypanosoma cruzi, the causative protozoan, is transmitted by contamination of the mucous membranes of the eye, mouth, and nose, or through skin abrasions by an infected bug. The infection is widespread in Central and South America. The highest incidence is in Brazil and Argentina, being most prevalent in areas where standards of living are poor.

The initial manifestation is a painful swelling in the eye or skin (the chagoma) together with enlargement of regional nodes. Fever follows and may persist for several weeks. In the young child, increasing debility progresses to cardiac failure and signs of meningeal irritation or encephalitis. The outlook is normally poor, with death supervening after many weeks. The disease may become chronic, especially in older children, with features of myocarditis persisting for variable periods of up to 10 years or more. Involvement of the alimentary tract, with dilatation and loss of muscle tone in the oesophagus and colon, may lead to dysphagia or constipation. Mental deficiency, speech disturbances, and involuntary movements indicate either ongoing CNS pathology or partial recovery after encephalitis in the acute phase.

Diagnosis depends on identifying the trypanosome in peripheral blood, but this may prove difficult in chronic cases. Laboratory-bred bugs, allowed to feed on a patient suspected of the disease, may be shown to have developing organisms in their gut after 2 weeks, and this can be helpful in confirming the diagnosis. Serological tests are not useful in endemic areas.

Treatment: If given in the acute stage, drug treatment may cure the disease:

Nifurtimox® (a nitrofurazone, not yet available in South Africa) 25 mg/kg/day orally in three divided doses for the first week, then 10–15 mg/kg/day for 2 months plus metronidazole 20 mg/kg/day for 1 month.

Benznidazole® (an imidazole not yet available in South Africa) 5–7 mg/kg/day given oarally for 2 months is an alternative therapy.

Preventive measures, which include improved housing and eradication of the vector, should be employed where possible.

Leishmaniasis

Caused by several different species of the protozoan leishmania, leishmaniasis is a collection of diseases which may involve the skin (cutaneous), skin and mucous membranes (mucocutaneous), and viscera (kala azar).

Phlebotomine sandflies are the vectors responsible for the spread of the infection, but this may also occur by direct contact through abraded skin, by blood transfusion, and even transplacentally from mother to fetus. Reservoir hosts such as rodents, dogs, and humans with inapparent infection also play a role in spreading infection.

The amastigote stage of the parasite occurs intracellularly in monocytes and endothelial cells of humans. After being taken up by the insect vector, the protozoa develop into flagellated extracellular promastigotes. These reach the salivary glands of the sandfly and are reinjected into the vertebrate host to complete the cycle.

There is a wide range of reactions to infection, which usually leads to a T lymphocyte-mediated response similar to that seen in tuberculosis and leprosy. The delayed hypersensitivity which results may be demonstrated by the leishmanin skin test. The majority of infections are not apparent. In others, absence of T cell-mediated immunity leads to diffuse cutaneous disease. Exaggerated delayed hypersensitivity is found in mucocutaneous forms, while depressed T cell response and an abnormal humoral immunity are present in visceral leishmaniasis.

Leishmania tropica causes infection confined to the skin. Predominantly a disease of children, it is endemic in large areas of south-west Asia, in southern Europe, and northern Africa. It also occurs in certain areas of southern Africa, such as Namibia.

The typical lesion, commonly referred to as 'oriental sore', but also as 'Baghdad boil' or 'Delhi boil', is an indolent granuloma. In rural areas the sore develops after a relatively short incubation period, ulcerates early, and heals within a year.

In urban areas there is a longer incubation period and a more protracted course.

Oriental sores are found on the exposed areas of the body and may be single or multiple. Initially presenting as irritating papules surrounded by erythema, they enlarge and are soon covered by brown scales or crusts which, when shed, reveal indolent ulcers with an offensive, purulent discharge. Satellite lesions may occur in the immediate vicinity of the sore. Secondary bacterial infection often occurs, and healing leads to scarring.

There are no constitutional symptoms.

Diagnosis is confirmed by demonstrating the parasite in smears or in biopsies of the ulcer.

Two unusual forms of cutaneous leishmaniasis are the result of abnormal host responses.

In **leishmaniasis recidiva** the delayed hypersensitivity response is exaggerated, but the infection is not eradicated. A chronic spreading lesion involves the face and resembles lupus vulgaris. A strongly positive leishmanin test establishes the diagnosis, but response to treatment is poor.

In **diffuse cutaneous leishmaniasis** little or no T cell response and very limited cellular reaction allow for widespread dissemination of the parasite in the skin. Chronic lesions about the nose continue to spread for many years. Large numbers of amastigotes are seen in macrophages, but the leishmanin skin test is negative.

Leishmania mexicana, found in Central America, causes a cutaneous lesion particularly involving the face and pinna of the ear (chiclero's ulcer).

Leishmania braziliensis has a wide distribution in South America, where it causes mucocutaneous disease (espundia). Fungating ulcers involve the nose, mouth, and even pharynx and tongue. Destruction of tissue leads to severe disfigurement and allows for secondary bacterial invasion. A positive leishmanin test distinguishes espundia from other causes of destructive lesions of the face.

Leishmania donovani, which is responsible for visceral disease (kala azar), has a wide distribution in areas in Asia, central Africa, southern Europe, and Central and South America. Kala azar affects all age groups, but in the Middle East and South America infants and young children are most commonly affected, while in India and the Sudan the older child is more commonly involved.

The incubation period is usually 2–6 months, and the onset insidious. Occasionally there is an abrupt onset with high fever, which later becomes undulant. Splenomegaly is almost invariably present. In certain areas lymphadenopathy is a prominent manifestation and simulates tuberculosis, leukaemia, and lymphoma. Anaemia, leucopenia, and thrombocytopenia occur later. In some cases hepatomegaly and jaundice appear. Gastrointestinal symptoms are said to be common in India. A picture similar to mucocutaneous leishmaniasis, with or without visceral involvement, may be seen in Africa.

In the untreated, progressive debility leads to intercurrent infection and death.

During or after treatment a depigmented macular rash or a papular lesion resembling leprosy may appear on the face and trunk.

Typically, large amounts of gammaglobulin are produced, but are non-protective against widespread dissemination of the parasite in liver sinusoids, spleen, bone marrow, and lymph nodes.

The **diagnosis** is established by identifying parasites in aspirates from these organs.

Treatment

Therapy is not indicated for oriental sores which are self-healing. When they involve the face, or are extensive or diffuse, chemotherapy should be given.

Sodium stibogluconate 20 mg/kg/day IV or IM is the medication of choice.

Systemic fungal infections

Of the thousands of known species of fungi, relatively few cause disease in man. Pathogenic fungi are divided into those causing superficial chronic disease of skin and nails (dermatophytosis, *see Chapter 24, Dermatological Disorders*), and the deep or systemic mycoses considered here. These may involve viscera such as lung, kidney, gastrointestinal tract, or meninges, but in some instances may also involve skin and mucous membranes.

Certain systemic fungal infections have a worldwide distribution but only cause serious infection in immunosuppressed hosts. Others have a limited geographic distribution, often infect many individuals in these areas, but cause disease only in a minority of those infected.

Table 8.15 Systemic fungal infections

World-wide distribution	Limited distribution
Actinomycosis*	Blastomycosis
Aspergillosis	Coccidioidomycosis
Candidiasis	Histoplasmosis
Cryptococcosis	Mucormycosis
Nocardiosis*	
Sporotrichosis	

* Actinomyces and nocardia are not true fungi, but filamentous micro-organisms related to mycobacteria or corynebacteria. Their characteristic branched mycelium growth makes them resemble fungi superficially, and for this reason they are included in this section.

Actinomycosis

The anaerobic causative organism, *Actinomyces israeli,* can be found on the teeth, pharynx, and tonsils of many normal individuals. Trauma from a tooth extraction, pyogenic infection, or possibly hypersensitivity to the organism is believed to precipitate the abscess formation, with multiple draining sinuses characteristic of the disease. Cervicofacial actinomycosis, presenting as a gradually enlarging, painless swelling of the neck and jaw, is the most common clinical form. Multiple sinuses form in the overlying skin, and pus contains typical 'sulphur granules'. Infection may spread to involve bone or meninges.

Abdominal actinomycosis, with the primary lesion in the caecum, appendix, or pelvic organs, presents as a hard, irregular, lower abdominal mass which may drain to the outside or progress to involve other abdominal organs.

Lung involvement leads to a chronic pulmonary infection, commonly of the lower lobes, which may extend to ribs, pleura, and subcutaneous tissues.

Treatment

Penicillin in massive doses (1–6 million units daily) required for several months. Surgical excision or drainage may be necessary adjuncts.

Nocardiosis

Nocardia belong to the same family as actinomyces but are aerobic and often acid-fast. This characteristic, and their ready fragmentation into bacillary forms, may make differentiation from *Mycobacterium tuberculosis* difficult, especially since suppurative disease of the lungs is a common manifestation of nocardiosis. The organisms are free-living in soil, and infection is by inhalation of contaminated dust. The initial presentation is an acute pneumonitis which has a marked tendency to become chronic in persons with lowered resistance. The lower lobes are involved most often. Fever, cough, dyspnoea, and chest pain are common clinical features, together with weight loss, night sweats, and radiological evidence of infiltration, suppuration, and cavitation. Localized spread to the pleural cavity or haematogenous spread to other organs may occur. A pustular skin eruption or multiple metastatic abscesses in many organs may simulate staphylococcal pyaemia. Meningitis and brain abscess may be complications.

The organism may gain entry through skin abrasions, leading to local chronic suppuration of subcutaneous tissues and bone, with draining sinuses. Discharging pus contains pigmented granules consisting of a tangled mass of hyphae.

The diagnosis of nocardiosis should be excluded in the presence of chronic lung suppuration in immunosuppressed children by repeated examination of sputum, microscopically and on culture.

Treatment
Sulphonamides or co-trimoxazole for several months.

Aspergillosis
Aspergillus fumigatus and other aspergillus may produce a variety of diseases in debilitated children and, rarely, in previously apparently healthy individuals.

Pulmonary aspergillosis usually complicates pre-existing chronic pulmonary disease. It may take the form of a hypersensitivity reaction with bronchospasm. Eosinophilia, elevated levels of serum IgE, and the recovery of *Aspergillus* organisms in secretions from the respiratory tract suggest the diagnosis.

Colonization of pre-existing lung cavities with the formation of fungal balls, or aspergillomata, may also occur. The lesion often causes no symptoms, and may only be found at necropsy. Recurrent haemoptyses and the finding of a cavitated lesion with a solid centre on chest radiograph are suggestive of the condition during life.

Rarely, diffuse pulmonary infiltration and the picture of a severe pneumonia unresponsive to antibiotics may occur. Lung biopsy may be the only means of establishing the diagnosis.

Any debilitating disease or immunosuppression may lead to dissemination of the fungus to lungs, kidneys, the brain, or endocardium.

Treatment
Amphotericin B.

Candidiasis
(See also Chapter 24, Dermatological Problems.)

Candida albicans may be a normal member of the flora of mucous membranes in the respiratory, gastrointestinal, and female genital tracts.

An oval, budding fungus which produces a pseudomycelium in tissues and exudates, it may cause lesions confined to mucous membranes, as in thrush or monilial vaginitis, or may be restricted to the skin and nails. Both skin and nails may be affected in mucocutaneous candidiasis. Rarely, invasion of the bloodstream gives rise to a candidaemia when multiple organs may be involved, or focal involvement of meninges, kidney, or endocardium may occur. Invasion is commonly via the gastrointestinal tract, but may be via the skin or renal tract.

Thrush has long been recognized as a common disease of early infancy, especially in pre-term neonates. The mother's vagina is thought to be the source of infection in most instances, but bottle teats and attendants' fingers may also spread infection. Trauma to the oral mucosa will increase the likelihood of thrush infection, and the use of broad-spectrum antibiotics has caused an increased incidence.

Characteristic greyish-white or cream patches on the oral mucosa, which when scraped have a raw, red area, are typical of thrush. Feeding problems are common as the result of oral discomfort, or are due to extension of the lesions into the oesophagus. Thrush oesophagitis has been shown to produce inco-ordination of swallowing, and an aspiration pneumonia as a sequel. Blood-stained vomiting may be a symptom. Monilial dermatitis of the perianal or buttock region is commonly present.

Pulmonary candidiasis in infants is a rare finding at autopsy. The rarity of lung involvement is attributed to the natural resistance of columnar epithelium to invasion by candida. Oral thrush is commonly but not invariably present. The diagnosis is difficult to make during life because there are no specific clinical or radiological features to distinguish the pneumonia as being of candidial origin. The isolation of candida in the mouth or pharynx is no proof of pulmonary candidiasis, but finding candida on blood culture in an infant with bronchopneumonia is strong presumptive evidence.

Disseminated candidiasis: Candidaemia is found in certain immunosuppressed or postoperative patients. A fluctuating fever is usual. Removal of intravenous catheters may abort the infection, but deep organ invasion such as endocarditis, urinary tract involvement, or meningitis may develop. Predisposing factors for dissemination include broad-spectrum antibiotic, AIDS or immunosuppressive therapy, diabetes mellitus, malignant disease, and surgery to the heart, brain, or gastrointestinal tract.

Candida endocarditis usually involves mitral and aortic valves, and may follow valve replacement or arise *de novo* in patients suffering from leukaemia. It should be considered in the presence of major arterial emboli and the finding of soft white retinal plaques.

Diagnosis

Candida may be cultured on Sabouraud's glucose agar. Repeated attempts to isolate the organism may be necessary. A variety of serological tests are available, but normal individuals show the presence of antibodies in low titre, and antibody formation is often defective in the immunosuppressed. A rising antibody titre is helpful in establishing the diagnosis.

Treatment

Thrush: Topical nystatin or amphotericin B.

Systemic candidiasis: Amphotericin B or flucytosine given IV.

Cryptococcosis

Also known as torulosis or European blastomycosis, cryptococcosis is caused by *Cryptococcus neoformans,* a simple, yeast-like, budding fungus which is free-living in soil and often found in pigeon faeces. The incidence in humans worldwide is not known because the majority of infections are asymptomatic. Disease is most commonly found in patients with neoplasia, collagen disorders, or those on steroid therapy. It has been seen in association with sarcoidosis, tuberculosis, and diabetes mellitus.

Infection occurs via the respiratory tract and pulmonary lesions may mimic tuberculosis, sarcoidosis or carcinoma. Involvement of skin, bone, joint, eye, kidney, or adrenal gland may occur, but the most common manifestation of dissemination is a chronic meningitis resembling a tuberculous infection. The subarachnoid space at the base of the brain is most frequently involved, but grey matter may also be affected.

Infrequently, a single granuloma may be found in the cerebellum or cerebrum, giving rise to a picture of encephalitis or a space-occupying lesion. The CSF in cryptococcal meningitis is under increased pressure and is generally turbid. Cells average 200–300 per cubic millimetre and are mainly lymphocytic, although in the early stages they may be neutrophils. An increased protein level together with a slightly decreased sugar and chloride are the usual findings. Organisms may be identified by Indian ink staining or on culture. The presence of cryptococcal antigen in the CSF or serum may be demonstrated by latex particle agglutination.

Cases of congenital cryptococcosis have been recorded, and the clinical picture is similar to that of other intrauterine infections such as toxoplasmosis.

Treatment

Amphotericin B on its own or with flucytosine.

Sporotrichosis

(See also Chapter 24, Dermatological Problems.) *Sporothrix schenkii,* a fungus of world-wide distribution in soil and on plants and timber, gains entry through an abrasion and commonly causes a characteristic skin lesion. A localized ulcerating granuloma at the site of infection is followed by thickening of draining lymphatic channels and the development of subcutaneous nodules, which may also ulcerate along the thickened lymphatic cord. Dissemination of the infection may occur in debilitated individuals and, rarely, the primary infection may be in the lung. Chronic inflammation and necrotic granulomas result.

Treatment

Potassium iodide by mouth is effective in skin lesions. Amphotericin B is indicated if systemic involvement occurs.

Blastomycosis

A systemic infection caused by *Bastomyces dermatitidis,* this disease is found in scattered areas of North America and Africa. Dogs and horses may be infected, but the organism is seldom isolated from the environment. The lung is believed to be the usual portal of entry, and infection gives rise to micro-abscesses resembling miliary tuberculosis. Dissemination may occur to any organ, but bone and skin are most commonly involved. Culture of the organism confirms the diagnosis. Serological tests are less reliable, being negative in 50% of the cases.

Treatment
Amphotericin B.

Coccidioidomycosis
Caused by *Coccidioides immitis,* a soil fungus, this condition is localized to south-western areas of the USA, and Central and South America. Infection is commonly by inhalation, and 60% of those infected show no symptoms. When present, they take the form of an influenza-type illness, together with skin eruptions such as urticaria, or erythema nodosum or multiforme. An allergic arthritis and phlyctenular conjunctivitis may be present. Pleural effusion may occur, and pulmonary involvement is frequently shown radiologically to be extensive, without obvious clinical signs. Diminished host resistance may lead to dissemination to the meninges or peritoneum.

The diagnosis is confirmed on culture, serology, or by demonstrating the fungus at biopsy.

Treatment
Amphotericin or miconazole given intravenously.

Histoplasmosis
This is common in the eastern-central USA, but sporadic cases occur in South America, Africa, Australia, and the Far East.

The causative organism *Histoplasma capsulatum* is found in soil contaminated by the excreta of birds and bats. Infection is by inhalation, and the majority of infections are asymptomatic, but massive infection leads to an acute febrile illness with cough, dyspnoea, and chest pain. Marked radiological changes are often present despite minimal clinical signs. Arthralgia and erythema nodosum or multiforme may occur. Most cases resolve with rest but, rarely, chronic pulmonary histoplasmosis supervenes and mimics pulmonary

tuberculosis. Acute disseminated disease may occur in infants or the immunosuppressed. The organisms multiply in the reticuloendothelial system, giving rise to weight loss, hepatosplenomegaly, and thrombocytopenic purpura and death unless treatment is given.

Culture of infected sites, histology, or serology establishes the diagnosis.

Treatment
Amphotericin B.

Mucormycosis
Mucormycosis is caused by organisms of the genera mucor, rhizopus, and absidia, which are widely distributed as bread moulds. It is characterized by the penetration of hyphae into the walls of blood vessels, leading to thrombosis, infarction, and necrosis. The gastrointestinal tract is a common site for serious infection in pre-term neonates and severely malnourished infants and children. The skin may be involved as a complication of burns. Diabetics are susceptible to infection, a characteristic site being the paranasal sinuses, from whence spread to the meninges may occur.

In leukaemia the lungs are often involved or the infection disseminates. Any severe debilitating illness such as chronic diarrhoea or uraemia and prolonged corticosteroid or chemotherapy predispose to the development of mucormycosis.

The diagnosis is frequently made only at autopsy, but should be suspected when an infection is associated with infarction. Culture or histology of a biopsy specimen confirms the diagnosis.

Treatment
Local excision or debridement is combined with amphotericin B given IV and as local irrigation (1 mg/ml). Ketoconazole is also effective, and can be given orally.

Parasitic helminths
Parasitic worms have a world-wide distribution, but are most prevalent in the tropics and subtropics where climatic conditions favour their spread. They multiply by laying eggs from which larvae hatch and mature to adult males and females. Most live in harmony with their human hosts, and they are seldom the only cause of poor nutrition in a

child. They may cause disease when they are present in large numbers, when infestations are repeated, and when the host defence mechanism is depressed.

Helminths are divided into nematodes (roundworms), cestodes (tapeworms), and trematodes (flukes).

Nematodes

The ova or larvae of most roundworms require an incubation period in warm, moist soil before they become infective. Children are very commonly infected because of their playing habits.

Table 8.16 lists some of the common roundworm infections in humans, and their usual modes of spread.

Ascaris lumbricoides

The ascaris is a soil-transmitted helminth with universal distribution, apart from regions with very hot, dry climates. As temperate and moist conditions are favourable for the worm ova, it is in these regions that ascaris infestation constitutes a public health problem. In some areas in the Pacific up to 94% of the population were found to be infested. Generally it is more prevalent among rural communities than those living in the cities, and young children are invariably the ones to be most heavily infested. The distribution is largely determined by the local habits of disposal of human excreta. The intensity of infestation in the individual corresponds roughly to the prevalence of the worm in the community.

The worm and its life cycle: Ascaris is the largest roundworm infesting humans, with the adult female reaching up to 400 mm in length. There is a wide variation in size depending on the age and worm-load. The worm is white-pink in colour, and tapers at both ends, with the posterior end of the male curved. The 200 000 ova which can be put out daily by the adult female are ovoid in shape and measure approximately $60 \times 40 \ \mu m$. In a favourable environment, e.g., moist clay soil, the ova can survive for up to two years. Dry heat, however, kills them within hours.

The ovum matures and becomes infective within 10–15 days of being passed. It is picked up by children playing in contaminated soil, or by eating vegetables treated with night-soil. The larvae hatch rapidly in the duodenum, penetrate into the bowel wall, and enter the portal or lymphatic circulation. On reaching the lung they burrow into the alveoli and make their way up the air passages into the pharynx. They are then swallowed and finally come to rest and mature in the gut. The cycle takes approximately 65 days and the adult worm lives 1–2 years.

Pathogenesis: Migration of the larvae through the lung is known to cause severe pulmonary eosinophilia *(see Chapter 13, Respiratory Diseases in Children)*. Focal or diffuse haemorrhage is said to occur in some children. The pulmonary phase is associated with an appreciable eosinophilia in the peripheral blood, and a subsequent rise in the IgE. Some authors claim that pre-existing asthma is aggravated by ascariasis.

Intestinal obstruction occurs as a result of an intertwined mass of worms blocking the bowel lumen. In addition, the worms stimulate intense spasm of the bowel around the worm bolus. Prolonged obstruction may result in necrosis of the

---

Table 8.16   Common nematode helminths and their usual mode of spread

Worms	Sources of infection	Mode of entry into human host
Ascaris	Faecal contamination of soil + vegetable	Eggs swallowed
Trichuris	Faecal contamination of soil + vegetable	Eggs swallowed
Enterobius*	Person to person. Contamination of families. Hands to anus to mouth	Eggs swallowed
Trichinella	Meat, especially pork	Encapsulated larvae swallowed
Hookworm	Damp ground, skin contact	Filariform larvae penetrate skin
Strongyloides*	Damp ground, skin contact	Filariform larvae penetrate skin
Filaria	Blood-sucking insects	Filariform larvae deposited through insect bites

* Auto-infection may occur. See life cycle in text.

bowel wall leading to perforation. A loop of bowel heavily laden with worms may twist, producing an intestinal volvulus, which will become ischaemic and gangrenous if left untreated. Intussusception and appendicitis are less common complications of ascariasis *(see Chapter 28, Surgical Problems).*

Worms often migrate into the common bile duct, causing biliary colic and cholangitis. Biliary strictures and calculi are uncommon complications, which usually occur if worms die within the biliary tree. The worms may penetrate into the liver parenchyma, stimulating a granulomatous inflammatory reaction; secondary infection will result in abscess formation. Obstruction of the pancreatic duct may cause pancreatitis.

There is well-documented proof that ascariasis interferes with the digestion and/or absorption of carbohydrates, proteins, fats, and vitamins, thus contributing to malnutrition of the host.

Clinical features: The history of worms escaping from the anus, mouth, or nose is common, but caution must be exercised in ascribing coexisting symptomatology to worm infestation.

There is no evidence that vague abdominal pain, fever, and convulsions can be caused by ascariasis.

Respiratory symptoms and signs are elicited by the migration of a large number of larvae through the lung *(see Pulmonary Eosinophilia, Chapter 13).* Abdominal symptoms and signs are due to partial or complete intestinal obstruction, characterized by abdominal pain and a palpable mass.

Biliary ascariasis is characterized by right upper quadrant abdominal pain and tenderness occurring in a patient with evidence of intestinal ascariasis. The gall bladder may be palpable, but jaundice is rare.

The features of acute pancreatitis due to ascaris infestation resemble those of biliary ascariasis with abdominal tenderness, and guarding extends towards the left upper quadrant and left lumbar region.

Diagnosis and investigations: Stool microscopy confirms the diagnosis of ascaris infestation. Plain X-rays of the abdomen will show worms and/or demonstrate signs of partial or complete intestinal obstruction. The 'whirlpool' or 'target' sign is produced by an intestinal volvulus. The vast majority of worms in the biliary tract can be demonstrated by intravenous cholangiography or ultrasound scanning. Barium meal examination

may demonstrate worms in the duodenum, and those entering the bile duct are sometimes identified. Occasionally endoscopic cholangiography is used. Diagnosis of pancreatic involvement is again confirmed by the above investigations and serum amylase estimations.

Prevention: As ascaris infestation depends on contamination of the soil by human faeces, public health measures must be directed towards providing adequate sanitation. The use of sludge from sewerage as fertilizer is inadvisable, as it almost certainly carries viable ova. Chemical treatment of contaminated vegetables is singularly unhelpful.

It has been recommended that older infants and children living in an environment where ascariasis is endemic should be given a vermifuge regularly every 3–6 months.

Treatment: *(Also see Chapter 28, Surgical Problems.)*
Antihelminth options are:
◆ piperazine citrate in syrup form, 3–4g. This may be repeated after 2 days
◆ mebendazole 100 mg bd for 3 days
◆ pyrantel 10 mg/kg in one dose
◆ albendazole: 2–5 years, 200 mg in one dose; over 5 years, 400 mg in one dose.

There is no specific treatment effective against the larval stage in the lungs.

No vermifuge should be given when there is any suspicion of the intestinal obstruction.

Trichuris trichiura

Also known as *Tricocephalus trichiura* or whipworm because of its whip-like anterior portion, this parasite is very common in children in southern Africa and in most warm, moist areas of the world.

Life cycle: Eggs mature within 3 weeks of being deposited in soil. Larvae hatch in the terminal ileum and caecum, and full maturation occurs in about 3 months. In heavy infestations, the ascending colon, sigmoid, and rectum are involved. Adult worms live for 3–5 years. Unlike most other intestinal parasites, visceral invasion does not occur.

Clinical picture: Most infections are mild and asymptomatic. Symptoms attributed to *Trichuris* are often due to coexisting bacterial or other parasitic infections.

Heavy infestations cause chronic diarrhoea with mucoid stools which may contain blood. Tenesmus is a common complaint. Rectal prolapse and iron deficiency anaemia are complications and are frequently the presenting features. Anaemia may be severe and lead to cardiac failure. Oedema, as a result of hypoproteinaemia, is also seen. Some children with heavy infestations fail to thrive and become marasmic.

Blockage of the appendiceal lumen can lead to acute appendicitis.

Diagnosis: In heavy infestations inspection of a prolapsed rectum or sigmoidoscopy will reveal multiple, flesh-coloured, fine, whip-like structures attached to the mucous membrane. The characteristic barrel-shaped eggs with bipolar prominences are found in the stool.

Treatment: Mebendazole 100 mg bd by mouth for 4 days, or albendazole 400 mg daily for 3 days by mouth.

Enterobius vermicularis

Synonyms: oxyuris, threadworm, pinworm.

Unlike most other helminths, *Enterobius vermicularis* is more prevalent in temperate climates. Transmission is favoured by lack of bathing, the wearing of excess clothing, and overcrowding. Pre-school and school children are very commonly infected, and the infection rapidly spreads to the whole family. Eggs contaminate bed linen, clothes, toilet seats, toys, the fur of domestic pets, and remain viable in dust for long periods if the atmosphere is cool, moist, and poorly ventilated. Re-infestation from anus-to-hand-to-mouth is very common.

Life cycle: Embryonated eggs are swallowed, larvae hatch and mature in the small intestine, and gravid females migrate to the perianal area at night to deposit their eggs. Embryonated eggs may hatch in the perianal area and crawl back into the anus before migrating higher up the bowel. This is known as retroinfection.

Clinical findings: Pruritus ani results from the gravid female's noctural wanderings and egg-laying in the perianal area. The irritation leads to scratching, secondary infection, and may interfere with sleep. Enuresis has been attributed to pinworm infection. Vaginitis, endometritis and, very rarely, salpingitis may be complications.

Diagnosis: Transparent adhesive tape applied to the perianal skin is the most satisfactory method of obtaining ova for identification. Ova are rarely found in stools, but the 10 mm enterobius female worm may occasionally be seen.

Treatment: Piperazine compounds, 75 mg/kg/body weight daily for 1 week, or mebendazole, 100 mg as a single oral dose repeated in 1 week, are effective. High infestation rates often require repeated treatment. The whole family should be investigated and treated accordingly.

Prevention: Frequent bathing and changing of underclothes help to control spread. Finger-nails should be kept short.

Hookworm

Ancylostoma duodenale and *Necator americanus* are widely distributed throughout the tropics and subtropics. Miners, agricultural workers, and children are most commonly infected. Seventy per cent of schoolchildren have been found to harbour hookworm in some localities in northern Zululand, but infection is negligible in many other areas of southern Africa, and when present is often light and asymptomatic.

Life cycle: Eggs deposited in the soil hatch within 24 hours. After maturation from rhabditiform to the infective filariform larvae, the latter penetrate the human host's skin and are conveyed to the heart and lungs, from whence they migrate up the respiratory passages to the pharynx and are swallowed. Maturation to adult worms occurs in the upper small intestine. Worms attach themselves to the mucosa and cause the loss of minute amounts of blood. Seven to ten weeks elapse from larval invasion to deposition of eggs in the stool.

Clinical findings: Most infections are asymptomatic. Larval invasion may cause an irritating papulovesicular dermatitis, commonly localized to the feet, and larval migration through the lungs may lead to bronchospasm and pneumonitis. Epigastric pain and tenderness suggestive of peptic ulceration are described, and believed to be caused by the worms' attachment to the upper intestinal mucosa. A ravenous appetite and pica may occur. The development of anaemia is dependent on the worm load and dietary iron intake. Symptoms and signs of anaemia develop slowly and patients may be in congestive cardiac failure when they first seek medical advice. Very heavy parasite loads also lead to diarrhoea with blood and mucus, and hypoproteinaemia which may aggravate oedema.

Diagnosis: Hookworm ova in the stool indicate infection, but unless the load is in the order of at least 20 000 eggs/gram of faeces there is no proof that these worms are the cause of the patient's symptoms and signs.

Treatment: Pyrantel 10 mg/kg is effective as a single dose. Mebendazole 100 mg bd for 3 days, or albendazole in mixed helminth infections.

Prevention: The wearing of shoes or protective clothing, and improved sanitation may help to reduce the incidence in highly endemic areas.

Strongyloides stercoralis

This roundworm has a world-wide distribution and is most prevalent in tropical areas where high humidity favours transmission.

Life cycle: Filariform larvae penetrate the skin and are conveyed to the lungs. They mature, migrate to the pharynx via the airways, and are swallowed. Adult worms settle in the upper small intestine. Eggs containing rhabditiform larvae may be passed in the stool to commence a free-living cycle in soil, or may undergo maturation in the intestine before reinvading their host's circulation. This autoinfection explains the persistence of the parasite in humans for long periods after having left endemic areas. The severity of infection appears to depend on the host's resistance and the parasite load. Immunosuppression which occurs in malnutrition, malignant disease, or during cytotoxic therapy predisposes to severe infections. Conditions such as megacolon or chronic constipation are thought to favour autoinfection.

Clinical picture: The majority of strongyloides infections are asymptomatic. Larvae found in various organs at necropsy are not necessarily responsible for the patient's death, nor for symptoms and signs.

A creeping eruption which is red and irritating and often found in the buttock or perianal area may occur within a week of exposure. Oedema and urticaria may also be seen. Skin lesions tend to recur for many years. Bronchitis or pneumonitis may follow skin lesions and become chronic.

Intermittent attacks of abdominal distension, diarrhoea, or malabsorption are described.

Shock, intercurrent bacterial infections, and acute respiratory failure may follow the use of steroids or immunosuppressive therapy in the presence of strongyloides infection, and can lead to a fatal outcome.

Strongyloides larvae have been blamed for conveying pathogenic bacteria from the bowel to the biliary tract and bloodstream.

Diagnosis: Larvae rather than eggs are present in fresh stool specimens. Aspiration of duodenal juice may be necessary to establish the diagnosis.

Treatment: Thiabendazole 25 mg/kg/day divided into 2 doses orally for 3 days. High doses of mebendazole or albendazole are successful in 80% of cases.

Preventative measures are similar to those for hookworm.

Filariasis

Five distinct species of filarial worms are important causes of disease in man. They are listed in *Table 8.17*. All are confined to the tropics and subtropics. Their larval stages require periods of maturation in blood-sucking insects. Minute, thread-like adult worms produce vast numbers of embryonated eggs. These uncoil to become microfilarial larvae, each species having a distinctive morphology which is used to differentiate one from the other.

Acute manifestations are seen in children, but the chronic effects are usually confined to adults.

Clinical syndromes

Lymphatic filariasis: Immunological responses to adult worms in lymphatics lead to acute lymphangitis. In *W. bancrofti* infections, the lower limbs and spermatic cord are commonly involved, leading to funiculitis, epididymitis, or orchitis. In chronic cases, hydrocele and elephantiasis occur. *B. malayi* and *B. timori* infestations tend to involve the upper limbs and cause more severe acute infections, with high fever and abscess formations.

Pulmonary eosinophilia syndrome: This syndrome is commonly caused by a hyperimmune response to *W. bancrofti* and brugia microfilariae, and is characterized by chronic cough, wheezing, and persistent eosinophilia.

Onchocerciasis: Adult worms become encapsulated to produce nodules. Microfilariae are

Table 8.17   Common filarial infections which cause disease in man

Filarial worm	Insect vector	Geographical distribution	Disease produced
Wuchereria bancrofti	Mosquito	Indian and other Asian countries, East Africa, Central and South America	Lymphatic filariasis
Brugia malayi	Mosquito	Indonesia, Far East	Lymphatic filariasis
Brugia timori	Mosquito	Indonesia	Lymphatic filariasis
Onchocerca volvulus	Simulium flies	West Africa, Central America, Yemen	Skin lesions, ocular lesions and blindness
Loa loa	Chrysops flies	West and Central Africa	Calabar swellings

responsible for more serious disease. Skin involvement initially causes an irritating eruption which may become secondarily infected with scratching. In chronic cases, loss of skin elasticity and atrophy leads to the appearance of premature ageing. Blindness as the result of a sclerosing keratitis is the most serious sequel to prolonged infection in hyperendemic areas.

Loiasis: Allergic reactions to the adult worms migrating through subcutaneous tissue causes recurrent calabar swellings. Adult worms may be seen migrating across the eyeball under the conjunctiva.

Treatment: Diethylcarbamazine, 75 mg/kg body weight, is effective in acute lymphatic filariasis. Heavily infected patients with *O. volvulus* and *Loa loa* infections should be given test doses of 25 mg/kg to avoid side-effects. Steroids are recommended before commencement of this therapy in heavy infections.

Prevention: Vector control and the wearing of protective clothing help to reduce the incidence of infections.

Trichinosis

Due to *Trichinella spiralis,* this condition occurs where poorly cooked pork containing encapsulated larvae is eaten. These larvae develop into adults in the upper small intestine. They penetrate the bowel wall and, having gained entry into the circulation, are deposited in muscle. Encapsulation of these larvae gives rise to acute inflammation. Fever, muscle pain, facial oedema, and a marked eosinophilia suggest the diagnosis. Invasion of the brain and myocardium has been described, but is rarely seen in children. Death may

occur in widespread infestation. The diagnosis is confirmed by identifying larvae on biopsy.

Toxocariasis (visceral larva migrans)

This is a zoonotic infection caused by the dog and cat nematodes, *Toxocara canis* and *T. cati,* which resemble human roundworms but do not develop beyond the second larval stage in man. Children in intimate contact with dogs, cats, or contaminated soil are infected by swallowing eggs.

Toxocara larvae produce eosinophilic granulomata in various organs. A tender hepatomegaly, marked hypergammaglobulinaemia and hypereosinophilia, in which up to 80% of the differential count consists of eosinophils, are the most characteristic findings; symptoms may be predominantly respiratory, with cough and wheezing. A perihilar pneumonitis is often demonstrated radiographically. Splenomegaly and lymphadenopathy may also occur. Anorexia, lassitude, failure to thrive, and intermittent fever may be the only manifestations. Rarely, encephalopathy with convulsions and coma, myalgia, or even myocarditis are seen.

In older children with no evidence of generalized disease, an ocular lesion involving only one eye may lead to visual deterioration, strabismus, and a central field visual loss. Retinal detachment, and occasionally chronic endophthalmitis with secondary glaucoma may follow. Eye involvement mimics retinoblastoma and the true diagnosis may only be made on histology of an enucleated eye *(see Chapter 25, Disorders of the Eye).*

Diagnosis: Eosinophilic leucocytosis is almost invariable in visceral larva migrans, and persists for up to 1 year. A marked increase in serum IgM and IgE is also a usual finding, but is rarely present in ocular toxocariasis.

Serological tests tend to be unreliable because of cross-reactions with antibodies of other nematodes, but high or rising titres of enzyme-linked immunoabsorbent assay and fluorescent antibody tests are suggestive of the infection.

Needle biopsy of the liver may demonstrate eosinophilic granulomas surrounding larvae, but failure to identify these granulomas does not exclude the diagnosis.

Management: Normally a self-limiting infection, the illness may last for weeks or months. Spontaneous improvement is usual.

Diethylcarbamazine is the most effective remedy (1 mg/kg body weight day l; 1 mg/kg weight tds day 2; 2 mg/kg body weight tds day 3; then 3 mg/kg body weight tds for 21 days). In ocular toxocariasis and seriously ill patients, prednisone should be given in addition. Mebendazole 100 mg bd for 3 days or thiabendazole 25 mg/kg body weight bd for 3 days may be effective.

Prevention: Deworming of puppies at 2 weeks of age and redosing twice at 2-weekly intervals, and yearly deworming of adult dogs and all newly-acquired puppies, will help to control the incidence of visceral larva migrans. Cats are less infective to children. Handwashing after the handling of animals should be encouraged.

Dog and cat hookworm infections

Ancylostoma ceylonicum, another pathogen of dogs, may cause clinical disease in humans. *A. caninum,* the common hookworm of dogs and cats, is an extremely rare parasite in man.

A. braziliense, a parasite of cats and dogs in the tropics, is the cause of cutaneous larva migrans (creeping eruption) and rarely, if ever, occurs as an adult worm in humans *(see Chapter 24, Dermatological Disorders).*

Tapeworms or cestodes

Tapeworms which cause disease in man are listed in *Table 8.18.*

These segmented flat worms consist of a head or scolex which becomes attached to the small bowel of the definitive vertebrate host, and segments or proglottids whose chief function is that of reproduction. Both male and female reproductive organs are present in proglottids. These proglottids and fertilized eggs may be found in the host's stools. Eggs are ingested by susceptible intermediate hosts. After hatching, larvae or oncospheres develop.

Variations occur in the oncospheres of different tapeworms. They penetrate the tissues of the intermediate host, which are eaten by the definitive host. Maturation of the larval stage to the adult worm in the definitive host completes the cycle.

Taeniasis

T. saginata is common in the Middle East and Africa, but is found world-wide. Human faecal contamination of grazing lands and the eating of rare beef or undercooked pork favours spread. *T. solium* is less common, but has a similar distribution to *T. saginata.* The larval stage or oncosphere consists of a small fluid-filled sac containing a single scolex, which is called a cysticercus and which, when present in numbers in the tissues of the intermediate host, gives rise to measly beef *(T. saginata)* or pork *(T. solium)* or cysticercosis in humans *(T. solium).*

Clinical findings: Adult worms may cause abdominal pain, but the passage of segments in the stool is the presenting complaint of most patients. Cysticercosis is discussed elsewhere *(see Chapter 15, Neurological Disorders.)*

Diagnosis: The eggs of the two species are identical, and examination of proglottids is necessary to differentiate them.

Diphyllobothriasis

This tapeworm occurs in cold regions of the world, such as the Scandinavian lakes, but is also found in certain parts of Africa. It has the ability to split the vitamin B_{12} intrinsic factor complex in the lumen of the host's bowel, thus preventing vitamin B_{12} absorption. Megaloblastic anaemia and neurological complications result.

Hymenolepiasis

Hymenolepis nana, or the dwarf tapeworm, commonly infects children in institutions, especially when overcrowding and unsanitary conditions are present. Humans act as both the definitive and intermediate host; the complete life cycle takes place in the bowel lumen and wall. This

Table 8.18   Tapeworms which may infect man

Worm	Definitive host	Intermediate host	Disease in humans
Taenia saginata	Humans	Cattle	Gastrointestinal
Taenia solium	Humans	Pig, humans	Cysticercosis
Diphyllobothrium latum	Humans, fish-eating animals	Fish	Megaloblastic anaemia
Hymenolepis nana	Humans	Humans	Gastrointestinal
Echinococcus granulosus	Dog	Humans, sheep, cattle	Hydatid disease
Multiceps multiceps	Dog	Herbivorous animals, humans	Central nervous system

autoinfection leads to an increasing population of adult worms. Irritation of the bowel wall causes abdominal pain and diarrhoea. The finding of typical double-membrane eggs in the stool establishes the diagnosis.

Treatment of intestinal cestodes

Niclosamide 2 g by mouth is given on an empty stomach. Small children should be given half this dose. Praziquantel 40 mg/kg in one dose or mebendazole 100 mg bd for 6 days also effective.

Hydatid disease

Sheep and cattle are the intermediate hosts of *Echinococcus granulosus*, and humans become accidentally involved by ingesting dog faeces containing eggs. Infections are most prevalent in sheep-farming areas.

Oncospheres penetrate mesenteric vessels and are carried to many organs, but the right lobe of the liver and the lung are most commonly involved. Cysts enlarge gradually and compress surrounding structures to produce symptoms and signs. Cysts usually remain intact for many years. Should they rupture, spread to many other organs follows.

The presence of an eosinophilia and a tumour mass should alert the clinician to the possible diagnosis. Serological tests, including the indirect haemagglutination and latex agglutination, may be of help in establishing the diagnosis. Aspiration of the cyst is contraindicated because of the danger of spread.

Treatment: Initial treatment should be with mebendazole 20–40 mg/kg/day for at least 8 weeks, or preferably albendazole 10–20 mg/kg/day for 6 weeks or longer. If a cyst causes serious pressure effects or involves the eye, sur-

gery is indicated, and drugs should also be given to prevent relapse or recurrence.

Multiceps multiceps

This is another dog tapeworm which has herbivorous animals as intermediate hosts, but the larval stage, known as a coenurus, may infect humans. Symptoms are neurological, and similar to those seen in cysticercosis.

Trematodes (flukes) schistosomiasis

Three major species of the genus schistosoma commonly infect man, *S. haematobium* being largely responsible for genitourinary disease, while *S. mansoni* and *S. japonicum* cause intestinal schistosomiasis.

Epidemiological features

It has been calculated that 200 million people world-wide are infected with bilharzia, while in South Africa 2 million are thought to harbour the parasite. Human schistosomiasis has an extensive distribution in the Middle East and Africa, with the exception of certain high mountain areas, the Sahara, and the western half of southern Africa. The popular belief that bilharzia only occurs in rivers flowing into the Indian Ocean in southern Africa is not strictly correct, as the Vaal catchment area is not free from infection.

There is evidence that the disease originated in the great lakes of Africa in prehistoric times. Bilharzia ova have been found in Egyptian mummies dating to 1 000 B.C. The presence of *S. mansoni* in the West Indies and north-eastern areas of South America is thought to owe its origin to Negro slaves. Brazil is estimated to have 12 million people with *S. mansoni* infection.

In southern Africa, the infection rate of schoolchildren with *S. haematobium* may be as high as

90% in certain rural endemic areas such as northern Zululand. A survey in 1964 showed that a quarter of the children attending the out-patient department at King Edward VIII Hospital in Durban, had *S. haematobium* ova on urine testing. Except for isolated pockets with a very high prevalence, *S. mansoni* is considerably less common in Natal. *S. japonicum* infections occur in certain areas of the Far East.

The distribution of infection is dependent on the presence of the intermediate snail host. These snails are found in permanent fresh water in streams, pools, canals, and particularly in storage dams and cement reservoirs. Boreholes and temporary pools of rain water are not their normal habitat, nor is sea water. *Bulinus (physopsis)* species harbours *S. haematobium,* bromphalaria sp. harbours *S. mansoni,* and oncomelaria sp., *S. japonicum.* Snails multiply rapidly by laying eggs which hatch after 10 –14 days, the young snail being susceptible to bilharzia at 1 day old and capable of reproduction by 6 weeks. Snails or their eggs are readily transported by insects, or on the feet of birds and animals, to a new habitat. They survive passage through water pumps and drying in sand or mud for months. Their most important habitats are collections of water near human habitation.

Wild animals have been infected with *S. mansoni* and, rarely, with *S. haematobium,* but it is doubtful whether animals play a role in the spread of schistosomiasis in southern Africa.

Urinary bilharzia is mainly a disease of children and young adults. Their fondness for swimming and their habit of urinating into the water in which they swim play major roles in the spread and prevalence of *S. haematobium. S. mansoni* disease occurs in a wider age range and is the result of increasing faecal pollution of water due to rising population density and inadequate sanitation.

Life cycle

The life cycle of the species is essentially similar. Miracidia hatch from eggs in water and enter the snail, where cercariae develop in sporocysts. Cercariae pass from the snail and swim in water until they penetrate the skin of their human host. They lose their tails, become schistosomules, and migrate to the portal vessels, where maturation to adulthood occurs. After mating, *S. haematobium* migrates to the vesical plexus, and *S. mansoni* to the tributaries of the inferior mesenteric vessels. Eggs pass through the tissues and enter the bladder or large intestine. The degree of reaction of tissues through which the ova pass varies greatly, and has resulted in a wide variety of opinions about the severity and clinical importance of bilharzia.

Pathology

This can be divided into three steps: the first coinciding with invasion by cercariae, the second with the onset of egg-laying, and the third or chronic stage with the consequences of the host's response to eggs in various organs. Immediate and delayed hypersensitivity reactions and immune complexes are responsible for the clinical findings of the first and second stages. Granulomatous response to the eggs, which is also a form of delayed hypersensitivity, leads to destruction of tissue and scarring. In *S. haematobium* infection, the urogenital tract and lower bowel are the principal sites of pathology. *S. mansoni* and *S. japonicum* disease affects mainly the gut and the liver.

Eggs may reach the lungs through collateral circulation, and may also get to the central nervous system. Multinucleated giant cells, histiocytes, and eosinophils surrounding eggs constitute the bilharzial granuloma.

A heavy parasite load, which is indicated by a high egg count in the stool or urine, is generally associated with more severe disease than is a light load and a smaller egg count. The host response plays an important role in pathogenesis, and accounts for differences in severity of disease in various race and population groups, even when exposure and egg loads are similar. In Zimbabwe schistosomiasis is regarded as a disease which produces severe complications, whereas in the coastal region of Natal, which is an area of high endemicity, serious disease is uncommon. In Brazil, whites develop severe disease more frequently than do African Americans with the same exposure and egg load. The hypersensitivity reactions characteristic of the first and second stages are very rarely seen in African children in coastal Natal, but occur in white children in the same area. A similar racial difference has been described in Zimbabwe.

Clinical features

An irritating, erythematous, papular rash referred to as 'swimmer's itch' may occur at the time and site of entry of cercaria. Four to six weeks later a high fever, urticarial rashes, oedema, lymphadenopathy and hepatosplenomegaly may be found. Complaints include severe headache, bronchospasm and rigors. Symptoms and signs of encephalitis and cardiac involvement are also described in this syndrome, which is most severe in *S. japonicum* infections (Katayama fever).

S. haematobium infection is often asymptomatic, or terminal haematuria may be the only symptom. Dysuria and suprapubic pain are less common and, rarely, precipitancy or dribbling incontinence occurs.

Obstruction of ureteric orifices or ureteric strictures may cause hydronephrosis or vesicoureteric reflux and obstructive uropathy may lead to renal failure. Bladder calcification follows heavy and repeated infections. Ureteric and bladder lesions, demonstrated radiographically, frequently regress after treatment and may do so spontaneously. Chronic renal failure, which is the consequence of chronic bacterial pyelonephritis, may supervene. In Egypt, *Salmonella* infections are often responsible for this complication. Cancer of the bladder is a rare complication.

The vagina, cervix, and uterus may be involved in females, and the urethra and prostate in males.

The diagnosis of *S. haematobium* infection is confirmed by finding terminal-spined ova in urine specimens. Maximum excretion of ova occurs at midday, and specimens collected at this time give the highest yield of ova. Bladder calcification revealed on plain abdominal radiographs may be the first indication of urinary bilharzia. Excretory urograms are indicated to exclude obstructive lesions when renal function is impaired. Rarely, cystoscopy and even biopsy may be needed to establish the diagnosis.

S. mansoni infection may cause abdominal pain and diarrhoea with dysenteric stools in the early stages. More chronic infection leads to nodular thickening, ulceration, and polyp formation, which are most marked at the rectosigmoid junction and in the lower colon. Blood and protein loss occurs, and anaemia, oedema, and ascites may be the consequences of these bowel lesions.

Lateral-spined eggs found in stools or histologically in rectal biopsy specimens confirm the diagnosis.

Hepatic and hepatosplenic bilharzia

Massive or repeated infections encourage carriage of eggs to the liver via the portal vein. Granuloma formation followed by portal fibrosis results in pre-sinusoidal portal hypertension, with passive congestion of the spleen, portosystemic collaterals, and oesophageal varices. Hypoproteinaemia, ascites, and oedema follow. Liver function tests usually remain normal. Patients with markedly abnormal liver function are often HBS Ag positive, and it is thought that this associated infection is responsible for the cirrhosis which has been described in bilharzia.

Patients with massive splenomegaly may develop portal hypertension. *S. mansoni* and *S. japonicum* infections commonly involve the liver, but *S. haematobium* may also do so.

Bilharzial nephrotic syndrome

Advanced *S. mansoni* infection has been associated with the nephrotic syndrome in Brazil and Egypt. Irreversible membrano-proliferative lesions are seen in Brazil, while in Egypt reversible proliferative lesions occur in association with co-existing salmonella infection. There is evidence that soluble immune complexes are formed and deposited on the glomeruli of these patients.

Pulmonary schistosomiasis

Eggs in the pulmonary circulation obstruct small arterioles and may cause necrosis of their walls, followed by thickening or fibrosis and obliteration of their lumens. If widespread and diffuse, this obliterative endarteritis leads to pulmonary hypertension and eventually to aneurysmal dilatation of the pulmonary artery. Right ventricular hypertrophy and failure follow, but respond to rest, digitalis, and diuretics. Patients with bilharzial cor pumonale may survive for many years. Heart failure in bilharzia may also occur as a result of rare myocardial granulomatous involvement.

Granulomas situated near bronchioles and alveoli may cause parenchymatous lung disease, fibrosis, and scarring, giving rise to chronic bronchitis, bronchiectasis and emphysema.

Pulmonary complications are rare in southern Africa. Most reported cases have been from South America and Egypt.

Central nervous system schistosomiasis

Eggs reach the nervous system via anastomatic vessels in the pelvis and vertebral venous plexuses. Spinal cord involvement is commonly due to *S. haematobium* and *S. mansoni,* whereas *S. japonicum* is more liable to cause encephalitis.

A bilharzial aetiology should be suspected when neurological symptoms and signs are associated with a marked eosinophilia. Cerebrospinal fluid shows a pleocytosis, raised protein level, and normal sugar.

Focal epilepsy, mental changes, visual defects, and upper motor neurone palsies have been described in bilharzial encephalitis; the presentation may be that of an intracranial space-occupying lesion.

Cord involvement often presents as an acute transverse myelitis or radiculitis. A granuloma of the cord may lead to paraplegia or weakness, together with sensory changes.

Treatment consists of antibilharzial therapy and corticosteroids. Surgery is indicated in certain instances, and the diagnosis is confirmed by surgical biopsy specimens.

Diagnosis of schistosomiasis

The presence of viable eggs in urine, stool, or biopsy specimen is proof of infection.

Bilharzia is a common cause of eosinophilia and should be excluded whenever this is found in patients in endemic areas or in visitors to such areas.

The finding of granulomatous lesions, black pigment, and portal fibrosis in liver biopsies is suggestive evidence of hepatic bilharzia — even in the absence of ova.

Advances in serological tests have increased their usefulness in diagnosis. The most helpful are an enzyme-linked immunosorbent assay based on schistosomal egg antigen, and fluorescent antibody test based on cercaria antigen.

Treatment of bilharzia

Praziquantel is the drug of choice, and is effective in all species, in a single oral dose (30 – 45 mg/kg). Side-effects are uncommon, but include abdominal colic for which antispasmodics may be necessary. Cure rates and reduction of schistosomal load are excellent.

Alternative drugs — niridazole, metriphonate and oxamniquine — are available in some countries, but have a number of contraindications and side-effects.

Prevention

Health education aimed at the avoidance of infection, and the provision of clean water and adequate sanitation are important public health measures.

Eradication of the snail host may be achieved by the use of molluscicides, in addition to improved irrigation practices.

Mass treatment with praziquantel in areas of high endemicity should be considered. The cost of mass treatment must be weighed against the cost of morbidity and mortality of bilharzia in the target community.

A.G. Wesley

9

Tuberculosis (TB)

Epidemiology

Tuberculosis (TB) ranks as one of the foremost infectious diseases in the Third World. Estimates indicate that there are about 10 million infectious cases throughout the world. It is a cause of considerable morbidity and mortality, especially among children; one million people die of TB annually, giving a death rate of 3–4 every minute. In terms of both past and current history it remains a prime indicator of the social and economic conditions of the community in which it is prevalent. Indeed the Dubos' noted that TB had become 'the social disease of the nineteenth century, perhaps the first penalty that capitalist society had to pay for the ruthless exploitation of labour'. The industrialized countries have paid this price and moved on. Today their economies have undergone massive expansion, are infinitely more sophisticated, and their standards of living have improved considerably. Therefore in these countries, the incidence of TB has been reduced to manageable proportions.

The disease is an ancient one: it dates back to some 4 000 to 5 000 years BC. However, it was only in 1882 that Robert Koch discovered the tubercle bacillus as the causative organism, thereby laying the foundation for a rational approach to this infection. Tuberculosis has been characterized by waves of epidemics followed by troughs of endemicity throughout the western world. This history is being repeated among some poor countries today. The epidemic in England began in the sixteenth century and peaked around the middle of the eighteenth century, when about half the population suffered from TB. The mortality at this time was exceedingly high, standing at about 500 for every 100 000 people; TB accounted for about 30% of all deaths among the working class. The reason for the marked concentration of TB during this period is linked to the rapid process of industrialization which was taking place in Europe. Industry was characterized by terrible working conditions, and residential areas were marked by an appalling lack of hygiene. Two important components of this damaging social environment which had a direct bearing on TB were malnutrition and overcrowding. Cramped living conditions increased both the risk of exposure and the burden of inhaled bacteria. This probably led to widespread infection. The immunoparesis of inadequate nutrition encouraged the progression from infection to overt disease. Frank illness caused more infection, plunging the poor into recurring cycles and widening circles of endemic and epidemic tuberculosis. In the nineteenth century epidemics continued to ravage western and eastern Europe, the east coast of North America, and South America. A quarter of all deaths in Paris during 1899 were due to TB.

The gradual elimination of tuberculosis as a major public health problem was brought about by attacking the 'unsanitary conditions' of the poor. It came through a process of improving social and economic conditions, enlightened public health legislation, and the accumulating benefits of industrialization. The incidence and death rate of TB were decreasing significantly long before the use of BCG and the advent of chemotherapy *(see Fig. 9.1)*.

Infectious illnesses disappeared in the richer world, as H H Scott says 'not because they were driven out by marvellous discoveries of medicine, they faded away before the general amelioration of the state of living as a result of improvements in sanitation — improvements in housing, drainage, refuse disposal — in education and elevation of the standard of living for the generality of the poor'. The overall incidence and mortality figures for North America now stand at 14 and 1.4 per 100 000 respectively.

In summary, therefore, the collective experience of the technically-advanced countries demonstrates that tuberculosis has been controlled through a combination of improved living conditions, distribution of financial, manpower, and technical resources, and chemotherapy.

In these richer countries of the north, TB persists or reappears among disadvantaged groups. For example it is found among Indians, Inuits, and inner-city groups in the USA, and in the United Kingdom among immigrants from developing countries within the Commonwealth. However, overall the figures are low: in parts of Britain and the Netherlands only 1–2% of children are infected. In developing countries between a third and two-thirds may be infected. Infection does not mean disease (*see below* for discussion on this). Much of the transmission of the bacterium occurs in early childhood.

Social upheavals have often been associated with the spread of tuberculosis. This is well illustrated by what has happened in South Africa. After the discovery of gold and diamonds, mining developed into a major industry, resulting in well over 200 000 rural peasant farmers becoming urbanized wage workers in less than thirty years. There was no TB among black people in pre-colonial times, and possibly up to the mid-nineteenth century. Northern Zululand was still free of this disease in 1907. There are probably many reasons for the absence of TB even after colonization, but one likely factor is the good nutritional state of the black population in this period.

Between 1820 and 1910 subsistence agriculture gave way to a thriving black peasantry which produced a surplus of food, and consequently enjoyed an adequate food intake. By 1920, however, the rural support system had collapsed because of the influence of mining, which led to the proletarianization of the peasantry and the emergence of a black working class. This created the conditions for the spread of TB.

The immigrants from Europe, especially Cornish miners who came during the early days of colonization, brought the disease with them. Tuberculosis was first reported among European colonizers at the end of the eighteenth century. In 1880, for

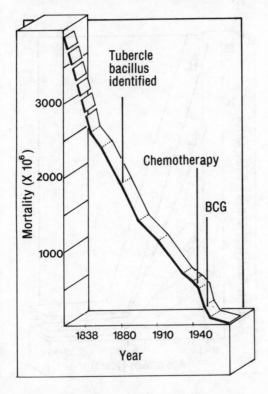

Fig. 9.1 Mortality from respiratory tuberculosis in England and Wales

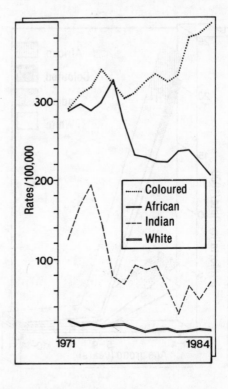

Fig. 9.2 Incidence of TB among different racial groups in South Africa (1971–84)

example, there was a high morbidity from TB among white people in South Africa, and little among blacks. Conditions in the mines resulted in spread of infection. By 1900 and thereafter, TB was rampant among blacks. Accordingly, it may be concluded that the specific factors which caused social dislocation and led to the spread of TB among blacks in South Africa were colonialism, political domination, taxation, land expropriation, the impact of traders, miners and mining, ecological disasters, and the drift of people away from the land to labour areas. Proliferation of peri-urban squatter camps, economic recession, and housing shortages continue to exacerbate the problem in modern times.

There are currently about 7 million infected people in South Africa (total population 28 million); there are estimated to be 100 000 infectious cases, and 6–10 people die every day of the disease. Eighty-two per cent of cases occur among blacks. The incidence of TB among different racial groups in South Africa is shown in *Fig. 9.2,* and the mortality rates in 1979 appear in *Fig. 9.3.*

The pattern shown is a reflection of the complex web of economic, social, and political factors which leave blacks the most disadvantaged group and whites the most privileged one. The probability of becoming infected with tubercle bacilli in the course of a year appears to be declining for most groups in South Africa, except among coloureds. The highest risk of infection exists for Africans in coastal areas, followed by coloureds, and then Africans in inland areas. Household contacts have the highest risk, with a 30% chance of becoming infected. The effect of socio-economic improvements on TB is illustrated in the mortality rates for white children between 1921 and 1979 *(see Fig. 9.4);* the marked decrease parallels improvements in standards of living. More than 2.5 million people in sub-Saharan Africa have TB coincident with Human Immunodeficiency Virus (HIV) infection. This association will reshape the epidemiology of TB in the Third World.

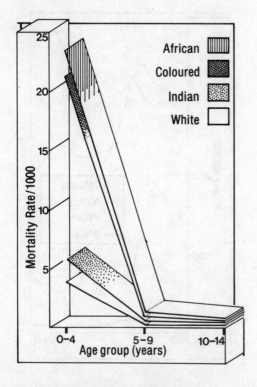

Fig. 9.3   TB mortality rates in children of different racial groups in South Africa (1979)

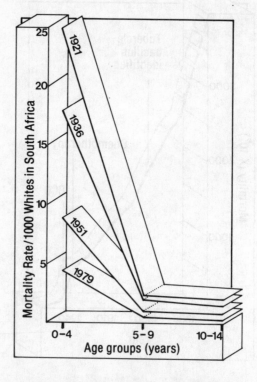

Fig. 9.4   TB mortality trend for white South African children (1921–79)

Pathogenesis

Clinical disease resulting from tuberculosis infection is determined by microbial as well as host factors. However, it must be remembered that *Mycobacterium tuberculosis* does not secrete exotoxins or possess endotoxins; it is harmful because several of its constituents provoke an immune response which is damaging to human tissues. Therefore TB may be considered an immunopathological disease, and in the account below, special note must be made of events which occur on first contact, and those which prevail after development of delayed hypersensitivity.

The bacillus is tough and able to evade rapid destruction in the human body because it possesses certain special properties: it multiplies slowly (about once a day), it is resistant to many drugs, it remains viable in macrophages by subverting macrophage-killing, and its waxy coat together with its many component substances depress immune responses against it.

Transmission is through minute moist droplets of sputum containing a few bacilli, which are expelled during speaking, coughing, or sneezing by an infected individual. The water in the droplet dries rapidly, but the desiccated droplet nuclei persist suspended in air for some time. In countries where bovine tuberculosis is prevalent and milk unpasteurized, the bacilli are swallowed and penetrate the tonsil or the intestinal mucosa. Rarely, the bacilli gain entrance through direct innoculation by infected needles, knives, and other instruments. Tonsillar enlargement and injection abscesses may therefore be tuberculous. The tiny infected droplet nuclei are inhaled to the terminal air spaces in the lung periphery, especially in the mid and lower zones. In the susceptible person they set up a pneumonitis characterized by exudation of polymorphonuclear leucocytes followed by monocytes. The mycobacteria are ingested by the polymorphs and are not destroyed, but rapidly released; they are then taken up by blood-borne monocytes/macrophages attracted to the site by the inflammatory process. This primary lesion is called the Ghon focus. Tissue destruction does not occur, and there are no clinical symptoms or signs.

The bacilli multiply and spread via the lymphatics to the regional lymph nodes, which enlarge. The Ghon focus and the original lymph node are together known as the 'primary complex'. This is followed by a 'silent' bacteraemia and establishment of minute metastatic foci in the apices of the lungs, anterior parts of vertebrae, the ends of long bones, meninges, other lymph nodes, and kidneys. During this process cellular immunity or 'delayed hypersensitivity' is gradually established. This is a complex phenomenon and the details are not known. It is likely that T cells are sensitized to specific antigens of the tubercle bacillus; these sensitized T cells liberate a number of soluble substances, rather like hormones, called 'lymphokines', which activate macrophages to kill any intracellular bacilli.

T cells (probably not the same as those responsible for macrophage activation) are also responsible for the delayed hypersensitivity response elicited on skin by purified proteins of the tubercle bacillus. This sensitization takes place between 3 and 6 weeks after pulmonary infection, and at its peak may infrequently become clinically evident as fever, erythema nodosum, and phlyctenular conjunctivitis *(see Fig. 9.5)*. At this stage, when the tuberculin test is positive, the immune response is effective, and most of the bacilli distributed throughout the body can be killed. It appears that the majority of infected children (i.e., those who are tuberculin-positive) destroy the bacilli and recover. However, between 5 and 10% of such children in Asia and South-East Asia develop overt clinical disease in about 4 months *(see Fig. 9.6)*.

Among the majority who control the bacillary multiplication, about 15% develop dormant or latent infection. A proportion of these may become reactivated in the ensuing years, causing clinical disease.

What happens during this period is influenced by a number of different factors:

◆ age
◆ nutrition
◆ immunocompetence
◆ overcrowding
◆ size of inoculum
◆ genetic endowment.

In the young (especially those under 5 years), in the malnourished, among those who are immunologically compromised (e.g., due to HIV, measles, malnutrition, malignancies, and drugs), and

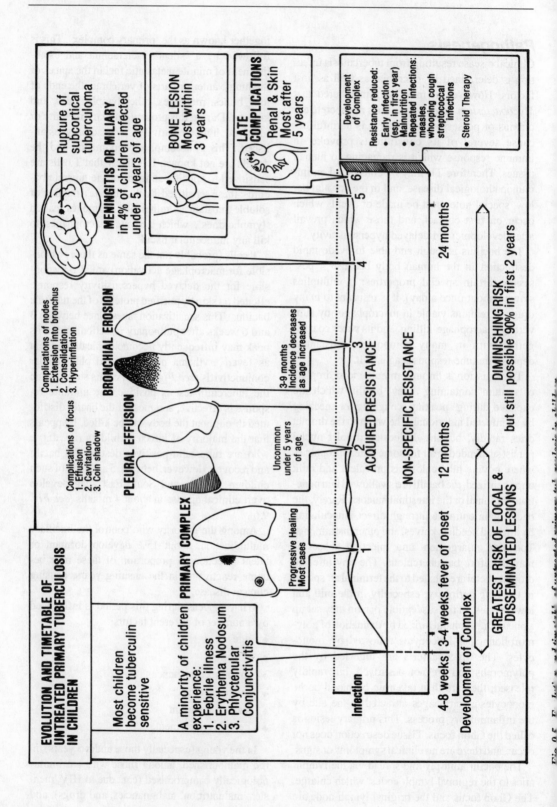

EVOLUTION AND TIMETABLE OF UNTREATED PRIMARY TUBERCULOSIS IN CHILDREN

Most children become tuberculin sensitive

A minority of children experience:
1. Febrile illness
2. Erythema Nodosum
3. Phlyctenular Conjunctivitis

PRIMARY COMPLEX

Progressive Healing Most cases

Complications of focus
1. Effusion
2. Cavitation
3. Coin shadow

PLEURAL EFFUSION

Uncommon under 5 years of age.

Complications of nodes
1. Extension into bronchus
2. Consolidation
3. Hyperinflation

BRONCHIAL EROSION

3-9 months Incidence decreases as age are increased

Rupture of subcortical tuberculoma

MENINGITIS OR MILIARY in 4% of children infected under 5 years of age

BONE LESION Most within 3 years

LATE COMPLICATIONS Renal & Skin Most after 5 years

Development of Complex
Resistance reduced:
• Early infection (esp. in first year)
• Malnutrition
• Repeated infections: measles, whooping cough streptococcal infections
• Steroid Therapy

Infection

4-8 weeks | 3-4 weeks fever of onset

Development of Complex

1   2   3   4   5 6

12 months | 24 months

ACQUIRED RESISTANCE

NON-SPECIFIC RESISTANCE

GREATEST RISK OF LOCAL & DISSEMINATED LESIONS

DIMINISHING RISK but still possible 90% in first 2 years

Fig. 0.5. Evolution and timetable of untreated primary tuberculosis in children.

among those from overcrowded homes (who presumably have a large infecting dose of bacilli), the risks of endogenous reactivation are quite high. Before chemotherapy, the lifetime risk of these dormant lesions reactivating was up to 15%; about 4% of children infected under 5 years of age developed miliary spread or meningitis within 2 years, and approximately 7% got bone or joint disease in about 3 years *(see Fig. 9.5)*. Twenty-five years ago 40% of Inuits infected with TB reactivated.

The immunopathological events which take place during ongoing primary disease or during reactivation are mainly due to sensitized T cells and macrophages. Lymphokines released by these T cells attract monocytes to the sites of inflammation, and activate them to destroy the mycobacteria. But the bacilli are able to survive in macrophages by inhibiting their bactericidal capacity, i.e., by preventing fusion of the lysosomes with phagosomes and becoming resistant to hydrogen peroxide. Bacterial cell wall components stimulate macrophages, causing the release of such

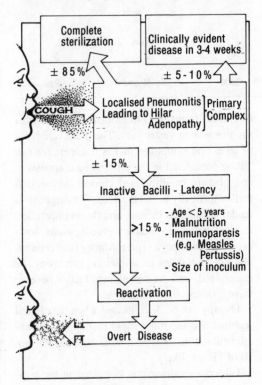

Fig. 9.6 Outcome following TB infection

soluble mediators as Interleukin I; this expands the population of sensitized T cells, and also has clinical effects such as fever. Accordingly, T cell proliferation, rapid macrophage turnover and activation, persistence of some bacilli and destruction of others, release of soluble mediators, and disintegration of cells occur simultaneously or in quick succession. This gives rise to the granuloma of tuberculosis, which is the prime cause of the disease state. It is evident that some of these processes are beneficial to the host (e.g., bacterial killing), while others are harmful (e.g., granuloma). It is likely that different subsets of T cells are responsible for the good and the bad effects of the immune response. The delayed hypersensitivity skin reaction to tuberculoprotein, for example, is produced by different types and subsets of cells, not only by cells responsible for protection. Therefore a positive skin test does not correspond to immunity. Indeed, delayed hypersensitivity can be disentangled experimentally from immunity: tuberculoprotein can induce delayed hypersensitivity without immunity, whilst mycobacterial RNA and ribosomes produce immunity without delayed hypersensitivity.

An individual with a positive tuberculin test must be assumed to have foci of inactive bacilli. These appear to possess antigens not present on actively-dividing bacilli, and therefore immune control over the former may be inadequate for the latter.

These dormant organisms are the root of a contradiction: they provide some degree of protection against further infection, but may under certain conditions (e.g., measles, malnutrition) escape immunological restraints, multiply, and cause disease.

Clinical and immunological spectrum of tuberculosis

In common with other chronic bacterial infections (e.g., leprosy), tuberculosis presents with a range of different clinical entities which are accompanied by a specific pattern of immune responses *(see Table 9.1)*. At one end there is aggressive cellular immunity, with few bacilli in granuloma and restricted clinical manifestations; at the opposite pole there is deficient cellular immunity, with a high bacterial load and disseminated disease.

227

Table 9.1 Spectrum of human tuberculosis

	Reactive	Intermediate		Unreactive
		Reactive	Unreactive	
1 Clinical	Localized small lung lesions	Localized small and large lung lesions	Diffuse small and large lung lesions	Miliary
		Lymph-adenopathy	Lymph-adenopathy	
		Serositis	Fistulae	
		Cavitation	Cavitation	
2 Immunological:				
Cellular immunity				
In vivo test: Tuberculin skin test	++++	+±	±	0
In vitro test: Leucocyte migration inhibition	++++	++	±	0
Humoral immunity:				
Antibodies to PPD	±	+++±	+++±	++++
3 Bacillary load				
(In sputum/tissues)	0	±	+++ ±	++++
4 Histological changes in lymph node				
B-dependent zones	±	±	++++	±
T-dependent zones	++++	++±	±	0
5 Response to treatment	Excellent	Good	Modest	Poor

Antibodies correlate inversely with cellular immunity. As shifts occur from one polar form to the other (due to treatment or the natural history), the varying concentrations of antigen and antibody produce hypersensitivity phenomena such as fever, arthritis, pleurisy, erythema nodosum, and phlyctenular conjunctivitis.

A number of unspecified, local immunological reactions occur during chemotherapy, produced by antigen-specific cells sequestered in selected sites. These may result in enlargement of cerebral tuberculomata, increase in lymph node size, and acute respiratory distress.

Clinical features

Introduction

Tuberculosis can affect virtually any organ in the body, and can therefore present in a multiplicity of clinical forms. It is to modern medicine what syphilis was to yester-year. The great variability of signs and symptoms makes it imperative that TB be considered in the differential diagnosis of any obscure or ill-defined clinical problem. A further difficulty is that the definitive diagnosis is made on bacterial culture, and this is impractical in most instances; ancillary investigations, however, play an important part. Among poor communities, a high index of suspicion must always be maintained, and treatment instituted whenever there is doubt about diagnosis.

Therapy can be discontinued when the clinical features and the more rapid resolution of non-tuberculous bacterial infections make the diagnosis of TB less likely.

Tuberculous disease is suspected in the presence of some or all of the following:

◆ residence in an endemic area

- poverty
- undernutrition
- chronic lack of well-being
- low grade fever
- gradual loss of weight, and
- long-standing pneumonia.

In the following diseases TB must be actively excluded, as the association is fairly frequent:

- HIV/AIDS
- kwashiorkor in an older child
- chronic otitis media
- post-measles state
- recurrent staphylococcal skin infections.

Tuberculosis is more severe among children in the Third World than it is in richer countries: there is frank kwashiorkor or marasmus; considerable lymphadenopathy, often with softening due to caseation; lung cavitation; and widespread dissemination to other sites, especially the meninges. Records suggest that TB was equally destructive in nineteenth-century Europe among impoverished working people: it was more frequent (especially among those under 5 years of age), it was accompanied by protein and vitamin A deficiencies, there was progressive primary disease, regional nodes caseated, meningitic involvement was frequent, hypersensitivity phenomena were uncommon, and tuberculin tests were often falsely negative.

Spread of primary infection

The primary complex which fails to resolve causes pulmonary disease. Initially the patient may be asymptomatic, but this is followed by an insidious deterioration in health and loss of weight. There is local extension of the lesions, with increasing lung destruction and lymph node enlargement. Swollen glands may:

- compress the airways, causing a brassy cough, stridor, or wheeze
- produce a ball-valve effect, resulting in obstructive emphysema
- occlude airways and cause collapse of a lobe
- interfere with venous return, and cause a superior mediastinal compression syndrome; vigorous coughing may force glands into the thoracic inlet and obstruct respiration; these glands may be palpated by inserting the fingers behind the manubrium

- perforate into the bronchus, and discharge caseous material into the peripheral lung, causing bronchopneumonia
- result in a pleural effusion.

The physical signs depend on the complications.

One point needs to be stressed: extensive bilateral bronchopneumonia may present with mild pyrexia, marked respiratory distress, and few (if any) adventitious sounds.

Radiological changes in pulmonary tuberculosis are given in *Table 9.2*.

Table 9.2   Types and frequency of radiological changes seen in pulmonary tuberculosis

	South Africa	
	Durban	Johannesburg
Mediastinal glands	42%	43%
Pleural effusion	13%	10%
Calcification	2%	8%
Parenchymal lesions:		
Segmental lesions	80%	90%
Cavities	5%	14%
Miliary	8%	9%
Primary complex	Unavailable	7%

Table 9.3   Miliary tuberculosis

Usually within 6 months of infection

Incidence reduced by BCG

Spread from lung focus causes generalized dissemination; spread from abdominal focus is first to liver

Dissemination leads to miliary tubercles in lungs, meningitis, choroidal tubercles (rare in African children), skin lesions, bacilluria, hepatosplenomegaly

Post-primary spread

This produces miliary tuberculosis and meningitis within a year of infection, and bone, joint, and kidney lesions some years later. Spread to lymph glands is common. In addition to local and bronchogenic extension in the lungs, there is haematogenous dissemination. This is due to erosion of a blood vessel by the primary complex. Gradual escape of bacilli into blood vessels, with seeding into distant tissues, may be followed by slow progression of infection or latency at these sites, such as bones, joints, and kidneys, with subsequent reactivation. This is disseminated TB. A sudden shower of bacilli into a blood vessel with concomitant disease is acute miliary TB *(see Table 9.3)*.

Reactivation tuberculosis

A small minority of children have adult-type disease: insidious onset of illness, with a cavity or opacity in the apical zones on chest radiograph. The types of tuberculosis, and common symptoms and signs in black children in Durban, are given in *Tables 9.4, 9.5, and 9.6.*

Table 9.4 Clinical types of tuberculosis in black children (Durban)

	%
Pulmonary	99
Lymph nodes	44
Meninges	15
Abdominal	8
Miliary	6
Pleurisy	3
Bones and joints	3
Genito-urinary; pericardium; eyes; erythema nodosum; ear, nose and throat; endocrine	< 2

Table 9.5 Common symptoms of tuberculosis in black children (Durban)

	%
Cough	63
Fever	40
Vomiting	31
Diarrhoea, anorexia	20
Weight loss	15
Weakness, night sweats, headache, fits	≤ 10

Table 9.6 Common physical signs of tuberculosis in black children (Durban)

	%
Hepatomegaly	56
Palpable lymph nodes	46
Respiratory distress	25
Splenomegaly	13
Clubbing, phlyctens	≤ 5

Lymph node enlargement

This is caused by regional lymphadenopathy as part of the primary complex. Thoracic lymph node complications have already been given above. Extrapulmonary sites of lymph node enlargement seen in Durban are (in descending order of frequency): cervical, axillary, submandibular, generalized, supraclavicular, and abdominal. Superficial nodes enlarge in one of two ways: either soon after the primary infection, or as part of reactivation. These glands often involve the neck and are visible, painless, firm, and occasionally adherent to each other and overlying skin, due to periadenitis. Nodes along the lymphatic channel are usually palpable. Nodes which have been infected for a long time and are calcified appear hard. Softening leads to abscess formation, and rarely to sinuses. Histological and bacteriological examination of lymph node contents may be necessary in the absence of other supporting evidence. The important diseases to consider in the differential diagnosis are:

◆ haematological malignancies, especially lymphoma
◆ acute pyogenic infections
◆ chronic fungal infection.

Skin tuberculosis

(See also Chapter 24, Dermatological Problems.) This occurs as small jelly-like nodules, papules with silvery scales, and ulcers. The skin may be the site of the primary complex, in which case the infection has been passed on through contact or injury. Blood-spread produces multiple miliary or papulonecrotic lesions, a single large plaque or ulcer, multiple abscesses, or a chronic, indurated, destructive lesion of the cheek, nose, or ear (lupus vulgaris). As has been indicated, tuberculous abscesses may develop after injections, or sinuses may develop over underlying adenitis. Erythema nodosum is a skin manifestation of hypersensitivity.

Bone and joint tuberculosis

(Also see Chapter 26, Orthopaedic Problems.) Pott's disease is discussed in *Chapter 26*. The hip is the second commonest site of involvement. There is pain over the hip, and this may be referred to the knee or inner aspect of the leg. In order to

reduce movement, muscle spasm occurs. The first presenting symptom may be a limp. In extreme cases there is shortening of the leg and dislocation of the hip. The child lies in bed with the hip externally rotated and semi-flexed, with the leg flexed at the knee. A cold abscess may be palpable anteriorly just below the inguinal ligament.

Cervical spine TB results in pain and spasm of neck muscles, which limit movement of the head in all planes. Dislocation causes the head to tilt to one side. Palpation of spinous processes may reveal an irregularity. Cold abscesses present in the retropharynx with a midline swelling, unlike acute pyogenic abscesses, which are unilateral.

Tuberculous dactylitis manifests as indurated, reddened fingers with thickened phalanges. The radiological features are of decreased density of bones, cysts, and periostitis. Syphilis, salmonella, and sickle-cell anaemia must be considered in the differential diagnosis.

TB of the knee presents with the signs of inflammation, and leads to lameness and occasionally a cold abscess in the popliteal fossa.

Liver and spleen tuberculosis

Hepatosplenomegaly is frequent, and occurs with or without acute miliary spread. It may be a non-specific reticulo-endothelial response to infection, or is due to tuberculous granulomas in these organs; these granulomas may calcify later. Symptoms include abdominal pain, fever, and weight loss. Rarely there is obstructive jaundice or acute hepatitis with progression to liver failure. An isolated tuberculoma may present as a hepatic nodule. Liver function tests will be abnormal in these instances. Occasionally the spleen enlarges in the absence of hepatomegaly. However, in endemic areas these physical signs are of little diagnostic importance, and liver biopsy is not a helpful procedure as tubercles are easily missed.

Adrenal tuberculosis

Infection of adrenals occurs, but is usually not associated with dysfunction. Addison's disease presents many years after bilateral infection, and is therefore mostly seen in adults.

Blood changes

In general there is no consistent pattern of blood changes in black children with TB.

Tuberculosis, especially when it disseminates to bone marrow, can result in a wide range of haematological abnormalities, including normocytic normochromic anaemia, aplastic anaemia, pancytopenia, neutrophil leucocytosis, and a leucoerythroblastic reaction and blood pictures resembling leukaemia and myelosclerosis. On rare occasions bone marrow biopsy picks up a tubercle.

Renal tuberculosis

In miliary spread, tubercle bacilli may be found in the urine. Chronic dissemination may result in more extensive lesions. This complication is often asymptomatic, and if sterile pyuria is detected incidentally, tuberculosis must always be excluded. Features rarely seen now are an aching loin pain, painless haematuria, nocturnal frequency, urgency, and renal colic.

Genital tuberculosis

Epididymitis is often associated with renal tuberculosis, and is caused by blood spread. Involvement is usually bilateral, with hard and irregular cords. Orchitis, rare before puberty, causes enlargement of the testicle. Penile tuberculosis has been recorded as a complication of circumcision. Vulval and vaginal involvement give rise to inguinal adenitis. Salpingitis causes abdominal pain, irregular menses and a lower abdominal mass. Sterility is frequent. Rectal examination may detect involvement of the prostate and seminal vesicles; pelvic examination in girls reveals adnexal masses.

Upper respiratory tract tuberculosis

Primary lesions of the mouth and tonsils have been noted, the latter especially after ingestion of contaminated milk. Submandibular and cervical adenitis is seen. Spread to the middle ear is by local extension along the Eustachian tube, or by haematogenous dissemination. Chronic, painless discharge, enlargement of the node between the mastoid and the mandibular ramus, and facial palsy occur.

231

Abdominal tuberculosis

Abdominal TB may arise in the following ways:

◆ secondary spread due to swallowed bacilli from pulmonary disease

◆ primary infection from cows' milk (rare in South Africa)

◆ extension from pelvic disease (post-menarche).

The infection spreads along the following pathway: intestinal mucosa, mesenteric glands, peri-adenitis and leakage of caseous material from glands, low-grade, sticky peritonitis, and infection of serosa and bowel wall. There are usually three clinical forms of abdominal TB:

◆ ascites

◆ palpable nodes

◆ gastrointestinal tract disease.

The main symptoms are swelling of the abdomen, fever, loss of weight, diarrhoea, and colic. Deep palpation reveals masses due to enlarged glands in the right iliac fossa, centrally or along both sides of the spine. Thickened adherent bowel, swollen omentum and glandular masses produce a doughy feel. Acute or subacute intestinal obstruction may be caused by stenosis or kinks in the bowel, or by external pressure from glands. Occasionally interluminal fistulae or an umbilical fistula are produced; a chronic fistula-in-ano may be tuberculous. Massive ascites can also occur. Obstruction of intestinal lymphatics can cause steatorrhoea and chylous ascites. In rare cases, strangulation of lymphatic channels produces chylous ascites with considerable abdominal distension, which is difficult to diagnose and goes on for many months. There is relentless wasting and inanition, despite antituberculous therapy. Compression of the inferior vena cava causes oedema of the lower limbs. Tuberculomas of the caecum may present as a tumour. An erosive gut ulcer can cause blood in the stools.

The differential diagnosis must include lymphoma for abdominal masses and other causes of intestinal obstruction, ascites, and blood in the stools.

Laparoscopy, bacteriology, and histology may be required for precise diagnosis.

Tuberculous meningitis (TBM)

This is the most dangerous of all the complications of tuberculosis, and is especially important in children, as it occurs more often in the young than in adults (see Table 9.7). About 20–40% of children with severe tuberculosis have extension of disease to the meninges. Infection at this site occurs in one of three ways: dissemination within 2 years of a primary infection, as a complication of existing

Table 9.7 Clinico-pathological features of TBM

Underlying pathology	Signs
Meningitis	Neck stiffness (infrequent under 2 years of age) Kernig's and Brudzinski's signs
Raised intracranial pressure	Vomiting, increasing head size, bulging fontanelle, sutural separation and 'cracked-pot' note, bradycardia, mild hypertension and occasionally papilloedema, impaired consciousness, fits
Vascular complications	Convulsions, hemiplegia, quadriplegia, cranial nerve palsies (especially 3rd, 4th, 6th and 7th, and occasionally 2nd), decerebrate rigidity
Encephalopathy	Abnormal behaviour, impaired alertness, dementia, spasticity, convulsions, and coma
Basal ganglia	Chorea, hemiballismus, athetosis, tremors, myoclonus, and ataxia
Space-occupying lesion	Asymptomatic, focal signs, raised intracranial pressure signs
Spinal arachnoiditis	Ascending or transverse myelitis: paraparesis, paraplegia, quadriplegia, sphincter disturbances

TB (miliary, tuberculoma, spine TB, and TB mastoiditis), and as a result of reactivation of a latent focus during intercurrent infection. Clinicians in developing countries have to maintain a high index of suspicion about the possibility of TBM in children, as the disease often begins insidiously with non-specific symptoms and signs. Even in the fully developed case the diagnosis can present difficulties. If there is doubt about the cause of any case of meningitis, it is safer to treat as for TBM until the problem is solved, as the outcome in TBM depends on the rapidity of diagnosis and institution of specific therapy. To ensure maximum recovery, therapy should begin within 10 days of onset of illness.

The prognosis can also be gauged according to the severity of the disease. In order to make this assessment, the degree of involvement is classified into three stages:

◆ *Stage I:* Signs of meningeal irritation; conscious, rational, no focal neurological signs, no hydrocephalus.

◆ *Stage II:* Confusion and/or focal neurological signs (squints, hemiparesis).

◆ *Stage III:* Stupor or delirium and/or neurological signs (paraplegia, hemiplegia).

The bacilli usually reach the brain and meninges through the blood stream; they lodge at these sites but do not immediately initiate inflammation. Meningeal infection is caused by rupture of a caseous focus in the sub-cortical region (Rich's focus) or in the spinal substance into the subarachnoid space, but rarely into the ventricles. The inflammatory response which ensues is probably due to hypersensitivity reactions to bacillary components (especially tuberculoproteins). The base of the brain becomes studded with tubercles, while the convex surfaces remain relatively unaffected. Thick exudate covers cranial nerves, blood vessels, and choroid plexus, and can lead to hydrocephalus. Arteritis affects blood vessels of all sizes, phlebitis occurs, and these changes lead to thrombosis and infarction of the brain. Once this has happened the neurological damage is permanent.

The inflammation can extend downwards to cause spinal arachnoiditis. Myelopathy may be due to this or to vascular complications. If untreated, TBM leads to death in 6–8 weeks.

The onset of the disease is gradual, with irritability, lassitude, headache, vomiting, and abdominal pain. Fits accompany vascular occlusion and brain infarction. The disease progresses through stages I – III. The different physical signs are grouped in the table according to underlying pathology.

Examination of the cerebrospinal fluid (CSF) is central to the diagnosis of TBM. The fluid is usually under pressure, but herniation of the brain stem does not occur, as cerebral oedema is uncommon; indeed lumbar puncture may provide some relief from intracranial tension. The fluid is clear and colourless, and forms a cobweb-like clot on standing. During the early stages of the disease and while on treatment, the cells in the CSF may be dominantly polymorphonuclears; however, lymphocytes usually predominate. Proteins are elevated considerably, and may give a xanthochromic appearance to the fluid. The sugar is modestly decreased, but can be very low in advanced cases. CSF chloride is reduced. It has been suggested that these changes occur in regular sequence: increase in cells, rise in proteins, decrease in sugar, and lastly a fall in chloride. One cautionary note must be sounded about these so-called 'typical' changes of TBM: the CSF often does not follow this overall pattern, and may in fact be quite normal. If it is remembered that the inflammatory reactions in the meninges may be likened to the tuberculin skin reaction, and that the latter may be negative in the presence of TB, then the variability of the CSF in TBM becomes understandable. If the CSF is normal but there is strong suspicion of TBM, a repeat lumbar puncture 48 hours later may reveal abnormalities.

Acid-fast bacilli may be seen on microscopy, but the success of this test depends on the amount of CSF, the number of samples scanned, and the time spent on searching for AFB. For these reasons, the range of positivity is wide — 10–85%, with the lower figure obtaining in the Third World. Culture of CSF is also not useful, as AFB are grown from only about 10–20% of samples, and results take 4 weeks or more. *The CSF takes about 4 months to return to normal.*

A large number of other methods have been evaluated for the diagnosis of TBM. These include biochemical tests (adenosine deaminase activity, lactate dehydrogenase, lactate, tryptophan colour

Table 9.8   Differential diagnosis of CSF in TBM

Condition	Distinguishing features
Pyogenic meningitis	Very low sugar, more neutrophils, bacteria detected; normal within 2 weeks of treatment
Viral meningitis or encephalitis	Normal sugar, slightly elevated proteins, mostly lymphocytes, no bacteria; normal very rapidly
Fungal meningitis	Organisms detected by special stains (especially Indian ink) or specific antisera
Brain abscess	Variable number of neutrophils (the closer abscess is to meninges, the higher the number of polymorphs). Slightly raised protein; normal or slightly reduced sugar

test, and AFB-specific compounds detected by gas chromatography), radio isotope studies (bromide partition test), and immunological tests (for detection of antigen, antibody, or acute phase reactants) using different assay systems. Polymerase chain reaction promises to be very sensitive and specific.

Computed tomography (CT) scanning with contrast enhancement is a valuable aid to diagnosis and prognosis, and should be undertaken when such facilities are available. It has been suggested that basal oedema and ventricular enlargement with basal enhancement are characteristic of TBM. Tuberculomas and infarcts may be demonstrated. CT scanning is particularly useful in the presence of raised intracranial pressure and focal neurological signs.

A myelogram should be done if there are spinal cord signs, in order to detect a compressive lesion or arachnoiditis.

The differential diagnosis includes a number of conditions such as meningitis due to viruses, bacteria, and fungi; neurocysticercosis; brain abscess; and brain tumours.

The most important conditions to be differentiated from TBM according to the CSF are given in *Table 9.8*.

If facilities for diagnosis are limited, the following scheme can be adopted to manage suspected cases of TBM:

◆ Take a careful history; noting especially contacts, and duration of illness.

◆ Detailed physical examination; especially other sites of TB, foci of pyogenic infections, exanthems due to viruses, pyrexia.

◆ Do a Mantoux test and chest radiograph.

◆ CSF — microscopy for bacteria and cells — sugar with Dextrostix®; if very low, treat for pyogenic meningitis (penicillin + chloromycetin) *and* tuberculous meningitis; if normal it is likely to be viral.

◆ Treat for TBM if still in doubt, and repeat CSF examination in 2 weeks; if CSF normal, unlikely to be TBM.

Eyes

TB causes conjunctival infection presenting as conjunctivitis, lacrymation, and swelling and reddening of the eyelids and sclera. The everted eyelid reveals thick granulation with yellow areas. Pre-auricular or tonsillar nodes enlarge. Phlyctens are uncommon; they are small, grey, soft nodules at the limbus, into which drains a leash of conjunctival vessels. Other sites involved include the cornea, lacrymal gland, iris, uvea, and retina (haemorrhages). Choroidal tubercles are exceedingly rare in black children.

Ears, mastoids

(Also see Chapter 14, ENT Problems.)
Tubercles appear on the ear drum and cause multiple perforations (especially in the lower half of the drum). This leads to a chronic painless discharge, and in primary infections to enlargement of the lymph node between the mastoid and angle of the mandible. There is an insidious development of conductive deafness and facial nerve palsy (especially in those below 2 years of age). The chief complication is spread to the brain and meninges.

Oropharynx

Painless dental ulcers with swollen submandibular and tonsillar glands represent one type of primary complex. The tonsils, adenoids, and larynx may also be infected.

HIV/AIDS
TB may present in unusual forms in adolescents with HIV/AIDS. The picture in children is still unclear.

Diagnosis of tuberculosis
The definitive diagnosis of tuberculosis is made on culture of *M. tuberculosis*. However, this takes 4–8 weeks and requires a modest degree of laboratory support, which may be unavailable in precisely those areas where TB is endemic. A further difficulty is that specimens for culture may be difficult to obtain. Children tend to swallow rather than spit out their sputum. Examination of stomach contents obtained by aspiration before the next feed is helpful for diagnosis. Laryngeal and tracheal swabs may also be used for this purpose. AFB may also be recovered from other infected tissues (e.g., pus, CSF, urine, pleural and ascitic fluids).

It is an interesting paradox that the disease which enabled Koch to lay the basis for scientific diagnosis of infectious diseases — founded on the culture of incriminating organisms — is now diagnosed by other means. These are:
- history of contact
- clinical features
- chest radiograph
- tuberculin skin testing
- evolution of disease
- special tests on CSF
- CT scan with contrast enhancement.

Management
Society: Development and health services
Community: Protection and prevention
Contacts: Detection and treatment
Case: Finding, holding, and treatment

Society
The following aspects are important:
- socio-economic development
- integrated health service
- strong primary care with adequate support and referral facilities

- appropriately trained health workers
- centrally co-ordinated TB control programme
- social welfare services.

Protection of the community
Protecting any specific community against TB should include:
- improvement of socio-economic status
- community participation in health care
- health education
- pasteurization of milk (tubercle bacilli do not grow in 'calabash' soured milk)
- BCG vaccination. This can give a false sense of security if not properly administered, and if its use is not correctly understood. An important study of BCG in Madras has tended to cloud the issue of its effectiveness in infants and children: the recommendations emanating from this project state quite clearly that BCG vaccination should be continued. BCG vaccination has produced variable results in vaccine efficacy studies throughout the world. A South African study indicated a protective effect in 58–65% of children. It produces immunity after 8 weeks or more, and therefore does not give immediate protection to a child who is exposed to a TB contact. Experimental evidence suggests that BCG reduces blood spread of bacilli from the site of primary infection. BCG vaccine is given at birth because of convenience and easy access to newborns. As this may not be the optimum period for immunization, BCG should be repeated between 4 and 6 months of age, or when the child is first seen by a health worker. It is given again on entering and on leaving school. *Table 9.9* gives alternative ages for BCG vaccination according to rate of infection in any community. It must be given intradermally or

Table 9.9 Age at which BCG should be administered, depending on prevalence of infection in older children

% of 10- to 14-year-olds infected	BCG given at:
> 5 %	Birth
2 – 5 %	School entry
< 2 %	12 – 13 years

Table 9.10 Investigation of TB contacts:[+] 0 – 14 years

Appears ill	Appears healthy
Refer for further investigation:	INH for 3 months, then Heaf test*:
Tuberculin test	Grade 0 – 1 +: BCG vaccination
Direct sputum	Grade 2+: No action
Clinical investigation	Grade 3+ or 4+: INH for further 3 months
X-ray	

[+]*Contact is defined as close prolonged and personal contact with an infectious case of pulmonary TB. Contact investigation is therefore limited to the immediate family of that case. This is the first priority. If a child is found to have a strongly positive Heaf reaction (3+ or 4+) on routine investigation, an infectious active case may be found within that child's family. The family of that child should therefore be investigated, as a second priority.*
* *Some contacts may be in the anergic phase of infection, i.e., recently infected, and not yet reactive to the tuberculin test.*

percutaneously, checking that the correct preparation for each method is used.

As the vaccine is destroyed by heat, the vaccination site must be kept out of the sun for a while, and vaccine itself must be kept cold while in use.

Limitations of BCG vaccination

◆ It cannot protect if given at birth only.

◆ It cannot protect if given to a child who has already been exposed to tuberculosis, i.e., to a known contact of an infectious case.

◆ It cannot protect if a vaccinated child is exposed to an overwhelming infection. It is by no means completely protective, but if tuberculosis develops, it helps to prevent serious complications (miliary TB, TB meningitis), and therefore reduces human suffering and death.

◆ BCG does not itself affect the transmission of infection.

Detection and treatment of contacts

This is very important, as most children are infected from an adult or child contact. Where there is one infectious case of tuberculosis there will be many more infected ones, some of whom may be ill. In high prevalence areas in South Africa, it has been shown that if contacts of infected children are traced, another positive case will be detected in

every fourth or fifth household visited. The yield is highest if the index case is under 5 years of age with a positive Mantoux test. All children in contact with an infectious case will have living tubercle bacilli within them, even though they may not be obviously ill. All must be given treatment. Any child under 5 years of age who has a significant Mantoux test (i.e., 10 mm, or 15 mm if BCG has been given), or an equivalent skin test, must be treated. All such children, and contacts, should receive the drugs listed in *Table 9.12* (regimen I for contacts ≥7 years; rifampicin, INH, and pyrazinamide for all those ≤ 6 years) *but* for 3 months only, once daily, Mondays to Fridays. This is called 'secondary chemoprophylaxis'. Trials of INH for prevention of overt tuberculosis have included more than 100 000 participants; most have shown at least a 50% reduction in the number of TB cases in the treated groups. The beneficial effect of this is believed to last many years (up to 20 years in the USA). Sick children can be detected by questioning of parents, and assistance given for urgent medical therapy of those who are affected. Many cases of TB meningitis could be prevented by this simple measure.

Tuberculin skin testing

Skin tests are used to detect delayed hypersensitivity to tuberculoprotein. A positive reaction indicates

Table 9.11 Skin tests for TB

Test	Method	Material	Application
Heaf	Percutaneous multiple puncture	Undiluted purified protein derivative (PPD)	For screening
Tine	Percutaneous multiple puncture	Old tuberculin impregnated on needles	For screening
Mantoux	Intradermal	PPD diluted to 2 or 5 test units (TU) Use 5 TU in the sick child	For 'doubtful' reactions

Reading of skin tests

Test	Read after (hours)	Negative	Non-specific	Doubtful		Specific
Heaf	72–96	No reaction	Smal discrete nodules	Larger papules uniting to form ring	Single dome-shaped area of induration	As with grade 3+ vesiculation or necrosis
			Grade 1	Grade 2	Grade 3	Grade 4
Tine	48–72	No reaction	1–2 mm induration per puncture site	3–4 mm		Coalesced
Mantoux (2 or 5 TU)	72	No reaction	< 10 mm induration			> 10 mm induration

If 'doubtful' after Heaf or Tine, do Mantoux.

that infection with the tubercle bacillus has occurred, but does not necessarily mean that active disease is present *(see Tables 9.10 and 9.11)*.

Grades 3 and 4 are indicative of tuberculosis, and require treatment. BCG vaccination can cause grades 1 and 2 Heaf reactions, and up to 10 mm induration on Mantoux testing.

Great care must be taken in doing the test, as it can easily be invalidated by careless technique, inactive PPD, and an ineffective Heaf gun. Prolonged treatment may result in a tuberculin test becoming negative, presumably due to destruction of all the bacilli.

A negative test does not indicate an absence of tuberculosis. It is negative in the presence of tuberculosis under the following conditions:

◆ poor technique

◆ when done soon after exposure. We do not know when exposure occurs, so all close child contacts must be treated, regardless of the reaction

◆ immunodeficiency:
  protein energy malnutrition
  measles

  overwhelming infection
  drugs – steroids.

Contact detection is time-consuming and tedious and requires great enthusiasm for its proper implementation, but is vital in the control of TB.

Case management

Case-finding

How do we seek out those children who have tuberculosis? There are four methods:

◆ detection when they present to a health service (passive)

◆ tracing contacts of patients with disease *(see above)*

◆ screening at-risk groups

◆ mass radiography (this is used in selected instances only).

Passive case-finding can be improved by health education to increase awareness of the common symptoms and signs of TB, and by providing health services which are accessible and appropriate.

Table 9.12 Recommended treatment regimens (Department of National Health and Population Development, 1990)
Children 7 years and over

Drug	Dose	Duration
REGIMEN 1		
Rifater ® (combination of rifampicin, INH, pyrazinamide)	1 tablet/10 kg	Once daily, Monday to Friday, for 6 months
REGIMEN 2*		
Rifampicin	10 mg/kg	As above
Isoniazid	8–10 mg/kg	
Pyrazinamide	20–25 mg/kg	
REGIMEN 3*		
Rifampicin	10–15 mg/kg	3 (or 2) x/week
Isoniazid	20 mg/kg	for 6 months
Pyrazinamide	30 mg/kg	

* In areas with known high incidence of INH resistance, ethambutol (20–30 mg/kg) may be added.

Children 6 years and under

	Dose	Duration
Rifampicin	10 mg/kg	Once daily, Monday to Friday, 6 months
Isoniazid	8–10 mg/kg	As above
Pyrazinamide	20–25 mg/kg	As above

Communities which are especially likely to be exposed to TB, such as the very poor, and those living in overcrowded conditions, can be investigated for TB.

Compliance
Where children are managed on an ambulatory basis, strict adherence to the treatment schedule can be assured through an extensive network of primary health care centres and trained community health workers or family members who can supervise therapy. Health professionals and local authorities should be encouraged to comply with national guidelines for diagnosis, treatment, and follow-up.

Case treatment
There are many drugs available for the treatment of tuberculosis *(see Tables 9.12, 9.13, and 9.14)*. Management may be affected by availability and cost of the drugs. Isoniazid (INH) must always be given; it is freely available, cheap, effective, and relatively non-toxic if used with reasonable care.

It is preferable to give rifampicin to all children with primary tuberculosis, because of the possibility of killing all tubercle bacilli in them.

Possible causes of failure to respond to treatment
Think of drug resistance last *(see below)*. First,
♦ check administration of medicine
♦ check that medicine is not being vomited
♦ check the ability of the child to absorb drugs. Try streptomycin or streptoneotizide, in case of malabsorption
♦ check possible anorexia due to ethionamide
♦ if there is nothing obvious, exclude other diseases, e.g., urinary tract infection.

The most important factor influencing response to treatment is adequate chemotherapy which is regularly administered. The severity of disease can influence outcome, but is relatively less important when compared to regular and sufficient drug treatment. Host factors such as age, sex, heredity, and intercurrent disease, while important, play a significantly diminished role in determining prognosis in this era of chemotherapy. Rest, accommodation, diet, nursing, climate, sanatoria, and psychological problems constitute an unimportant set of elements affecting response to treatment. Inactivation of INH and adverse response to PAS, thiacetazone, and other drugs can be related to host factors, but in general play a marginal role in influencing the outcome of treatment.

Drug resistance
Populations of tubercle bacilli contain at least two different groups of organisms: an overwhelming

majority susceptible to antituberculous drugs, and a small minority which is not susceptible. Drug treatment kills off susceptible bacteria, thereby allowing the resistant organisms to proliferate and replace the former. Development of resistance in this manner, through the use of drugs, is termed 'acquired' or 'secondary' resistance. It is most often the result of inadequate chemotherapy. Patients who have had no prior anti-TB therapy and who have been infected by drug-resistant bacilli from a case with acquired resistance have 'primary' resistance. Strains of tubercle bacilli in which drug resistance is inherent or natural, as opposed to drug-induced, do occur, but are not important in management.

In a population of tubercle bacilli the average frequency of INH-resistant mutants is about 1 per 10^5 bacilli, streptomycin-resistant mutants about 1 per 10^6 bacilli, and doubly-resistant mutants about 1 per 10^8 bacilli. The frequency of drug-resistant mutants is determined by the origins of the strain, the total number of bacilli, the type of drug used, and its concentration.

More drug-resistant tubercle bacilli develop within larger populations of organisms and at lower concentrations of drugs. Accordingly, large tuberculous lesions penetrated by low concentrations of a single drug will rapidly lead to excessive multiplication of drug-resistant organisms,

whereas even low concentrations of two drugs can inhibit such growth.

Primary resistance to INH and streptomycin among TB patients has been of the order of 5.8% and 6.6% respectively in India, 3.7% and 9.4% in Japan, and 1.3% and 2.8% in the United Kingdom. In the USA, among new patients with TB, primary resistance to INH has been 0.9%, to streptomycin 1.5%, to INH + streptomycin 0.4%, and to all three drugs 0.3%

Testing for sensitivity of tubercle bacilli to currently-used drugs, before instituting chemotherapy regimens, is not indicated, as this simply increases costs and inconvenience without materially altering overall success rate.

Treatment guidelines

♦ Treatment must be supervised.
♦ Rifampicin and INH must be used (unless absolutely contra-indicated).
♦ Minimum course is 6 months.

Supervision (whether ambulatory or in-patient):

♦ No drugs given to the patient to take home.
♦ No self-administration of drugs.
♦ Supervisor (reliable lay or professional person with a strong sense of responsibility) must give drugs to patient.

Table 9.13 Recommendations for the treatment of childhood tuberculosis in the United Kingdom (British Thoracic Society)

	Initial phase		Continuation phase	
	Drugs	*Months*	*Drugs*	*Months*
Pulmonary	RHZ	2	RH	4
	or RH	2	RH	7
Non-pulmonary				
Meningitis	RHZ	2	RH	10
Pericarditis	RHZ	2	RH	4
Lymph node	RHZ	2	RH	4
Bone, joint, other sites	RHZE	2	RH	4
	or RHE	2	RH	7
Chemoprophylaxis	H	6		6
	RH	3		3

R = Rifampicin   H = Isoniazid
E = Ethambutol   Z= Pyrazinamide

◆ Drugs should be pre-packed in individual dosages.

Points to remember
◆ Drug toxicity is less common in children than in adults. Hepatotoxicity is especially rare.
◆ There is a ten-fold decrease of tubercle bacilli in the first 2 days of treatment. Accordingly, risk of cross-infection is negligible after a fortnight of therapy.
◆ If the child cannot swallow tablets or capsules, crush the former and empty the latter in a spoon, flavour with acceptable vehicle, and administer. This is preferable to using available syrups.

Monitoring progress
The following are useful indicators:
◆ appetite
◆ temperature
◆ weight gain
◆ chest radiograph on admission, and after 60 days. If abnormal, repeat at 180 days; avoid frequent x-rays.

Treatment of different types of TB
HIV/AIDS: These patients require standard drugs, but probably for longer periods. In Africa there may be a case for putting all HIV-positive children on prolonged prophylactic INH.

Simple primary tuberculosis does respond to treatment with INH alone, but because of the risk of infection with an already-resistant organism, it is better to use at least two drugs.

Disseminated tuberculosis: In extensive pulmonary TB, organ TB, and miliary TB, start treatment with three first-line drugs: INH, streptomycin, and either rifampicin or ethambutol. With improvement, discontinue streptomycin, and use oral drugs for 2 years. Most patients become non-infective within 4 weeks on adequate therapy.

Bone and joint TB: General principles of treatment are followed, including keeping the affected joint at rest by splinting, extension, etc.

Lymph node TB: Responds to usual treatment, but may require incision and evacuation.

Pericarditis: Responds to usual treatment of tuberculosis with or without aspiration for tamponade. Steroids are indicated. Watch for constriction which requires surgical decortication.

Abdominal tuberculosis: Presents other complications such as diarrhoea, peritonitis, and intestinal obstruction, all of which can cause impaired absorption. Intramuscular drugs are essential (streptomycin or streptoneotizide).

TBM: If in doubt, treat for pyogenic and TBM together until diagnosis is clear (usually in 2–3 weeks). **N.B.** Start treatment at once — delay is dangerous. It is important to use drugs that enter the theca freely, are relatively non-toxic, and available. Of all drugs that are available, INH is the most important.

Drugs used in TBM
(See Table 9.14)
◆ INH, ethionamide, ethambutol (not < 7 years of age), rifampicin, cycloserine, pyrazinamide
◆ ACTH gel. Use in all cases: 20 IU 12-hourly; maximum 50 IU/day with added potassium. Prednisone 2 mg/kg/day may achieve a similar anti-inflammatory result, except that its use exposes the child to severe effects of other common infectious diseases.

Intrathecal therapy:
Drugs:
◆ Dexamethasone 4 mg IT for 5 days (can be substituted by hydrocortisone).
◆ Streptomycin 50–100 mg/daily (calcium or sulphate preparation). Indications:
— clinical deterioration, despite adequate treatment. Frequent fits
— incipient spinal block (high rising CSF protein, low CSF pressure)
— high CSF cell count, very low CSF sugar, many TB bacteria in CSF.

Duration of treatment
The children are kept under supervised treatment (hospital and settlement) for 18 months. Children kept for shorter periods have often relapsed or died.
◆ INH (or neotizide) is given IM until the patient is able to take it satisfactorily by mouth. The dose must be increased as the child gains weight. It is continued for at least 1 year after discharge; longer if possible, as calcification can appear at the base of the brain after about 2 years, and the calcium of

Table 9.14 Drug treatment for primary TB

Drug	Dose	Action	Transport across blood–brain barrier	Major toxicity	Miscellaneous
Isoniazid (INH)	Infancy: 20–30 mg/kg/day 1 year: 200 mg/day 3 year: 300 mg/day > 3 years: 10–15 mg/kg/day ID$_3$ 15 mg/kg/day	Cidal	Crosses uninflamed meninges	Fever, rash, neuritis, anxiety, fright, hallucinations, convulsions, liver damage, haemolysis in G6PD deficiency	Neurotoxicity prevented with pyridoxine 50 mg/day IM x 1 week Effective against intracellular and extracellular organisms Inactivation under genetic control — 2 types: i. rapid—polyneuritis uncommon ii. slow — polyneuritis more often Give in TBM initially
Streptomycin	20 mg/kg/day IMI ID$_3$ 20 mg/kg/day	Static in low doses; cidal in big doses on extra-cellular bacteria	Does not cross blood—brain barrier	VIIIth cranial nerve toxicity — (vestibular and auditory), nephrotic, skin reactions	Useful in malabsorbtion Effective against extracellular organisms only Must be used in combination with other anti-TB drugs to obviate resistance

Streptoneotizide per ampoule

Streptomycin	1 g
Neotizide	600 mg
	Dose as for INH

Drug	Dose	Action	Transport across blood–brain barrier	Major toxicity	Miscellaneous
Ethambutol	25 mg/kg/day ID$_3$ 30 mg/kg/day ID$_2$ 35 mg/kg/day	Static	Does not cross uninflamed meninges, but crosses in meningitis	Retrobulbar neuritis, peripheral neuritis	Use in combination only Acts on intracellular + extra-cellular bacteria
Rifampicin	10 mg/kg/day ID$_3$ 15 mg/kg/day	Cidal	Does not cross uninflamed meninges, but crosses in meningitis	Liver damage, anorexia, vomiting, haemolytic anaemia, thrombo-cytopenia, renal failure	Acts on intracellular + extra-cellular bacteria In TBM: use higher doses, use if deterioration, use if drug resistance Stains urine orange
Ethionamide	15–20 mg/kg/day	Static	Cross uninflamed meninges	Liver damage, anorexia, vomiting	Related to INH Use in combination only
Pyrazinamide	35 mg/kg/day ID$_3$ 50 mg/kg/day ID$_2$ 75 mg/kg/day	Cidal	Crosses uninflamed meninges	Liver damage, anorexia, arthralgia, hyperuricaemia	Effective against extracellular organisms
Cycloserine	5–10 mg/kg/day	Static	Crosses uninflamed meninges	Neurotoxic	

healing tuberculosis may contain live tubercle bacilli.

◆ Ethionamide/pyrazinamide/rifampicin is continued until discharge. South African health authorities recommend higher once-daily doses in TBM: ethionamide 20 mg/kg, pyrazinamide 40 mg/kg, rifampicin 20 mg/kg, INH 20 mg/kg.

◆ ACTH is continued until the CSF is normal and has remained so for 2–3 weeks (this may be a period of 3 months). Prednisone is given for as short a period as possible in children, replacing it with ACTH as soon as this is feasible.

◆ Intrathecal streptomycin is continued until the CSF has been normal for 1–2 months, or if there is a dramatic clinical response to treatment with this drug.

It is most important that once an adequate schedule has been introduced, it should not be modified, except in accordance with weight gain or drug toxicity. Dosage should *not* be reduced for loss of weight.

Special procedures

◆ Decompression by lumbar puncture. This does not cause coning in TBM, and can give dramatic relief.

◆ Ventricular puncture.

◆ Ventricular drainage — if there is raised intracranial pressure and a failure to improve after an initial good response. When used correctly it has produced excellent results.

◆ Laminectomy is used by some units for arachnoiditis with paraplegia; others prefer supportive and antituberculous treatment with steroids.

H.M. Coovadia

10

AIDS

Introduction

AIDS (Acquired Immunodeficiency Syndrome) was observed as a clinical entity in homosexual men and intravenous (IV) drug users in 1981, and in children in 1983. The causative agent, a retrovirus known as the human immunodeficiency virus (HIV), was discovered in 1983. HIV infection impairs immune function by destroying T4 lymphocytes and predisposing to overwhelming opportunistic infections and early death.

Unfortunately early speculation regarding the origin of AIDS was inherently racist, and Africa was implicated without adequate scientific evidence. It appears that cases of AIDS were recognized in Africa in the late 1970s and early 1980s, a pattern similar to that in the United States and Haiti. To date the origin of HIV remains controversial.

AIDS/HIV infection is now recognized as a major global health problem, and in some African countries has reached epidemic proportions. At present there is no vaccine or curative therapy available for HIV infection.

Epidemiology

AIDS was first recognized in the USA among white middle-class homosexuals, which attracted considerable public attention and led to extensive research into various aspects of the disease.

AIDS has now become pandemic. It is estimated that several million people world-wide have been infected with HIV. In Africa many thousands of suspected cases are unreported, and many are not recognized due to lack of health and testing facilities as well as policy regarding notification and reporting.

Geographical patterns

Three patterns of spread of HIV have been recognized, and each pattern reflects different sexual and social behaviour.

Geographical patterns

Pattern I   Homosexual and bisexual men (now spreading into heterosexual population)
            Use of unsterile needles by IV drug users
Countries: North America, Western Europe, parts of Latin America, Australia and New Zealand
M/F ratio: M > F
Cases reported in the late 1970s.
Pattern II   Mainly heterosexuals
            Babies born to infected mothers
            Prostitutes at risk
            Use of unscreened blood for transfusion, and related products
Countries: Mainly Africa, parts of Latin America and the Caribbean
M/F ratio: Equal
Cases first reported in the late 1970s.
Pattern III   Homosexual and heterosexual
            Imported blood products
Countries: Mostly Asia, Oceania (excluding Australia and New Zealand)
Spread in the late 1980s.

Epidemiology in Africa

In most parts of Africa the male to female ratio of HIV infection is approximately 1:1. Sexual transmission in adults occurs mainly among the 20–40 years age group. In Africa HIV transmission follows the same pattern as other sexually transmitted diseases such as syphilis or gonorrhoea. Unscreened blood and blood products, and unsterile needles and syringes still play a role in those parts of Africa with limited resources.

Paediatric AIDS cases are increasing in Africa and in other parts of the world. In the majority the transmission is vertical from mother to child, and therefore is most common in those under 5 years of age. Mother-to-child transmission may occur before birth, at birth, or after birth through breast-feeding. However, the latter is not an argument against breast-feeding, as in developing countries the change from breast-feeding to artificial feeding has resulted in substantial increases in infant mortality.

The rate of mother-to-child transmission ranges between 13% and 40%. The European collaborative study found a low transmission rate of 13%, whilst in Zambia and Zaire it was estimated to be 39%. The high rate of transmission was partly explained by greater frequency of symptomatic mothers in African studies compared with the European study. A combination of fetal, maternal, and viral factors may result in predisposition to HIV infection.

Routes of transmission of HIV infection
Sexual contact
> sexually promiscuous adults/adolescents
> prostitutes
> homosexuals
> bisexual men
> sexual abuse

Perinatal
> mother-to-child infection

Intravenous routes
> unscreened blood and blood products
> infected syringes and needles
> IV drug users – sharing unsterile needles and syringes

Groups at high risk of infection
prostitutes
uniformed service men
prisoners
truck drivers (long-distance)
people with STD
promiscuous adolescents and adults
barmaids

Problems in Africa
AIDS is spreading rapidly in Africa. Important socio-economic factors which have contributed to the spread include:
◆ migrant labour, especially country to country, and from rural to urban areas
◆ erosion of traditional values and breakdown of family life
◆ poor access to health and educational services.

A higher prevalence of HIV has been noted in urban areas, along truck routes used by long-distance drivers, and in adults with sexually transmitted disease, especially genital ulcerative disease.

Aetiology
HIV is a retrovirus. Some members of the retrovirus group have been known to cause immunodeficiency and central nervous system degeneration in animals.

The family of human immunodeficiency virus currently contains two members, HIV-1 and HIV-2. HIV-1 has a wide geographical distribution, whilst HIV-2 appears to be limited to certain areas such as West Africa and Mozambique.

The core of the HIV *(Fig. 10.1)* contains RNA and the enzyme reverse transcriptase. The outer coat contains lipid and glycoprotein 120 (gp 120). HIV invades a cell, where it is replicated within the nucleus *(see Fig. 10.2).*

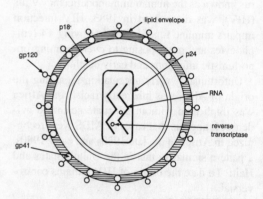

Fig. 10.1 Human immunodefiency virus (HIV)
The glycoproteins (gp) and proteins (p) are important, as they are the antigens which stimulate the immune systems to generate specific antibodies.
(Adapted from 'Explaining the nature of the virus that causes AIDS', AIDS Action, issue 3.)

The HIV infects the helper-inducer T4 or CD4+ subset of T lymphocytes, macrophages, and other cells such as bowel epithelium and microglial cells. The external envelope glycoprotein gp 120 of HIV has great affinity for the CD4 molecule which is present on the surface of these cells. HIV irreversibly infects and often destroys cells. Since T4 cells play an important role in many facets of the immune system, depletion of these cells causes profound immunosuppression and clinical manifestations of AIDS.

Immunology
Most of the immunological abnormalities characteristic of HIV infection occur relatively late in the course of infection.

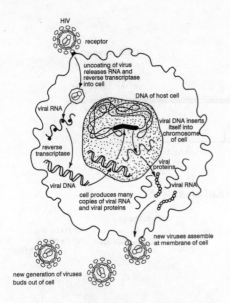

HIV
receptor
uncoating of virus
releases RNA and
reverse transcriptase
into cell
viral RNA
DNA of host cell
reverse
transcriptase
viral DNA inserts
itself into
chromosome
of cell
viral
proteins
viral DNA
viral RNA
cell produces many
copies of viral RNA
and viral proteins
new viruses assemble
at membrane of cell
new generation of viruses
buds out of cell

Fig. 10.2 Host cell invaded by HIV: Viral RNA forms viral DNAs by means of reverse transcriptase. Viral DNA inserts itself into ribosome where viral proteins are generated so

Prognosis

Infant mortality and morbidity due to common childhood illnesses such as pneumonia and gastro-enteritis appear to be much higher in children infected with HIV than in the non-infected.

Survival of children with AIDS depends on:

Age at diagnosis of AIDS: Children below 1 year of age with AIDS have a much higher mortality than other age groups. These children acquire the infection from their mother, and they survive approximately 2 years.

Disease pattern at the time of diagnosis: *Pneumocystis carinii* pneumonia carries a high mortality with first infection. Children presenting with candida oesophagitis, encephalopathy, or renal disease have a median survival time of less than 1 year. Survival up to 4 years has been observed in children with recurrent bacterial infections and lymphocytic interstitial pneumonitis. Opportunistic infections are the cause of death in the majority of children with AIDS.

Immunological abnormalities in paediatric aids

T cells	total lymphopenia
	T4 lymphopenia
	reversal of T4:T8 ratio
B cells	hypergammaglobulinaemia (early abnormality)
	abnormal antibody response to variety of antigens
PMN*	neutropenia
	chemotaxis and phagocytosis

*PMN = Polymorphonuclear cells

Natural history

See Figs 10.3 and 10.4.

Incubation

Children with perinatal infection are assumed to be infected *in utero* or at birth. The incubation period is between 4 and 6 months, but in some instances has been found to be as long as 7 years. The incubation period for transfusion-acquired disease is approximately 17 months.

Clinical spectrum of the disease

(See Table 10.1.)

Table 10.1 Clinical features and presentation in 185 children with symptomatic HIV-related disease (Zimbabwe)

Clinical features	%
Lymphadenopathy	52.4
Pulmonary infiltrates	45.4
Failure to thrive	37.8
Hepatomegaly	34.6
Splenomegaly	26.0
Oral candidiasis	23.2
Chronic/recurrent diarrhoea	4.3
Chronic mucopurulent rhinitis	4.3
Meningitis (purulent)	2.1
Symptomatic thrombocytopenia	1.6
Cardiomyopathy (CCF)	1.1
Kaposi sarcoma	1.5
Encephalopathy	1.6

Source: Central African Journal of Medicine, Vol. 36, No. 5, 1990.

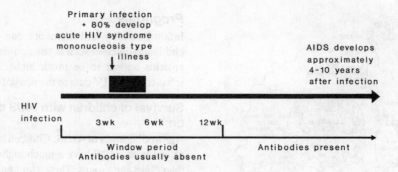

Fig. 10.3   Natural history of HIV infection in adolescents and adults

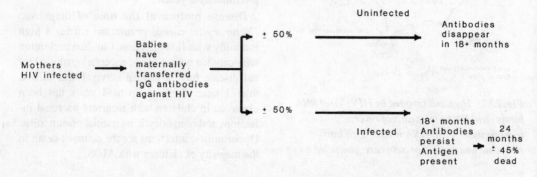

Fig. 10.4   Natural history of mother to child HIV transmission

The clinical manifestations of HIV infection range from subclinical to severe forms. The course of the disease is variable.

AIDS has an earlier onset in children and infants compared to adults. Approximately 50% of paediatric cases are diagnosed during the first year of life, and up to 80% by 2 years of age.

HIV infection causes a multisystem disease. The accompanying immune deficiency leads to various opportunistic infections, bacteraemia, and increased frequency of malignancies.

Bacterial infections

Common problems such as septicaemia, meningitis, pneumonia, and abscesses frequently occur before any other features of HIV infection are evident in children. These infections are recurrent and severe. Infecting organisms include *Streptococcus pneumoniae*, *Haemophilus influenzae*, *Staphylococcus aureus*, and Gram-negative organisms including salmonella. Chronic suppurative otitis media is a very common complication in HIV-infected children.

Opportunistic and viral infections

These cause late complications in children with HIV disease. Candida, *Pneumocystis carinii*, cytomegalovirus (CMV), *Herpes simplex*, adenovirus, and cryptosporidium have been isolated from these patients. CMV infection has been reported to cause pneumonitis, hepatitis, and gastrointestinal ulcerations.

Generalized lymphadenopathy/ hepatosplenomegaly

Generalized lymphadenopathy, with or without hepatomegaly, was the commonest presentation in 185 children with symptomatic HIV-related disease in Zimbabwe. Lymphadenopathy was marked in the majority of children, with particular involvement of cervical and axillary nodes.

Respiratory system

Pulmonary disease is a frequent presentation in childhood HIV disease, and often the first manifestation of the HIV infection. It is associated with high morbidity and mortality.

Bacterial pneumonia is frequent in children, and may be associated with bacteraemia.

Tuberculosis: In developing countries, pulmonary tuberculosis is frequently found in adults and children with HIV infection.

Lymphoid interstitial pneumonitis (LIP): LIP is a chronic progressive pulmonary disorder usually presenting after the first year of life. It is uncommon in adults. Coughing is present, with normal auscultatory findings. Hypoxia is frequently present. Digital clubbing occurs as the disease progresses.

Generalized lymphadenopathy and parotid and other salivary gland enlargement are usually present. The pathogenesis is unclear. A diffuse nodular pattern, with or without hilar or paratracheal lymph node enlargement, may be present on the chest X-ray.

Pneumocystis carinii, a protozoan spread by water droplets, causes opportunistic infection in immunosuppressed patients, especially those with AIDS and malignancies. In the USA, it is the most common opportunistic infection in children with HIV-related disease. However, reports from some parts of Africa suggest that *Pneumocystis carinii* may be a less frequent cause of pneumonia in children with AIDS. A common presentation is acute onset of tachypnoea, fever, and nonproductive coughing. Hypoxaemia is frequently present.

At present, definite diagnosis can only be made by identifying the organism in respiratory secretions or lung tissue.

Failure to thrive

Failure to thrive is a major feature of the disease. Growth faltering or severe malnutrition was seen in approximately 40% of the children with symptomatic HIV infection in Zimbabwe.

Gastrointestinal tract

HIV disease as well as other associated infections cause gastrointestinal symptoms. Oral candidiasis is frequently present, and may be associated with candida oesophagitis. Recurrent and chronic diarrhoea is common, and contributes to malnutrition.

Neurological syndromes

Approximately 50% of children with HIV infection will have neurological involvement. Features are as follows:
- microcephaly
- developmental delay or loss of motor milestones
- encephalopathy — which may be static, progressive or intermittent
- paresis, cerebellar ataxia, abnormal muscle tone
- secondary CNS infection, e.g. bacterial meningitis; cryptococcal meningitis, although frequent in adults with AIDS, is uncommon in children.

Computerized axial tomography scan findings include cerebral atrophy, enlargement of subarachnoid space and ventricles.

Haematological abnormalities

Several abnormalities have been reported. Immune thrombocytopenia is the most serious haematological abnormality seen. Other features include moderate anaemia, lymphopenia and neutropenia.

Cardiovascular system

HIV-associated cardiomyopathy and pericardial effusion have been reported in children, as well as conduction abnormalities.

Renal disease

Abnormal urinalyses are a frequent finding. HIV-associated nephropathy is uncommon, but the prognosis appears to be poor.

Malignancies

Malignancies such as Kaposi's sarcoma appear to be more frequent in adults than in children.

Differential diagnosis

HIV infection often presents with common child-hood infections such as respiratory infections, diarrhoea and malnutrition. However, HIV infection should be suspected if in addition to any of the above, the child has generalized lymphadenopathy, hepatosplenomegaly, oral candidiasis, chronic otitis media, or neurological symptoms.

Congenital immunodeficiency syndromes and congenital infections can usually be differentiated by their characteristic clinical and laboratory features.

Paediatric case definition

The Centre for Disease Control (CDC) in the USA has established strict criteria for the definition of paediatric AIDS. These include immunological tests, identification of opportunistic infections, and histological diagnosis of LIP and malignancies. These criteria are of limited use in developing countries due to the unavailability of sophisticated technology.

The World Health Organization (WHO) has proposed a much simpler case definition of paediatric AIDS, which can be used where laboratory facilities are limited *(see Table 10.2)*. This is at present being evaluated in various countries. It is

Table 10.2   WHO clinical case definition of AIDS in children

Major signs
    weight loss or failure to thrive
    chronic diarrhoea (> 1/12)
    prolonged fever (> 1/12)
Minor signs
    generalized lymphadenopathy*
    oropharyngeal candidiasis
    repeated common infections (otitis, pharyngitis, etc.)
    persistent cough (> 1/12)
    generalized dermatitis
    confirmed maternal HIV infection

Paediatric AIDS is suspected in an infant or child presenting with at least two major signs associated with at least two minor signs, in the absence of a known cause of immunosuppression.
* Generalized lymphadenopathy = lymph nodes measuring at least 0.5 cm and present in two or more sites, with bilateral lymph nodes counting as one site.

important to note that AIDS case definition is not a substitute for clinical judgement.

Diagnosis

(See Table 10.3)

Children exposed to known risk factors (including maternal factors) who present with clinical features suggestive of AIDS should be completely evaluated for HIV-related disease. The clinical diagnosis is confirmed by documenting infection with retrovirus. The Enzyme Linked Immunosorbent Assay (ELISA) antibody test, which detects antibodies to viral proteins, is commonly used as an initial screening test. Western blot assay, which detects antibodies to specific viral proteins, is used to confirm the initial ELISA result. Before performing laboratory tests, it is important that parental consent is obtained and confidentiality is maintained at all times. Pre-test and post-test counselling of the patient/parents is an essential part of the diagnostic testing.

Infants born to infected mothers acquire maternal antibodies to HIV transplacentally, whether or not the infants themselves are infected. Maternal antibodies (1gG) may persist up to 15 or 18 months, and therefore antibody tests are not diagnostic of a true infection in that age group. At present tests for 1gM antibody to HIV are unreliable; PCR is promising in western countries.

Table 10.3   Serodiagnosis of HIV infection

1 **Antibody detection**
    a. **ELISA**
        measures antibodies to viral proteins
        sensitive test
        used for screening donated blood for transfusion
    b. **Western blot assay**
        detects antibodies to specific viral proteins
        more specific than ELISA
        most common confirmatory test in clinical use
2* **Antigen detection**
    a. P24 antigen ELISA
    b. PCR (polymerase chain reaction) to detect HIV-specific DNA.
3* **Viral cultures**

* Not widely available and at present used mainly for research.

Other supportive laboratory tests

Polyclonal hypergammaglobulinaemia occurs very early in the disease and is a strong indicator of AIDS. The level found in HIV infection is much higher than in malnutrition and tuberculosis.

Decreased numbers of CD4 and inverted CD4:CD8 ratio are the hallmarks of HIV infection. In children, severe bacterial and opportunistic infections may occur with normal numbers of CD4.

Management

Management consists of a multidisciplinary effort, with special emphasis on emotional support for the patient and family whenever the need arises.

Counselling

Pre-test and post-test counselling are an integral part of management of HIV infection. Counselling has two major components:

a. *Educational aspect,* which includes modes of transmission, safer sex practices, treatment available, and follow-up.

b. *Psychosocial component,* which consists of assessment of family support and coping mechanisms of the family and child. This information is used to help the family cope with the illness and its social and moral ramifications.

Support groups in various developing countries have been a very valuable asset in helping families with AIDS cope with various aspects of the disease. Confidentiality of the results should be assured at all times.

Clinical management

General

Nutrition: Advice on high calorie diet and other essential nutrients should be given to the mother as soon as the child is found to have HIV infection. Breast-feeding should be encouraged in developing countries irrespective of the presence of HIV in the mother, because of the costs and hazards of artificial feeding. Growth should be monitored regularly. Patients with oesophagitis may need to be fed by nasogastric tubes.

Hydration: Oral rehydration therapy, and in some instances intravenous fluids, may be needed during severe diarrhoeal episodes. Mothers should be taught about diarrhoeal management at home.

Immunization: Recommendations for immunization in HIV-infected children have been controversial, largely because of the immunosuppression which accompanies the disease. However, with the high prevalence of infectious diseases in developing countries, it is advisable to continue with the present policy of immunization, including BCG, until information is available to the contrary.

Specific

Bacterial infections: Fever is common in HIV-infected children, and it is difficult to distinguish fever due to underlying HIV infection from that due to bacterial or other infections. Antibiotics are therefore used frequently. Antibiotics should cover common childhood organisms, but as disease progresses, antibiotic coverage should include Gram-negative organisms.

Mycobacterium tuberculosis: In a child with suspected tuberculosis, an appropriate regimen of anti-tuberculous therapy should be used. Some have recommended INH prophylaxis in children with AIDS in view of the increased risk of infection with tuberculosis.

Candidiasis: Oral candidiasis is common and recurrent. Recommended treatment is gentian violet, nystatin, or ketoconazole.

Pneumocystis carinii: Currently trimethoprim-sulfamethoxazole is the drug of choice. Clinical response to treatment is slow, and may take up to 7 days. Relapses are frequent.

Lymphocytic interstitial pneumonitis (LIP): Short-term steroids have been used in progressive disease with good effect. It is important to exclude superadded infection during exacerbation.

Retroviral drugs: At present trials are underway for azidothymidine (AZT) in children. It is virostatic and reduces levels in the blood, but it does not eradicate the virus. The drug is expensive, and therefore beyond the financial reach of developing countries.

HIV vaccine: Extensive research is in progress at present to find an effective vaccine against HIV.

▶ ## Management in the community

AIDS epidemics have begun to overburden traditional hospital-based health care services. There is an urgent need to reorientate the present health services towards primary health care. Health workers should be trained to provide the following services to the community:

◆ education and information regarding HIV infection and its prevention
◆ early detection
◆ counselling
◆ care of the infected child at home and clinic level
◆ care of the dying child.

Prevention

In the absence of a cure or vaccine, prevention is the only method available at present to help reduce the spread of AIDS. Prevention programmes should take into account local cultural beliefs and attitudes.

The majority of childhood AIDS is acquired through mother-to-child transmission. Prevention of heterosexual transmission in young adults and adolescents would therefore reduce childhood AIDS.

Health education

Health education programmes should be designed to influence sexual and other risk behaviours so that transmission is reduced. Health education should include the following:

◆ facts about AIDS
◆ facts about routes of transmission
◆ warning about the risks of indiscriminate sex
◆ advice on the use of condoms to reduce the risk of transmission
◆ facts about how AIDS is *not* spread, for example casual contact at school and hand-shaking.

These programmes need to be innovative, taking into consideration that thus far education has had minimal impact on the AIDS epidemic — irrespective of level of education or standard of living of the target groups. Amongst other things, cultural beliefs and practices, the behaviour patterns of the community, and epidemiological imperatives have to be considered in the design of these programmes. The successes and failures of

AIDS education programmes in other parts of the world must clearly be taken into consideration. Existing structures such as civic organizations, schools, and churches will have to be mobilized in an all-out effort to change sexual practices.

HIV-infected women should be counselled about the risks of infection to the newborn. HIV transmission through breast milk may occur. However, due to unavailability of safe alternatives in developing countries, breast-feeding is still recommended.

Use of unsterile needles and equipment should be strongly discouraged. Health centres, private practitioners, traditional health workers, and the general population should be educated about the risks associated with this.

Health workers and care-givers should treat all blood as if it is infected. Contact with blood should be minimized, and open sores on the skin should be covered with waterproof plasters. Laundry and infected equipment should be sterilized by soaking for 20 minutes in household bleach diluted with 10 parts water.

Screening of all blood donors and blood products is essential, in addition to exclusion of donors with at-risk behaviour patterns.

Implications of paediatric AIDS
The family

Some of the important psychosocial issues faced by the infected child and the family are:

◆ coping with a potentially fatal illness
◆ emotional and financial demands of chronic ill health
◆ disruption of normal family life
◆ guilt, anxiety, and depression
◆ ostracism by the community and other family members
◆ early death of the infected parent/parents.

Easy access to counselling services and ready support from other groups such as social workers, psychologists, and the religious fraternity may help the family to cope better.

Day-care/school attendance

HIV is not spread by casual contact. With the exception of children with oozing skin lesions or biting behaviour, children with asymptomatic infections should be allowed to attend normal school, day-care and other institutions. Acts of discrimination against HIV-infected children and their families due to ignorance and fear in the community should be discouraged by appropriate health education.

Infant mortality trends

Paediatric AIDS is a major threat to child survival, despite recently-improved primary health care programmes in developing countries. In Zaire it is estimated that HIV infection may be responsible for a 15% increase in infant mortality. Similar trends may exist in other countries with high or increasing seroprevalence of HIV in adults.

Death of young adults

Young adults, the potential work-force in all fields, are at risk of HIV infection and therefore early death. This will have an impact on various aspects of the national economy and on family life. Loss of parents, family members, and teachers has a profound effect on children.

Orphans

The WHO has estimated that there will be 10 million orphans of HIV-infected parents in Sub-Saharan Africa by the year 2000. Some children who have lost both parents are being looked after by their elderly grandparents with limited or no income, while others have become 'street children' and therefore are constantly at risk of STD and HIV.

Health workers and national policy-makers need to formulate plans to care for these children.

R.G. Choto
K.J. Nathoo

11
Gastrointestinal disorders

Vomiting and regurgitation

Introduction

Vomiting is a common complaint in the paediatric age group. It is a centrally-controlled, complex interaction between the gastrointestinal and neurological systems. It is often associated with nausea and autonomic symptoms, and with signs such as salivation, pallor, sweating, tachycardia and anorexia. Usually it is preceded by retching, which culminates in sustained contraction of the abdominal muscles, when the contents of the stomach are ejected forcefully. In contrast, regurgitation is a simple, passive process, not associated with muscular contraction or autonomic symptoms. Regurgitation is a characteristic feature of gastro-oesophageal reflux.

Approach to the child with vomiting

The following comments apply to those children in whom vomiting is persistent or recurrent; acute abdominal emergencies will not be dealt with in this section *(see Chapter 28, Surgical Problems)*.

History

A good, detailed history from the child or the accompanying parent is an important aspect. This alone will frequently establish the cause of vomiting, and can prevent unnecessary investigations. Points in the history which should be established are as follows:

♦ **Duration of symptoms:** The age of onset of vomiting may help to indicate the most likely cause *(see Table 11.1)*.

♦ **Frequency and quantity of vomitus:** This gives some indication of the seriousness of the condition. The infant who frequently spits up small amounts of milk after feeds is less likely to have a serious problem than one who has two or three large vomits each day. One way of establishing the quantity is to compare its volume to the size of the meal ingested prior to the episode.

♦ **Character of vomitus:** This information helps to establish whether the patient has vomiting as opposed to regurgitation of gastric contents.

♦ **Associated symptoms:** The presence of nausea, sweating, pallor, and salivation is further evidence for vomiting as opposed to regurgitation, and usually suggests a more serious cause for the symptom. Associated diarrhoea or constipation should be asked about.

♦ **Contents of vomitus:** A description of the contents should establish whether the food was unaltered or mixed with gastric juice, whether it contained fresh blood, 'coffee ground', or bile. It is helpful to establish whether the vomitus contains food that was ingested more than six hours previously.

♦ **Relationship to other events:** Establishing a temporal relationship between vomiting and events such as mealtimes or the time of day is helpful.

♦ **Additional information:** It is essential to enquire about any medications the patient may be taking. Toxic effects of drugs such as theophylline and digitalis may manifest initially with vomiting.

Examination

Infants who are thriving despite a parent's description of prolonged, severe vomiting are unlikely to have a serious underlying disease. Conversely, failure to thrive — as assessed by weight loss and stunting — is far more worrisome, and suggests a more serious condition. Clinical features of dehydration are indicative of severe vomiting.

The sclera should always be carefully examined for jaundice. Acute infectious hepatitis is frequently accompanied by persistent vomiting. Thrush, pharyngitis, and otitis media can all account for vomiting, and should be actively excluded by inspection. Generalized or localized distension of the abdomen, and peristaltic waves are suggestive of intestinal obstruction in the small or large bowel. Thus, peristaltic waves emerging from the left subcostal margin and moving to the right in early infancy suggest hypertrophic pyloric stenosis. Hernial sites should be examined to exclude incarcerated hernias. Palpation of the abdomen should exclude a pyloric tumour where appropriate, or other abdominal masses and visceromegaly. On auscultation, increased bowel sounds may accompany infectious gastroenteritis and intestinal obstruction, while decreased sounds

suggest an ileus *(see Chapter 28, Surgical Problems)*.

Examine for signs of meningeal irritation and raised intracranial pressure. Persistent or paroxysmal coughing as seen in pertussis or some asthmatics may precipitate vomiting. Vomiting can be the presenting symptom in congestive cardiac failure. Bradycardia and hypertension are features

---

Table 11.1 Causes of vomiting in infancy and childhood

A. Vomiting in the first week of life

Common causes

- Gastric irritation:
  Ingestion of blood/mucus. idiopathic
- Feeding faults:
  Overfeeding/underfeeding

Less common causes

- Infections:
  Gastroenteritis, oral thrush, urinary tract infection (UTI), meningitis, septicaemia, necrotizing enterocolitis
- Raised intracranial pressure:
  Hydrocephalus, intracranial bleeding, kernicterus
- Intestinal malformation and obstruction:
  Hiatus hernia, intestinal atresia, malrotation, meconium ileus, volvulus, intestinal duplication, annular pancreas, Hirschsprung's disease
- Toxic and metabolic disorders:
  Cardiac failure, drugs (e.g., digoxin), inborn errors of metabolism

B. Vomiting in early infancy

Common causes

- Gastro-oesophageal reflux
- Feeding faults:
  Overfeeding/underfeeding
- Emotional deprivation
- Common infections:
  Upper respiratory tract infection, gastroenteritis, oral candidiasis

Less common causes

- Infections:
  UTI, meningitis, encephalitis, hepatitis, pertussis
- Intestinal malformation and obstructions:
  Hypertrophic pyloric stenosis, lactobezoar, malrotation, volvulus, intestinal duplications, Hirschsprung's disease
- Intracranial pathology:
  Hydrocephalus, kernicterus
- Toxic and metabolic disorders:
  Cardiac failure, drugs, uraemia, hypercalcaemia, inborn errors of metabolism

C. Vomiting in late infancy

Common causes

- Infections:
  Gastroenteritis, respiratory tract infection, UTI

Less common causes

- Infections:
  Meningitis, hepatitis, encephalitis, pertussis
- Intestinal malformation and obstruction:
  Intussusception, malrotation, gastro-oesophageal reflux
- Food intolerance:
  Cows' milk protein sensitivity, coeliac disease
- Toxic and metabolic disorders:
  Poisoning, drugs, uraemia, Reye's syndrome

D. Vomiting in childhood

Common causes

- Acute causes:
  Gastroenteritis, upper respiratory tract infection, food poisoning
- Acute dietary indiscretion

Less common causes

- Infection:
  UTI, meningitis, hepatitis, encephalitis
- Digestive tract disorders:
  Peptic ulcers, appendicitis, intussusception, malrotation, childhood Menetrier's disease, achalasia
- Toxic and metabolic disorders:
  Drugs, poisons, Reye's syndrome, uraemia, diabetes mellitus, hypercalcaemia
- Raised intracranial pressure:
  Hypertensive encephalopathy, tumours, hydrocephalus
- Psychogenic and other:
  Migraine, cyclic vomiting, bulimia

---

which should suggest the possibility of raised intracranial pressure.

Investigations

The common causes of vomiting in childhood *(see Table 11.1)* seldom need special investigations, but if necessary, these should be based on the most likely diagnosis as determined by the history and physical examination.

In exceptional cases the patient may require referral. The primary care professional should ensure that the patient is haemodynamically stable and breathing adequately prior to transfer *(see Chapter 28, Surgical Problems)*.

Gastro-oesophageal reflux
(Also see Chapter 28, Surgical Problems).

Definition

Gastro-oesophageal reflux (GOR) represents the retrograde flow of the gastric contents from the stomach into the oesophagus. During the neonatal period, reflux is regarded as a physiological phenomenon. GOR severe enough to cause problems and require treatment is estimated to occur in 1:300 to 1:1 000 children.

Ninety per cent of patients with problematical GOR present with symptoms before 6 weeks of age. The majority resolve spontaneously by 1–4 years of age, with the introduction of solid food and the assumption of the upright posture. Untreated, 10% will have complications such as failure to thrive, recurrent pneumonia, and peptic oesophagitis with oesophageal strictures.

Clinical presentation

The infant with GOR can present in any of the following ways:
♦ **Simple regurgitation of feeds:** In the vast majority of cases, infants with GOR will present with frequent regurgitation shortly after a milk feed as the only complaint. On examination there is no physical abnormality, and the infant generally shows satisfactory growth.
♦ **Overt regurgitation with failure to thrive:** This accounts for a small number of cases, and is more common in patients with GOR associated with cerebral palsy (Sandifer's syndrome). In these, the volume of feeds regurgitated is of such

magnitude that the patient retains insufficient calories for growth.
♦ **Regurgitation with respiratory symptoms:** GOR in these patients is associated with recurrent pneumonia, frequent attacks of wheezing, persistent coughing, and occasionally apnoeic spells. Pneumonia and coughing may be due to aspiration of milk into the trachea and lungs, and the apnoea may follow laryngo-spasm due to regurgitation of acid contents into the pharynx. In some cases aspiration occurs during the swallowing process and is due to pharyngeal inco-ordination, suggesting that the GOR is merely part of a more diffuse disturbance of motility. Recurrent wheezing associated with GOR is more controversial: in some, this is believed to be secondary to aspiration of milk, but in others it may be a vagus-nerve-mediated reflex bronchospasm that is triggered by acid reflux into an inflamed oesophagus. In these, vigorous treatment of the oesophagitis may abolish the wheezing episodes entirely.
♦ **Regurgitation with a complication of GOR:** Acid-induced oesophagitis may result in frank or occult bleeding and, if left untreated, can result in stricture formation *(see Chapter 28)*.

Diagnosis

In most cases a positive diagnosis of GOR can be made on the basis of history alone. If there are features suggestive of a complication, it is necessary to confirm the presence of reflux and investigate the associated problems. A thorough assessment and treatment plan is best performed at a referral centre with the following: Upper G.I. barium series, intra-oesophageal pH monitoring, radio-nuclear scintography, oesophagoscopy and biopsy.

Treatment

The majority of children who have benign GOR and continue to thrive need minimal symptomatic therapy. Often reassurance alone is sufficient. Additional therapeutic manoeuvres should be designed to minimize regurgitation while awaiting spontaneous resolution. These measures include changing the feeding pattern to provide small, frequent meals, thickening the formula feeds with cereals (Nestargel® or Infant Gaviscon®), nursing the infant prone, with the head of the crib slightly

Table 11.2   Conditions causing recurrent abdominal pain in childhood.

Common causes

Parasitic infestations	Ascaris, giardia
Chronic non-specific abdominal pain (CNAP) of childhood	
Faecal loading of the colon	

Less common causes

Infections	Abdominal TB, yersinia
Inflammatory	Peptic ulcer, oesophagitis, inflammatory bowel disease
Metabolic	Disaccharide intolerance
Renal	Pyelonephritis, hydronephrosis

Unusual causes

Obstructive	Malrotation, intussusception, biliary colic, renal stones, hernias
Inflammatory	Chronic pancreatitis
Metabolic	Diabetes, cystic fibrosis, coeliac disease, hyperlipidaemia
Gynaecological	Ovarian cyst, salpingitis
Miscellaneous	Lead poisoning, acute intermittent porphyria

elevated and, occasionally, administering prokinetic agents such as cisapride and metoclopramide.

Patients with complicated GOR require aggressive medical management. If this fails, surgery is indicated.

Recurrent abdominal pain
(Also see Chapter 28, Surgical Problems.)

Introduction
Abdominal pain is one of the most common complaints in childhood and adolescence.

The pain may be visceral or somatic in origin. Visceral pain is caused by distension of a hollow, muscular organ. It may be periumbilical, epigastric, or lower abdominal, and either colicky or a non-specific discomfort which is vague and poorly localized. Somatic pain originates from the skin, muscles, or parietal peritoneum. It is usually confined to a specific area, and is aggravated by palpation over that region. Occasionally, abdominal pain is referred from a lesion involving some other site such as the spine or peripheral nerve root.

Aetiology
There are numerous causes of recurrent abdominal pain in childhood. These can be broadly divided into common, less common, and unusual causes *(see Table 11.2)*.

Parasitic infestations
Ascaris infestation may cause abdominal pain either by obstruction of the intestine or by migration of a worm up the biliary tract *(see Chapter 28, Surgical Problems)*.

Pain due to giardiasis is usually described as a diffuse discomfort. It may be accompanied by anorexia, nausea, abdominal distension, and diarrhoea. These symptoms may fluctuate in severity, and even disappear completely for variable periods of time.

Chronic non-specific abdominal pain of childhood (CNAP)
This condition may also be referred to as functional abdominal pain, or the irritable bowel syndrome of childhood. It typically affects children between 5 and 14 years of age. There is a gradual onset of a vague, typically constant pain, located peri-umbilically or in the mid-epigastrium with minimal radiation, rather than colic. The pain is unrelated to meals, activity, or particular foods. It may occur in the evenings and delay onset of sleep, but does not awaken the patient at night.

Pain periods occur in clusters lasting from days to weeks, with pain-free periods varying from weeks to months. Episodes of pain may occur as often as several times a day or as little as once a week. The intensity of pain is variable; some episodes are severe enough to interfere with activity briefly, others cause the patient to double over and cry. Episodes last less than one hour in 50% of patients and less than three hours in a further 40%.

At least one of the following occurs in 50–70% of cases: headache, pallor, nausea, dizziness, tendency to fatigue, and low-grade fever.

The patients often have obsessive, compulsive personalities, and are driven to achieve. The family history is strongly positive for functional disorders, including spastic colon, irritable bowel syndrome, anxiety attacks, mental disorders, and migraine. These children are usually well-grown and appear healthy. Nail-biting, cold extremities, and dilated pupils are described but are not consistently present. The abdomen is not distended, and is soft to palpation. There is no guarding, and complaints of tenderness on deep palpation are often out of keeping with the physical findings. Apparent tenderness may disappear transiently if the child is distracted during palpation of the abdomen. Examination of the other systems is normal.

Diagnosis

Unnecessary investigations increase parental and the patient's fears of serious underlying disease, which further increase the stressful environment that provokes symptoms.

▶   Where the clinical features suggest CNAP, investigations must be kept to a minimum, viz., FBC, ESR, urine analysis, and stool analysis for parasites and occult blood.

Negative investigations, together with a suggestive history and examination, should lead to a firm diagnosis of CNAP.

Table 11.3   Features suggesting an organic cause for childhood abdominal pain

Age of onset: < 5 years or >14 years of age
Pain localization: Well away from region of umbilicus
Nocturnal pain: Particularly if it awakens patient
Food intake: Aggravates or relieves pain
Associated features: Fever, arthralgia, rash, jaundice
Loss of appetite: Particularly with documented weight loss
Alteration in bowel habit: Diarrhoea, constipation, frequency
Positive family history: Peptic ulcer, inflammatory bowel disease
Abdominal distension, mass, or visceromegaly
Faecal soiling
Anal skin tags
Occult blood-positive stools

Features that should alert the physician to the possibility of an organic disorder for the pain, are listed in *Table 11.3*. If any of these are present at the initial or subsequent examination, the diagnosis of CNAP should be considered and investigated.

Management

The management of the child with CNAP begins with a positive diagnosis of a functional disorder and an acknowledgement by the physician that the pain experienced by the patient is real. It is essential to reassure the patient and parents that no serious organic pathology exists. By accepting this, the patient is better able to cope with the symptoms in the future. Parents should combine sympathy with firmness, and discourage the child from using the symptoms to manipulate his/her environment.

Medications have very little place in the management of the child with CNAP. Symptoms in some patients have improved with dietary modification which includes more fibre. Conversely, too much fibre may cause increased gas production in the large bowel, which can aggravate pain. Finally, regular follow-up by the physician, with continued reassurance, serves to reinforce the belief that there is no serious organic pathology.

With firm reassurance by the physician, complete resolution of symptoms occurs in 30–50% of children within six weeks of presentation. The remainder continue to have symptoms, but with decreased frequency and severity. In the majority of these cases, symptoms resolve after some years, but recur in adulthood and become more consistent with the adult irritable bowel syndrome.

Faecal loading of the colon

The retention of large amounts of faeces in the rectum and colon may be more common than CNAP as a cause of recurrent abdominal pain in childhood. It follows repeated episodes of incomplete evacuation of the bowel. This may have been initiated by a period of voluntary stool withholding early in the child's life, when the urge to defecate was resisted. The causes of this are multiple, and include fear of pain on defecation due to anal fissures, rebellion against rigorous toilet training, refusal to use school toilet facilities, and disinclination to interrupt pleasurable activity.

The condition may be aggravated by a sedentary way of life, and poor eating habits with diets containing little natural fibre. There is progressive accumulation of stool until, in severe cases, the entire colon is filled with solid faecal matter. The pain — described as cramping followed by a dull ache — is believed to result from strong colonic contractions aimed at clearing the faeces, and usually occurs after a meal due to the gastro-colic reflex.

Presentation

On physical examination these children are well grown and appear healthy. The abdomen is usually flat and soft to palpation. Abdominal distension should alert the physician to the possibility of some underlying condition such as Hirschsprung's disease. There is often some tenderness to deep palpation in the mid-epigastrium, and not uncommonly over the region of the caecum and descending colon as well. Frequently faeces are palpable in the left iliac fossa over the region of the sigmoid colon. In advanced cases faeces might also be felt in the caecum. Faecal soiling is highly suggestive of faecal loading, as is the finding of an anal fissure or a large amount of faeces on rectal examination (*see Chapter 30, Behavioural and Psychological Disorders*). A straight X-ray of the abdomen in the supine position demonstrates a large amount of faecal matter throughout the colon.

Causes

Organic causes that should be considered include hypothyroidism, anorectal malformations, Hirschsprung's disease, neuronal intestinal dysplasia, and intestinal pseudo-obstruction syndromes. These are all relatively rare, and have abdominal distension with constipation rather than pain as the major presenting symptom.

Treatment

Continued therapy and regular follow-up are needed for many months. Anal fissure should be treated with applications of anaesthetic creams to the anal verge. Thereafter treatment is designed to clear the entire colon and then prevent re-accumulation of stool.

Initial clearance is best achieved with oral administration of large volumes of a balanced electrolyte/polyethylene glycol solution if available, and bowel wash-outs or repeated Fleet® or Microlax® enemas three times a day for 3 days. Clearance can be checked clinically, and if necessary confirmed with repeat abdominal X-rays.

Preventing the re-accumulation of stool involves three steps:

◆ Dietary modification to increase the intake of foods rich in natural fibre (bran, fruits, and vegetables), or supplementary fibre.

◆ Daily evacuation of stool by means of a regular toilet regimen. These children frequently do not sense the need to defecate and it takes time for normal rectal sensation to return.

◆ Medication to aid defecation.

Initially stool lubricants (mineral oil) and stool softeners (Duphalac®) are necessary to help establish regular bowel habits. Occasionally in difficult cases there is a need for stimulant laxatives (Senokot® and Dulcolax®) as well. These should not be continued for more than 6 – 8 weeks, as they might cause permanent damage to the myenteric plexus and smooth muscle atrophy in the colon.

Regular follow-up to ensure compliance and monitor progress is recommended.

Other causes of recurrent abdominal pain (RAP) in childhood

Occasionally, other causes of RAP (listed in *Table 11.2*) have to be differentiated from CNAP and faecal loading of the colon. The following is a brief outline of features which may help to identify these disorders.

Primary peptic ulcer disease (PUD)

The incidence of this condition is not known, but with greater use of endoscopy in childhood it is being increasingly diagnosed. Children over 8 years of age are more likely to complain of pain with PUD. Prior to this age, many children with ulcers first present with a complication such as bleeding or perforation. Pain is typically intermittent, and localized to the epigastrium in about 50% of cases. In others, it is described as periumbilical or diffuse. Pain which wakes the patient at night, or is present on rising in the morning, is highly suggestive of PUD. Symptoms may be related to meals and may be relieved by vomiting or antacid ingestion. A positive family history of PUD, particularly if in a first-degree relative, is an important diagnostic clue. Examination of the abdomen often reveals marked tenderness to deep palpation in the epigastrium. Anaemia and occult blood-positive stools are supportive findings. If the history and physical examination suggest PUD, the patient should be referred for further evaluation.

Inflammatory bowel disease (IBD)

Ulcerative colitis, Crohn's colitis, and the various other microscopic colitis syndromes have pain localized typically to the lower abdomen. The pain is usually maximal prior to defecation and is relieved by the passage of a stool. Colitis is frequently associated with a bloody, mucoid diarrhoea. Small intestinal Crohn's disease can have pain localized to the right iliac fossa or the periumbilical region. IBD is commonly associated with systemic manifestations such as anorexia, weight loss, fever, lethargy, joint pains, or a rash. Examination may reveal a palpable mass in the region of the terminal ileum in Crohn's disease. Other noteworthy findings are anaemia and a raised ESR.

Disaccharide intolerance

Abdominal pain due to disaccharide intolerance is most commonly secondary to dietary lactose malabsorption. Pain in these patients is often accompanied by abdominal bloating, flatulence, and diarrhoea. The stools may test positive for reducing substances. The diagnosis can be confirmed simply by eliminating the offending disaccharide from the diet with prompt and complete resolution of all symptoms.

Intestinal obstruction

See Chapter 28, Surgical Problems.

Metabolic causes

Abdominal pain may be a prominent feature of diabetic ketoacidosis. This is usually accompanied by features of polyuria, polydipsia, vomiting, and dehydration, with a fruity odour to the breath *(see Chapter 20, Endocrine and Metabolic Disorders).*

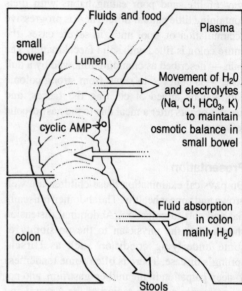

NORMAL STATE

Fig. 11.1 Movement of water and electrolytes through and from the gut. Normal state

Diarrhoea

Diarrhoea is one of the most common symptoms of children. It may be due to enteral or parenteral infections, inherited or acquired disorders of digestion and absorption, motility disturbances, and self-administered substances such as enemas or laxatives.

Pathophysiology

Under normal circumstances a large amount of fluid enters the upper small bowel daily. Some is from ingestion, but the majority is from secretions by salivary glands, stomach, pancreas, and small intestine. The small bowel is normally highly efficient, and reabsorbs about 90% of this fluid. A further 8–9% is reabsorbed by the colon, which in health can reabsorb three times this amount *(see Fig. 11.1).*

Diarrhoea results when the amount of fluid in the colon exceeds its absorptive capacity. This may be due to the following mechanisms:

Colonic absorption normal

When colonic absorption is normal but the volume of the fluid entering it is excessive, possible causes include:

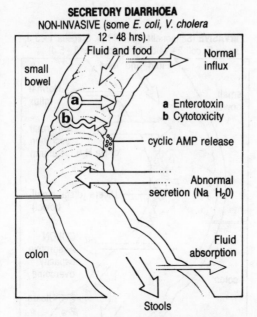

Fig. 11.2 *Movement of water and electrolytes through and from the gut in secretory diarrhoea*

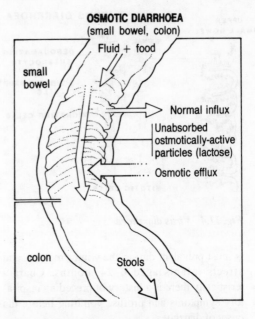

Fig. 11.3 *Movement of water and electrolytes through and from the gut in osmotic diarrhoea*

◆ toxin-induced secretory diarrhoea, e.g., cholera *(see Fig. 11.2)*

◆ osmotic diarrhoea, e.g., lactose intolerance *(see Fig. 11.3)*

◆ small intestinal mucosal damage with secretion-absorption disequilibrium, e.g., virus diarrhoea *(see Fig. 11.4)*

◆ motility disturbance with intestinal hurry.

Colonic absorption impaired

When colonic absorption is impaired, it is usually as a result of inflammatory colitis, e.g., shigella, *Entamoeba histolytica (see Fig. 11.5).*

Acute infective diarrhoea

Acute diarrhoea is one of the leading causes of childhood mortality in developing countries. It is primarily a disease of poverty. Overcrowding, and poor sanitation and waste disposal lead to a heavily contaminated environment. Lack of hygiene and an unsafe and insufficient water supply results in faecal-oral spread of infection. Susceptibility to the disease is further increased by early weaning from exclusive breast-feeding and by malnutrition.

Aetiology

It is possible to identify a recognized stool pathogen in about 70% of cases of acute diarrhoea. A large number of viruses, bacteria, parasites, and fungi have been implicated as causes of diarrhoea *(see Table 11.4).*

In developed countries, human rotavirus (HRV) is the most common cause of acute diarrhoea. This

Table 11.4   Pathogens causing acute diarrhoea in childhood

A	Viruses	Human rotavirus, enteric adenovirus, norwalk-like viruses, astrovirus, calicivirus, coronavirus, small round viruses
B	Bacteria	*Escherichia coli, Vibrio cholerae,* salmonella, shigella, campylobacter, *Clostridium difficile,* yersinia, pseudomonas, klebsiella, staphylococcus
C	Parasites	Protozoa: Giardia, cryptosporidium, *Entamoeba histolytica, Balantidium coli*
		Helminths: Schistosoma, trichuris, strongyloides, trichinella, trematodes

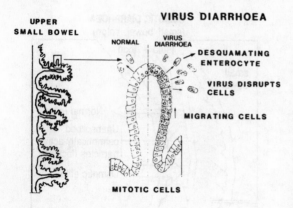

Fig. 11.4   Virus diarrhoea

is most prevalent during the winter months, and affects infants aged 6–24 months. Characteristically there is a history of preceding respiratory symptoms and profuse vomiting before the onset of diarrhoea.

In developing countries, diarrhoea peaks in summer. This is presumably due to climatic factors leading to a greater bacterial contamination of the environment. Bacteria are frequently isolated — at times multiple pathogens from the stool of a single patient. It commonly affects infants under six months of age. An abrupt onset of diarrhoea with prominent neurological symptoms, a high fever, and no vomiting is seen in shigella enteritis, in which the stools are often blood-stained.

Pathogenesis
HRV invades the mature intestinal mucosal cells at the tips of the villi. This results in rapid shedding of these cells, to be replaced by less mature cells migrating up from the crypts *(see Fig.11.4)*. These not only have lower disaccharidase activity for carbohydrate digestion, but are also less efficient in absorbing fluids and electrolytes. Other viruses probably exert their effect in much the same way.

Bacteria produce diarrhoea in many ways. Some adhere to the mucosal cell and produce an enterotoxin which stimulates the secretion of large amounts of fluid and electrolytes *(see Fig. 11.2)*, (e.g., *Vibrio cholerae* and toxigenic *E. coli*). Others invade the mucosal cell directly *(see Fig. 11.5)*, e.g., shigella, campylobacter, entero-invasive *E. coli*; yet others produce a cytotoxin, e.g., entero-haemorrhagic *E. coli*. The mucosal damage in

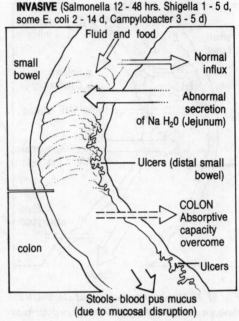

Fig. 11.5   Invasive enteropathogens with incubation periods

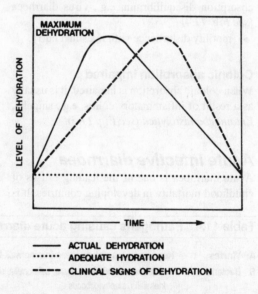

Fig. 11.6   Gastroenteritis. Slow development of signs of dehydration

these cases results in a decreased absorptive surface, and the secondary inflammatory response causes increased secretion of fluid into the gut lumen.

Effects of diarrhoea

These are the same in all cases, irrespective of the pathogenesis. In the acute case, the disease results in loss of water and electrolytes from the body. This leads to dehydration and electrolyte disturbance. In addition, dysfunction of the gut causes impaired digestion and absorption of nutrients, and therefore diarrhoea has an effect on the nutritional state of the patient.

Dehydration

The stool water in diarrhoea is primarily derived from the circulation and secreted by the intestinal mucosa. Thereafter adaptive fluid shifts occur. These cause the symptoms and signs of dehydration, which always lag behind the real fluid loss. In fulminant secretory diarrhoea such as cholera, it is thus possible for the patient to be clinically shocked before signs of dehydration are evident *(see Fig. 11.6)*. The clinical features of dehydration are listed in *Table 11.5*.

The volume of water lost cannot be estimated confidently by assessing the signs of dehydration, as the sequence and severity of signs may vary from patient to patient. In particular, the skin tissue turgor is influenced by factors besides dehydration. It is assessed by lifting a fold of skin on the anterior abdominal wall between thumb and forefinger. On releasing the fold, a delayed return of the skin signifies a decreased tissue turgor. In severely wasted children, the turgor may be decreased even though there is no dehydration. Conversely, obese or oedematous patients may not show a decrease in tissue turgor despite being dehydrated. In hypernatraemic dehydration the skin turgor is similarly maintained, making the assessment of dehydration more difficult.

Dehydration is dangerous if it leads to **circulatory failure** which kills the patient, or which may be followed by complications such as acute renal failure, cerebral complications including hypoxic ischaemia or cerebral vascular thrombosis, necrotizing enterocolitis, and shock lung.

Accordingly, the most important assessment in any case of dehydrating diarrhoea is that of the state of circulation. Shock may be either compensated or uncompensated. In the early stage the

Table 11.5   Degrees of dehydration: clinical features and management

	Potential dehydration I	Dehydration II	Circulatory failure (shock) III
Sequence of symptoms	Thirst	Irritability	Apathy
Signs	Decreased secretions (urine, saliva, sweat, tears) Dry mouth Sunken eyes Decreased skin turgor Sunken fontanelle Acidotic breathing Peripheral vasoconstriction Tachycardia Altered level of consciousness Hypotension Coma and convulsions		
Management principles	Maintain hydration Continue feeds	Rehydration	Resuscitation

body is still able to maintain a normal blood pressure and perfusion of the vital organs by peripheral vasoconstriction under the influence of catecholamines. Clinically these patients appear weak and apathetic, and may have a decreased level of consciousness. There is tachycardia, the skin may appear mottled, and the extremities feel cool to touch. The capillary filling time is prolonged to more than four seconds. In the phase of uncompensated shock, the patient will also have a low blood pressure, manifest clinically as impalpable peripheral pulses.

Biochemical disturbances

These are very common, and occur as a result of direct losses and adaptive responses. The principal electrolytes lost are sodium, potassium, chloride, and bicarbonate.

Sodium disturbances should be suspected when CNS features such as drowsiness or apathy, irritability with a high-pitched cry, jitteriness, and convulsions are worse than expected on the basis of the patient's state of dehydration.

Hyponatraemia: A serum sodium below 130 mmol/l is more common in malnourished patients, but is also seen in cases of severe secretory diarrhoea. A sodium level below 120 mmol/l should be corrected with a fluid containing a higher sodium content than half-strength Darrow's solution, especially if it occurs in a patient with large fluid losses.

Hypernatraemia: A serum sodium level above 150 mmol/l may be suspected if the patient has severe acidosis out of keeping with the degree of clinical dehydration. (Salicylate toxicity can cause similar clinical features.) It is more common in well-nourished or obese infants, often under six months of age, but can also be seen in malnourished patients when there has been inadequate fluid replacement of some days' duration. In treatment, a rapid decline in serum sodium can result in cerebral oedema with raised intracranial pressure and convulsions, and should be avoided.

Hypokalaemia: A serum potassium below 3.5 mmol/l is frequently seen in diarrhoea. Even when the serum potassium concentration is normal, malnourished patients often have depletion of the total body potassium. Severe hypokalaemia causes an ileus, hypotonicity, and, rarely, bradycardia or other arrhythmias. In older children, a characteristic feature is an inability to hold up the head.

Hyperkalaemia is less commonly encountered, but is life-threatening in patients who remain anuric despite rehydration. Additionally, acidosis causes a transfer of intracellular potassium to the extracellular space, causing the serum level to be spuriously normal or elevated. When a potassium level above 6.5 mmol/l is associated with characteristic ECG changes (peaked T waves, flattened P waves, prolongation of the P-R interval and progressive widening of the QRS complex), this should be considered an emergency for active management.

Metabolic acidosis is invariably present in dehydrated patients with diarrhoea due to loss of base in the stools, increased reabsorption of hydrogen ion in the gut, poor tissue perfusion, starvation, and decreased renal hydrogen clearance. Active management is required only in profound acidosis, or when the patient is in shock.

Blood sugar disturbances are frequently observed. *Hypoglycaemia* is seen in malnourished, septicaemic, hypothermic infants, as well as in those who have been starved for some time. Some patients develop hypoglycaemia as a consequence of hepatic insults such as Reye's syndrome or toxic herbal medication.

Hyperglycaemia is usually due to stress-related catecholamine release. It is often associated with hypernatraemia. The differentiation from diabetes mellitus is made by the presence of severe ketoacidosis and polyuria in the latter condition. With correction of dehydration and electrolyte disturbance, the blood sugar returns to normal and insulin is usually not required.

Uraemia is usually due to prerenal factors, but may accompany intrinsic acute renal failure in severe dehydration with shock. In such cases the serum creatinine is elevated. A urine specimen should be tested for the presence of cells, casts, and protein.

Diarrhoea can also lead to depletion of **calcium, magnesium, and zinc**, particularly if it is prolonged.

Convulsions

These are relatively common in patients with diarrhoea, and may be due to cerebral venous thrombosis, fever, metabolic encephalopathy, meningitis, and encephalitis, as well as cerebral oedema secondary to rapid intravenous infusion of hypotonic fluid. An attempt must be made to find a cause before assuming that the convulsion is due to dehydration. Where convulsions are associated with hypernatraemia and occur before the start of treatment, this may indicate cerebral infarction and irreversible neurological damage.

Protein-losing enteropathy

The altered mucosal permeability of acute infection is associated with intestinal protein loss, occasionally severe enough to result in hypoproteinaemia with oedema. Such patients may be misdiagnosed as suffering from kwashiorkor, but do not have other features of malnutrition, and are often under six months of age. The hallmark of the condition is a panhypoproteinaemia, with both albumin and globulin being reduced.

Ileus and necrotizing entercolitis (NEC)

Abdominal distension may be due to gut dilatation occurring with hypokalaemia, septicaemia, or toxaemia, but may also be due to anatomical obstruction such as intussusception or volvulus. The distinction is sometimes difficult, and requires X-ray of the abdomen and investigation of electrolyte and coagulation status as well as bacterial cultures. NEC is a rare complication, sometimes seen in shocked, malnourished babies, especially if feeds were continued in the face of severe dehydration and shock. The patients are clinically septicaemic and have acute abdominal distension, with blood in the stools. X-rays show bowel wall thickening with intramural gas (pneumatosis intestinalis), or even gas in the portal venous system. Perforation and free peritonitis may occur. The mortality rate is high *(see Chapter 28, Surgical Problems).*

Diagnosis

The history must include information about the onset and severity of the diarrhoea and any associated symptoms. One should enquire about any home management, including the type and quantity of oral fluids and feeds, and prescribed or traditional medications. An attempt should be made to identify any predisposing factors amenable to intervention.

The assessment of the case must focus on the possible causative agent and the presence of any complications.

Early vomiting is a feature of small intestinal disease, frequently virus-induced, and also of food poisoning. The stools in virus and enterotoxin diarrhoea are often very watery. Dysenteric stools with blood and mucus are seen with bacterial infection of the large gut, such as *shigella* and with amoebiasis. Older children also often complain of cramp-like abdominal pain. Mild abdominal distension and tenderness are frequently found.

Management
See Table 11.5.

The main aim of management in the early stage is to *prevent* dehydration and to continue feeds in such a way as to allow maximal digestion and absorption of nutrients.

Preventing dehydration
(See Fig. 11.7.)

Water absorption is a passive process, following the movement of solute — especially sodium — across the mucosa. Sodium uptake is stimulated by the presence of glucose and certain amino acids in the luminal fluid. This process is energy-dependent and can work against a concentration gradient. The absorptive capacity of the gut is such that maintenance of hydration by mouth is possible even in the face of large losses, provided the fluid given contains glucose at a concentration of approximately 2–2.5% (or 4–5% in the case of sucrose) in addition to sodium.

The amount of fluid lost in each vomit or stool is the additional amount that the child should get, preferably before the next feed. This usually amounts to approximately 15–30 ml/kg per stool passed.

A successful home-made solution consists of

  8 level teaspoons cane sugar

  ½ level teaspoon salt

  1 litre clean or boiled water.

However, the type of fluid is not critical in the early stage, and any available clear fluid can be used. It is important to give this fluid in small doses, to avoid gastric distension and vomiting. Babies frequently become thirsty because of early dehydration and may drink too much too fast, resulting in vomiting.

Continuing feeds

Maintaining nutrient intake is important for recovery, especially if the child is already nutritionally compromised at the onset of diarrhoea. It is not necessary to change the milk feed at this stage; but in the case of solids, select those items of the usual diet which are easily digestible, bland, and soft, such as starchy porridge or mashed banana. Give small quantities at a time, as frequently as tolerated, and aim to restore the normal intake by the second or third day.

Oral rehydration

The dehydrated patient requires fluid for the replacement of the deficit, for continuing stool losses, and for normal maintenance.

Most patients are successfully rehydrated by the oral route, but the following circumstances indicate the need for intravenous fluids:

♦ peripheral circulatory failure
♦ severe acidosis with vasoconstriction
♦ encephalopathy
♦ significant abdominal distension: ileus or obstruction
♦ deterioration or lack of improvement after adequate oral fluids for 2–4 hours
♦ persistent severe vomiting after 2–4 hours adequate oral fluids.

See Table 11.5.

Once dehydrated, the patient has sustained significant losses of base and potassium. The oral rehydration solution (ORS) should therefore contain potassium and base in addition to sodium and glucose. The World Health Organization (WHO) has recommended an ORS with a sodium content of 90 mmol/l. This is particularly appropriate for patients with secretory diarrhoea such as cholera, but for most patients, a sodium content of approximately 60 mmol/l (equivalent to the concentration in half-strength Darrow's solution) is adequate *(see Table 11.6).*

ORS is offered in small, frequent quantities, e.g., by teaspoon. The aim is to give as much as the child wants, guided by his thirst, offering about 15–30 ml/kg per hour, until he is stronger and more alert, passing urine, and showing signs of wanting food again. At this stage, the patient can be offered a small feed, and thereafter needs ORS only for additional stool losses, as described above.

The majority of dehydrated patients will respond to this regime and do not require further investigations.

Vomiting is not a contraindication to oral rehydration. It is due to impaired gastric emptying, and often also to starvation ketosis, and usually settles within a few hours provided care is taken to avoid gastric distension (by administering small quantities of rehydration solution frequently).

Resuscitation

Shock is a medical emergency and is an absolute indication for intravenous (IV) fluids. If an IV line cannot be established quickly, a needle may be inserted under strict aseptic precautions into the

---

Table 11.6 Composition of the SAPA* and WHO recommended ORS formulas, and half-strength Darrow's solution

Ingredient	SAPA-ORS	Formula WHO-ORS	$^1/_2$ strength Darrow's
Sodium (mmol/l)	64	90	61
Potassium (mmol/l)	20	20	17
Chloride (mmol/l)	54	80	51
Bicarbonate (mmol/l)**	30	30	27
Glucose	2%	2%	5%

* South African Paediatric Association

** Lactate is being used in place of bicarbonate in half-strength Darrow's solution. Citrate is replacing bicarbonate in ORS powder mixtures, as it increases the shelf-life and is equally effective as a base.

antero-medial aspect of the tibia for intraosseous infusion. The fluid chosen to treat shock should contain a sodium content similar to normal plasma, such as Ringer's, Haemacell®, normal saline solution, or even stabilized human serum or plasma. Initially, 20 ml/kg is infused as rapidly as possible. Sodium bicarbonate, 2 mmol/kg, is administered as a slow IV bolus because of the associated severe metabolic acidosis. After this initial resuscitation, the patient should be reassessed, and if the circulation has not improved, a further 10 ml/kg of the initial fluid may be given rapidly. If the patient remains in shock thereafter, cardiogenic or vasogenic causes of shock must be considered. At that stage, a central venous pressure reading should be obtained, to decide on the need for inotropic support or further fluid requirement.

Once shock is corrected, the rate of IV fluid administration is adjusted to 10 ml/kg/hour. At this stage a blood sample is taken for estimation of electrolytes, and urea and blood gas analysis. The patient must be reassessed within 4 hours to determine urine output, the rate of ongoing stool losses, and the adequacy of the fluid rate. The fluid can usually be changed to half-strength Darrow's solution at this stage, before oral fluids are reintroduced.

In patients who require **intravenous fluids for reasons other than shock**, half-strength Darrow's can be chosen from the onset, at a rate of 10–15 ml/kg/hour. Early assessment is indicated within 4–6 hours to confirm improvement in the clinical state.

Metabolic management includes the administration of potassium chloride, 3 mmol/kg/day, to all patients who require rehydration. Potassium-containing ORS supplies the normal maintenance requirement if given at a rate of 100 ml/kg/day, but does not provide for the correction of deficits. In patients with hypokalaemia, the oral dose of potassium can safely be doubled, provided the patient is passing urine normally.

Patients on IV fluids for more than 24 hours need calcium and magnesium supplementation also.

Drug therapy is the least important aspect of acute diarrhoea management.

Antibiotics are not required in the majority of cases of acute diarrhoea in children. However, they are indicated for those with blood and mucus in their stools; those who are thought to be septicaemic on clinical grounds; and those who are immunocompromised because of very young age, low birth weight, severe malnutrition, or HIV infection.

Antidiarrhoeal medications have no real place in the management of most cases of acute diarrhoea. Adsorbents such as kaolin hide the true extent of water loss, and thus remove the most important guide to the need for additional fluids. Antisecretory drugs such as loperamide have a small place only, as the majority of cases of diarrhoea (such as those due to rotavirus) have a mixed osmotic and secretory component, and do not respond.

Antiemetics are not indicated, as the vomiting is due to local factors in the gut or starvation ketosis, and responds well to simple measures of fluid therapy. The usual antiemetic drugs also have significant side-effects.

Outcome

In well-nourished children, acute diarrhoea is a self-limiting condition of 3–5 days' duration in the vast majority of instances. Provided adequate fluids are given and judicious nourishment is carried out, complications and deaths are rare. In a small proportion of cases, the mucosal insult is severe and the diarrhoea does not settle, becoming persistent or chronic.

In malnourished children, acute infective diarrhoea is a much more serious disease. These patients recover more slowly; recurrent attacks are more likely, and are associated with a further decline in the nutritional state. Associated infections such as pneumonia are common. Such patients have a high mortality rate.

Prevention

In practical reality, the essential public health measures of housing, water supply and sanitation, waste disposal, and environmental control will not be available to a large proportion of impoverished people in the foreseeable future. Similarly, hygienic standards are difficult to achieve in the face of shack-living and overcrowding.

In the interim, it is still possible to lower the incidence of diarrhoea significantly by an increased emphasis on the following aspects of the GOBI FFF policy advocated by the WHO:

◆ exclusive breast-feeding for at least 4 months

◆ early identification of, and nutritional intervention for, malnutrition

◆ immunization, especially against measles, which is frequently complicated by diarrhoea

◆ maternal education to promote an understanding of hygiene and optimal use of available resources.

(Also see Chapter 4, Community Paediatrics.)

Chronic diarrhoea

Chronic diarrhoea is usually defined as the passage of abnormal, unformed stools for 14 days or more.

Aetiology of chronic diarrhoea

Numerous conditions have been implicated as causes of chronic diarrhoea in infants and young children *(see Table 11.7)*. It is useful to categorize the patients with chronic diarrhoea into one of three broad groups as follows:

a. with failure to thrive plus excessive stool water losses

b. with failure to thrive, but without excessive stool water losses

c. without failure to thrive.

The term 'malabsorption' applies to a wide variety of disorders of small intestinal function, in which one or more constituents of the diet are inadequately absorbed. This leads to abnormally loose or frequent stools in the majority of cases. Patients with chronic diarrhoea and failure to thrive can therefore be considered to have malabsorption.

A: Patients with chronic diarrhoea and failure to thrive plus excessive stool water losses

This group includes most cases of chronic diarrhoea in infants and young children in developing countries. It accounts for about 10% of patients who require admission for treatment of acute dehydrating diarrhoea. What is more, over half of all deaths due to diarrhoeal disease occur within this group.

Table 11.7 Disorders associated with chronic diarrhoea in childhood

Mucosal damage	Anatomical abnormalities
Infections (viral, bacterial)	Short bowel syndromes
'Post-enteritis enteropathy'	Intestinal lymphangiectasia
Malnutrition	Congenital crypt hypoplasia
Bacterial overgrowth	Malrotation
Coeliac disease	
Protein-sensitive enteropathy	**Enzyme deficiencies**
Eosinophilic gastroenteropathy	Secondary disaccharidase deficiencies
Hirschsprung's disease	Adult-type lactase deficiency
Immunodeficiency syndromes	Congenital disaccharidase deficiency
Dermatitis herpetiformis	Enterokinase deficiency
Secretory disorders	**Metabolic abnormalities**
Congenital chloridorrhoea	Acrodermatitis enteropathica
VIP-oma	Abetalipoproteinaemia
Zollinger-Ellison syndrome	Wolman's disease
Systemic mastocytosis	Hypoparathyroidism
Carcinoid tumours	Hyperparathyroidism
	Pancreatic insufficiency
	Cystic fibrosis
	Schwachman-Diamond syndrome
	Congenital lipase deficiency

It is associated with failure to gain weight, or progressive loss of lean body mass. In addition, stool water losses are of such severity that the child will become dehydrated unless additional fluids are provided over and above the normal daily maintenance requirements.

Pathogenesis *(See Fig. 11.8)*: The central problem in these patients is prolonged small intestinal mucosal injury with ineffective villus repair. The sequence of events leading up to this state is

incompletely understood. The onset of the disease is initially indistinguishable from other episodes of acute infective gastroenteritis. However, unlike the majority — in whom the disease is an acute self-limiting illness — in these patients the abnormal watery stools persist.

By the time the disease is fully established it is usually no longer possible to identify a specific bacterial or viral agent. One of the factors implicated is non-specific small intestinal bacterial

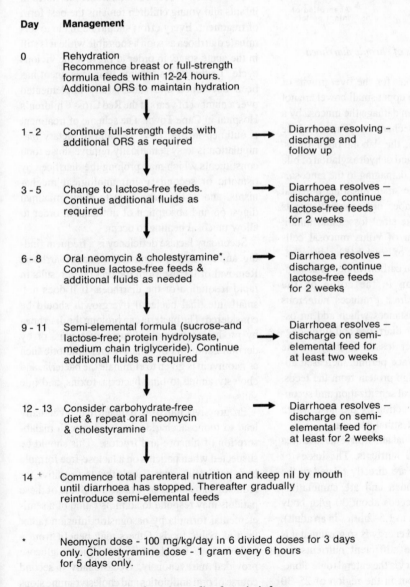

Day	Management	
0	Rehydration. Recommence breast or full-strength formula feeds within 12-24 hours. Additional ORS to maintain hydration	
1 - 2	Continue full-strength feeds with additional ORS as required	Diarrhoea resolving – discharge and follow up
3 - 5	Change to lactose-free feeds. Continue additional fluids as required	Diarrhoea resolves — discharge, continue lactose-free feeds for 2 weeks
6 - 8	Oral neomycin & cholestyramine*. Continue lactose-free feeds & additional fluids as needed	Diarrhoea resolves – discharge, continue lactose-free feeds for 2 weeks
9 - 11	Semi-elemental formula (sucrose-and lactose-free; protein hydrolysate, medium chain triglyceride). Continue additional fluids as required	Diarrhoea resolves – discharge on semi-elemental feed for at least two weeks
12 - 13	Consider carbohydrate-free diet & repeat oral neomycin & cholestyramine	Diarrhoea resolves – discharge on semi-elemental feed for at least for 2 weeks
14 +	Commence total parenteral nutrition and keep nil by mouth until diarrhoea has stopped. Thereafter gradually reintroduce semi-elemental feeds	

* Neomycin dose - 100 mg/kg/day in 6 divided doses for 3 days only. Cholestyramine dose - 1 gram every 6 hours for 5 days only.

Fig. 11.7 Management of persistent diarrhoea in infants

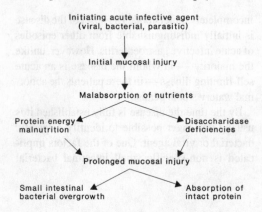

Fig. 11.8 Pathogenesis of chronic diarrhoea

overgrowth. The reasons for the overgrowth of micro-organisms in the upper small bowel are not known. The bacteria can damage the mucosa by a number of possible mechanisms. These include direct mucosal invasion, the elaboration of toxins, and the deconjugation and dehydroxylation of bile salts, which are in turn damaging to the mucosa.

Once established, the small intestinal mucosal damage causes a number of secondary events which further aggravate stool losses and inhibit repair. The destruction of villus mucosal cells causes progressive loss of brush border disaccharidases, which results in carbohydrate malabsorption. Bacterial action in the colon on the malabsorbed carbohydrate produces numerous osmotically-active substances which add an osmotic component to the diarrhoea and further aggravate the stool water losses. Damage to the intestinal mucosal surface permits increased absorption of intact foreign protein from the feeds. This in turn leads to local sensitization and secondary immunological reaction by the host, which further damages the intestinal mucosa.

The decreased intestinal absorptive surface area affects retention of all nutrients. The losses of nutrients in the stools are directly related to the severity of the diarrhoea and are cumulative. When stool output exceeds about 30 g/kg body weight/day (equivalent to 1.5–2 litres in an adult), the loss of nitrogen and energy is so great that it is impossible to provide sufficient nutrients for growth and tissue repair via the enteral route alone. Clinically a stool output in the region of 25–30 g/kg/day represents a level above which dehydra-

tion will occur unless additional fluids over and above maintenance requirements are provided.

Eventually a vicious cycle develops, in which diarrhoea causes progressive malnutrition which further aggravates the diarrhoea. The condition has been described as a post-enteritis enteropathy. Treatment of patients at this stage can be extremely difficult, and may require prolonged hospitalization. It is best carried out in a centre which has experience in dealing with such problems.

Treatment: Prevention of chronic diarrhoea in infants and young children remains the best form of treatment. Every effort should be made to terminate diarrhoea as soon as possible while it is still in the acute stage, in order to prevent the vicious cycle. To this end a scheme of management has been developed and successfully implemented over a number of years at the Red Cross Children's Hospital in Cape Town. The scheme of treatment is outlined in *Fig. 11.7*. The aim of dietary manipulation is to systematically remove those food constituents which may prolong the diarrhoea by osmotic or secondary immunological mechanisms, and at the same time to allow maximal digestion and absorption of nutrients in order to allow mucosal healing to occur.

Secondary lactase deficiency is a frequent finding, and can cause a significant osmotic diarrhoea. Removal of lactose from the diet often results in rapid resolution of the diarrhoea. If it does not, small intestinal bacterial overgrowth should be considered. The bacteria can prolong the diarrhoea by producing mucosal damage or toxins, or by deconjugation of bile salts. An oral antibiotic such as neomycin is given to eliminate the bacteria, and cholestyramine to bind bacteria, toxins, and bile salts.

Progressive mucosal damage can eventually lead to monosaccharide intolerance with malabsorption of glucose and fructose. This should be suspected when patients on a lactose-free formula have persistent watery stools that test positive for reducing substances on Clinitest®. Some of these patients may respond to administration of a semi-elemental formula by nasogastric infusion rather than as bolus foods. Others may benefit from a carbohydrate-free feed with additional glucose provided intravenously. Occasionally a second course of oral antibiotics and cholestyramine stops the diarrhoea.

Ultimately, cumulative losses of nitrogen and energy result in significant deterioration of nutritional status, so it is appropriate therapy to consider total parenteral nutrition for cases where diarrhoea persists for more than two weeks. If, however, the diarrhoea resolves following a diet change, the patient should not be discharged home to his usual diet without instructions for appropriate feeding. This should be done only when a satisfactory weight gain has been demonstrated.

B: Patients with chronic diarrhoea and failure to thrive, but without excessive stool water losses

Diarrhoea in these cases may be associated with either very poor weight gain or progressive weight loss, but stool water losses are not severe enough to cause dehydration. In the majority this is due to a malabsorption of dietary fats or carbohydrates.

Fat malabsorption: Malabsorption of dietary fats should be suspected from the history and physical findings. Typically the stools are described as loose, bulky, pale, greasy, and very offensive-smelling. Frank oil may be seen surrounding the faeces. Examination of the child reveals decreased subcutaneous tissue and muscle wasting, best demonstrated over the buttocks, thighs and arms. The abdomen is usually distended and there may be hepatomegaly.

Fat malabsorption may be due either to intraluminal factors affecting digestion, or to factors affecting uptake across the mucosa and subsequent transport in the lymphatics. Intraluminal digestion is largely dependent on delivery of adequate exocrine pancreatic enzymes and bile salts. In white populations, cystic fibrosis is by far the most common cause of exocrine pancreatic insufficiency in childhood. Deficiency of bile salts is most commonly associated with chronic liver disease. World-wide, coeliac disease is the most common cause of a mucosal abnormality causing fat malabsorption in children. In disadvantaged communities, other conditions which should be considered are heavy infestation with *Giardia lamblia*, and abdominal tuberculosis, which can cause obstruction to lymphatic flow from the gut.

Carbohydrate malabsorption: Congenital disaccharidase deficiencies are extremely rare. The acquired forms are most commonly secondary to mucosal injury following an acute infectious insult *(described in A, above)*. Carbohydrate malabsorption may be suspected from the description of the stools, which characteristically are watery and expelled forcefully, together with a lot of gas. The older child may describe abdominal cramps which are relieved by the passage of a stool, while the young infant may be irritable and cry a lot just prior to stooling. The stools are acidic and may cause severe excoriation of the patient's buttocks. The diagnosis is confirmed by demonstrating a stool pH less than 4, positive reducing substances in the faecal water, and an abnormal breath hydrogen test following ingestion of the specific dietary sugar. Where facilities for doing these tests are unavailable, a therapeutic trial of removing the carbohydrate from the diet should be instituted. If carbohydrate malabsorption is causing the symptoms, there will be an abrupt resolution following removal of the offending sugar from the diet.

Treatment involves dietary modification to completely exclude the specific sugar. If the disaccharidase deficiency is secondary to a previous infectious insult, it may be possible to reintroduce the sugar into the diet at a later stage without recurrence of symptoms.

C: Patients with chronic diarrhoea, but without failure to thrive

Despite the description of frequent loose or liquid stools, these patients remain otherwise healthy and continue to show satisfactory weight gain and growth. In the infant or young child, this is most frequently due to the entity variously known as chronic non-specific diarrhoea, toddler's diarrhoea, irritable bowel syndrome of childhood, or functional diarrhoea. The characteristic features of this condition are as follows:

♦ The diarrhoea first starts after 6 months of age and usually resolves spontaneously by 4 years.

♦ Diarrhoea is intermittent, with variable periods of relatively well-formed stools.

♦ The stool water losses are never severe enough to cause dehydration.

♦ The stools are passed only during the day when the child is awake, and never at night.

♦ The first stool of the day tends to be large and relatively well-formed. Thereafter the stools become smaller in volume but more liquid in consistency.

◆ Stools may contain some mucus and frequently have recognizable undigested food particles.

◆ There is often a positive family history of bowel disturbance, such as spastic colon or adult-type irritable bowel syndrome.

Physical examination of these patients fails to reveal any abnormality, and special investigations are usually unrewarding. The diagnosis can be made on the history alone, and is supported by the normal physical findings and growth parameters. Investigations should be limited to urine analysis and culture, and examination of the stools for ova and parasites. Look particularly for giardia infestation, which can mimic the condition, and which responds very rapidly to treatment with metronidazole.

Treatment consists of reassurance, and explanation of the functional nature of the disturbance, which probably represents a motility disorder that corrects itself with maturation. Dietary manipulation should be strongly discouraged, as it may aggravate the condition and lead to malnutrition through elimination of multiple foods erroneously thought to be implicated in the pathogenesis.

I.D. Hill
D.F. Wittenberg

12
Liver disorders

Introduction

The liver is susceptible to a wide variety of diseases in childhood. Most commonly the child will present with jaundice and hepatomegaly due to a viral infection of the liver. The incidence of hepatitis A, which is the most common viral cause of hepatitis, is closely related to the socio-economic status of the population.

The exact incidence of hepatitis A is almost impossible to determine, as most cases, particularly in childhood, are asymptomatic, and in many areas cases are not reported. Nevertheless, in endemic areas such as parts of India and Africa the prevalence of antibodies to hepatitis A is nearly 95% by the age of 5 or 6 years. Infection with hepatitis A is controlled by effective sewerage disposal and improved general hygiene. In a developed country such as the United Kingdom, the incidence of hepatitis A has been found to be a marker of inner city deprivation.

Hepatitis B chronically infects more than 200 million people world-wide. There is considerable geographic variation, but the prevalence is particularly high in parts of Africa. Surveys of black South African mine-workers reveal a 10% incidence of hepatitis B surface antigen. It is estimated that there are 2 million hepatitis B carriers in South Africa. In a study of rural black South Africans, the incidence was significantly lower amongst the inland South Sotho as compared to the coastal Nguni people in areas such as KwaZulu and Transkei. The incidence of hepatitis B amongst urban black children in Soweto has shown a decline, indicating a positive effect of urbanization on the disease.

In southern Africa traditional healers in certain areas use herbal remedies which contain substances toxic to the liver. Fulminant hepatic failure may follow the administration of traditional remedies. Veno-occlusive disease, which is relatively common in certain areas of South Africa, is closely related to exposure to senecio species, which grow wild in the veld. Exposure to organic solvents, as for instance in the practice of glue-sniffing, may result in liver damage.

Health workers should be aware of those forms of liver disease that are prevalent in their area. Improvement of general living conditions and health education will significantly reduce the incidence of liver disease in a community. Specific problems such as the use of traditional remedies will require tactful consultation with traditional healers in an attempt to dissuade them from these life-threatening practices.

Hepatitis

The term hepatitis implies an inflammatory process of the liver. Histologically there is an inflammatory mononuclear cell infiltrate and varying degrees of damage to the hepatocytes. The latter may result in swollen hepatocytes with a granular appearance, or in shrunken or loss of hepatocytes, as indicated by disruption of the normal reticulin network. This can be caused by factors such as infections, toxic substances (including drugs), and metabolic disorders *(see Table 12.1)*. In some instances the cause is not apparent and the hepatitis is termed idiopathic or cryptogenic. The overwhelming majority of children develop hepatitis as a result of infection with hepatitis A or B viruses.

Hepatitis A (HAV)

Epidemiology

HAV is spread by faecal-oral transmission via contaminated water supplies and foodstuffs. For this reason HAV infection is common amongst children in developing areas where there is inadequate or no sewerage disposal. In developed areas HAV infection occurs less frequently and at a later age, when it often results in a more severe illness.

Table 12.1   Causes of hepatitis in childhood

Infection

Viral

   Hepatitis A (HAV)

   Hepatitis B (HBV)

   Hepatitis C (HCV formerly non-A, non-B)

   Hepatitis D (HDV or Delta Agent, occurs with HBV)

   Hepatitis E (HEV)

   Infectious mononucleosis (Ebstein Barr virus)

   Cytomegalovirus (CMV)

   Herpes simplex

   Human immunodeficiency virus (AIDS)

Parasites

   Toxoplasma gondii

   Entamoeba histolytica

   Schistosoma mansoni (bilharziasis)

Bacterial

   Leptospirosis

   Pyogenic bacteria

Physical agents

   Burns

   Irradiation

   Hypothermia

   Metabolic errors

   Wilson's disease

Toxins and drugs

Toxins

   Senecio alkaloids

   Aflatoxins

   Amanita mushrooms

Drugs

   Antimicrobials – wide variety including

     tetracyclines

     erythromycin

     ampicillin

     sulphonamides

   Antituberculous drugs

     isoniazid

     rifampicin

     pyrazinamide

     ethionamide

     ethambutol

   Cytotoxic and immunosuppressives including

     methotrexate

     azathioprine

     cyclophosphamide

   Anticonvulsants including

     sodium valproate

     carbamazepine

   Analgesics and anti-inflammatory agents including

     paracetamol

     salicylates

     phenylbutazone

     indomethazine

   Anaesthetic agents including

     halothane

Virology

HAV is a small (27 nm) cubic ribonucleic acid (RNA) virus classified as a picorna of the enterovirus genus *(see Fig. 12.1)*. HAV, which is antigenically distinct, multiplies in several human cell lines. The liver, which is the principal site of viral replication, may be damaged directly by the virus but also by the immune response that it elicits. Once infected the individual develops life-long immunity.

Incubation is usually 2-4 weeks, but may be as short as a few days. The virus multiplies in the liver and is shed via the bile into the stools within 1–2 weeks of exposure *(see Fig. 12.2)*. Infectivity is maximal at the onset of the non-specific prodromal symptoms and before there is biochemical evidence of hepatitis. IgM antibodies appear in the serum at this stage and result in a rapid fall in the concentration of the virus in the stool. IgG antibodies, which persist for many years, result in permanent immunity and there is no chronic carrier-state of HAV.

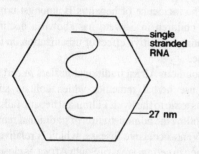

Fig. 12.1   Hepatitis A virus

Clinical features

The illness is usually mild, and in young children is frequently asymptomatic. Prodromal symptoms include nausea, vomiting, diarrhoea, fever, and at times right upper quadrant abdominal pain. These are followed within a few days by the onset of jaundice. With the appearance of jaundice the prodromal symptoms generally resolve in young children, although in older children there may be a transient exacerbation of the prodrome with the onset of jaundice.

On examination there is a tender hepatomegaly in most cases, and splenomegaly in about 30% of cases. The urine is dark and the stools are pale if there is significant cholestasis. In the majority jaundice resolves within 2 weeks, although unusually it may persist for months.

Investigations

Serum transaminases rise a few days before the onset of jaundice and peak shortly afterwards at 10–30 times above the normal levels *(see Fig.*

12.2). The serum alkaline phosphatase is usually only moderately elevated. Bilirubin levels rise and peak several days after the transaminases. The prothrombin time is usually normal, and abnormality may be indicative of liver necrosis. The diagnosis is confirmed by the presence of IgM antibodies to HAV.

Management

As there is no specific treatment, the management is supportive. Uncomplicated cases are best managed at home. The diet should be tailored to the child's own preferences to ensure an adequate intake of fluids and energy. It is neither possible or desirable to enforce bed-rest. Corticosteroids are not indicated, and paracetamol and salicylates are contraindicated.

Prevention

Since the majority of cases are asymptomatic and those that develop symptomatic hepatitis are most

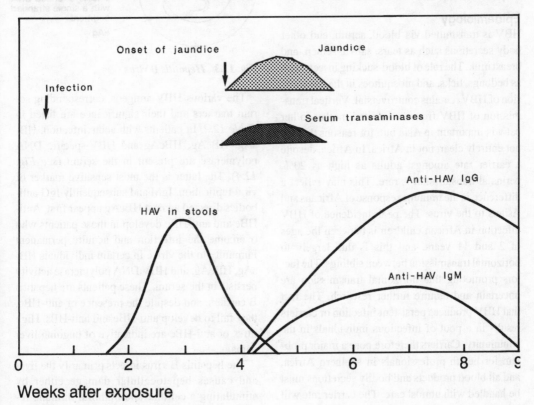

Fig. 12.2 Features of hepatitis A infection

infective in the prodromal phase, it is impossible to isolate them from the general population. For this reason it is imperative to ensure adequate sewerage disposal, safe drinking water, and encourage basic personal hygiene such as washing hands after defecation and before handling food. In many areas this is not possible, and for this reason the disease is endemic. Normal immunoglobulin contains sufficient antibodies to HAV to give passive immunity for about 3 months at a dose of 0.02–0.04 ml/kg.

Complications

Complications are rare. Fulminant hepatic failure is the most serious complication, with an incidence of about 5 per 1 000 cases. Aplastic anaemia is a very rare complication but has a high mortality. There is no chronic infection or carrier status.

Hepatitis B (HBV)

Epidemiology

HBV is transmitted via blood, serum, and other body secretions such as tears, saliva, semen, and breast milk. The role of blood-sucking insects such as bedbugs, ticks, and mosquitoes in the transmission of HBV remains controversial. Vertical transmission of HBV from an infected mother to her baby is important in Asia but, for reasons that are not entirely clear, not in Africa. In Africa, despite a carrier rate amongst adults as high as 20%, perinatal transmission is rare. This may reflect a difference in the immune response of Africans and Asians to the virus. The peak incidence of HBV infection in African children is between the ages of 2 and 11 years, and this is due largely to horizontal transmission between siblings. The factors promoting this horizontal transmission are uncertain and require further research. The fact that HBV produces persistent infection or carriers results in a pool of infectious individuals in the community. Carriers therefore pose a major problem for health professionals in southern Africa, and all blood products and bodily secretions must be handled with utmost care. The carrier rate will be reduced only by a significant improvement in the living conditions of communities in the region.

Virology

Hepatitis B is a 42 nm spherical deoxyribonucleic acid (DNA) virus occurring primarily in humans *(see Fig. 12.3)*. The whole virus, or Dane particle, consists of an outer lipoprotein coat (hepatitis B surface antigen HBsAg) and an inner nucleocapsid core (Hepatitis B core antigen HBcAg). The hepatitis B virus has been subdivided further into four HBsAg subtypes (adw, ayw, ayr, and adr) but these subtypes do not appear to affect the course of the disease. An additional antigen, the 'e' antigen (HBeAg), which is probably part of the core, and HBV-specific DNA polymerase are indicators of acute infection.

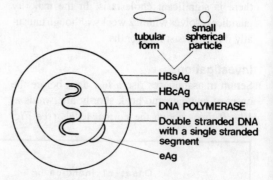

Fig. 12.3   Hepatitis B virus

The various HBV antigens, corresponding serum markers and their significance are listed in *Table 12.2*. In patients with acute infection, HBsAg, HBeAg, HBcAg and HBV-specific DNA polymerase are present in the serum *(see Fig. 12.4)*. The latter is the most sensitive marker of viral replication. IgM and subsequently IgG antibodies directed against HBcAg appear first. Anti-HBe and anti-HBc develop in those patients who overcome the infection and acquire permanent immunity to the virus. In certain individuals HBsAg, HBeAg, and HBV DNA polymerase activity persists in the serum. These patients are hepatitis B carriers, and despite the presence of anti-HBc, they fail to develop anti-HBe and anti-HBs. High titres of anti-HBc are indicative of ongoing liver damage.

The hepatitis B virus infects primarily the liver and causes hepatocellular damage either by stimulating a cellular and humoral immune response directed against the infected hepatocytes, or possibly by a direct effect on the hepatocyte.

Table 12.2 Markers of HBV infection and infectivity

Marker	Acute infection	Past infection	Carrier High risk*	Low risk*
HbsAg	Present	Absent	Present	Present
HbsAb	Absent	Present	Absent	Absent
HbeAg	Present	Absent	Present	Absent
HbeAb	Absent	Present	Absent	Present
HbcAbIgM+	Present	Absent	Absent	Absent
HbcAbIgG	Absent	Present	Present	Present
Liver enzymes	Increased	Normal	Mildly increased	Normal

+ Marker of active infection
* Refers to likelihood of transmitting the virus

Clinical features

The clinical features of hepatitis B infection are variable, depending to a large extent on the immune response. Up to 50% of patients have anicteric subclinical infections. Symptoms suggestive of a minor 'flu-like illness are common in children. The acute hepatitis resulting from hepatitis B is clinically indistinguishable from that

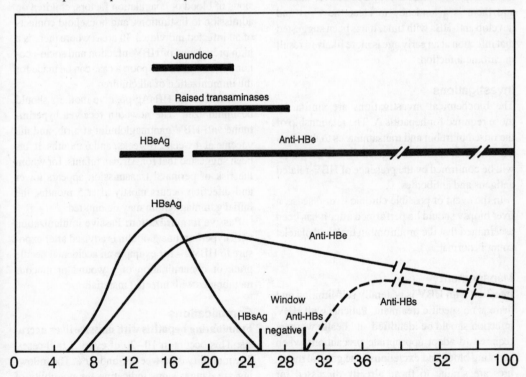

Fig. 12.4 Features of hepatitis B infection

caused by hepatitis A. Clinical features such as prolonged prodromal period, arthralgia, and skin rashes are not reliably associated with HBV infection in children. The course of the illness, however, is somewhat prolonged.

Chronic hepatitis may follow an acute episode, but often may be discovered incidentally due to the detection of the HBsAg in the blood. It may present with non-specific complaints such as malaise, lethargy, and failure to thrive, indicative of underlying chronic liver disease and cirrhosis. Liver biopsy is often the only method of determining the degree of liver involvement.

Glomerulonephritis may result from HBV circulating immune complexes. These children develop a membranous glomerulonephritis and present with a nephrotic syndrome. Arthritis and pericarditis may also result from these circulating immune complexes.

Carriers are a unique feature of hepatitis B infection. In these patients the indicators of active infection persist without evidence of liver disease and there is a tendency to clear the virus and develop anti-HBs with time. It has been suggested that infection at an early age is more likely to result in chronic infection.

Investigations

The biochemical investigations are similar to those required for hepatitis A. The relationship of the raised bilirubin and transaminases to the clinical course is shown in *Fig. 12.2*. The diagnosis will be confirmed by the presence of HBV-related antigens and antibodies.

In the event of possible chronic liver disease, a liver biopsy should be performed after it has been ascertained that the prothrombin time and platelet count is normal.

Management

Infection with HBV is generally self-limiting and there is no specific treatment. Patients with HBV infection should be identified and health workers required to adopt appropriate precautions when handling blood and excretions. The general measures are similar to those already discussed for hepatitis A. The risk of horizontal transmission is quite high in Africa, and it is standard practice to isolate patients with acute hepatitis B.

The role of steroids, antiviral drugs, and interferon in chronic infection remains uncertain, although encouraging results have been reported in some clinical trials.

Prevention

The prevention of HBV infection is a priority, and all blood and blood products such as antihaemophiliac globulin should be carefully screened. HBV-positive patients should be identified, and in high-risk areas pregnant women should be screened to enable preventive measures to be taken to protect their offspring. Improvement of general standards of hygiene will serve to reduce the number of carriers in the community; in parts of the United States and countries of northern Europe the carrier rate is as low as 0.1%.

Active immunization: A safe and effective vaccine against HBV is available. It is expensive, and at present recommended only for the protection of children and newborns at risk. Risk groups include those children requiring repeated transfusions of blood or coagulation factors, children on admission to institutions, and household contacts of an infected individual. In areas where there is a high prevalence of HBV infection and socio-economic conditions are poor, a case can be made for the immunization of all children.

All infants of HBsAg-positive mothers should be immunized. The newborn receives hyperimmune anti-HBV gammaglobulin at birth, and the vaccine at 4 weeks, 8 weeks, and 6 months. It has been suggested that for African infants, for whom the risk of perinatal transmission appears lower and infection occurs mostly after 5 months, the initial gammaglobulin may be omitted.

Passive immunization: Passive immunization with hyperimmune globulin is advised after exposure to HBV — for example an accidental needle prick or contamination of a wound or mucous membranes with infected material.

Complications

Fulminating hepatitis with massive liver necrosis: This occurs in 10–20 of every 1 000 cases. The mortality is between 80 and 90%. The following are danger signs indicating the possibilty of this complication:

◆ deepening jaudice with persisting prodromal symptoms or a decrease in liver size

◆ sleepiness, confusion, or abnormal behaviour indicative of impending hepatic encephalopathy
◆ bleeding tendency, particularly if this fails to correct after administration of vitamin K.

These patients require immediate referral and admission to hospital for intensive supportive management. This will include maintenance of an adequate fluid and energy intake, total exclusion of protein from the diet, clearance and sterilization of the gut, and administration of clotting factors by means of fresh frozen plasma.

Aplastic anaemia: This is a rare but often fatal complication.

Chronic hepatitis: This is defined as hepatitis persisting for more than 3 months, and it is unclear whether the child is a carrier or has chronic disease. If a child remains HBsAg-positive for 6 months, a liver biopsy is indicated. These patients should be referred to a regional hospital for further assessment. The histology may be normal or show features of chronic persistent hepatitis, chronic active hepatitis, or established cirrhosis.

Hepatocellular carcinoma: The highest incidence occurs in areas where chronic infection with HBV is endemic. The tumour can occur in children, but is unusual.

Other forms of viral hepatitis

Hepatitis C (HCV)
Viruses other than HAV and HBV were previously designated as non-A, non-B (NANB). It is now believed that the major NANB virus is hepatitis C, and that it is a significant cause of post-transfusion hepatitis. There is evidence of perinatal transmission from infected mother to her newborn baby.

HCV is a relatively small RNA virus and is present in low titres in the serum. There is an enzyme-linked immunosorbent assay (ELISA) test for the antibody. World-wide 80% of patients with post-transfusion NANB hepatitis have antibodies to HCV, which is detected on average 15 weeks after the onset of hepatitis. HCV cannot be excluded in serum-negative patients until 6 months after the onset of symptoms.

At present it is recommended that all HCV antibody-positive individuals should be excluded from blood donor pools. There is no specific treatment, and although encouraging results have been obtained using interferon, patients tend to relapse on cessation of treatment.

Hepatitis D or delta agent (HDV)
This is a small, incomplete RNA-containing virus which requires HBV for infectivity and replication. HDV worsens the prognosis of acute HBV hepatitis and increases the risk of fulminant hepatitis in carriers. Children, including neonates, are susceptible, but infection with HDV is much more common in adults. The diagnosis is made by finding the HDV in liver or serum or by testing for IgM and IgG HDV-specific antibodies. No treatment is available, although vaccination against HBV should limit its spread.

Hepatitis E (HEV)
A second NANB hepatitis virus has been described and designated HEV. It is an RNA virus and is transmitted by the faecal-oral route. As yet details regarding its distribution and significance for children are uncertain.

Hepatitis F (HFV)
This infection may arise sporadically or in epidemics, resulting in severe hepatitis. Patients frequently develop an encephalopathy up to 3 months after the onset of jaundice. The prognosis is poor, and the only option for many patients may be liver transplantation.

Hepatitis G (HGV)
HGV is a recently-described cause of giant cell hepatitis with a poor prognosis.

Chronic liver disease

Chronic hepatitis can be simply defined as hepatitis where the course is prolonged beyond the normal. In children this is generally defined as more than 3 months. For this reason a liver biopsy should be considered in all children at this stage, and the child referred. Not all patients have an initial acute episode. Many present for the first time with symptoms and signs of chronic liver disease. Chronic hepatitis can be divided into chronic persistent and chronic active hepatitis.

Chronic persistent hepatitis

This is a relatively benign condition. The child has persistently elevated liver transaminase enzymes after acute viral hepatitis. The diagnosis is confirmed by biopsy which demonstrates a periportal inflammatory cell infiltrate but otherwise normal histology.

No specific treatment is required, and in the majority the condition will resolve with time. In the event of the patient being HBsAg-positive, there is an increased risk of developing cirrhosis.

Chronic active hepatitis

Chronic active hepatitis is a more serious condition, which is fortunately relatively uncommon. It is an autoimmune disorder that occurs in adolescents and young adults, and is an important cause of chronic liver disease in this age group. The same histological picture occurs as a result of HBV infection, but this is relatively uncommon in younger patients.

Clinical picture

The clinical features vary from those of acute hepatitis to non-specific complaints such as malaise. On examination most patients have jaundice, hepatosplenomegaly, and cutaneous features of chronic liver disease such as spider angiomata, striae, acne, and palmar erythema. Extrahepatic manifestations of the autoimmune process such as arthritis, haemolytic anaemia, thyroiditis, glomerulonephritis, enteropathy, and inflammatory bowel disease may be present.

Investigations

The bilirubin and liver transaminases are raised whilst there is hypoalbuminaemia and a prolonged prothrombin time. The gammaglobulin fraction, particularly IgG, is raised. In HBsAG-negative patients autoantibodies such as antinuclear antibody and rheumatoid factor are often positive.

The diagnosis is confirmed on liver biopsy. Typical histology is an inflammatory cell infiltrate extending from the portal tracts into the liver parenchyma with piecemeal necrosis and bridging fibrosis.

Table 12.3   Causes of childhood cirrhosis

Biliary cirrhosis
  Biliary atresia or hypoplasia
  Choledochal cyst
  Cystic fibrosis
  Bile duct stenosis or obstruction
  Ascending cholangitis

Post-necrotic cirrhosis
  Post hepatitis:
    neonatal hepatitis
    viral hepatitis
    chronic hepatitis
    drugs, toxins, or poisons
  Venous congestion:
    constrictive pericarditis
    congestive heart failure
    Budd-Chiari syndrome
  Veno-occlusive disease

Genetic causes
  Wilson's disease
  Galactosaemia
  Alpha-1-antitrypsin deficiency
  Glycogen storage disease

Management

These patients will be managed optimally in a referral hospital. Once the diagnosis has been established, steroids are recommended. The aim is to control the inflammatory process as indicated by the serum biochemistry, with a minimum of side-effects. Patients are weaned slowly from the steroids, but over half will relapse, and a significant number will eventually develop cirrhosis. Interferon has proved effective in patients with HBV-positive disease, but it is uncertain whether it affects the long-term prognosis significantly.

Cirrhosis

In patients with cirrhosis the normal liver architecture is destroyed and replaced by nodules of regenerating tissue surrounded by prominent fibrous tissue. The resulting fibrosis and abnormal porto-systemic vascular connections cause ongoing damage. Once established, cirrhosis will progress to involve the whole liver, resulting inevitably in liver failure. The progression is variable, and children may survive with normal growth and development for years.

The most simple and practical classification of the causes of cirrhosis is a division into biliary cirrhosis, due to bile duct obstruction, and postnecrotic cirrhosis, where the lesion is primarily hepatocellular *(see Table 12.3)*. Cirrhosis is the end stage of many conditions, and once established it may be impossible to determine the original cause.

Clinical features
The clinical features may be those of the underlying condition, portal hypertension, or chronic liver disease. It is important to remember that despite significant cirrhosis there may be no physical signs on examination.

Investigations
The serum albumin is low, whilst liver enzymes and gammaglobulins are raised. Alkaline phosphatase and serum cholesterol are characteristically raised in biliary cirrhosis. A biopsy should be performed to determine the degree of cirrhosis, provided that the clotting profile is normal.

Management
The management is essentially supportive. When possible the underlying condition should be addressed. Maintenance of general nutrition is important. Complications such as fat malabsorbtion and ascites may require attention. Liver transplantation can be offered where health budgets provide for such services.

Portal hypertension
The most important causes of portal hypertension in childhood are chronic hepatitis and portal venous thrombosis. An approach to the causes of portal hypertension is outlined in *Table 12.4*.

Clinical features
These children may present with a gastrointestinal haemorrhage from oesophageal varices, asymptomatic splenomegaly, or ascites and abdominal distension. At a late stage there may be hepatic decompensation and encephalopathy.

Investigations
Where possible the primary cause of the portal hypertension is determined by serology, specific biochemical tests, liver scan, or biopsy. Liver function tests and a clotting profile are indicated in most patients. Oesophageal varices are identified by endoscopic examination.

Table 12.4   Causes of portal hypertension in childhood

Extrahepatic

Presinusoidal:	Portal or splenic vein obstruction
Postsinusoidal:	Budd-Chiari syndrome
	Inferior vena caval obstruction
	Veno-occlusive disease
	Pericarditis or heart failure

Intrahepatic
Cirrhosis
Schistosomiasis
Congenital hepatic fibrosis
Acute or chronic hepatitis

Management
The management of portal hypertension in childhood is essentially conservative. Ascites can be effectively controlled by manipulation of the sodium intake and use of diuretics. Despite the fact that massive splenomegaly may occur, there is very seldom any reason to consider splenectomy. Bleeding oesophageal varices can be controlled by endoscopic injection sclerotherapy, but in the event of catastrophic haemorrhage surgical intervention may be necessary. A gastrointestinal haemorrhage is always a serious complication, and any child affected should be referred as an emergency to a centre capable of managing the complication. It is vital that the child be adequately resuscitated before such a transfer.

Hepatic schistosomiasis (bilharzia)
In southern Africa infestation with *Schistosoma mansoni* occurs frequently in certain areas amongst schoolgoing children. The intermediate host is a freshwater snail, and cercaria released from the snail penetrate the skin to produce infection. The parasites migrate to the liver, where further development takes place. As a result of deposition of eggs there is an intense inflammatory response, with healing by fibrosis. In the liver

the lesions involve the portal tract and result in marked fibrosis, although not the nodular regeneration typical of cirrhosis. The hepatic fibrosis causes portal venous obstruction which results in the splenomegaly typical of hepatic schistosomiasis.

Clinical features

The clinical features of the hepatic involvement include hepatomegaly in the early stages and manifestations of portal hypertension. Firm splenomegaly, which may be an incidental finding in an apparently-well child, is present in many patients. Other findings include ascites and oesophageal varices in the event of longstanding portal hypertension. Hepatic decompensation, resulting in ascites and signs of liver failure, is rare in South Africa, but does occur in Brazil and Egypt.

Investigations

The diagnosis may be made by the identification of ova in the urine, stool, or on liver biopsy. A specific ELISA test has been developed which may facilitate the diagnosis.

Liver function tests remain normal or minimally deranged until late in the course of the disease.

Management

Prevention of the disease is important in the light of potentially-serious hepatic involvement (see Chapter 8, Infectious Diseases).

The recommended treatment is a single dose of praziquantel (40 mg/kg). The efficacy of treatment depends on the degree and duration of infection as well as the severity of complications.

Veno-occlusive disease

This is a form of hepatic vein obstruction which occurs most frequently in children. In southern Africa the disease follows the ingestion of alkaloids from the senecio plant species. This plant is found growing wild in many parts of Africa, and is used in traditional procedures administered either orally or by enema.

The lesion is initially in the central vein of the hepatic lobule and smaller branches of the hepatic vein. Initial endothelial oedema is followed by fibroblastic proliferation and ultimate occlusion of the vessel. Venous congestion and necrosis of hepatocytes eventually result in cirrhosis.

Clinical features

Veno-occlusive disease is most common under the age of 6 years. The onset is sudden, with hepatomegaly and severe ascites in the absence of jaundice. In endemic areas the picture is typical and the diagnosis is often clinically apparent.

Management

There is no specific treatment, and management is directed towards controlling the ascites. Some patients will die in the acute phase, and those who survive may progress to cirrhosis with portal hypertension.

Education of the population regarding the risks of herbal enemas and traditional medicines is essential for the prevention of this condition.

Approach to the infant with persistent jaundice

There are various causes of persistent jaundice in the first few months of life. An important first step is to determine whether the jaundice is due to an unconjugated or conjugated hyperbilirubinaemia.

Unconjugated hyperbilirubinaemia is mainly due to haemolysis or inadequate hepatic conjugation and will not be further discussed here (see Chapter 5, Newborns).

Conjugated hyperbilirubinaemia by definition is when the conjugated bilirubin fraction is greater than 20% of the total bilirubin. Important causes of a conjugated hyperbilirubinaemia are neonatal hepatitis and obstruction of the biliary tree (see Table 12.5).

Clinical features

All these infants present with jaundice, dark urine, and pale or light yellow stools. The jaundice has often been present from the neonatal period and has initially been thought to be physiological. On examination usually there is hepatosplenomegaly, and growth retardation may be present. There may be a bleeding tendency.

Diagnosis

The first priority is to identify treatable conditions. For this reason thyroid function, serology for syphilis, reducing substances in the urine for galactosaemia, and urine culture are a priority. The most important differential diagnosis is between the hepatitis syndrome and biliary atresia, which

Table 12.5 Causes of hyperbilirubinaemia in infants

A. **Infective**
  Viral:
    Cytomegalovirus
    Herpes simplex virus
    HIV (AIDS)
    Hepatitis B virus
  Bacterial:
    Syphilis
    Urinary tract infection
  Protozoal:
    Toxoplasma gondii
B. **Mechanical biliary tract obstruction**
  Biliary atresia, extra- and/or intrahepatic
  Biliary hypoplasia
  Choledochal cyst
  Bile plug syndrome
C. **Genetic or metabolic**
  Galactosaemia
  Alpha-1-antitrypsin deficiency
  Cystic fibrosis
  Hypothyroidism
  Hyperalimentation
  Chromosomal abnormalities:
    Trisomy 21
    Turner syndrome
D. **Idiopathic neonatal hepatitis**

Table 12.6 Differential points between the hepatitis syndrome and biliary atresia

Hepatitis syndrome	Biliary atresia
Pigmented stools	No stool pigment
AST, ALT raised	AST, GGT, ALP raised
GGT/AST ratio < 2	GGT/AST ratio > 2
Positive serology/cultures	Negative serology/cultures
Butyl-IDA isotope scan	Butyl-IDA isotope scan
No biliary obstruction	Biliary obstruction

together cause 90% of cholestatic jaundice in infants. The differential factors are outlined in *Table 12.6.*

Unfortunately there is no single investigation which will differentiate reliably between the hepatitis syndrome and biliary atresia. Observation of the stools for 7 days is a simple and relatively reliable method of determining whether there is biliary obstruction present. This can be undertaken at a peripheral clinic or by a general practitioner. Stool without pigment is white, but any yellow or green discoloration is indicative of bile drainage from the biliary tree. No bile drainage for 7 days indicates total biliary obstruction, an almost certain diagnosis of biliary atresia, and the urgent need to refer.

Management

Treatable causes such as syphilis or a urinary tract infection are managed appropriately. Neonatal hepatitis, with a typical giant cell histology, is confirmed on liver biopsy. In most cases no definite cause for the hepatitis will be determined, and management will be supportive.

Infants in whom biliary atresia is suspected require an explorative laparotomy and intra-operative cholangiogram. Intrahepatic biliary atresia is inoperable, but extrahepatic biliary atresia can be successfully palliated by a portoenterostomy procedure which allows the bile to drain directly from the liver into the bowel *(see Chapter 28, Surgical Problems).*

Approach to the child with hepatomegaly and hepatosplenomegaly

It is useful for health professionals to have a logical and practical approach to the problem. It must be remembered that the liver and spleen may be palpable due to chest pathology such as asthma or bronchiolitis which depress the diaphragm. In this event the liver and spleen are not enlarged, but simply displaced downward.

There are many ways to approach the problem, but the clinical and investigational approach to the causes of hepatosplenomegaly outlined in *Table 12.7* is used by the author. Portal hypertension will result in splenomegaly in many conditions discussed below.

From the history and examination there will be clues as to the possible cause of the enlarged liver and spleen. In the **inflammatory** group jaundice is often present. Evidence of tuberculosis or other generalized infection may suggest the possibility of **reticulo-endothelial (Kupffer) cell hyperplasia** as the cause. Examination of the cardiovascular system is essential to exclude the

Table 12.7   Causes of hepatomegaly and hepatosplenomegaly in childhood

(Possible investigations indicated after each heading)

Inflammation: Abnormal liver function tests, specific
   biochemical, serological, and other tests.
Infection
   Neonatal and congenital: Cytomegalovirus, herpes
   simplex, rubella, toxoplasmosis, syphilis, listeriosis
   Viral hepatitis: Hepatotropic and other general viral
   infections
   Parasitic infection: Hydatid disease, amoebiasis
Auto-immune liver disease
Toxic and and drug reactions
Biliary tract obstruction

Reticulo-endothelial cell hyperplasia (Kupffer cells
   comprise 10% of the normal liver): Blood cultures,
   chest X-ray, biopsy if uncertainty.
Septicaemia
Malignant disease – not involving the liver
Granulomatous response – tuberculosis

Venous congestion (portal hypertension will result in
   splenomegaly in many of the conditions causing
   hepatomegaly): X-ray chest, cardiac ultrasound
   examination.
Congestive heart failure
Pericardial effusion or constrictive pericarditis
Budd-Chiari syndrome

Space-occupying lesions: CT scan or isotope scan.
Abscess
Secondary and primary neoplasms

Infiltrations: Haematological investigations, liver or bone
   marrow biopsy.
Erythroblastosis – Rh incompatibility, thalassaemia
Lymphoma
Leukaemia
Histiocytosis syndromes

Storage disorders: Liver or other tissue biopsy.
Glycogen storage disease (liver only)
Mucopolysaccharidoses
Lipid — Gaucher's, Niemann-Pick, and Tay-Sachs diseases

Fat accumulation (liver only): Clinical diagnosis, liver
   biopsy if in doubt.
Malnutrition
Hyperalimentation
Cystic fibrosis
Galactosaemia
Uncontrolled diabetes mellitus
Hepatotoxic drugs

Metabolic disorders: Specific diagnostic tests.
Wilson's disease
Cystic fibrosis
Galactosaemia

possibility of a cardiac condition resulting in **venous congestion.** The Budd-Chiari syndrome is characterized by marked ascites and the absence of filling of the jugular veins, with pressure over the liver. A **liver abscess** is suggested by local tenderness and swelling in an acutely ill child. A bleeding tendency, lymphadenopathy, severe or unusual infections, and anaemia (amongst other signs) may indicate an **infiltrative process** involving the liver and possibly the spleen. **Storage diseases** are often associated with an abnormal appearance, neurological signs, and marked firm enlargement of liver and spleen. **Glycogen storage disease** affects only the liver and is often associated with mental retardation and a history of unexplained metabolic acidosis in the neonatal period. **Fatty infiltration** of the liver is typical of kwashiorkor, and malnutrition is one of the commonest causes of hepatomegaly in childhood in southern Africa. **Metabolic disorders** are

generally identified by the associated clinical features of the particular condition.

Investigations

The special investigations will be determined by the clinical appraisal of the patient. In many cases the diagnosis can be made clinically and confirmed by relatively simple laboratory investigations. Liver function tests will be required in all cases, and the inflammatory conditions will result in a marked rise of the hepatic transaminases (AST, ALT). X-rays of the chest may indicate cardiac or pulmonary pathology, and in many instances a liver, bone marrow, or other tissue biopsy will confirm the diagnosis. CT or technetium scans may be necessary to exclude space-occupying lesions, and in this event the patient will have to be referred.

K.C. Househam

13

Respiratory disorders

Introduction

Acute respiratory infections (ARI) are fast replacing acute diarrhoea as the leading cause of death in children living in the Third World. The World Health Organization estimates that 15 million children under 5 years of age will die every year. ARI are estimated to cause between 25 and 33% of these deaths, with acute pneumonia causing approximately 75% of the deaths from ARI. Mortality in developing countries is 10–50 times greater than that in the First World.

ARI mortality is highest in those under 2 years, the malnourished, early weanlings, and those with poorly-educated parents or who have no easy access to health care.

ARI is generally responsible for between 20 and 60% of all outpatient visits, and for 12–45% of hospital admissions.

The majority of deaths can be prevented by immunization and case control programmes in community health centres.

Acute respiratory infections in South Africa

In South Africa ARI are responsible for 20% of deaths under the age of 5 years, the commonest cause being acute pneumonia, which is responsible for about 90% of these fatalities. The death rate from ARI for black children in South Africa is as much as 270 times higher than for whites, but the rate for white and Asian children is still 7 times higher than it is for children in the industrialized countries. In the Western Cape the incidence of pulmonary tuberculosis is among the highest in the world, with 576 new cases per 100 000 children per year.

Factors influencing the incidence of respiratory tract infections

Children normally develop four to eight episodes of ARI per year, the rate being inversely related to age. Most infections are of the upper respiratory tract, with about 30% affecting the lower respiratory tract. The following factors have a bearing on the incidence of ARI:

◆ **Poor nutritional status:** Pneumonia is twelve times more common in malnourished children. Vitamin A deficiency and low birth weight also increase the incidence.

◆ **Poor socio-economic status:** Poverty, crowding, and the indoor use of wood or coal fires for heating and cooking.

◆ **Parental smoking:** The number and seriousness of ARI and the number of asthma attacks increase in children who passively inhale tobacco smoke.

◆ **Parasitic infection:** The inflammatory changes in the lung associated with infiltration by ascaris larvae or eosinophils predispose to bacterial superinfection.

◆ **Breast-feeding and early weaning:** There is a decreased incidence of ARI and case fatality rate in breast-fed children, whilst early weaning is associated with increased incidence and mortality from ARI.

◆ **Immunization:** Up to 25% of ARI deaths can be prevented by measles, diphtheria, pertussis, and BCG vaccination.

Clinical features

Symptoms

The common symptoms pertaining to the respiratory tract are cough, stridor, wheeze, and dyspnoea. A full history includes the circumstances and the time of onset of symptoms, whether they are of acute onset or recurrent, and the degree of disability they engender.

Physical examination

The following features in the physical examination are important in assessing respiratory disease:

◆ **Nose and throat:** Repeated bacterial infections tend to cause enlarged tonsils. However, in the malnourished patient with reduced thymolymphatic response to infection, tonsillar hypertrophy is minimal. Alae nasi flare indicates breathlessness from any acute respiratory disease. Obstructed nasal passages due to allergic rhinitis suggest additional respiratory pathology with an allergic basis.

♦ **Tachypnoea** accompanies obstructive airway disease (bronchopneumonia or asthma) and non-obstructive conditions (pleural effusion, pneumothorax, pulmonary fibrosis). Dyspnoea (retraction of intercostal and subcostal spaces and of the sternum) indicates airway obstruction.

♦ Nature of **cough** should be noted during the examination: productive (bronchitis, bronchiectasis), wheezy (lower airway obstruction, e.g., asthma), croupy (laryngo-tracheobronchitis, foreign body), or aphonic (laryngitis, laryngeal papillomata, or foreign body).

♦ **Chest deformity:** A barrel- or funnel-shaped chest, marked Harrison's sulcus, and rounded, high shoulders, all indicate that respiratory disease — usually airway obstruction — has been present for some time.

Table 13.1   Causes of wheezing

Continuous	From birth	Vascular anomalies
		Laryngeal or tracheal lesions
		Sequelae of prematurity:
		Bronchopulmonary dysplasia
		Wilson-Mikity syndrome
	Late onset	Congenital lobar emphysema
		Bronchial anomalies
		Tracheal or laryngeal foreign body
Episodic	Infrequent	Bronchiolitis
		Acute pneumonia
		Pulmonary infiltrates and eosinophilia
		Primary tuberculosis
		Congestive cardiac failure
	Recurrent	Asthma
		Obliterative bronchiolitis (Macleod's syndrome)
		Bronchiectasis
		Cystic fibrosis

♦ **Clubbing** of the fingers indicates, among other conditions, the presence of suppurative lung disease. Bronchiectasis is a common cause of chronic pulmonary symptoms in underprivileged children, but clubbing usually takes several years to develop.

♦ **Chest movements:** During inspiration both the chest and abdomen expand, and the reverse occurs in expiration. If there is paralysis of either the intercostal muscles or diaphragm (e.g., polio), 'see-saw' breathing occurs, in which the two parts move in opposite directions.

♦ **Chest percussion:** Hyper-resonance (emphysema, pneumothorax), dullness (consolidation, atelectasis, pleural thickening), stony dullness (effusion or empyema).

♦ **Position of trachea,** if shifted, will indicate either pulling, after collapse of a lung segment, or pushing, as by fluid or tension pneumothorax. This sign must be interpreted in conjunction with findings on percussion and auscultation.

♦ **Auscultation of thorax:** Nature of breath sounds: distant (intrathoracic fluid, pneumothorax, pleural thickening); bronchial breathing (consolidation of underlying lung). Additional sounds: wheezes, especially expiratory, indicate lower airway obstruction (see Table 13.1); crackles arise from equalization of pressure in small and medium airways constricted by peribronchial fluid and other pathology.

♦ **Restlessness, drowsiness, pallor, or central cyanosis** give an indication of deranged gas exchange and respiratory failure.

Classification of respiratory infections

The upper respiratory tract is separated from the lower respiratory tract at the base of the epiglottis. Common respiratory infections and their aetiology are shown in Table 13.2. The lower respiratory tract is also involved in about 20–30% of the upper respiratory tract infections.

Treatment of ARI in community health centres

The WHO has developed a protocol for treatment of children who have limited access to health care.

The programme is based on the diagnosis and treatment of ARI in health care centres, and is

Table 13.2   Acute respiratory tract infections

	Diagnosis	Common aetiology
Upper respiratory tract	Rhinitis	Viral
	Otitis media and tonsillitis	Bacterial *(S. pneumoniae, H.influenzae)*
	Pharyngitis	Bacterial (streptococcus) Viral
Lower respiratory tract	Laryngotracheobronchitis	Viral (measles, para-influenza)
	Tracheobronchitis and bronchiolitis	Viral (RSV)
	Pneumonia	Bacterial *(S. pneumoniae, H. influenzae)*

designed to be administered by community workers with limited training. In addition, an ARI programme requires support from district and regional hospitals. When introduced, ARI case management programmes have resulted in an 84% reduction in mortality from ARI.

A simple system for assessing the severity of ARI depends on respiratory rate at rest, intercostal and sternal recession, and ability to drink *(see Table 13.3)*.

Co-trimoxazole or amoxycillin are the antibiotics used, because they are cheap, given orally, and effective against the bacteria of community-acquired respiratory tract infections, viz., *Streptococcus pneumoniae* and *Haemophilus influenzae*.

The following measures should be carried out before and during transfer to hospital:

♦ antipyretics where necessary

♦ oxygen (40%) by mask or nasal prongs

♦ clearing the nasal passages (secretions are sucked out with a syringe or suction apparatus after softening with drops of sodium bicarbonate or saline)

♦ a stomach tube is necessary to decompress the stomach from swallowed air and to give fluids (50–80 ml/kg/day) if needed. If the child is severely distressed, fluids are given intravenously.

All children with ARI being treated at home require regular visits by community health workers. If there is deterioration in the child's symptoms, or if the cough persists after 14 days, the child should be referred to exclude chronic respiratory problems such as pulmonary tuberculosis, foreign body inhalation, or complications of pneumonia (empyema, lung abscess, or bronchiectasis).

Upper respiratory tract infections

See Chapter 14, Ear, Nose, and Throat Disorders.

Table 13.3   Acute respiratory tract infections: Classification and management

Severity	Criteria	Management
Mild	Cough, fever Respiratory rate < 50/minute	Supportive measures Antipyretic *No antibiotics*
Moderate	Cough, fever Respiratory rate > 50/minute No rib or sternal retraction	Supportive measures Antipyretic (paracetamol) Antibiotics
Severe	Cough, fever Respiratory rate > 50/minute Recession Unable to drink Cyanosis	Supportive measures Antibiotics Refer to hospital

Table 13.4   Aetiology and treatment of pneumonia in special groups of children

Group	Organisms	Antibiotic
Immunocompromised	Gram-negative organisms	Ampicillin
	Staph. aureus	+
	Opportunistic organisms	Cloxacillin
	Pneumocystis carinii	+
	M. tuberculosis	Aminoglycoside
Less than 3 months	Gram-negative organisms	Ampicillin
	Group B streptococcus	+
	Staph. aureus	Aminoglycoside
Hospital-acquired pneumonia	Gram-negative organisms	Aminoglycoside
	Methicillin-resistant	+
	Staph. aureus	?Fucidic acid
		+
		Cephalosporin (3rd generation)

Pneumonia in children

Aetiology

In developed countries childhood pneumonia is usually caused by viral infections, and has a low morbidity and mortality. In developing communities bacteria are responsible for about 65% of pneumonia cases, probably due to children often carrying a high bacterial load, and the mortality from pneumonia can be 300 times higher than in developed communities.

S. pneumoniae, H. influenzae, and Staph. aureus are the organisms most commonly involved. Viral infections are responsible for approximately 35% of pneumonia in children. The precise role of other organisms such as *Mycoplasma pneumoniae, Chlamydia trachomatis* and *Pneumocystis carinii* is as yet uncertain.

In developed communities respiratory syncytial virus, adenovirus, para-influenza and influenza viruses are the most common causative organisms. *Mycoplasma pneumoniae* is common in older children. Bacteria cause only between 5 and 10% of pneumonia, with *S. pneumoniae* and *H. influenzae* being the most common. Over and above the common causative organisms in the general childhood population, there are special circumstances which make certain groups of children more susceptible to pneumonia and/or in need of different treatment. These are outlined in *Table 13.4*.

Clinical picture

The clinical picture for pneumonia is determined by the age of the child and the causative organism. Neonates present only with lethargy, fever, and tachypnoea, and sometimes with apnoea *(see Chapter 5, Newborns)*. Older children often begin with an upper respiratory tract infection followed by a cough, fever, and tachypnoea. Fever, tachypnoea, and crackles are present in most children. The classical signs of lobar consolidation — dullness to percussion, and bronchial breathing — are found in the minority. Occasionally pneumonia will progress to respiratory failure, which is clinically recognized by severe tachypnoea, tachycardia, grunting, recession, restlessness, and central cyanosis.

Sudden deterioration during the course of pneumonia is suggestive of pneumothorax or pyopneumothorax, requiring immediate drainage.

Radiological picture

Bacterial pneumonia in children is normally characterized by widespread, poorly-demarcated, alveolar opacities with air bronchograms. The classical lobar or segmental opacification with air bronchograms is less common. Viral pneumonia, in contrast, usually causes perihilar streaking and air trapping. Mucus plugging results in lobar or segmental collapse which is easily confused with alveolar opacification. One cannot differentiate with certainty between viral and bacterial pneumonia using radiological features alone.

Radiological aetiological clues:

◆ Staphylococcal pneumonia often progresses to pneumatocele formation, lung abscesses, empyema, or pyopneumothorax.

◆ Klebsiella, anaerobes, *H.influenzae*, and tuberculosis can cause cavitating pneumonia.

Pneumatoceles are thin-walled, air-filled spaces with or without an air-fluid level. They can rupture, causing a pneumothorax, or become so large that they compress the rest of the lung, causing respiratory failure. The majority clear spontaneously within 3 months. Other causes of pneumatoceles are *H. influenzae* pneumonia, hydrocarbon inhalation pneumonia, and lung contusion.

Diagnosis

A high white cell count with a leucocytosis and positive C-reactive protein are often indirect evidence of bacterial pneumonia. However, viral pneumonia can also cause a high white cell count, and children very ill from a bacterial pneumonia often fail to show these features. Blood cultures before treatment may isolate the causative organism, which may also be cultured from any pleural fluid. Sputum culture, throat swabs, or pharyngeal aspirates are not specific, as the specimen is usually contaminated by upper respiratory tract organisms. Transtracheal and lung aspirates are specific tests, but should only be performed in institutions with the necessary expertise. Bacterial antigens can also be isolated from the urine. A tuberculin skin test should always be done. Viruses can either be cultured from throat swabs or demonstrated using immunofluorescent techniques.

Treatment

Correct antibiotic choice: Co-trimoxazole or amoxycillin is given *at primary level.* Referral is essential if the child shows evidence of respiratory distress or failure.

District and regional hospitals: Amoxycillin (200 mg/kg/day in 4 divided doses), unless staphylococcal pneumonia is suspected, when cloxacillin (100 mg/kg/day in 4 divided doses) is added. In children over 5 years parenteral penicillin can be used, as *S. pneumoniae* is the most likely cause. Once the child is fever-free for 3 days, the antibiotics can be given by mouth for a total of 7–10 days. Patients with a lung abscess or empyema should be treated for 21–42 days.

Children under the age of 3 months, severely malnourished children, children with hospital-acquired pneumonia or with severe immune suppression will require different antibiotics *(see Table 13.4).*

Supportive therapy:

◆ *High fever:* Paracetamol (30 mg/kg/day) in 4–6 divided doses.

◆ *Nasal passages* kept clear with sodium bicarbonate or saline nasal drops.

◆ *Hydration maintained:* If unable to take feeds, a nasogastric tube can be passed, but in severely distressed children intravenous fluid (50–80 ml/kg/day) is required.

◆ *Hypoxaemia:* Administration of oxygen by a head box, face mask, or nasal prongs. A child who is not pink in oxygen should be transferred to a hospital where arterial blood gases can be measured, as assisted ventilation may be required.

◆ *Haematocrit below 30%:* A blood transfusion (10–20 ml/kg) must be given to improve oxygen transport.

Failure to respond to therapy

Reasons:

◆ Incorrect choice of antibiotic, or the dose is inadequate.

◆ The pneumonia is not caused by the suspected organism, or the organism is resistant to the antibiotics used. Knowledge of the local antibiotic sensitivity patterns of organisms is helpful.

◆ Development of an empyema.

◆ The pneumonia is caused by *M. tuberculosis.*

◆ Suppressed immunity (often due to malnutrition or HIV infection) may lead to infection by an opportunistic organism.

◆ Underlying cause for the pneumonia, e.g., foreign body aspiration or bronchiectasis.

◆ Left-sided cardiac failure commonly masquerades as pneumonia.

The child should be referred to a higher grade hospital if the temperature has not settled after 3–5 days and the cause has not been identified.

Prognosis

Most children recover from pneumonia without any residual damage. Incorrectly treated, pneumonia can lead to tissue destruction and bronchiectasis. About half of the children who develop pneumonia secondary to measles or adenovirus have persistent airway obstruction and reduced lung function as the result of small airway disease.

Other causes of pneumonia

(See Table 13.5.)

Pulmonary tuberculosis

(See Chapter 9, Tuberculosis.)

This should always be excluded, due to the high incidence of tuberculosis in developing communities. Tuberculosis should be suspected specifically if pneumonia does not respond to treatment, if it occurs in an immunocompromised child, or in cases of bronchiectasis. Radiological changes include hilar or mediastinal lymphadenopathy, lobar collapse or hyperinflation, cavitation, and pleural effusion.

Hydrocarbon inhalation pneumonia

Paraffin, petrol, and other hydrocarbons used for cooking and heating purposes are often stored in unmarked bottles. Children sometimes accidentally drink from these bottles or inhale the contents, and 20–40% will develop chemical pneumonitis. Within 30 minutes the child develops signs of respiratory distress, which can get progressively worse over the next 24–48 hours. Secondary bacterial pneumonia often follows chemical pneumonitis if it is not prevented by prophylactic antibiotics. Ingestion of large amounts of hydrocarbons may cause neurological signs (confusion, loss of consciousness, convulsions). Other complications are pneumothorax and pneumatocele formation. The chest radiograph shows widespread alveolar opacification, which often appears worse than the clinical picture of the child. *(Also see Chapter 27, Poisoning.)*

Treatment: Oxygen and observation are essential, as extensive involvement may require mechanical ventilation. Induced vomiting is absolutely contraindicated, as this can lead to increased hydrocarbon aspiration. Antibiotics are indicated only if a secondary bacterial infection is

Table 13.5   Other causes of pneumonia*

Pulmonary tuberculosis
Hydrocarbon inhalation
Atypical pneumonia
      Mycoplasma pneumoniae
      Chlamydia trachomatis
Pneumonia eosinophilia (Loeffler's)
Aspiration
      Premature infants
      Neurological defects
        Palatopharyngeal incoordination
      Gastro-oesophageal reflux
      Anatomical defects
        Tracheo-oesophageal fistula
        Cleft palate
Infectious diseases
      HIV disease
      Pneumocystis carinii
      Lymphocytic interstitial pneumonia
      Measles with secondary bacterial and viral infection
      Pertussis
      Legionnaires' disease

* See text for the common causes of pneumonia.

suspected. Steroids do not change the course of the disease.

Pulmonary eosinophilia

Pulmonary infiltrates with eosinophilia in peripheral blood (PIE) occur fairly frequently in children in poor living conditions, with an increased chance of worm infestation.

Classification:

◆ *Simple PIE (Loeffler's):* Symptoms lasting less than a month.

◆ *Prolonged PIE:* Definite, recurrent pulmonary symptoms of 2–6 months' duration; but with eventual recovery.

◆ *Tropical eosinophilia:* Applied to cases where eosinophilic lung granulomas contain degenerating microfilaria.

◆ *Polyarteritis nodosa:* Patient is usually ill with asthmatic symptoms and a poor prognosis.

◆ *Drugs* can cause fleeting lung infiltrates and a blood eosinophilia, e.g., nitrofurantoin, penicillin, imipramine.

◆ *PIE with asthma:* Some asthmatics have pulmonary infiltrates which may be shifting in nature.

In many cases an aetiological agent cannot be demonstrated. Type I (Löeffler's) occurs more often in children with a personal or family history of allergy. If a specific cause is found, it is usually a nematode (ascaris or toxocara), but amoebiasis, trichinosis, hookworm infestation, and strongyloidiasis may cause PIE.

Diagnosis: The child coughs or wheezes, with occasional crackles, the chest radiograph shows migratory and transient pulmonary infiltrations, and occasionally atelectasis. The blood eosinophil count is 10–50% of white cells. It is difficult to establish a definitive diagnosis, as symptoms may occur before ova or adult ascaris appear in the stools; larval toxocara become encysted in tissue (including lung) and never reach the gut to produce ova.

Management: Treatment is symptomatic, as the disease is self-limiting, but giving a broad-spectrum vermicide (mebendazole) may help. If symptoms are troublesome, a short course of prednisone will accelerate resolution of pulmonary infiltrates, but tuberculosis must first be excluded.

Legionnaires' disease

Legionella pneumophila causes lower respiratory infection of varying severity. Epidemics have occurred in institutions as well as sporadic cases in the community. Subjects who get pneumonia are usually immunodepressed or debilitated. Disease in the young child is rare, although serological surveys of children show that half may develop antibodies to legionella by 4 years of age.

Extrapulmonary signs are relatively frequent: encephalopathy, microscopic haematuria, and raised liver enzymes may suggest the diagnosis, which can be confirmed by culture of lung tissue or by serology.

The organism, a Gram-negative rod, has been found in building sites, air-conditioning systems, water, and elevator shafts. No patient-to-patient spread has yet been demonstrated .

Clinical response to erythromycin is often dramatic, and the drug should be continued for 3 weeks. Relapses are possible in the immunocompromised, and pulmonary fibrosis has been described long after recovery.

Approach to a child with recurrent or persistent pneumonia

See Table 13.6 for causes of recurrent and persistent pneumonia.

Diagnostic pointers when assessing a child with recurrent or persistent pneumonia

The diagnosis of **asthma** is suggested by nocturnal cough, a positive family history, recurrent wheezing, and the child improving when given bronchodilators. *(See PIE, above, and Chapter 22, Common Allergic Disorders.)*

The **damaged airways** group give a history of pneumonia followed by recurrent chest symptoms. Chest radiograph shadows usually persist in the same position, if not to the same severity. Antibiotics are of no use unless there is pyrexia due to superadded infection, but chest physiotherapy is helpful. Airways are often 'hyperactive', and the child sometimes improves on a bronchodilator.

In the **aspiration** group there is a history of feeding difficulties, drooling, vomiting, and wheezing. Chest radiograph changes are usually in upper lobes in the infant under 6 months. *(See Chapter 11, Gastrointestinal Disorders, and Chapter 28, Surgical Problems.)*

Mucociliary defect due to bronchopulmonary dysplasia follows mechanical ventilation as a neonate.

When **immune deficiency** is suspected, a weekly differential white blood count is recommended to detect cyclic neutropenia or reduced numbers of lymphocytes. Further investigation is confined to specialist centres.

Extrathoracic airway obstruction
(See Table 13.7 and Fig. 13.1.)

Acute laryngotracheobronchitis (croup)
Acute laryngo-tracheo-bronchitis (LTB) is the commonest cause of stridor in children between 6 months and 2 years. It is almost always caused by viral infections, commonly para-influenza viruses. In developing countries measles and *herpes simplex* infection of the larynx are the commonest

Table 13.6 Causes of recurrent or persistent pneumonia

Diffuse

Allergy

Undiagnosed asthma

Pulmonary infiltrates with eosinophilia

Inflammation

Airways damaged by viral, bacterial, or fungal infections

Recurrent aspiration

Sucking or swallowing abnormalities:

Cerebral palsy

Brainstem or cranial nerve lesion

Tracheo-oesophageal fistula (H-shape)

Partial thoracic stomach (hiatus hernia)

Achalasia of cardia

Muco-ciliary clearance defects

Following pertussis, mycoplasma, and viral infections

Immotile-ciliary syndrome (Kartagener's syndrome)

Cystic fibrosis

Broncho-pulmonary dysplasia

Immune deficiencies

T-lymphocyte deficiency

Agammaglobulinaemia (Bruton's disease)

Neutrophil deficiency:

Defective phagocytosis, cyclic neutropenia

Complement defects

Immunosuppressive drugs

Lymphoproliferative malignancy

Malnutrition

Selective IgA deficiency

Localized

Foreign body

Extrinsic airway compression, e.g., lymph nodes

Bronchiectasis

Lobar sequestration

Table 13.7 Common causes of extrapulmonary airway obstruction

Age	Condition
Neonate	Choanal atresia
	Pierre-Robin syndrome
	Paralysis of vocal cord
	Aspiration of meconium in liquor
	Laryngomalacia
Infants and children	Infections:
	Laryngotracheobronchitis
	Diphtheria
	Epiglottitis *H. influenzae* type b
	Bacterial tracheitis
	Retropharyngeal abscess
	Paratracheal lymph node enlargement
	Mechanical:
	Foreign body
	Laryngeal papillomatosis
	Subglottic trauma (post intubation)
	Hypertrophied tonsils, adenoids
	Allergic:
	Angioneurotic oedema
	Trauma:
	Thermal and chemical

causes of severe croup. *Herpes simplex* virus infection of the larynx is difficult to diagnose, as only about 50% of these children have herpetiform lesions in their mouths.

Clinical picture

Two to three days after an acute upper respiratory tract infection the child develops stridor, with a characteristic bark-like cough and a hoarse voice. The children do not have a high fever, nor appear to be toxic. As the upper airway obstruction (UAO) worsens, the child becomes hypoxic, which causes tachycardia, restlessness, and confusion. The child can also become exhausted from the effort of breathing, which results in the stridor being less prominent, with no improvement in airway obstruction. With increasing obstruction the child develops both inspiratory and expiratory stridor, then followed by a pulsus paradoxus and the use of abdominal muscles in expiration.

Treatment

Treatment is instituted according to the grading system of Klein *(see Table 13.8)*. It should be stressed that this grading is only applicable to acute LTB. A child with grade 2 airway obstruction should be transferred to a hospital where nebulized adrenaline can be administered.

Nebulized adrenaline (1:1 000 solution 1 ml in 1 ml saline) should be repeated every 20–30 minutes in grade 2 and worse obstruction. Parenteral steroids (dexamethasone 0.6 mg/kg as a single dose) may benefit children with grade 2 or worse airway obstruction, but are contraindicated in measles and herpes LTB.

Table 13.8 Acute laryngotracheo-bronchitis: Grading and treatment

Grade	Criteria	Treatment
Grade 1	Inspiratory stridor	Observe
Grade 2	Inspiratory and expiratory stridor	Nebulzied adrenaline
Grade 3	Inspiratory and expiratory stridor + pulsus paradoxus	Continuous nebulized adrenaline. If no improvement, intubate
Grade 4	Impending apnoea	Intubate

Children with grade 3 stridor should be referred to a hospital where nasotracheal intubation or tracheotomy can be performed. Children with grade 4 obstruction should be intubated immediately before transfer to a hospital where high-level care is available. Nasotracheal intubation is the treatment of choice, but where intensive care is not available, tracheotomy is preferred.

Other differences found in the course of LTB in the Third World, as compared to that found in children in developed communities, are that:

◆ The obstruction is severe enough to warrant relief by intubation in 60% of cases, compared with only 2–18%.

◆ Significant lower respiratory tract infection may co-exist with UAO, and is much more common than the 3–6% reported from the First World.

◆ The frequency of complicating pneumonia is probably related to immune depression from malnutrition, measles, and iron deficiency anaemia — all common concomitants of LTB in a developing country.

◆ The ultimate result of these adverse factors is a mortality rate of 6–20% of children who require intubation, compared with Western series of less than 2%.

Acute bacterial epiglottitis

This is an uncommon cause of airway obstruction, but the mortality is extremely high if the disease

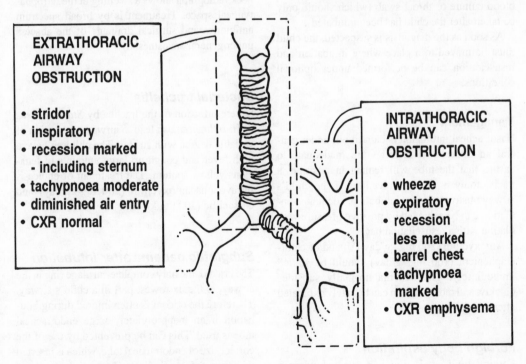

EXTRATHORACIC AIRWAY OBSTRUCTION

- stridor
- inspiratory
- recession marked
  - including sternum
- tachypnoea moderate
- diminished air entry
- CXR normal

INTRATHORACIC AIRWAY OBSTRUCTION

- wheeze
- expiratory
- recession less marked
- barrel chest
- tachypnoea marked
- CXR emphysema

Fig. 13.1. Differences between upper and lower airway obstruction

is not immediately recognized. It occurs mainly in 2- to 5- year-old children and is mostly caused by *H. influenzae* type b.

The most important clinical signs are severe dysphagia, drooling, and airway obstruction, with a high fever, and toxicity due to *H. influenzae* septicaemia. The airway patency is protected by sitting in a characteristic position with the head forward, the cervical spine held straight, and the child supports his or her upper body with the arms. Any disturbance of this position during examination of the throat or positioning the child for neck radiographs can lead to immediate complete airway obstruction.

► Acute epiglottitis is a medical emergency. The characteristic 'cherry red' swollen epiglottis confirms the diagnosis, but is not always readily visible. Further examination must then be avoided, as complete obstruction or vomiting may be precipitated. A lateral neck radiograph shows a swollen epiglottis and aryepiglottal folds, giving the appearance of a 'hitch-hiker's thumb'. The hypopharynx is over-distended with air, and the cervical vertebrae held in a straight position.

The causative organism can be isolated from a blood culture or throat swab (which should only be taken after the child has been intubated).

As soon as the diagnosis is suspected, the child must be moved to a place where intubation and resuscitation can be performed under optional conditions.

Management

Nasotracheal intubation is carried out under general anaesthesia. If facilities are inadequate to ensure that the tube will remain in position, a tracheotomy is a safer procedure. If the child's airway obstructs before intubation, adequate ventilation can be achieved by positive pressure ventilation with a resuscitation bag.

Amoxycillin (200 mg/kg/day IV) and/or chloramphenicol (100 mg/kg/day) should be started immediately. The oedema normally subsides quickly, and most children can be safely extubated after 36–48 hours.

Foreign body aspiration

Foreign body aspiration is suspected when a healthy child suddenly develops stridor and severe airway obstruction, requiring immediate therapy. If life-threatening airway obstruction is present and the foreign body is not removed by a Heimlich manoeuvre, or by placing the child over the knee and giving a few hard thumps on the back, the child must be intubated immediately and the foreign body forced into one of the bronchi. This relieves the laryngeal obstruction, and the child can be transported safely to a hospital where removal by a bronchoscopy can be performed.

Oesophageal foreign bodies also cause stridor by displacing the tracheo-oesophaegeal membrane anteriorly into the lumen of the trachea.

Retropharyngeal abscess

Lymph nodes in the prevertebral space drain the nasopharynx and posterior nasal passages. Abscess formation in these glands can lead to obstruction of the upper airways. The children are toxic, have dysphagia, hyperextension of the head, noisy breathing, and enlarged submandibular and cervical glands. On examination of the throat the large retropharyngeal mass is visible. A lateral neck radiograph shows a swelling in the retropharyngeal space. Treatment is by broad spectrum antibiotics and surgical drainage of the abscess under general anaesthesia.

Bacterial tracheitis

Severe infection of the trachea by *Staph. aureus* or *H. influenzae* can lead to airway obstruction of variable degree with stridor. The children have a high fever and cough up large amounts of tenacious yellow sputum. The treatment of choice is intravenous amoxycillin (200 mg/kg/day) and cloxacillin (100 mg/kg/day).

Subglottic oedema after intubation

The cricoid, the only complete cartilage ring in the airway, is the narrowest part in a child's airway. Therefore the cricoid is often injured during intubation if an inappropriately large endotracheal tube is used. This can be prevented by use of the correct size of endotracheal tube, which is inserted without any force (indicated by an air leak around the tube after it has been inserted).

Smoke inhalation (thermal trauma)

Acute upper airway obstruction (UAO) from laryngeal or tracheal oedema can occur following inhalation of hot air, smoke, or chemical fumes, especially if the patient is confined in a closed space. Various noxious gases may be generated from the material burnt. Combustion of wood generates carbon monoxide, which combines with haemoglobin, resulting in low arterial oxygen content in the absence of cyanosis, which may cause hypoxaemic cerebral damage. Other gases (e.g., aldehydes) cause local pulmonary tissue damage. Bronchiolitis and alveolitis may also occur, with wheezing and crackles. There may be an interval of some hours between smoke inhalation and onset of respiratory manifestations.

Management

Breathing pure oxygen will reverse carbon monoxide intoxication. If burns of the face and mouth are present, UAO is very likely to develop, and early intubation of the trachea is recommended. If respiratory insufficiency supervenes from thermal trauma to the lung, mechanical ventilation is also needed. Bronchodilators by nebulization may be helpful, but anti-inflammatory action of corticosteroids has not been shown to be useful.

Laryngeal papillomatosis

Warty tumours may grow in any portion of the larynx, and usually involve the vocal cords. Airway obstruction may occur, especially if viral upper respiratory infection is superimposed. These symptoms are usually preceded by a period of hoarseness or aphonia.

Intrathoracic airway obstruction

Lower airway obstruction is characterized by expiratory wheezing, and can be caused by obstruction of the small airways (bronchioles) or of larger airways *(see Table 13.9 and Fig. 13.1)*. The most common cause of lower airway obstruction in children under 1 year is acute viral bronchiolitis, while asthma is the commonest cause in older children.

Table 13.9   Intrathoracic airway obstruction

Large airways	Small airways
Foreign body inhalation	Acute viral bronchiolitis
TB gland obstruction	Asthma
Congenital abnormalities	Pneumonia with eosinophilia
Anomalous artery	Aspiration pneumonia
Bronchogenic cyst	Cardiac failure
Tracheomalacia	Cystic fibrosis
	Bronchiectasis

Acute viral bronchiolitis

Infection of the bronchioli, usually by the respiratory syncytial virus (RSV), has a peak incidence in children between 3 and 4 months of age in developed countries, and a few months later in developing countries, but it can occur up to 2 years of age. Adenovirus bronchiolitis is also common in poor communities. Bronchiolitis occurs most in autumn and winter, especially in overcrowded homes and crèches.

RSV infection causes mucosal oedema and epithelial desquamation of the bronchioli, leading to small airway obstruction with increased airway resistance and air trapping.

Clinical picture

The infection starts with an upper respiratory tract infection (URTI), especially when other family members have a cold. The child develops a cough, tachypnoea, a low-grade fever, and in severe cases feeding difficulties.

On examination, the child has a barrel chest as a result of air trapping, widespread expiratory wheeze, and bilateral crackles. Only children with severe tachypnoea (> 50/minute) or feeding difficulties require admission to hospital. Severe airway obstruction resolves within 3–5 days.

Diagnosis

Diagnosis is clinical, with identification of the virus being of little practical importance. A chest radiograph will exclude other causes of airway obstruction, and the picture of acute bronchiolitis is that of air trapping — as illustrated by flat diaphragms and air visible in the retrosternal space on a lateral X-ray. Mucus plugging can cause segmental and lobar collapse, which is often confused with the radiological picture of broncho-pneumonia. The severity can be determined by checking arterial blood gases.

Treatment

The treatment is supportive:

◆ Enough oxygen to prevent hypoxia.

◆ Fluids given by mouth or nasogastric tube, except in the tachypnoeic children. Intravenous fluid is restricted to 60 ml/kg/day to prevent development of inappropriate ADH secretion.

◆ A trial with nebulized ipratropium bromide is warranted, as 40% of children benefit. Nebulization is discontinued in those who do not respond. Steroids are not helpful.

◆ Antibiotics are not indicated unless:

— white cell count is > 15.0 x 10^9/l

— temperature is 38.5 ^{o}C

— there is patchy opacification on chest radiograph.

◆ Ventilation for respiratory failure (rarely required).

Long-term sequelae

◆ About 50% of affected children will have further attacks of lower airway obstruction.

◆ A greater percentage of children who had acute bronchiolitis will develop asthma than of those who did not have symptomatic bronchiolitis.

◆ Bronchiolitis obliterans develops in a small proportion, especially following adenovirus infection. These children remain symptomatic for months after the acute attack, with constant expiratory wheezing and bilateral crackles. The chest radiograph shows air trapping with perihilar streaking. Some children present with repeated attacks of pneumonia. The diagnosis can be confirmed by means of a radioisotope ventilation scan. These children sometimes respond to oral prednisone (1 mg/kg/day), and inhalated steroids and bronchodilators. In certain cases bronchiolitis obliterans leads to bronchiectasis.

Cardiac failure

(Also see Chapter 17, Cardiac Disorders.)
Children with left-sided cardiac failure, especially those younger than 2 years, may present with an expiratory wheeze which results from bronchial mucosal oedema causing increased airway resis-

tance. Narrowing of the left main bronchus by an enlarged left atrium may contribute. The expiratory wheeze and alveolar opacification from cardiac failure is difficult to differentiate from infection.

Cystic fibrosis

Cystic fibrosis (CF) is one of the commonest genetic defects in Caucasian children, occurring in 1:2 000 live births. In developing countries the CF gene, situated on the short arm of chromosome 7, is not common (*see Chapter 3, Genetics and Congnital Disorders*). The children normally start with chronic respiratory symptoms in the first year of life, but this can be considerably delayed. There is persistent cough, recurring pneumonia, chronic upper respiratory tract infections, and chronic airway obstruction. Eventually bronchiectasis develops. Accompanying or preceding the respiratory symptoms children develop malabsorption due to pancreatic insufficiency. These children have bulky, foul-smelling stools containing large amounts of fat and protein. Obstruction of the biliary tree due to viscid secretions leads to prolonged jaundice in neonates, who may also present with meconium ileus.

Diagnosis

The diagnosis is confirmed by a positive sweat test (> 60 mmol/l chloride) or demonstration of the genetic deletion (fragment delta F508 on chromosome 7), which is present in 70% of children with CF.

Treatment

The treatment of cystic fibrosis is specialized, and it is advisable to refer the child to a treatment centre. The cornerstones of treatment are:

◆ regular home chest physiotherapy with postural drainage

◆ aggressive treatment of respiratory tract infections

◆ pancreatic enzyme replacement

◆ high-calorie and high-protein diets

◆ education of the parents and children.

The pulmomary disease is progressive, leading to chronic respiratory failure and cor pulmonale. The mean survival in cystic fibrosis clinics is between 20 and 30 years.

Foreign body inhalation

Although children of all ages inhale foreign bodies, it is most common in boys under the age of 3 years.

History

The typical history is that of a healthy child who choked while playing, started coughing, turned blue, and was short of breath for a period of time. The classical clinical triad of unilateral wheeze, decreased unilateral ventilation, and lung collapse is found in the minority, although in most children an area of decreased ventilation is found.

A normal physical examination does not exclude the diagnosis.

Foreign body inhalation should be considered in the differential diagnosis of the following clinical pictures:

- stridor not responding to therapy
- asthma not responding to bronchodilators
- pneumonia not responding to treatment
- repeated episodes of pneumonia occurring in the same lobe
- unexplained respiratory failure of sudden onset
- chronic cough
- localized bronchiectasis.

Radiology

Only 10–30% of foreign bodies are radio-opaque. Indirect evidence of foreign body aspiration is lobar collapse, lobar hyperinflation, no difference in the volume of a lung on radiographs taken in inspiration and expiration, and decreased vasculature in a lung as a result of hypoxic vasoconstriction.

Treatment

Rigid bronchoscopy is essential for diagnostic and therapeutic reasons.

Suppurative lung disease

The two main causes of chronic suppurative lung disease are bronchiectasis and lung abscess, both of which are uncommon in children.

Bronchiectasis

Bronchiectasis occurs when there is permanent destruction of the bronchial walls due to chronic infection, and is caused by one of three mechanisms:

- Bronchial lumen obstruction, e.g., TB glands and foreign bodies.
- Parenchymal destruction from necrotizing pneumonia, usually caused by bacteria (staphylococci, klebsiella, anaerobes, *Bordetella pertussis*, tuberculosis) and respiratory viruses, especially measles and adenovirus.
- Repeated respiratory tract infections are an important cause in malnourished children, those with cystic fibrosis, generalized immune deficiencies and aspiration pneumonia. At least 50% of children suffering from dyskinetic cilia, a condition associated with dextrocardia (Kartagener's syndrome), develop chronic sinusitis and bronchiectasis.

Clinical picture

These children are seen repeatedly or admitted to hospital with lower respiratory tract infections. Characteristically they have a cough productive of copious amounts of infected sputum. Haemoptysis is rare in children. The history of sputum production is difficult to ascertain, as children swallow sputum immediately after coughing it up. On examination, only those with severe, long-standing involvement have clubbing, halitosis, and are growth-retarded. On ausculation of the chest, widespread crackles and wheezes are heard, although in some cases the signs can be localized to the affected lobe. The expiratory wheeze does not always respond to bronchodilators, because of airway destruction. A sign of advanced disease is pulmonary hypertension, which eventually leads to cor pulmonale.

Diagnosis

The diagnosis is made from the clinical picture, suspected on chest radiography, and confirmed by either bronchography or computer tomography.

The chest radiograph can be non-specific, or show an area of opacification which fails to resolve. Alternatively there may be widespread destruction of the lung, with fibrosis and loss of volume. A honeycomb appearance (small cysts) may be seen in the affected area, which is the result of destroyed bronchi and parenchyma. Bronchography or computer tomography is indicated if there is uncertainty about the diagnosis, or if surgery is planned.

Treatment

Bronchiectasis can be prevented by the correct treatment of pneumonia, early detection and treatment of tuberculosis, and immunization of children. The cornerstone of medical treatment is physiotherapy with postural drainage, continued daily at home. Appropriate antibiotics must be prescribed for lung infections, and the child immunized against influenza each winter. Some children benefit from bronchodilation.

Surgical treatment is indicated if the disease is unilateral, pulmonary hypertension is not present, and the lung function is not so compromised that the child will be a respiratory invalid after the surgery. Clinical indications of compromised lung function are tachypnoea and hypoxia in room air.

Lung abscess

Lung abscesses usually follow *Staph. aureus, H. influenzae, Klebsiella pneumoniae, M. tuberculosis*, and sometimes *S. pneumoniae* infections. The children are toxic, have a high swinging fever, produce foul-smelling sputum, and respond poorly to antibiotics. Amphoric breathing is often heard over the abscess. Chest radiography shows a cavity with a fluid level which must be differentiated from a loculated pyopneumothorax, diaphragmatic hernia, and echinococcus cyst.

Treatment

Treatment consists of postural drainage and intravenous antibiotics (penicillin, cloxacillin, and aminoglycoside). If the lung abscess does not drain, the child must be referred to a tertiary hospital to exclude an obstruction of the bronchus.

Chronic cough

(See Table 13.10.)
A cough that lasts longer than 30 days is regarded as a chronic cough. The cough is a symptom of an underlying disease, and therefore should not be suppressed if the cause has not been determined.

The most common cause of a chronic cough is undiagnosed or untreated asthma. Pulmonary tuberculosis is a frequent cause in developing countries.

Wood fires used for heating and cooking may cause chronic bronchitis and repeated attacks of pneumonia. A chest radiograph is mandatory in all children with a chronic cough.

If no diagnosis can be made, a trial with a bronchodilator for a month, combined with erythromycin, often solves the problem.

Lobar and segmental collapse

Lobar collapse is clinically suspected when dullness to percussion and decreased air entry is present, and the trachea is displaced to the same side. Segmental collapse is seldom diagnosed clinically. On chest radiography there is lung volume loss, displacement of the fissures, and a dense opacification without air bronchograms. The most common causes of lobar and segmental collapse are seen in *Table 13.11*.

Treatment

A foreign body calls for urgent bronchoscopy. Other causes of collapse are treated by physiotherapy, with specific treatment for the primary cause. Most cases of collapse resolve with physiotherapy; bronchoscopy is indicated where this does not occur.

Diseases of the pleural cavity

Pleural fluid

Fluid in the pleural cavity can be either a transudate or an exudate. These require differentiation as their causes differ, and an exudate might need to be drained.

Exudates

An exudate has one or more of the following characteristics:
◆ the ratio of protein in the pleural fluid to the protein in serum is greater than 0.5
◆ the ratio of lactic dehydrogenase (LDH) in the pleural fluid to that in serum is greater than 0.6
◆ the LDH in pleural fluid is greater than 250 IU/l.

Table 13.10   Chronic cough: Causes and associated features

	Aetiology	Other signs, symptoms	Radiograph
Upper airway	Allergic rhinitis	Enlarged tonsils, adenoids	Normal, or bronchi thickened at bases
	Pharyngitis	Post-nasal drip	Normal
	Sinusitis	Post-nasal drip	Opaque sinus
Lower airway	Asthma	Wheezy, night cough, expiratory wheeze, chest deformity	Hyperinflation
	Bronchitis (viral)	Wheeze	Normal, or increased basal bronchial markings
	Aspiration	Wheeze	Increased bronchial marking common
	Cigarette smoke	Nil	Normal
	Pulmonary TB	Loss of weight	Peripheral and hilar opacity, mediastinal glands
	Pertussis	Apnoea in infants, paroxysmal cough	'Shaggy heart'
	Mycoplasma pneumoniae	Paroxysmal cough, often clinical clear chest	Diffuse sub-segmental or patchy consolidation
	Chronic lung disease: Bronchietasis	Crackles, wheezes, clubbing	Hyperinflation, ring shadows
	Obliterative bronchiolitis	Wheezes	Hyperinflation, segmental atelectasis
	Cystic fibrosis	Failure to thrive, chronic diarrhoea, clubbing	Hyperinflation, disseminated densities, lobar atelectasis
	Focal lesions: Foreign body	Onset with choking, localized wheeze	Radio-opaque foreign body, atelectasis, localized emphysema
	Mediastinal mass	Localized wheeze	Mediastinal mass, atelectasis
Psychogenic		Honking cough, ceases with sleep	Normal

A diagnostic tap to determine the nature of the fluid is necessary, and aspiration is done over the point of maximal dullness after confirmation of effusion by a chest radiograph. Other causes of an opaque chest X-ray, such as total lung collapse,

Table 13.11   Lobar collapse: Common causes

TB gland obstruction
Mucus plugging in asthma
Mucus plugging in pneumonia
Foreign body inhalation
Aspiration pneumonia
Bronchial stenosis (acquired and congenital)
Bronchiectasis

pneumonectomy, diaphragmatic paralysis, and diaphragmatic hernia should be considered.

Causes of an exudate: Bacterial pneumonia and pulmonary tuberculosis. Common causes of subsequent empyema are staphylococcus, haemophilus, or anaerobic pneumonia. Subdiaphragmatic pathology (amoebic liver abscess or a subphrenic abscess) less commonly causes empyema. Most of the cells in the exudate caused by a bacterial infection are polymorphonuclear leucocytes, whilst in tuberculosis lymphocytes predominate.

Most children with empyema are successfully treated with antibiotics and intercostal drainage. If in spite of this treatment the fever does not resolve or the empyema is loculated, an open drainage under general anaesthesia is needed.

Tuberculous effusions do not need intercostal drainage. If the child is very short of breath, drainage by needle aspiration is usually sufficient *(see Chapter 9, Tuberculosis)*.

Transudates

A transudate is usually associated with conditions of fluid overload or severe hypoproteinaemia. The most common causes are left-sided cardiac failure, nephrosis, and renal and liver failure. Transudates have very few cells in them, and do not need drainage unless the patient is very short of breath.

Pneumothorax

Spontaneous pneumothoraces occur during staphyloccal pneumonia, acute asthma attack, pneumatocele rupture, or following hydrocarbon inhalation pneumonia. Chest wall trauma or mechanical ventilation injury to the lung may cause a pneumothorax. Clinical signs are sudden dyspnoea, tympanic note to chest percussion, with decreased air entry and shifting of the trachea to the opposite side. A tension pneumothorax is present when shock results from a decrease in venous return to the right side of the heart. The diagnosis is confirmed on chest radiograph. Treatment is by inserting an intercostal tube with an underwater seal *(see below)*.

Congenital abnormalities of the respiratory system

Congenital abnormalities should be considered in children who present with:
♦ unexplained stridor
♦ unexplained shortness of breath
♦ repeated respiratory tract infections, especially if cavities are seen on the chest radiograph
♦ expiratory wheeze not responding to bronchodilators
♦ unexplained opacification on chest radiograph, especially if it has been present since birth.

The commonest congenital abnormalities are choanal atresia, subglottic stenosis, congenital lobar emphysema, bronchogenic cyst, lobar sequestration, diaphragmatic hernia, and eventration of the diaphragm.

More detail on congenital abnormalities of the respiratory system is given in *Chapter 5, Newborns*.

Long-term effects of respiratory disease

Children suffering from respiratory disease in developing countries have a 50% chance of developing long-term symptoms and radiological abnormalities, especially following post-measles pneumonia.

Ten years after hydrocarbon inhalation and acute viral bronchiolitis, small airway disease persists, making these children vulnerable to any further insults to their lungs. A high proportion of adults suffering from chronic bronchitis have symptoms dating back to childhood.

Long-term effects can be prevented by immunization of children, parental education about acute respiratory infections, limiting the use of biofuels for heating and cooking by electrification of homes, limiting environmental pollution, making parents aware of the hazards of smoking, and having health care available and accessible so that children with acute respiratory infections can receive immediate attention.

Respiratory emergencies

Tension pneumothorax

Tension pneumothorax requires immediate needle aspiration of pleural air. The needle is inserted into the second or third intercostal space, between midclavicular and anterior axillary lines. This is followed by chest tube insertion and underwater seal.

Near drowning

Hypoxaemia begins within seconds of submersion; ineffective circulation follows within 2–4 minutes, and irreversible central nervous system changes about 5 minutes later. Laryngospasm initially prevents aspiration, but when this relaxes, water enters the lungs.

On-the-spot first aid

Remove any foreign material from mouth and pharynx with a finger, and initiate ventilation by mouth-to-mouth breathing. If no palpable heart beat is present, external cardiac massage is started and mouth-to-mouth breathing continued in transit to hospital. In hospital, cardiopulmonary resuscitation is undertaken as outlined in 'Respiratory arrest' *(see below)*.

All patients should be kept in hospital at least overnight. Stiff, surfactant-deficient lungs may occur, and mechanical ventilation with positive end-expiratory-pressure is then indicated.

Respiratory arrest

Respiratory arrest may result from the many causes of respiratory failure *(see Table 13.12)*.

Two vital factors in emergency care and resuscitation of such cases are:

◆ adequate preparation and maintenance of equipment

◆ an organized response by personnel involved.

Steps

◆ Clear the airway with laryngoscope and suction catheter. If equipment is not immediately available, turn head to side and sweep out mouth with a finger. Keep head turned to prevent re-accumulation of material in hypopharynx.

◆ Carry out 5-second, external cardiac massage (15 compressions).

Table 13.12 Causes of respiratory failure

Newborn problems *(see Chapter 5, Newborns)*
Older children
   Respiratory
      Laryngotracheobronchitis
      Acute epiglottitis
      Pneumonia
      Pneumothorax, pyopneumothorax
      Status asthmaticus
      Aspiration of vomit, blood, foreign body
   Central nervous system
      Encephalitis
      Status epilepticus
      Cerebral tumour, raised intracranial pressure
      Infective polyneuritis
      Poliomyelitis
      Tetanus
   Cardiovascular
      Haemorrhagic shock
      Acute cardiac failure
      Arrhythmias (including digitalis poisoning)
   Trauma
      Head and chest injury
      Drowning

◆ Then ventilate by mouth-to-mouth or bag and mask method.

◆ One worker performs external cardiac massage, while the other ventilates the patient. If the bag and mask or mouth-to-mouth breathing does not produce good chest movement, or if rapid restoration of spontaneous breathing does not occur, endotracheal intubation is carried out immediately. Ventilation is then given by bag with oxygen-enriched gas.

◆ Cardiac massage is continued with sufficient force to produce palpable femoral pulsation until a good spontaneous heart beat occurs.

◆ Cardiac stimulants are indicated if heart action is not restored promptly:

Adrenaline 1:10 000 solution: 1–3 ml IV or into the endotracheal tube;

Calcium gluconate 10%: <5 kg 1 ml, >5 kg 1 ml/10 kg IV;

or

Calcium chloride 10%: 0.2 ml/kg to a maximum of 10 ml;

Sodium bicarbonate mmols: 0.3 x body weight (kg) x base deficit;

Dopamine 5–10 µg/kg/min can be added by the IV route.

Management of sequelae

Prompt recovery: Assistance should not be withdrawn too rapidly after recovery from apnoea, since respiration may be inadequate for a short period.

Delayed recovery: Prolonged mechanical ventilation may be necessary before there is recovery of adequate spontaneous ventilation.

Measures to prevent or minimize reactive cerebral oedema should be instituted early: IV dexamethasone, IV mannitol, fluid restriction, head-up position, and hyperventilation.

Status asthmaticus

See Chapter 22, Common Allergic Disorders.

Inhaled foreign body

See above.

Anaphylactic shock

See Chapter 22, Common Allergic Disorders.

A.G. Wesley
R.P. Gie

14

Ear, nose, and throat disorders

Introduction

Diseases of the ear, nose, and throat form a significant portion of the diseases seen in paediatric practice. There are differences in the nature and extent of disease amongst the various race groups, which are due mainly to diverse socio-economic circumstances: the acute, severe, infective conditions as well as the associated complications are more prevalent amongst the lower socio-economic groups.

The ear

Wax and foreign bodies

Occlusion of the external ear canal with wax is a common problem, presenting with a history of deafness and echoing of the voice in the head. The younger child often rubs the affected ear continuously. Injudicious use of ear buds by the mother often results in impaction of the wax. Wax can be removed either by direct manual intervention or by irrigation. The former method should only be used by a trained person; the latter method is the treatment of choice providing there is no other pathology, i.e., a perforation of the eardrum, or otitis externa. This type of wax should be softened with local applications of either warm olive oil or proprietary preparations available for dissolving wax, e.g., Cerumol® or Waxsol®. After the wax has softened, the ear may be syringed.

Foreign bodies are often inserted into the ear by children. They may be organic or inorganic. Organic foreign bodies, e.g., beads or stones, should be carefully removed manually, with a right-angled pick or burette. Should these not be available, an 18 gauge needle can have the tip bent by pressing it against a solid object, thus fashioning a pick. Attempted grasping with crocodile forceps may force the object against the tympanic membrane and damage it *(see Fig. 14.1)*. Loose inorganic objects may be syringed out of the ear.

Organic foreign bodies are hygroscopic and produce swelling of the external canal, with

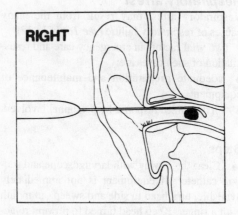

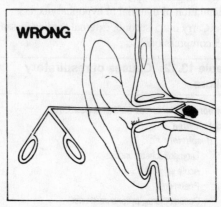

Fig. 14.1   Removal of a foreign body from the ear

infection. These should be removed directly, or if there is difficulty in removing them and they are impacted, the patient should be referred. Care must be taken not to damage the eardrum or ossicles.

Otitis externa

This is an acute or chronic inflammation of part, or the whole, of the skin of the external ear canal, arising from either local or generalized skin disease, or a combination of both. It can be divided into two broad groups:

a. **The dermatoses**, e.g., psoriasis, eczema, etc. Dermatoses should be treated like dermatological conditions elsewhere on the body.

b. **Infections:** There are numerous aetiological factors for infective otitis externa:

◆ the underlying cause of dermatosis elsewhere in the body

◆ trauma, e.g., attempted cleaning of the external canal with a solid object

◆ contamination, e.g., as a result of swimming

◆ allergy, e.g., chlorine in the swimming pool water

◆ maceration

◆ hot, humid climate

◆ structural and anatomical abnormalities of the external canal

◆ chronic drainage of chronic otitis media.

Over 55% of otitis externa seen at King Edward VIII Hospital (Durban) is of fungal origin.

Table 14.1   Otitis externa

Predisposing factors	Treatment
Dermatoses	Aural toilet
Trauma	for diagnosis
Contamination	and treatment
Allergy	Glycerine and ichthammol
Maceration	wick, Kenacomb® cream
Humidity	with clotrimazole for fungi
Anatomical abnormality	Antiseptic drops
Chronic discharge	

Clinical features

These include deafness, itching of the ear, and pain on mastication or moving the jaw. Discharge is minimal, and like wet blotting paper. The ear canal has a beefy-red, swollen appearance. The tympanic membrane is normal.

Treatment

This consists of:

◆ cleaning the ear

◆ drying the ear to reduce the oedema

◆ treating the infection.

The author's approach is to use a bland hygroscopic preparation, such as glycerine and icthammol, which dries out the ear. This is applied on a 1cm gauze wick. Once the oedema has settled, the ear is packed with gauze impregnated with Kenacomb® ointment, or some substitute. Where obvious fungal otitis externa is present, the ear may be packed with a gauze strip impregnated with clotrimazole (Canesten®) or clotrimazole plus steroid (Lotriderm®), or a substitute. Ear drops can now be applied locally – either a bland preparation, e.g., tincture of Merthiolate®, or drops which alter the pH of the ear, e.g., mild acetic acid eardrops, aluminium acetate or Burrow's solution, or one of many antibiotic drops on the market. These are also used for mild infections. Oral antibiotics are only indicated if there are signs of systemic disease such as fever, cellulitis of the auricle, or tender postauricular nodes.

Furunculosis of the external ear canal

Furunculosis is a staphylococcal infection of the hair follicle in the cartilagenous portion of the external canal. Initially there is oedema and redness; later a small, localized abscess may form, with almost total occlusion of the external canal. The condition is exquisitely painful and is noted for pain and tenderness on moving the ear or opening the jaw.

Treatment

In the early stages, when there is only oedema and redness, treatment consists of packing with glycerine and ichthammol on a daily basis until the swelling is receding. Treatment is then continued with topical antibiotic ointment or drops. In the later stages, when the abscess can be seen to be pointing, incision and drainage are carried out, followed by topical antibiotics, e.g., Kenacomb®, Neosporin®. Systemic antibiotics are used only when there is spread of infection to produce postauricular lymphadenitis, cellulitis, or perichondritis.

Congenital ear anomalies

Congenital ear anomalies are relatively common. They vary from pre-auricular sinuses which may become infected, through to agenesis of the external canals, or abnormalities of the ossicles and inner ear. As hearing impairment is commonly

301

associated with congenital ear malformations, patients should be referred for assessment and treatment where necessary.

Otitis media

Acute or chronic ear infections are among the most common conditions affecting children, particularly those of the lower socio-economic groups. Acute otitis media may arise from blood-borne infection, or spread directly from the external canal through a perforation of the middle ear, or spread up the eustachian tube.

▶ Over 70% of infections arise from eustachian tube involvement.

Factors causing a predisposition to eustachian tube obstruction and inflammation are:

◆ upper respiratory tract infections, with adenoiditis and retrograde spread of infection up the eustachian tube

◆ allergic rhinitis

◆ tonsillitis

◆ sinusitis (not to be confused with allergic rhinitis)

◆ deviated nasal septum, with resulting recurrent nasal infection

◆ acute exanthema of childhood, such as measles

◆ poor feeding technique. Bottle-feeding babies in the horizontal position can cause aspiration of milk into the eustachian tube to the middle ear, producing otitis media. This is because the eustachian tube in neonates and infants is straighter, shorter, and wider, relative to skull size, than in older children or adults

◆ pre-existing middle ear effusion may become infected

◆ cleft palate leading to eustachian tube dysfunction

◆ immunodeficiency syndromes

◆ chronic systemic disorders, e.g., diabetes, anaemias, cystic fibrosis, leukaemias, and nephritis

◆ primary ciliary dyskinesia, or in Kartagener's syndrome.

Acute otitis media

(See Table 14.2.)
This has a progression which occurs in four stages, each with distinctive clinical features:

Stage 1: Eustachian tube occlusion: Results in absorption of air from the middle ear cavity, with the patient complaining of a feeling of blockage and deafness of the ear on the affected side. The drum is slightly retracted.

Stage 2: Inflammation: The tympanic membrane becomes inflamed and reddened.

Stage 3: Suppuration: Transudation and exudation occur, resulting in pus formation in the middle ear. The drum bulges prominently. There is extreme pain, which is relieved on rupture of the tympanic membrane, with a gush of pus from the ear.

Stage 4: Resolution, which may be complete or incomplete. Resolution may occur at any stage. Incomplete resolution leaves the patient with either a chronic discharge, chronic perforation or serous otitis media.

Treatment of acute otitis media is always medical.

Stage 1: The patient requires analgesics and decongestants.

Stages 2 and 3: In addition to the above, antibiotics are added. The organism in small children is often *Haemophilus influenzae*, whereas in the

Table 14.2   Acute otitis media

Stage	Presentation	Treatment
Tubal occlusion	Sensation of pressure in the ear Deafness	Decongestant
Inflammation	Pain, deafness	Antibiotics Decongestant
Suppuration		
a. without perforation	Intense pain in ear Deafness	Antibiotics Myringotomy if pain still present after 24 hours of therapy
b. with perforation	Sudden relief from pain on perforation Deafness Purulent discharge	Antibiotics Aural toilet e.g., suction, dry mopping
Resolution		
a. incomplete serous otitis	Deafness	Myringotomy
b. complete	No symptoms	

older child it is pneumococcus or streptococcus. Appropriate antibiotics are therefore amoxicillin or ampicillin as the first choices, but co-trimoxazole and cefaclor have also been shown to be very effective and should be used if penicillin-based antibiotics cannot be used.

Myringotomy should be considered if there is a markedly bulging drum and there has been no response to medical treatment, i.e., decongestants, analgesics, and antibiotics over a period of 24 hours. All patients should have a trial of conservative treatment before embarking on myringotomy and drainage of the middle ear. Myringotomy has not been shown to be of great value, and in a series of cases in which patients were treated with antibiotics alone, antibiotics plus myringotomy, and myringotomy alone, the patients who did best were those treated with antibiotics alone. The patients who did worst were those treated with myringotomy alone.

In a Third World environment we recommend the use of antibiotics, analgesics, and decongestants. A 7-day course of antibiotics and follow-up examinations are essential to ensure complete healing.

Recurrent otitis media

Recurrent infections of the middle ear occasionally cause great problems in paediatric practice. Each individual attack is treated as above. A careful search is made for predisposing factors as mentioned above, and where possible these are corrected. Adenotonsillectomy is indicated where no other cause can be found. Results are unpredictable, but surgery does often help, especially where tonsillitis and otitis occur together. Prophylactic antibiotics may be considered in resistant cases.

Chronic suppurative otitis media

This presents as a painless, continuous or intermittent otopyorrhoea, associated with a perforation of the tympanic membrane and a variable amount of conductive hearing loss. There are two types of chronic suppurative otitis media (*see Fig. 14.2*).

Safe or tubotympanic disease: This is the end result of acute suppurative infection acquired in infancy or early childhood. The perforation is central in type and may be any size or shape. There are episodes of acute infection. The discharge is initially mucoid and stringy, but later becomes copious and purulent during acute exacerbations or if there is any osteitis (*see Table 14.3*).

Treatment: The infected middle ear should be viewed as an abscess, and the basic principle of draining the pus should be adhered to by:

◆ Aural toilet with cotton wool buds. (These buds can be made by twirling ordinary cotton wool onto an orange stick or metal applicator. They are carefully screwed on clockwise so that they can be unscrewed anticlockwise). Care should be taken to dry-mop the ear regularly and adequately so that topical applications do not float on the pus.

◆ Regular suction using a 5 FG paediatric nasogastric feeding tube, if available. Alternatively, the tube should be attached to a 20 ml syringe and the ear sucked out carefully. This treatment is preferable to dry mopping. Syringing

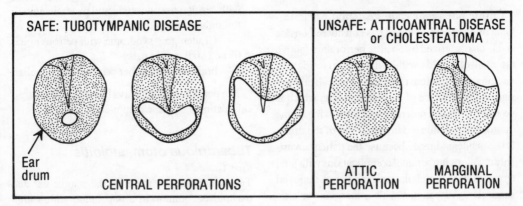

Fig. 14.2 Chronic suppurative otitis media

Table 14.3 Chronic otitis media

Safe
Chronic non-specific suppurative otitis media
Diagnosis:Central perforation (from small to sub-total)
Purulent discharge
Longstanding history
Treatment:1. Medicala. Aural toilet
b. Local astringent drops with or without antibiotics
2. Surgery fora. Failure to dry on conservative treatment
b. Deafness
c. Chronic perforation
d. Extension of disease beyond

confines of mastoid
Unsafe
*Cholesteatoma*Primary
Primary acquired or attico-antral abcess
Secondary

Diagnosis:Foul-smelling discharge
Attic or marginal perforation

Treatment:Surgery only

---

the ear, during an episode of acute otitis media is *not* recommended.

Concurrently, topical antibiotic ear-drops are helpful in drying up the secretions. Systemic antibiotics are valueless, as are ear swabs for culture and sensitivity. Surgery is reserved for those patients developing complications of the condition, such as:

◆ persistence of the discharge, despite adequate treatment

◆ deafness, due to failure of the eardrum to heal, or due to erosion of an ossicle

◆ extension of the disease to involve facial nerve, labyrinth, or intracranial structures

◆ the development of acute mastoiditis.

Unsafe disease or cholesteatoma: Cholesteatoma or attico-antral disease is considered unsafe and is characterized by an attic perforation (above the malleolar folds within the pars flaccida), or marginal perforation *(see Fig. 14.2)*. It always signals the presence of a cholesteatoma, which is no more than an epidermoid cyst growing in the mastoid cavity, due to faulty healing of the drum. It is considered unsafe because the patient invariably develops intracranial complications with fatal termination if the cholesteatoma is not removed surgically. All patients with a marginal or attic perforation should be referred for surgical management *(see Table 14.3)*.

Complications of otitis media
The spread of infection beyond the bony walls of the middle ear cleft and mastoid may occur during acute or chronic otitis media. Complications are most often seen during acute exacerbations of chronic suppurative infections, frequently associated with cholesteatoma.

Types of complications that occur are:

◆ subperiosteal abscess (this is the classical acute mastoiditis)

◆ facial paralysis

◆ labyrinthitis

◆ intracranial extension with:

— subdural, extradural abscess

— acute meningitis

— thrombophlebitis of the sigmoid sinus, with resultant septicaemia and pyaemic emboli throughout the body

— Gradenigo's syndrome with petrous apicitis and sixth nerve palsy

— brain abscess, either cerebral or cerebellar.

The patient should always be referred for surgical treatment of these complications.

Tuberculous otomastoiditis
(See Table 14.4.)
Tuberculous involvement of the middle ear and mastoid is common in a population with a high incidence of tuberculosis. It is secondary to tuberculosis elsewhere and reaches the ear

through the bloodstream or via the eustachian tube.

Presentation: Tuberculous otitis presents initially with a series of tubercles on the tympanic membrane; tubercles occur on the mucosal middle ear cleft at the same time. Breakdown of the tubercles on the tympanic membrane results in the formation of multiple perforations. Progression of the disease results in coalescence of the perforations into a large perforation, through which pale pink granulations protrude. Facial paralysis and cold subperiosteal abscesses occur. Secondary bacterial invasion is common.

Onset of conductive deafness and otorrhoea are so insidious that often the first presentation is that of a serious complication.

Any child of two years or less with a discharging ear and an ipsilateral facial paralysis should be considered to have tuberculous otitis until proved otherwise.

Diagnosis is made on detection of tubercle bacilli in the discharge, or on biopsy of the aural granulations.

Treatment consists of:

- systemic anti-tuberculous chemotherapy
- regular aural toilet
- surgical intervention for serious complications, or for the removal of bony sequestra from the mastoid.

Table 14.4   Tuberculous otomastoiditis

Diagnosis:	Multiple perforations
	Pale granulations with watery
	discharge
	Facial paralysis under 2 years of age
Treatment:	Antituberculous treatment

Otitis media with effusion *(serous otitis media)*

Acute otitis media with effusion (acute serous otitis media)

Transient eustachian tube obstruction may occur in the absence of infection. This may follow on upper respiratory tract infections or allergy. The patient complains of a blocked ear or of a full sensation in the ear. Otoscopy reveals serous fluid in the middle ear, with an air fluid level or scattered air bubbles. Treatment consists of oral antihistamine decongestants. The process resolves in 4–7 days.

Chronic otitis media with effusion (Chronic serous otitis media)

The alternative name for this condition is 'glue ear'. Although the cause is not known, several causative factors have been implicated:

- unresolved otitis media
- eustachian tube obstruction
- viral infections of the middle ear cleft
- allergy or allergic rhinitis
- supine position in bottle-feeding
- hypothyroidism
- certain congenital anomalies. It is seen in 90% of children with cleft palate and 40% of children with submucous cleft palate, and in very many children with Down's syndrome.

Otitis media appears to be the most significant of the above. Some studies have shown that after the first attack of otitis media, 70 % of children still had an effusion at 2 weeks, 40 % at 4 weeks, 20% at 8 weeks, and 10 % at 12 weeks. It has been further reported that recurrent attacks of acute otitis media increase the risk of middle ear effusion. The risk of persistent disease is increased about seven times in children who have had one or two prior episodes of acute otitis media, eight times in children with three to six episodes, and 166 times in patients with more than six episodes. Otitis media with effusion is more common in males, and persistent disease occurs more frequently in children under the age of 2 years. The prevalence of otitis media is very high: some studies in the USA and UK report up to 50% of children developing this complication during the course of a year.

Presentation: Patients present with conductive deafness. This may be reported as disobedience, poor learning ability, or inattention at school. On examination, the tympanic membrane is dull, bears a cartwheel vascular pattern, and may be brownish in colour. The tympanic membrane may be retracted or bulging, but there is decreased movement on Seigelization.

Treatment is problematic; repeated studies using decongestants and antihistamines have failed to demonstrate any efficacy. Similarly steroids or steroid–antihistamine combinations have also failed to show any benefit. Mucolytic agents have been used with equivocal benefits. Autoflation can be tried, but seldom helps chronic cases. Amoxicillin has been shown to be of marginal benefit in controlled trials. This supports a possible infective aetiology.

The mainstay of treatment is surgical, which consists of myringotomy and the insertion of tympanostomy tubes (grommets). The benefit of this operation is that it produces immediate relief from the deafness. However, the long-term benefits of this operation have not been clearly demonstrated. The operation is sometimes combined with adenoidectomy, which appears to reduce recurrence, but long-term benefits are unclear. Children with grommets *in situ* should preferably not swim. Alternatively, silicone ear plugs or a substitute must be inserted.

In summary, the only treatment to improve hearing is myringotomy with tympanostomy tubes. The short-term benefits are inestimable, particularly in school children. Most children improve spontaneously, and the condition is very rare beyond the age of 12 years. Tympanostomy tubes are extruded 4–6 months after insertion. Repeated myringotomies and grommets may be needed in some patients.

Ear trauma

Severe ear injuries can result from head injuries, motor vehicle accidents, or blast injuries. Damage to the eardrum may follow a blow to the ear or sudden impact with water, or the insertion of pointed instruments into the ear. One study showed that 50% of penetrating wounds of the tympanic membrane were due to cotton-tipped swabs.

If there is a perforation of the eardrum alone, the treatment is one of watchful expectancy. The bloodclot is not removed, eardrops are not used, and the patient is advised not to allow water to get into the ear. In the majority of cases, the perforation heals on its own. Surgery is reserved for those patients in whom the traumatic perforation does not heal in 8–12 weeks, or in whom there is severe deafness, suggestive of ossicular disruption.

Deafness

It has been stated that 2% of school children have some degree of hearing loss. This varies from the presentation of learning difficulty to the child who has no speech or hearing at all. More than 90% of hearing loss is due to middle ear problems which are partially or completely curable.

There are two basic types of hearing loss:
♦ conductive
♦ sensorineural.

As conductive hearing loss involves damage to the conducting mechanism, these patients have a lesion which is surgically correctable.

Sensorineural hearing loss involves the organ of Corti and the VIIIth nerve system, and these children may be helped with hearing aids.

Detection of hearing loss

The main role of health professionals in hearing problems is to detect the problem as early as possible and institute therapy as soon as possible.

The most critical period for learning language is the first 2 years of life. If a child has not acquired language by the age of 5, it is unlikely that he will develop it.

If hearing problems are not detected early, lost ground in language development is never fully regained. Hearing aids can be fitted from 6 months of age. The ideal system is to have newborn screening, based on some form of high-risk register, or assessment at the regular under 5s clinic. Children at risk who should be assessed are those with:
♦ a family history of hearing loss
♦ a history of possible intra-uterine infection e.g., German measles
♦ congenital anomalies, e.g., cleft palate
♦ very low birth weight, i.e., below 1 500 g
♦ a history of neonatal jaundice
♦ hypoxia or low Apgar score at birth
♦ evidence of neonatal infection, especially meningitis or treatment with ototoxic drugs.

Before any child is labelled as having mental retardation, autism, auditory agnosia or developmental speech delay, a hearing test is required. Verbal communication depends on hearing; in the past many children have been labelled with one of the above conditions without proper assessment. Any child suspected of deafness should be referred to a competent otologist for assessment and early treatment, in order to allow for proper development.

Communication sets humans apart from other animals, and hearing is an integral part of communication. Hearing puts us in contact with the animate world and with abstract thought. Adequate development of communication skills is severely handicapped by poor hearing in the child. All children who are at risk of deafness, or where there is parental suspicion of deafness, or who have failed to acquire speech by 2 years, or who have a very indistinct speech between 2 and 3 years of age, must be referred to a competent professional for assessment and management.

For screening procedures *see Chapter 2, Growth and Development*. Any patient failing simple screening tests must be referred to a professional audiologist for further assessment.

Facial paralysis

Facial paralysis is one of the most distressing conditions which can affect people. Because the facial nerve passes through the mastoid bone, many otological problems produce a lower motor neurone facial paralysis. The most common cause of a lower motor neurone paralysis is Bell's palsy, which is an idiopathic condition which presents without warning. Often there is a history of having had a draught on the ear of the affected side a few hours before, or of having had pain in the affected ear. Apart from the facial palsy, there are no clinical signs.

Treatment is controversial, and in controlled trials no treatment has been shown to be superior to placebo. Nevertheless, a modified Tavener regime may be of value: decreasing doses of prednisone adjusted to the patient's weight are given over a period of two weeks. Not all facial palsies are Bell's palsy, and the other causes of facial paralysis should be borne in mind, lest the treatment do more harm than good. The other common causes of facial palsy are:

- otitis media and mastoiditis
- trauma
- tumours, either of the mastoid or cerebellopontine angle
- herpes zoster oticus or Ramsay Hunt syndrome

- tuberculous mastoiditis.

Otological opinion should be sought for any of the above conditions, as surgery may be indicated to improve the condition or facilitate the return of normal function.

The nose

Congenital malformations

The most important congenital malformation is that of congenital choanal atresia or atresia of the posterior nares. This is said to be due to the persistence of the primitive bucconasal membrane. It may be bony, membranous, or mixed. Commonly it is bilateral.

Clinical features: Unilateral atresia may present with nasal obstruction, which goes unnoticed for many years, accompanied by an excessive nasal discharge which is tenacious and glue-like on the obstructed side. Bilateral atresia is evident at birth, presenting as cyclical dysphyxia, consisting of a quiescent period, followed by one of asphyxia which is relieved by mouth breathing. Often the presentation is one of a child who goes blue at rest and pink on crying. There may be delayed symptoms of failure to develop taste and smell.

At birth all children should have their nasal passage patency tested by the passage of a nasogastric tube through the nares and postnasal space. If there is an obstruction, contrast radiography should be performed.

Unilateral atresia may also present with persistent rhinorrhoea from the affected side.

Early supportive **treatment** consists of strapping an airway into the mouth or passing an orolaryngeal tube. Surgical correction of the defect should be undertaken as soon as possible. Tube-feeding through an orogastric tube is essential until the baby can swallow normally.

Blockage of the nose

Acute viral rhinitis

The common cold is the most frequent infectious human disease, with its highest incidence in early childhood. It is a viral infection, conveyed by contact or airborne droplets, and is usually complicated by secondary bacterial infection. In a non-complicated case, full resolution occurs in

5–10 days. Secondary infection may spread through the mucosal lymphatics to the whole of the respiratory tract, including the middle ear cleft, resulting in otitis, sinusitis, or bronchitis.

Treatment

Prophylactic: contact with known cases should be avoided.

Therapeutic: analgesics and decongestants, of which oral antihistamines, with or without ephedrine, are of value.

Antibiotics should be reserved for the treatment of secondary infections.

Steam inhalations and vasoconstrictive nose drops may give temporary relief, but should not be abused. Acute viral rhinitis is a serious problem in the neonate, particularly in those of low birth weight. Because of obligatory nose-breathing, feeding becomes a problem, causing choking and consequently pneumonia. Lower respiratory infections are thus common complications of acute viral rhinitis in this group. Avoiding contact with affected individuals is thus of prime importance.

Persistent rhinitis in newborns

This must be differentiated from persistent noisy breathing, which may be obstructive in origin or due to choanal atresia or rhinitis. Most newborns are nasal breathers, and if there is nasal congestion they may become irritable and dyspnoeic. Babies gradually learn to become mouth breathers as well as nasal breathers by the age of 5 – 6 months.

Rhinitis can be due to various causes, including:
♦ transient, idiopathic, stuffy nose of the newborn, with a mucoid or clear nasal discharge, is a condition which lasts about 3 weeks. Treatment consists of normal saline nose drops which can be instilled and after several minutes removed with cotton-tipped applicators or sucked out with a mucus extractor. If there are feeding problems, 0.25% ephedrine nose drops may be given just prior to feeding
♦ the effect of a drug the mother is taking, e.g., beta-blocker
♦ chemical rhinitis (rhinitis medicamentosa) from irritative nose drops
♦ pyogenic rhinitis. Babies may develop a clear or mucoid discharge with infection, rather than a

purulent discharge, and diagnosis is made on culture of the discharge
♦ congenital syphilis. The discharge presents before 6 weeks of age. Diagnosis is made on serology of the mother
♦ hypothyroidism
♦ nasal fractures secondary to birth trauma.

Chronic recurrent viral rhinitis

Changing social and economic patterns have resulted in more and more families with both parents working and the children left in day-care centres, crèches and nursery schools from a very early age. Chronic rhinitis is very common amongst this group of children. There are a large number of viruses which cause infective rhinitis, and rhinoviruses have many different antigenic serotypes. Adenovirus may chronically infect lymphoid tissue and explain the chronicity of symptoms and failure of antibiotic therapy. Recurrent infection is the commonest cause of chronicity. Secondary bacterial infection often supervenes. The close proximity of children in these groups results in continuous reinfection and chronicity.

Treatment is symptomatic, and prevention of repeated infection can be attained by removing the child from the group temporarily.

Allergic rhinitis

See Chapter 22, Common Allergic Disorders.

Mouth breathing

Children are often brought in with the complaint of mouth breathing or snoring. The common causes are allergic rhinitis and large adenoids. Only rarely do nasal polyps or tumours block the passages. The former appear as glistening grey or pink jelly-like masses just inside the external nares, either singly or in clusters, and must be distinguished from swollen turbinates.

The diagnosis can be made on the history, which will allow one to exclude allergic rhinitis.

Large adenoids can be diagnosed on lateral X-rays of the sinuses. If allergic rhinitis and large adenoids are excluded by history, examination, and X-ray, then the patient should be referred to an otolaryngologist for further evaluation and management.

Epistaxis

Epistaxis is a very common complaint, and most children have a few isolated nosebleeds. Recurrent nosebleeds usually warrant treatment. The most common cause is mild trauma to the anterior part of the nasal septum in Little's area, caused by rubbing the nose, nose-blowing, nose-picking, or some other form of local trauma. It is very rare for children to develop a severe blood loss as a result of nosebleeds, unless there is some underlying cause for the bleed. In such cases, the contributive factor should be ruled out:

- allergic rhinitis
- chronic bleeding disorders
- vascular malformations
- hypertension
- juvenile angiofibroma. (This is a tumour which occurs only in males at puberty, and they present with nasal obstruction, a mass in the post-nasal space, a frog-face deformity, and repeated epistaxis.)

Treatment: In mild cases, the nose can be pinched in such a way that Little's area is pressed for up to 10 minutes. If bleeding persists, pressure is not being applied to the right spot, and the pressure point should be changed. If local pressure is inadequate, nasal packing with 5% cocaine and 1:1 000 adrenalin is recommended. If these methods fail to control bleeding, the patient should be referred for further packing and other measures if necessary.

In recurrent epistaxis, the best treatment is chemical cautery of Little's area, doing one side at a time with silver nitrate crystals or glacial acetic acid. Electrocautery may be used if this fails.

Sinusitis

Sinusitis is one of the most overworked diagnoses in medical practice. Sinusitis refers only to infections of the sinuses and to a specific pattern of signs and symptoms. Most cases of rhinitis are misdiagnosed as sinusitis, and care must be taken before labelling a patient as a sinus sufferer. Allergic and infective rhinitis are by far the commoner conditions.

Acute sinusitis

This is a very common condition. There are several predisposing factors:

- acute infective rhinitis
- swimming or diving
- dental extraction
- trauma
- local nasal obstruction or neighbourhood infections.

Common organisms are pneumococci, streptococci, staphylococci, and *H. influenzae*. Anaerobic organisms have been shown to be particularly important in sinusitis.

Clinical features:
- pain over the affected sinus
- percussion tenderness over that sinus
- nasal discharge with postnasal drip
- nasal obstruction
- oedema in the overlying soft tissues is occasionally seen
- constitutional symptoms, i.e., pyrexia, malaise, mental depression, cough, and foetor.

Diagnosis is made on the history of facial pain, postnasal drip, pain aggravated by bending over, stuffiness of the nose, and on examination, finding pus under the middle turbinate and eliciting percussion tenderness over the sinuses. Diagnosis is confirmed on X-ray.

In the infant, acute ethmoiditis may go undiagnosed for several days, with a fever of unknown origin. In older children it may be confused with headaches due to other causes.

Complications: Acute sinus infections may spread beyond the confines of the sinus to produce a subperiosteal abscess at the inner canthus of the eye, or forehead. The infection may spread intracranially to present with an extradural abscess, subdural abscess, meningitis, or brain abscess. Uncommonly, cavernous sinus thrombosis may occur.

Treatment: All sinuses should be viewed as individual cavities which, when full of pus, can be regarded as abscess cavities. The basic principle involved in the management of any abscess is drainage, plus antibiotics and analgesics. Antibiotics of choice are amoxicillin, co-trimoxazole or cephalosporins, such as cefaclor. Metronidazole should be added. Alternatively, amoxicillin and clavulanic acid (Augmentin®) can be used.

Medical decongestion consists of the use of topical decongestants, applied to the nose every 4 hours to produce decongestion of the sinus ostium. Nose drops should not be continued for more than 7 days, because of the risk of rebound oedema. Oral decongestants, combined with antihistamines, may be used.

Surgery is indicated if there is no improvement within 24 – 48 hours.

Surgical management consists of lavage of the sinuses. An antral washout is carried out with a trocar and cannula. In children it is usually performed under general anaesthetic. For patients with resistant infections who require more than two lavages, or for patients with any of the complications of sinusitis, external drainage is mandatory. This procedure and fronto-ethmoidectomy or other operation should be carried out by an ENT surgeon.

Recurrent sinusitis

The most common cause is allergic rhinitis, but other causes are diving, deviated nasal septum, nasal malformations, polyps, or foreign bodies. In the case of recurrent pyogenic sinusitis, referral is essential.

Chronic sinusitis

Chronic, non-specific, purulent sinusitis may follow a single or repeated attack(s) of acute sinusitis, and may be associated with allergic rhinitis or vasomotor sinusitis as a predisposing factor. It is due to chronic inflammation of the mucosa of the sinuses, and all stages from a hypertrophic to an atrophic mucosa may be found at the same time. Oedema of the tissues may exist, and may be mild or lead to nasal polyposis. Fibrosis of the mucosal lining makes the condition incurable. The organisms are mixed, with streptococci, pneumococci, and anaerobes being the most common. Gram-negative organisms are often secondary invaders.

Clinical features consist of a purulent postnasal drip, chronic nasal obstruction, and headache (especially frontal and periorbital). Anosmia may be present.

Current thinking is that anterior ethmoid infection is the key to the whole disease. Functional endoscopic sinus surgery of the ethmoid is coming into is own as a cure for this condition. Patients should be referred to an ENT surgeon for assessment and management.

Foreign bodies in the nose

Any child presenting with a unilateral, purulent, nasal discharge should be considered to have a foreign body. Foreign bodies are often noted by parents soon after insertion. Care should be taken in their removal. They must be adequately visualized, and care should be taken not to push the foreign body into the postnasal space, as it can be aspirated and the patient may asphyxiate.

The procedure is to pass an instrument beyond the back of the foreign body and tease it out. Irregular objects may be grasped using crocodile forceps. Alternatively, a Foley's catheter may be passed beyond the foreign body, the balloon may be blown up and the Foley's catheter pulled back, teasing the foreign body out. Children with compacted foreign bodies should be referred.

Nasal polyps

Nasal polyps are pale, grape-like masses appearing in the middle meatus. They may be secondary to infection and/or allergy. They also occur in aspirin hypersensitivity and in mucoviscidosis. Nasal polyps are rare in children. All cases should be referred for management.

Fractured nose

The nose is very commonly injured in children who often fall or suffer a blow to the nose. The majority of blows to the nose result in swelling and haematoma without a fracture. Persistent nosebleeding, instability of the bones, or a sensation of crepitus suggests that a fracture is present. Marked deviation of the nose or marked depression of the nose confirms the diagnosis of a fracture. Furthermore, if the parents feel the nose looks abnormal after the oedema has settled, a fracture must be suspected.

Examination of the nose may reveal a septal injury with a fracture or a dislocation. X-rays are not usually helpful. Any patient with a suspected nasal fracture should be referred for treatment. The fracture should be set within the first seven days. Failure to set the fracture can result in severe deformity, which becomes progressively worse as the child grows up, and is accompanied by a severe septal deviation and nasal obstruction.

A greenstick fracture may result in a similar deformity. It is important to note that the fracture can be set within the first week, but that where there has been a delay, one may have to wait until the child is 15 or 16 years of age to perform a rhinoplasty. It is therefore absolutely essential to straighten the nose as soon as possible after the injury.

The throat

Tonsillitis and adenoiditis

The majority of cases of sore throat and fever in children are due to viral infections, which may have a secondary bacterial infection.

Tonsillitis and adenoiditis go through five definite phases of infection. The first stage is that of mucosal inflammation. At this stage 90% are due to viral infection. The second stage is one of cellulitis, in which the infection penetrates the tonsil, which becomes angry, red, and inflamed. The next stage is the follicular stage, in which there is production of pus in the crypts. The fourth stage is membranous, in which these follicles coalesce to form a membrane. The final stage is that of resolution.

The patient complains of a sore throat with fever, difficulty with swallowing, earache, and referred pain.

In infancy tonsillitis presents with refusal of feeds, drooling, fever, and diarrhoea.

Treatment of choice is antibiotics, preferably penicillin, with analgesics and throat lozenges to relieve the pain on swallowing.

Acute rheumatic fever is long known to have been a sequela of ß-haemolytic streptococcal infection of the tonsil. Extensive use of antibiotics in tonsillar infections has been shown to have reduced the incidence of rheumatic fever in the underprivileged. Early use of appropriate antibiotics in tonsillitis is recommended to prevent this condition.

Peritonsillar abscess or quinsy

Peritonsillar abscess may follow tonsillitis. It is thought that the underlying reason for the development of peritonsillar abscess is the presence of an abnormally large crypta magna in the tonsil. The presentation is one of increasing pain, trismus, drooling of saliva, and dysphagia. The patient becomes toxic and very ill. On examination, there is a huge swelling of the affected tonsil; soft palate

and uvula are pushed over to the opposite side (*see Fig. 14.3*).

A serious complication of inadequately treated peritonsillar abscess is a lateral pharyngeal abscess. This presents with a fullness and tenderness of the neck. Without intervention, the lateral pharyngeal abscess eventually threatens life by airway obstruction or carotid artery erosion.

Treatment:
♦ antibiotics, preferably intravenous
♦ incision and drainage, which can be done without an anaesthetic in the clinic
♦ tonsillectomy, six weeks thereafter.

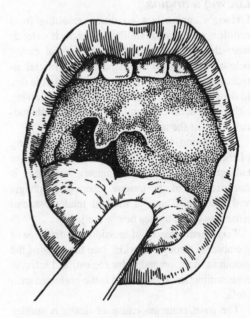

Fig. 14.3 Peritonsillar abscess (quinsy)

Acute retropharyngeal abscess

Fifty per cent of cases occur in children under 2 years of age, due to inflammation and breakdown of infection in the retropharyngeal nodes which drain the adenoids and nasopharynx.

The patient presents with fever, dyspnoea, hyperextension, dysphagia, and a retropharyngeal swelling lateral to the midline. Diagnosis is made on lateral X-ray and confirmed on palpation. A retropharyngeal abscess is a surgical emergency and should be incised and drained in theatre, as

311

soon as possible. Drainage is performed through the mouth.

Tuberculous retropharyngeal abscess

This must be differentiated from the pyogenic retropharyngeal abscess. It is caused by a cold abscess forming deep into the prevertebral fascia, due to tuberculous osteitis of the cervical spine. It presents as a midline swelling.

Treatment: Anti-tuberculous treatment, drainage and stabilization of the cervical spine.

Ludwig's angina

Ludwig's angina is a condition resulting from cellulitis of the submandibular space. It extends from the mucous membrane of the oral cavity below the tongue to the muscular and fascial attachment of the hyoid bone. The infection is due to dental disease in over 50% of cases, following either an abscess or dental extraction. Streptococcus is one of the most common organisms.

Presentation is one of fever and marked swelling of the floor of the mouth. The tongue becomes enlarged, tender, and oedematous, and there is displacement of the tongue, causing dysphagia and drooling. There is marked tenderness and tenseness of the tissues below the jaw.

Treatment consists of incision and drainage of the abscess through the skin, into the floor of the mouth in the submandibular region, and intravenous antibiotics. Amoxicillin is the preferred antibiotic.

The most common cause of death is sudden airway obstruction. All patients with Ludwig's angina should be admitted and the airway observed carefully. Incision and drainage is mandatory where obstruction is suspected. Tracheostomy may be necessary in severe cases.

Salivary gland disorders

Acute suppurative parotitis is a condition which occurs at the extremes of life, particularly in dehydrated and debilitated patients. The patient presents with a red, tender, swollen parotid gland. The diagnosis is made by the palpation of tenseness over the parotid gland and by expressing pus from the parotid duct.

Treatment consists of rehydration and antibiotic therapy. The organism is staphylococcus. A sialogogue such as lemon should be used to promote copious secretion from the parotid gland, to improve the salivary flow and clear up the infection. Incision and drainage may be required if a parotid abscess develops.

Recurrent parotitis

Some children experience repeated episodes of parotid swelling with pain and tenderness. The pain is usually mild. The condition may be unilateral but may alternate sides. The cause is often unknown. Sialectasia may be present, which may be primary or secondary. An autoimmune process may be present in some cases.

Treatment consists of analgesia and the use of a sialogogue such as lemon or acid drops. A short course of corticosteroids may be necessary. Sialography should be performed if silectasia is present; meatotomy of the duct may be necessary. Where calculi are present, removal of the calculus may be necessary. Sialography often helps as a treatment modality. The dilatation produced by the sialogram often cures the condition and may prevent recurrences.

Tumours of the parotid

Any tumour of the parotid must be referred to a surgeon for management. Mesothelial tumours, i.e., haemangiomas and lymphangiomas, are the commonest tumours of the parotid in the paediatric age group. Hard or persistent masses suggestive of a glandular or epithelial origin should be referred to a surgeon for treatment, as 50% are malignant in childhood.

Rannula

A rannula is a pseudo-cyst of the sublingual salivary glands, found in the floor of the mouth, to one side of the frenulum. The name rannula is derived from the frog, and it is a thin-walled bluish cyst. Referral for excision of the sublingual gland is essential.

Tongue tie

See Chapter 28, Surgical Problems.

Stomatitis
Inflammatory lesions of the oral mucosa can be produced by a number of different local and systemic causes.

Traumatic ulcer
This can occur due to injury to the mouth with toys or other sharp objects.

Treatment is oral hygiene, i.e., washing out the mouth with peroxide, betadine, or povidone iodine mouthwashes. Severe lacerations may need to be sutured.

Aphthous ulcer
This is a very common condition with soft, white ulcers in the oral mucosa which occur in crops throughout the year. They can be pin-point size, but can enlarge to 2–3 cm, have a sloughing base with an erythematous margin, are markedly painful, and have a tendency to recurrence. There is a minor and major form. The minor form presents with a few small, single ulcers; the major form can lead to marked ulceration of the mouth.

Treatment:
- oral hygiene
- analgesic lozenges
- topical steroids, such as Kenalog and Orobase®.

Herpetiform ulcers
Herpetiform ulcers form a small percentage of ulcers. They are pin-head size to begin with but when coalesced they form large ulcers. They go on for several years.

Treatment is with acyclovir and oral hygiene.

Oral thrush
This is common in paediatric practice, particularly in small children and infants. Antibiotic therapy or immune deficiency may result in oral thrush.

Treatment is with oral nystatin.

Lingual thyroid
This may present in paediatric practice as a mass at the back of the tongue. On protruding the tongue a mass is seen rising into the oropharynx. This is more common in females and may be the only thyroid present. Thyroid scans must be performed

to ascertain if any normal thyroid is present. If none is present, no treatment is undertaken, as the patient will be hypothyroid after the operation.

Tonsillectomy and adenoidectomy
(See Table 14.5.)
The tonsillectomy and adenoidectomy operation has fallen into disrepute because of its abuse. In the USA, 30% of children have the operation, with only 1–2% having adequate medical indications.

Table 14.5 Indications for tonsillectomy and adenoidectomy

General	Local
Cor pulmonale due to nasal obstruction	Recurrent acute tonsillitis
Rheumatic fever	Chronic tonsillitis
	Peritonsillar abscess
	Recurrent pyogenic cervical adenitis
	Otitis media
	Sinusitis
	Mouth breathing
	Persistent nasal obstruction
	Snoring
	Sleep apnoea
	Suspected tonsillar tumour

Indications for tonsillectomy
General: These are very few and far between. The most commonly accepted is the rare condition of cor pulmonale with adenoid hypertrophy. Chronic hypoxia leads to pulmonary hypertension and right-sided heart failure.

Rheumatic fever if exacerbated by recurrent tonsillar infections, or the danger of subacute bacterial endocarditis are also indications for tonsillectomy.

Local:
- recurrent attacks of tonsillitis; either more than 4 – 5 attacks per year, or persistent lymphadenopathy associated with tonsillitis
- chronic tonsillitis, i.e., patients with small fibrosed tonsils with symptoms of general malaise and halitosis and in whom pus can be expressed from the crypts on pressure
- peritonsillar abscess *(see above)*

◆ recurrent pyogenic cervical adenitis

◆ otitis media associated with recurrent tonsillar infection

◆ mouth breathing, with or without dental caries, which can be related to large adenoids and tonsils

◆ the sleep apnoea syndrome.

Contraindications for tonsillectomy and adenoidectomy

◆ Submucous cleft palate or cleft palate. Removal in this condition aggravates the velopharyngeal incompetence and produces nasal speech.

◆ Bleeding disorders.

◆ Patients with acute upper respiratory tract infections should have their operations postponed. Patients with infectious mononucleosis should not have the operation performed at the time.

◆ During polio epidemics, tonsillectomy and adenoidectomy should not be performed because of the increased incidence of bulbar polio.

A number of invalid reasons which account for the removal of the large majority of tonsils and adenoids are:

◆ Large tonsils — the size of the tonsils is not an indication for tonsillectomy, unless they are so large that they produce respiratory problems and dysphagia.

◆ Recurrent colds and sore throats — tonsillectomy and adenoidectomy do not decrease the incidence of viral pharyngitis, and patients should be warned that after tonsillectomy, the incidence of viral upper respiratory tract infection will be much the same.

◆ Miscellaneous conditions, such as poor appetite, allergic rhinitis, asthma, unexplained fevers, and halitosis are not indications for tonsillectomy.

The larynx
Stridor

Respiratory stridor in the neonate may be due to laryngo- or tracheomalacia, congenital webs, mass lesions of the larynx, or neurological lesions of the larynx.

The patient with an aphonic cry or neonatal stridor should be carefully examined and a direct laryngoscopy performed. Direct laryngoscopies can be performed on children up to 6 months of age without anaesthetic. The majority of cases are due to laryngomalacia or tracheomalacia.

Treatment of choice is a 'wait and see' attitude. In laryngomalacia, the stridor is usually inspiratory and clears up by the age of 2 years. All cases of stridor should be referred for assessment, as no decision on treatment can be made without adequate visualization of the larynx.

Hoarseness

The older child may present with hoarseness and should be presumed to have an acute upper respiratory tract infection in the initial phase. This should be treated with inhalations, antibiotics, and decongestants. If this does not clear within 2 weeks, the patient should be referred for assessment.

Juvenile laryngeal papillomatosis

This is a condition affecting young children, who present with multiple papillomas of the larynx, resulting in hoarseness, stridor, and upper respiratory tract obstruction. There may be a history of maternal *condyloma acuminatum*. All patients suspected of this condition should be referred for management.

C.M.C. Fernandes

15

Neurological disorders

Infections of the central nervous system

Infections of the central nervous system account for the majority of cases of neurological diseases admitted to paediatric wards. Most of these are life-threatening, and the prognosis depends on the rapidity of diagnosis and of therapy with appropriate antibiotics and supportive measures.

Bacterial infections

Acute bacterial meningitis

Despite the introduction of effective antimicrobial agents and the advent of new diagnostic and treatment methods, bacterial meningitis remains a serious illness which is associated with significant morbidity and mortality in both First and Third World countries. In the western world nearly 10% of affected children die, and permanent neurological sequelae are present in over 30% of cases. In developing countries the figures are much higher (mortality 20% and morbidity ranging between 20 and 50%). However, with the advent of bacterial vaccines and recent advances in the understanding of the pathogenesis and pathophysiology of meningitis, the future prognosis for this devastating illness looks promising.

Epidemiology: There are striking regional and geographical differences in the prevalence of the most common bacteria which cause meningitis: in the United Kingdom *Neisseria meningitidis* predominates at present; while in the USA and in most developing countries except those in the meningococcal belt, *Haemophilus influenzae* is the predominant organism.

The organisms accounting for the majority of cases of pyogenic meningitis in Durban after the newborn period, in order of frequency, are *Haemophilus influenzae, Streptococcus pneumoniae,* and *Neisseria meningitidis. Haemophilus influenzae* becomes uncommon after the first few years of life, while pneumococcus is the predominant organism in older children. In the immuno-compromised child, less familiar organisms such as salmonella, shigella, proteus, pseudomonas and other Gram-negative organisms may be responsible.

In neonates *Escherichia coli* and group B haemolytic streptococci are the usual causative organisms. Occasionally klebsiella, *Listeria monocytogenes,* and staphylococci are the infecting organisms.

Pathogenesis: The most frequent route of meningeal infection is via the bloodstream, but the factors responsible for haematogenous spread and for meningeal localization of the bacteria are poorly understood. Bacteria can also gain direct access to the meninges via congenital neuroectodermal defects, osteotomy sites, compound skull fractures, and from infections in adjacent tissues, e.g., the middle ear and paranasal sinuses. Occasionally meningeal infection may follow lumbar or ventricular punctures or the insertion of a ventriculo-peritoneal shunt for relief of hydrocephalus. In these situations the infecting organisms are usually Gram-negative or staphylococci.

Early inflammatory changes: The clinical features of meningitis were previously attributed to a direct toxic effect of bacterial products such as cell walls and endotoxin on tissues exposed to them. However, recent studies in animals and in humans have shown that specific cells such as macrophages or astrocytes within the CNS, if exposed to these bacterial products, can synthesize and release cytokines such as interleukin 1 (IL-1), and cachetin or tumour necrosis factor (TNF), which are responsible for much of the brain damage seen in meningitis. IL-1 is an important endogenous pyrogen, and it acts synergistically with TNF in amplifying the inflammatory response. This would include increasing vascular permeability, inducing CSF pleocytosis, increasing prostaglandin synthesis, and a host of other changes associated with the acute phase response, such as complement activation and release of leucotrienes and platelet-activating factor. This intense inflammatory response results in the well-known breakdown of the blood–brain barrier, and may in itself be responsible for the frequent occurrence of subdural effusion, vascular obstruction, brain oedema, and raised intracranial pressure which occur in association with severe meningitis.

Subpial encephalopathy: Although the causative organisms themselves are not seen to penetrate the brain parenchyma, ischaemic cell changes and neuronal loss occur deep in the perivascular inflammation. The extent and severity of this subpial encephalopathy are probably related to the effectiveness of the host's immune response in eliminating the invading organism.

Subpial encephalopathy accounts for the occurrence of seizures in bacterial meningitis.

Vasculitis and infarction of major vessels: Vasculitis is a common feature of bacterial meningitis, and can be considered an extension of the inflammatory reaction in the pial-arachnoid layer to meningeal and intracerebral blood vessels. Both arteries and veins are involved, but the phlebitic process is severe, and frequently complicated by thrombosis and complete occlusion. Although vasculitic changes occur early, they only become prominent by the second and third week after onset of meningeal infection. Major cerebral arterial infarction, as opposed to pial arteriolar occlusion, is less common in bacterial than in tuberculous meningitis. Cortical venous thrombosis, however, appears to occur with greater frequency in the former.

Extensive venous or arterial infarction results in clinical signs such as hemiplegia, decorticate or decerebrate rigidity, cortical blindness, and stupor or coma with or without seizures.

Moderate to marked elevation in CSF pressure is characteristic of acute bacterial meningitis in children, and the factors responsible include:

◆ impaired circulation of CSF resulting from the accumulation of purulent material in the ventricles and the subarachnoid space

◆ cerebral oedema

◆ brain engorgement.

Clinical features: *(See Table 15.2.)* The clinical picture will vary according to the infecting organism and the age of the child. In an older child, mild to moderate fever, headache, vomiting, photophobia, irritability, neck stiffness, convulsions, change in

Table 15.1 Causes of pyogenic meningitis

Neonates	Coliform bacteria
	Group B streptococcus
	Staphylococcus
	L. monocytogenes
Infants and pre-school children	*H. influenzae*
	Meningococcus
School-age children	Pneumococcus
	Meningococcus
Immune-deficient/ CNS defects	Pneumococcus
	Coliform bacteria
	L. monocytogenes
CSF shunts	*Staph. epidermidis*
	Staph. aureus
	Coliform organisms

level of consciousness, cranial nerve palsies, and, rarely, papilloedema may be the presenting picture. In the very young the diagnosis of meningitis is difficult, and the only signs may be irritability or incessant crying. Low-grade fever, lethargy, vomiting, convulsions, and a bulging fontanelle should raise suspicion of meningitis, and examination of the CSF in these circumstances becomes mandatory.

Table 15.2 Clinical features of pyogenic meningitis

Meningitic	Neck stiffness
	Kernig's sign
	Brudzinski's sign
Encephalitic	Change in behaviour
	Altered level of consciousness
	Convulsions
	Paralysis (cranial nerves, limbs)
Raised intracranial pressure	Headache
	Vomiting
	Neck stiffness
	Bulging fontanelle
	Sutural separation
	'Cracked-pot' note
	Papilloedema (uncommon in infants)
	CSF under pressure on lumbar puncture
Vascular	Focal neurological signs
	'Encephalitic' signs/symptoms

Table 15.3 Features helpful in diagnosis of aetiology

Age	Neonates and early infancy	*E. coli*
	Late infancy and early childhood	*H. influenzae*
	Late childhood	Pneumococcus
Nutrition	Adequate	*H. influenzae*
	Poor	*E. coli*
Associated findings	Purpura	Meningococcus
	Arthritis	Meningococcus
	Subdural effusion	*H. influenzae*
	Convulsions	*H. influenzae*
	Infarction	*H. influenzae*
		Pneumococcus
	Cerebral oedema	TBM unlikely
	History of fractured skull; splenectomy	Pneumococcus
	Congenital CNS lesion	Pneumococcus Coliform orgs.
	Good outcome	Meningococcus

Neck stiffness, and Kernig's and Brudzinski's signs are often absent in the young infant until the disease has reached an advanced stage.

Diagnosis: A high index of suspicion must be maintained at all times. The definitive diagnosis is made by examination of CSF obtained by lumbar puncture.

Careful examination of the *Gram-stained centrifuged deposit of CSF* is crucial in the evaluation of a patient with suspected bacterial meningitis. Organisms are seen in over 80% of patients who have positive bacterial cultures. The sensitivity of the Gram's stain decreases to about 60% in patients with partially treated bacterial meningitis.

The cell count and the concentration of glucose and protein are helpful but not diagnostic, as these may be similar to those in viral, tuberculous, and fungal meningitides. However, bacterial meningitis is very likely if the CSF is cloudy or turbid, shows more than a 1 000 polymorphs per mm^3, a glucose concentration of less than half that in plasma, and raised protein. On rare occasions the CSF may be normal, but if the clinical features suggest meningitis, antibiotics should be commenced while awaiting CSF and blood-culture results, and the CSF should be re-examined within 12–24 hours.

Other rapid diagnostic tests such as counter immunoelectrophoresis (CIE), ELISA, and latex agglutination tests detect specific bacterial antigens in the CSF. These tests are currently used for *H. influenzae* type B; *N. meningitidis* groups A, B, C, Y, and W135; group B streptococci; pneumococci; and *E. coli*. The latex agglutination test appears to be more sensitive than the CIE test, and has the advantage of rapid performance with results available within a few minutes. The latex test may be particularly useful in peripheral units because neither specialized equipment nor detailed technical expertise is required. Quantification of the antigen content by CIE may have some prognostic value, as it has been shown that in children with high concentrations of antigen there is a greater risk of developing neurological sequelae. The rapid antigen tests are most helpful in patients with negative CSF and blood cultures, especially those patients who have received prior antibiotic treatment.

Culture of CSF and blood is mandatory in all patients with suspected bacterial meningitis, because identification of the agent can assist in selecting the appropriate antimicrobial therapy.

In areas poorly served by laboratory facilities, the diagnosis of bacterial as opposed to viral meningitis is made on the basis of:

♦ frank pus on lumbar puncture
♦ turbid or opalescent CSF
♦ low CSF sugar (determined by Dextrostix®).

If in doubt, treat according to clinical criteria and CSF findings (*see Table 15.3*). Although lumbar punctures (LP) in children are generally safe, in patients with shock or clinical evidence of raised intracranial pressure LP can be hazardous, and it is safer to commence appropriate antibiotics once blood cultures have been taken. The LP can

Table 15.4 Indications for CT scans in meningitis

Focal neurological deficit
Prolonged obtundation, irritability, or seizures
Enlarging head circumference
Persistent elevation of CSF protein and/or pressure
Relapse after initial response
Associated purulent otitis media

be undertaken 24–48 hours later, when raised intracranial pressure and shock have subsided.

The indications for CT scans in meningitis are given in *Table 15.4*.

Treatment is directed at:

◆ eliminating the organism by antibiotic therapy

◆ preventing and treating associated complications

◆ general care of the child with impaired consciousness, e.g., tube-feeding, turning, care of eyes, etc.

Antibiotic therapy: The aim is to choose the correct antibiotic in sufficiently high dosage to achieve effective bactericidal CSF concentrations. The choice of antibiotic will depend on the causative organism *(see Tables 15.5 and 15.6)*, but

before this is known all patients over the age of 4 weeks are treated intravenously with either a combination of penicillin and chloramphenicol, or high dose ampicillin and chloramphenicol or third generation cephalosporin *(see Table 15.7)*. Once the organism is isolated and the sensitivities are determined, the appropriate antibiotics are instituted.

If no organism is detected, penicillin and chloramphenicol are continued. The current recommended duration of treatment for uncomplicated *S. pneumoniae* and *H. influenzae* meningitis is 10 days, while for *N. meningitidis* it is 7–10 days. Improvement is evident within 72–96 hours if the appropriate antibiotics have been used. The temperature settles and the child's general condition improves.

Table 15.5 Specific treatment by organism

	First choice	Second choice
Meningococcus	Sol. penicillin 6-hourly <12.5 kg 1 mu 6-hourly IV >12.5 kg 2 mu 6-hourly IV	Chloramphenicol IV/orally Sulphadiazine 150 mg/kg/day given qid
Pneumococcus	Sol. penicillin 6-hourly IV <12.5 kg 1 mu 6-hourly IV >12.5 kg 2 mu 6-hourly IV	Chloramphenicol IV/orally 3rd generation cephalosporins Vancomycin
H. influenzae Beta lactamase +ve	Chloramphenicol 6-hourly IV 100 mg/kg/day in 4 divided doses	3rd generation cephalosporin (e.g., cefotaxime) 200 mg/kg/day given 6-hourly
Beta lactamase -ve	Ampicillin 4-hourly IV 150–400 mg/kg/day given 4-hourly	3rd generation cephalosporin (e.g., cefotaxime)
L. monocytogenes	Ampicillin 4-hourly IV 150–400 mg/kg/day given 4-hourly	Co-trimoxazole 50 mg/kg/day in 3 divided doses, or chloramphenicol

Table 15.6 Antibacterial drugs useful in childhood meningitis

Drug	Dosage	Organisms
Benzyl penicillin	4–8 x 10^6 units/day	Meningococcus, *Strep. pneumoniae*, *Strep. faecalis*
Chloramphenicol	100 mg/kg/day	*H. influenzae*, meningococcus, *Strep. pneumoniae*
Ampicillin/amoxycillin	150–400 mg/kg/day	*H. influenzae*, *E. coli*, *L. monocytogenes*
Carbenicillin	100–600 mg/kg/day	*Pseudomonas aeruginosa*
Flucloxacillin	50 mg/kg/day	Penicillinase-producing *Staph. aureus*
Vancomycin	40 mg/kg/day	Penicillin-allergic patient with *Staph. aureus* infection
Gentamicin	8 mg/kg/day	Pseudomonas, *E.coli*, proteus, klebsiella
Cefotaxime	200 mg/kg/day	*H. influenzae*, *Strep. pneumoniae*, meningococcus, *E. coli*, klebsiella, proteus
Ceftazidime	60–90 mg/kg/day	*H. influenzae*, *Strep. pneumoniae*, meningococcus, *E. coli*, klebsiella, proteus
Ceftriaxone	100 mg/kg/day	*H. influenzae*, *Strep. pneumoniae*, meningococcus, *E. coli*, klebsiella, proteus

318

Table 15.7 Recommended antibiotic regimens for initial treatment of meningitis in different age groups

Age group	Drug
Neonates and infants <3/12	Ampicillin and 3rd generation cephalosporin (cefotaxime, ceftazidime)
Older infants and children	Ampicillin or penicillin and choloramphenicol or 3rd generation cephalosporins (cefotaxime, ceftazidime)

In general, a repeat LP is not necessary for patients who show a good clinical response. However, in those who have persistent fever *(see Table 15.8)* and those who do not respond appropriately, repeat LP during, and at the conclusion of, therapy are recommended. Antibiotic therapy should be continued for an additional 7–10 days if:

♦ the percentage of polymorphonuclear leucocytes in the CSF at the conclusion of therapy exceeds 25% of the total CSF leucocyte count

♦ the CSF glucose concentration is less than 1.1 mmol/l and is less than 20% of the concomitant serum glucose

♦ the CSF protein concentration exceeds 10% or is more than that noted on the initial CSF evaluation.

Corticosteroids and bacterial meningitis: Despite the advent of potent antimicrobial agents, the morbidity and mortality from bacterial meningitis have remained largely unchanged in the last 20 years. In the past this was thought to be the result of microbial virulence, but recent animal and human studies of the pathogenesis of meningitis have shown that much of the damage in bacterial meningitis is due to the release of cytokines (IL-1 and TNF) by the host cells, triggered by bacterial cell wall fragments and endotoxin. Studies done in the USA have shown that the release of cytokines can be reduced by concurrent treatment with corticosteroids. Children treated with dexamethasone (0.15 mg/kg 6-hourly for the first 4 days) were febrile for a shorter period and had a significantly lower incidence of sensorineural deafness 12 months later. Although the evidence to date is encouraging, its routine use in all patients with pyogenic meningitis should await the results of further clinical trials.

Table 15.8 Causes of persistent fever in meningitis

Drugs	Inappropriate drugs
	Inadequate dosage
	Inappropriate route of administration
	Irregular administration of drugs
	Drug fever (penicillin and sulphonamides)
Abscess or phlebitis at injection sites	
Suppurative complications	Septic arthritis
	Osteomyelitis
	Pericarditis
Neurological complications	Subdural empyema
	Subdural effusion
	Brain abscess (rarely)
Hospital-acquired viral or bacterial infection	
Other infections	Otitits media
	Mastoiditis
	Sinusitis
	Pulmonary infections
	Urinary tract infections,
Incorrect diagnosis	e.g. TBM or fungal meningitis

Complications:
Cerebral oedema is a characteristic feature of the acute stage of bacterial meningitis. In the mild case, fluid restriction is all that is required. When antibiotics are given intravenously, it is important to monitor the quantity of fluids. In those cases with severe raised intracranial pressure, hyperventilation, intravenous mannitol and/or dexamethasone may be life-saving. Mannitol is given as a slow infusion, once over 30 minutes at a dose of 7 ml/kg of the 20% solution, and repeated after 20 minutes if necessary. There is a risk of rebound cerebral oedema developing. Dexamethasone is given at a dose of 1 mg/kg/day in three divided doses for a period of 2–3 days only.

As cerebral oedema causes poor cerebral perfusion, it is important to monitor cardiovascular status and to correct shock and hypotension if present.

Subdural effusions: Approximately 15% of children with bacterial meningitis will develop subdural effusions. In the great majority of cases these are secondary to *H. influenzae* infections, followed by pneumococcal and meningococcal infections. Subdural effusions are infrequent in children over 2 years, and are suspected if:

♦ temperature fails to settle after 48–72 hours of appropriate treatment

♦ focal or persistent convulsions occur

♦ focal neurological signs develop

♦ signs of raised intracranial pressure persist after 48 hours

♦ clinical condition deteriorates after initial response

♦ bulging fontanelle or progressive enlargement of the head occurs.

The diagnosis is confirmed by transillumination and CT scan.

Small or moderate-sized effusions need not be aspirated, especially if the clinical course is improving.

Subdural aspiration is indicated if:

♦ the patient's clinical condition remains static or is deteriorating

♦ the effusion is suspected of being an empyema

♦ the effusion is very large and is displacing the ventricle

♦ there are focal neurological signs or signs of raised intracranial pressure.

A single aspiration is all that is necessary; multiple aspirations are not recommended, as even large effusions tend to subside spontaneously. Furthermore, multiple aspirations may actually aggravate the problem by causing bleeding into the subdural space, thereby increasing the volume of the collection.

Rarely, large volumes of fluid continue to accumulate in the subdural space and cause increased intracranial pressure. In this situation the fluid can be aspirated on a daily basis. Neurosurgical intervention is advisable if after two weeks of repeated aspiration the symptoms continue.

Convulsions occur in almost half of the patients with haemophilus meningitis, in a quarter of those with pneumococcal meningitis, and in only 10% of those with meningococcal disease. The management consists of immediate rectal or IV diazepam. Phenytoin or phenobarbitone is used for maintenance in the short term only, as recent studies have shown the risk of epilepsy to be high only for those children who have persistent neurological deficits.

Hydrocephalus requiring definitive treatment appears to complicate bacterial meningitis in about 10–15% of cases. Any pyogenic meningitis can cause hydrocephalus, but it is particularly common after *H. influenzae* infections. In most cases hydrocephalus following meningitis is communicating, and results from occlusion of CSF pathways by the infective exudate. This is most common in the region of the basal cisterns and tentorial hiatus. In about 10–20% of cases the aqueduct of Sylvius or the outlets of the 4th ventricle become obstructed by reactive gliosis and fibrosis, causing non-communicating hydrocephalus. Treatment consists of relieving pressure initially by ventricular drains, and when CSF is sterile by means of a ventriculo-peritoneal shunt if hydrocephalus has not resolved by then.

Syndrome of inappropriate ADH secretion: Hyponatraemia occurs in about 20% of children with bacterial meningitis, due to inappropriate ADH secretion. Symptoms are those of water intoxication: restlessness, irritability, and convulsions. Treatment consists of fluid restriction.

Cerebral infarction from vasculitis occurs most often with haemophilus or pneumococcal infections. It results in focal neurological signs, e.g., cranial nerve palsies, hemiplegia, etc.

Deafness: Sensorineural hearing loss is not an uncommon persistent neurological abnormality. It occurs in about 10–20% of children with bacterial meningitis, and seems to occur more frequently in cases of pneumococcal meningitis.

Subdural empyema and brain abscess: Subdural empyema is an uncommon complication of acute bacterial meningitis, and brain abscess almost never occurs. Whenever subdural empyema or brain abscess and meningitis coincide, a thorough search must be carried out to exclude a primary source of suppuration arising from the paranasal sinuses or mastoid cavities.

Prognosis: Many factors influence the outcome of patients with bacterial meningitis:

♦ virulence and concentration of organisms in the CSF

♦ age of the child

♦ duration of illness before treatment is instituted

♦ nutritional status of the child.

Coma on admission, shock, or convulsions after therapy suggest a poor prognosis. The highest mortality and morbidity are from Gram-negative bacillary meningitis, followed by pneumococcal and haemophilus infection. Meningococcus produces the lowest number of deaths and sequelae.

Mortality is high in children under the age of 2 years. Late diagnosis and treatment due to inadequate primary health care facilities are the most important factors amongst black children.

Of those who survive, about 16% have various neurological sequelae on discharge from hospital. The proportion having complications which manifest later (e.g., mental retardation, seizure disorders, behaviour disorders, deafness, visual loss, etc.) remains unknown.

Prophylaxis: Since close contacts of patients with meningitis caused by *N. meningitidis* and *H. influenzae* type B are at a substantially increased risk of contracting the disease, they should be treated with prophylactic antibiotics *(see Table 15.9).*

Table 15.9   Prophylactic antibiotics for bacterial meningitis

Drug	Age of contact	Dosage
Meningococcal disease		
Rifampicin	1 month–12 years	10 mg/kg bd for 2 days
	< 1 month	5 mg/kg bd for 2 days
H. influenzae disease:		
Rifampicin	1 month–12 years	20 mg/kg once a day for 4 days
	< 1 month	10 mg/kg once a day for 4 days

Prevention of bacterial meningitis by vaccines has been the subject of intense research for many years. Effective vaccines are now available against meningococcal groups A, C, Y, and W135, but not for the group B strains.

For *H. influenzae* type B a polysaccharide vaccine has been in existence for a few years now, but it has decreased immunogenicity in children under 2 years of age — the group that is predominantly affected. However, recent trials in young children of an *H. influenzae* type B polysaccharide antigen conjugated to diphtheria toxoid has been very encouraging.

Recurrent meningitis

Recurrent bacterial meningitis is an uncommon problem in children, but when it occurs a thorough investigation is required to exclude congenital and acquired anatomic defects, and defects in the immune system. Conditions which may be associated with recurrent meningitis or mimic recurrent meningitis are listed in *Table 15.10.*

Neonatal meningitis
See Chapter 5, Newborns.

Chronic bacterial meningitis
See Chapter 9, Tuberculosis.

Brain abscesses
Associated clinical circumstances: Brain abscesses represent the most common form of intracranial suppurative disease in infants and children. The bacteria commonly reach the brain by direct spread from an adjacent cranial site of infection. The most common sites are in the middle ear,

Table 15.10   Conditions associated with recurrent meningitis

Bacterial infections
  Gross anatomic defects
    Traumatic: Skull fracture involving paranasal sinuses, cribriform plate, or petrous bone
    Congenital: Meningomyelocele, midline cranial or spinal dermal sinus, petrous fistula, neuroenteric cysts
Parameningeal focus of infection
  Mastoiditis
  Paranasal sinusitis
  Brain abscess, extradural abscess, subdural empyema
Defective immune mechanism
  Hypogammaglobulinaemia
  Splenectomy
  Sickle-cell anaemia
Idiopathic recurrent bacterial meningitis
Fungal infections (cryptococcal)
Intracranial and intraspinal tumours
Sarcoidosis
Idiopathic Mollaret's meningitis (benign recurrent aseptic meningitis)

mastoids, and paranasal sinuses. Direct spread may also occur:

♦ from contaminated compound skull fractures and penetrating head injury
♦ from facial/orbital cellulitis and dental sepsis
♦ from metastatic spread from a distant focus
♦ through a midline congenital dermal sinus
♦ very rarely from bacterial meningitis.

Brain abscess can also develop as a complication of cyanotic congenital heart disease and infective endocarditis.

Brain abscesses arising from parameningeal foci are usually single and are located in the frontal, fronto-parietal, or temporal lobe, and occasionally in the cerebellar hemispheres. Those arising via haematogenous spread from a distant focus tend to be multiple and occur throughout the brain substance.

Brain abscesses are seen in all age groups, with a peak incidence between the ages of 4 and 8 years. At least 25% of the children have cyanotic congenital heart disease. In black children ear and sinus infections appear to be the most common predisposing factors.

Microbiology: There is a wide variety of organisms isolated from brain abscesses, but the most frequent are microaerophilic streptococci. Other organisms include haemolytic streptococci, *S. pneumoniae, Staph. epidermidis, Staph. aureus,* and Gram-negative organisms. Rarely fungi (nocardia, candida, aspergillus) and amoebae may cause cerebral abscesses.

Clinical symptoms and signs (in order of frequency):

♦ headache
♦ vomiting
♦ fever
♦ lethargy
♦ seizures
♦ focal neurological signs
♦ papilloedema
♦ neck stiffness.

Investigations: Haematological studies usually show an elevated WCC and ESR.

If a cerebral abscess is strongly suspected, and especially if papilloedema is present, a **lumbar puncture** should **not** be attempted because of the danger of coning of the brain stem.

In up to 10–15% of cases the CSF is normal. In the remainder there is a lymphocytic response with normal levels of glucose and a slightly raised protein ('neighbourhood syndrome'). Gram's stain and culture will not reveal micro-organisms unless the abscess has ruptured into the subarachnoid space, or there is accompanying meningitis.

Skull X-rays may show signs of raised intracranial pressure, evidence of cranial injury, osteomyelitis, or occasionally a gas-containing abscess cavity. Sinus and mastoid X-rays may show evidence of infection.

In the absence of CT scan a radio nuclide brain scan provides the most reliable non-invasive means of localizing a supratentorial brain abscess.

CT scanning is the neuroradiologic procedure of choice for confirming the diagnosis, localizing the lesion, and monitoring progression of the abscess after treatment has been instituted.

Treatment: The treatment includes surgical drainage or repeated aspirations, and the use of appropriate antimicrobial therapy. The initial empiric antibiotic therapy for brain abscesses includes penicillin and chloramphenicol by the intravenous route. Metronidazole can be added for infections due to anaerobic organisms. For *Staph. aureus* infections cloxacillin, fucidin or vancomycin is necessary. It should be emphasized that the treatment in the case of brain abscess or subdural empyema does not end with drainage of the abscess, but must include attention to the predisposing cause, e.g., mastoidectomy, clearance of sinuses, etc.

Prognosis: There are few data on the residual morbidity associated with brain abscesses in children. In most American series neurological sequelae were present in from 40–50% of patients. Seizure disorders occurred in over a third of these cases.

The major factor determining ultimate outcome is the condition of the patient at the time of initial presentation.

Subdural empyema

Subdural empyema is less common than brain abscess, but is a life-threatening condition. In the pre-antibiotic era it was usually fatal, but with the advent of effective antimicrobial agents and modern diagnostic and treatment methods, the mortality rate has been reduced considerably.

Pathology: Infections of the middle ear and paranasal sinuses constitute the most common predisposing conditions leading to spread of bacteria into the subdural space. This may result from either thrombophlebitis of emissary veins or by contiguous spread from sites of infection (osteomyelitis, mastoiditis). In black patients paranasal sinusitis appears to be the most common predisposing factor.

Trauma and neurosurgery are less common factors.

Clinical presentation: In infants symptoms and signs are non-specific and include:
♦ fever
♦ lethargy
♦ poor feeding
♦ bulging fontanelle
♦ focal neurological signs.

The common features in the older child are shown in *Table 15.11.*

Table 15.11 Common clinical features of subdural empyema in children

Headache	Universal complaint
Vomiting	Common
Fever	Most cases
Neck stiffness	80% of cases
Focal neurological signs	80–90% of cases

Investigations: Haematological investigations show leucocytosis and a raised ESR.

CSF examination is contraindicated if subdural empyema is suspected, especially if there are focal neurological signs and papilloedema.

Radiological investigations:
♦ Skull X-ray frequently shows associated sinus and mastoid infection.
♦ CT scan is the investigation of choice for confirming the diagnosis and localizing the lesion.

Treatment: Successful treatment of subdural empyema entails a combination of medical and neurosurgical therapy. High-dose penicillin G, chloramphenicol, metronidazole, and the new third generation cephalosporins are the most effective agents. Prophylactic anticonvulsants are

advocated because seizures complicate more than 60% of cases.

Methods of surgical drainage include trephination, burr-holes, craniotomy, or needle aspiration through the fontanelle in small infants.

Prognosis: All patients should have repeat CT scans about 5–7 days after surgery to demonstrate adequate drainage, as reaccumulation of pus is a common complication.

Late seizures complicate adequately-treated subdural empyema in about 30–40% of cases, but the majority show a remarkable recovery from major neurological deficits.

Viral infections

Acute illness:
♦ viral meningitis
♦ encephalitis, meningoencephalitis, and encephalomyelitis
♦ acute transverse myelitis
♦ poliomyelitis.

Chronic illness (chronic progressive viral infections of the CNS):
♦ subacute sclerosing panencephalitis
♦ Creutzfeldt-Jakob disease

Table 15.12 Causes of aseptic meningitis syndrome

Bacteria
   M. tuberculosis
   Partially treated bacterial meningitis
   Brucellosis
   M. pneumoniae
   Borrelia burghdorferi (Lyme disease)
Parameningeal Infection
   Brain abscess
   Subdural empyema
Fungi
   Cryptococcus neoformans
   Candida
Parasites
   Cysticercosis
Malignancy
   Leukaemia
   CNS tumours
Miscellaneous
   Collagen vascular disease
   Chemical meningitis secondary to intrathecal injections
   Sarcoidosis
   Mollaret's meningitis

- progressive multifocal leucoencephalopathy
- progressive rubella panencephalitis.

Viral meningitis

Viral meningitis is the most frequent cause of the aseptic meningitis syndrome, which is characterized by:

- an acute illness with signs and symptoms of meningeal irritation associated with CSF pleocytosis (usually mononuclear)
- variable increases in protein content
- normal glucose level
- an absence of organisms on Gram's stain, routine culture of the CSF, and assays for bacterial antigens in the CSF.

The most common viruses associated with meningitis include enteroviruses, mumps, lymphocytic choriomeningitis, the herpes viruses, varicella, human immunodeficiency virus, and the arboviruses. *Table 15.12* gives the other causes of the aseptic meningitis syndrome.

Clinical features: Fever, headache, vomiting, malaise, drowsiness, and photophobia are the usual presenting signs. Fever, irritability, and lethargy are the most conspicuous features in infants. Generalized convulsions and focal neurological deficits are uncommon in cases of viral meningi-

Table 15.13 Non-neurological signs

Parotitis	Mumps, rarely Coxsackie virus, lymphocytic chloriomeningitis, Epstein-Barr virus, HIV
Rash	Echovirus, Coxsackie virus, Herpes zoster
Vesicular lesions	Herpes simplex
Myalgia	Coxsackie virus
Hepatosplenomegaly	Epstein-Barr virus, cytomegalovirus, HIV

tis. Whereas it is impossible to differentiate the various aetiological agents of viral meningitis clinically, non-neurological signs occasionally accompany the illness and provide a clue to the causative agent *(see Table 15.13)*.

Diagnosis: The diagnosis of viral meningitis depends upon the examination of the CSF. The typical picture consists of a cellular response

(predominantly lymphocytic) ranging from 10 to over 1 000 per mm^3, a protein level which is slightly raised, and a normal glucose level. However, in about 75% of patients with viral meningitis (especially enteroviral infections), a predominance of polymorphonuclear leucocytes will occur during the first 24–36 hours. Moreover, a mild reduction in the CSF glucose content can occur with certain viral infections such as mumps, lymphocytic choriomeningitis, *herpes simplex,* infectious hepatitis virus, and the enteroviruses. Occasionally patients with these infections may even have CSF protein levels in the region of 1–2 g/l. For these reasons it may be impossible to differentiate viral from bacterial meningitis on the basis of a routine CSF examination.

Therefore in patients who have an aseptic meningitis syndrome and who do not appear seriously ill, antimicrobial therapy can be withheld, even when polymorphonuclear leucocytes predominate in the CSF. In such instances the CSF has to be re-examined within 8–12 hours, when the shift from polymorphonuclear leucocytes to mononuclear cells will be demonstrated in at least 80% of cases.

The definitive diagnosis of viral meningitis depends upon the isolation of a virus from CSF, stool, or throat swab, and/or a fourfold increase in serum and CSF antibody.

Management is symptomatic and supportive. The illness usually lasts 1–2 weeks, and most children recover completely.

Encephalitis

Encephalitis is an inflammatory process that affects the cerebral hemispheres. However, many patients with encephalitis also have meningeal involvement, and in this situation meningo-encephalitis may be a more appropriate term. Encephalitis may occur during the acute phase of the viral illness, or several days or weeks later. In the latter case, the pathogenesis is thought to be immunological. In some viral infections, encephalitis manifests years later as a progressive neurological disorder, e.g., subacute sclerosing panencephalitis, progressive rubella panencephalitis.

Aetiology: Encephalitis is caused by a wide variety of infective agents *(see Tables 15.14 and 15.15),* but despite exhaustive investigations most cases (up to 80%) remain unexplained. Of the recorded viral infections, enteroviruses account for almost 90% of cases.

Table 15.14   Viruses causing encephalitis

Enteroviruses	Myxoviruses	Others
Coxsackie	Influenza	Viral hepatitis A,
Echo	Measles	B, and C
Polio	Mumps	HIV
	Rubella	
	Rabies	
Herpesvirus	Poxvirus	Arbovirus
Herpes simplex	Vaccinia	Mosquito-borne
Varicella/zoster		Tick-borne
Cytomegalovirus		
Epstein-Barr virus		

Clinical features: The onset is usually heralded by fever, headache, nausea, vomiting, lethargy, and various degrees of alteration in level of consciousness (drowsiness, confusion, stupor, deep coma). Convulsions (both generalized and focal) and focal neurological signs are frequent, and occasionally abnormal movements may occur, with basal ganglia involvement.

With brain stem involvement, pupillary changes, multiple cranial nerve palsies, and pyramidal tract signs may be present. If the spinal cord is involved (encephalomyelitis), loss of sphincter (bladder and anal) control, limb paresis, and segmental sensory loss may occur. The syndrome of 'acute cerebellar ataxia' may complicate viral infections, and is particularly associated with varicella infections.

Diagnosis: The diagnosis can be made on clinical grounds, especially when signs of mild infection (fever, headache, nausea, vomiting, lethargy) are associated with obvious evidence of diffuse, multifocal or focal neurological abnormalities. The clinical features of encephalitis alone cannot establish an aetiological diagnosis. However, on occasions certain non-neurological signs which accompany the illness may provide a clue to its aetiological nature, e.g., an associated rash might indicate encephalitis due to measles or varicella; a fulminant progressive clinical course or the

presence of a vesicular rash or ulcers on the tongue may indicate herpes encephalitis.

The CSF may be normal in encephalitis, but usually shows a lymphocyte pleocytosis with a normal or slightly elevated protein level and a normal sugar content. A definitive diagnosis is made by isolating the virus from the CSF, stool, or throat swab. As there is an appreciable delay in obtaining the results, these tests are of limited value in most cases. Early diagnosis may be necessary (e.g., herpes encephalitis) where specific

Table 15.15   Non-viral causes of encephalitis

M. tuberculosis
M. pneumoniae
Rickettsiae
Coccidiodes immitis, Cryptococcus neoformans
Atypical presentation of acute bacterial meningitis, brain abscess
Collagen vascular diseases

treatment is being considered. Polymerase chain reaction (PCR) techniques have recently been applied for the detection of enteroviral and herpetic infections of the central nervous system, and are proving to be promising.

Differential diagnosis includes:

♦ other intracranial infections (*see Table 15.15*)
♦ encephalopathy.

When changes in the level of consciousness, seizures, and neurological signs are caused by certain infective, toxic, metabolic, and vascular diseases and the CSF is acellular, the condition is diagnosed as encephalopathy. In an encephalopathic process focal or multifocal neurological signs and neck stiffness are uncommon findings.

Management: Specific antiviral treatment is presently available only for herpes encephalitis. In all other cases therapy is largely symptomatic and supportive, and consists of careful fluid and electrolyte therapy, anticonvulsants for seizures, and treatment of cerebral oedema.

Despite the above, the mortality remains at about 15–20%, and a third of the survivors show severe neurological defects. Many of these patients with neurological defects have had seizures.

Herpes encephalitis

Herpes simplex virus (HSV) encephalitis is the most common cause of fatal sporadic encephalitis in children, and residual brain damage is common in those who recover. HSV accounts for between 5 and 20% of all cases of proven viral encephalitis. Two types of HSV exist: type 1, which mainly infects non-genital sites, and type 2, which is primarily found in the genital region. After the neonatal period HSV type 1 is the principal cause of encephalitis, whilst type 2 tends to cause aseptic meningitis. HSV type 1 has a striking predilection for the fronto-temporal areas of the brain, causing a focal haemorrhagic necrosis in these areas. The hippocampus, cingulate gyrus, and insular cortex are also frequently affected. Occasionally other areas may be involved, including the brain stem.

Pathogenesis: It is not entirely clear how HSV infects the brain. During primary infection it may reach the brain via hematogenous spread, or it may spread from infected nasopharyngeal mucosa in a retrograde fashion along the olfactory tract to the basal regions of the frontal and temporal lobes. In most patients (especially in adults) it is thought to result from reactivation of latent HSV in the trigeminal ganglia, following an earlier primary infection of the mouth.

Neonates are infected during passage through an infected birth canal (genital herpes — HSV type 2), or from ascending infection after prolonged rupture of membranes.

Clinical features: Clinical features are similar to those of other encephalitides. In the newborn, vesicular skin lesions may precede the onset of encephalitis. In many cases skin lesions are absent, and in these situations the clinical presentation is similar to that of other severe intrauterine infections. Outside the newborn period herpes encephalitis (HSE) can present with or without skin and oral lesions. In the latter situation the diagnosis is difficult, but the presence of fever, focal neurological signs (hemiparesis, cranial nerve palsies, and focal seizures) and a CSF pleocytosis with many red cells (because of the haemorrhagic necrosis) should make one suspect herpes encephalitis. Without specific therapy the course of HSE is progressive, terminating in deep coma and death.

Investigations to establish the diagnosis are given in *Table 15.16*.

Diagnosis: Definitive diagnosis is made by isolating the virus or antigen on brain biopsy. However, with the advent of effective and relatively safe antiviral agents, many will question the necessity for routine brain biopsy before treatment is begun. Some clinicians believe that in any patient with encephalitis and focal clinical features, and especially in those with focal findings on non-invasive investigations, treatment with acyclovir (10 mg/kg 8-hourly x 10 days) should be commenced immediately. Acyclovir therapy does not prevent the diagnostic CSF anti-HSV antibody response. The diagnosis of HSV can then be confirmed retrospectively from evidence of specific antibody production in the CSF.

Treatment: The availability of effective and relatively safe antiviral agents for HSV infection emphasizes the need for making an early diagnosis, as prompt treatment reduces the high morbidity and mortality associated with this disease. PCR and viral antigen detection in CSF should lead to early, accurate diagnosis of HSE in the future.

Table 15.16   Investigations in suspected herpes encephalitis

1. Microscopic examination of mucocutaneous lesions: multinucleated giant cells and intranuclear inclusions.
2. Serology: HSV haemagglutinating antibody titres -
3. CSF: Routine examination — ↑WBC especially lymphocytes
   — ↑RBC (75% of cases)
   — ↑or N protein
   — N glucose, rarely ↓
   HSV haemagglutinating antibody titres:
   A serum to CSF haemagglutinating antibody titre ratio of 20 or less makes HSV infection likely.
   HSV culture — rarely positive.
   HSV antigen (ELISA or immunoblot): sensitivity after 1 week of illness 100%, <1 week of illness 60%
4. EEG: Periodic temporal spike and slow wave discharge.
5. CT scan: Localized low density or haemorrhagic lesion in fronto-temporal regions.
6. MRI — most sensitive radiologic test.
7. Brain biopsy: Virus isolation
   Routine histopathological examination
   Electron microscopy
   Detection of HSV antigen (immunofluorescence or immunoperoxidase staining).
8. Polymerase chain reaction (PCR) — high sensitivity and specificity.

In Third World countries, malnutrition and the post-measles state, either singly or in combination, predispose towards dissemination of herpes infection. Therefore if there is a strong clinical suspicion of HSV encephalitis in a predisposed patient, antiviral therapy with acyclovir should be instituted immediately in order to reduce the high morbidity and mortality. Furthermore, as the level of consciousness is the single most important prognostic factor in HSV infection, the decision to treat must be made early, before any deterioration in mental status occurs.

Subacute sclerosing panencephalitis (SSPE)

SSPE represents a prototype neurodegenerative disease of childhood, caused by a measles or measles-like virus. Measles immunization does not appear to produce SSPE.

Epidemiology: The estimated world-wide prevalence is about 1 per million cases of natural measles; in the USA the annual incidence among persons under 20 years of age is 0.35/million, and in the UK, 0.2/million of the total population. The incidence is slightly higher in certain population groups, such as the Sephardic Jews in Israel, and Arabs in the Middle East. It is higher still among the coloured population in the Cape Province of South Africa. Recent studies in Durban indicate that SSPE is more common among black children than has hitherto been realized. In the rest of Africa, despite the high incidence of measles in young children, surprisingly few cases have been reported. The highest incidences have been from Kenya, Nigeria, Tanzania, and Ethiopia.

The vast majority of SSPE patients have had measles at an early age — before the second birthday in 45% of cases, and before the third year of life in about 80% of cases. SSPE can occur as early as 3 months after the initial attack of measles, and as late as 20 years later, but the usual latent period is between 8 and 12 years. Males are affected more than females, and until recently whites more than blacks.

Pathology: The typical pathological findings include perivascular infiltration by mononuclear and plasma cells in both grey and white matter of both cerebral hemispheres. The basal ganglia, brain stem, and spinal cord are also involved. The cerebellum is usually spared. Eosinophilic intranuclear and intracytoplasmic inclusions are the histopathological hallmarks of the disease.

Clinical features: The illness evolves in several stages (*see Table 15.17*). The course is usually progressive, ending in death within 1–3 years. Rarely, there are one or more spontaneous remissions.

Diagnosis: The diagnosis of SSPE is based on a combination of clinical and several laboratory studies:

♦ The serum and CSF measles antibody titres are high: titres of 1:64 to 1:2 048 in serum, and 1:8 to 1:64 in CSF.

♦ CSF immunoglobulins are also elevated. A typical clinical presentation and elevated CSF measles antibody titre are sufficient to establish the diagnosis.

♦ The EEG may show characteristic periodic bursts of 2–3 H^z high voltage slow waves followed by a relatively flat pattern ('suppression burst' pattern). This is characteristic of the second stage of the disease, and usually disappears later in the course of the illness.

♦ *Brain biopsy* is no longer necessary for diagnosis, but in atypical cases it can be useful.

Table 15.17 Subacute sclerosing panencephalitis: Clinical features

Stage I	Gradual impairment of higher cerebral function, poor school performance, forgetfulness, indifference, lethargy, personality change, aggressive behaviour, paucity of speech. Duration 1 week to 2 months.
Stage II	Mental deterioration beomes progressively more obvious; seizures (both focal and generalized), myoclonic jerks, hypertonia, choreoathetoid movements. Duration 1 month to 1 year.
Stage III	Dementia is severe, child is bedridden, decerebrate or decorticate posture, hyperthermia, progressive bulbar palsy, choreoathetoid movements, myoclonic spasms may continue and show flinging character in the limbs, progressive alterations in level of consciousness, respiration may become irregular and death may supervene.
Stage IV	Vegetative state, spastic quadriparesis, no bladder or bowel control.

Eosinophilic inclusions in the cytoplasm and nucleus of neuronal and glial cells are the cardinal features of this infection.

Differential diagnosis includes the various childhood neurodegenerative diseases.

Treatment: There is no effective treatment other than symptomatic and supportive measures. Carbamazepine, sodium valproate, and diazepam have proved effective in the management of myoclonic, generalized, and psychomotor seizures. Attempts at treatment have been directed at the hypothesized defect in immune response or at the viral pathogen, using therapeutic agents such as levamisole, amantadine, inosiplex and interferon, but to date none of these has been shown to be of value.

Fungal infections

In children fungal infections of the CNS are very much less common than bacterial or viral infections. They may occur in normal individuals, but the majority of infections occur in patients with impaired immunity. The fungi most commonly affecting children, in order of frequency, are *Cryptococcus neoformans*, *Candida albicans*, *Coccidioides immitis*, aspergillus, and histoplasma.

Cryptococcosis (torulosis)

Cryptococcus neoformans is the most common fungal infection of the central nervous system. It is a simple, yeast-like, budding fungus which is free-living in soil and often found in pigeon and other avian faeces. Infection occurs via the respiratory tract and pulmonary lesions may mimic tuberculosis or sarcoidosis.

The majority of cryptococcal infections are asymptomatic. Disease usually occurs when there is a serious underlying condition such as lymphoma, leukaemia, AIDS, sarcoidosis, collagen vascular disease, tuberculosis, or diabetes mellitus. Occasionally it may occur in patients who are on steroid therapy.

Pathology: The usual pathology is a chronic basilar meningitis resembling tuberculosis. Occasionally lesions occur throughout the brain in the form of granulomas (cryptococcomas) or abscesses. The spinal cord may be involved and show granulomas. Rarely intracranial calcification develops.

Clinical features: The most common symptoms and signs are headache, fever, nausea, vomiting, mental changes, and neck stiffness. Less common are visual disturbances, cranial nerve palsies, papilloedema, cerebellar signs, seizures, and aphasia. Hydrocephalus occurs with regularity and necessitates shunting procedures. As some patients with cryptococcal meningitis are asymptomatic, the CSF must be examined if the organism is isolated from the lungs (most common site) or elsewhere in the body.

Diagnosis: The CSF picture suggests a chronic lymphocytic meningitis. Characteristically the CSF pressure is high, the protein level is increased, and the glucose level is decreased. In over 95% of cases CSF cell counts are abnormal, with the majority having less than 200 white cells. In over 60% of cases the encapsulated organism can be demonstrated by an Indian ink preparation of the spinal fluid.

The most useful serological test is the latex agglutination test for cryptococcal antigen, which can be positive even when CSF cultures and Indian ink preparation are negative.

The definitive diagnosis is made by isolating the organism from the CSF. Cultures are positive in over 90% of cases.

CT and MRI scans will reveal basal enhancement, hydrocephalus, and mass lesions caused by cryptococcus.

Treatment: Cryptococcal meningitis is invariably fatal if not treated. Amphotericin B combined with 5-flucytosine has been shown to be superior to amphotericin B alone. Amphotericin is given parenterally (0.3 mg/kg/day), in combination with 5-flu cytosine (150 mg/kg/day divided into 6-hourly doses). In general therapy should be continued for at least 6 weeks. In addition, weekly CSF samples should show declining antigen titres and be sterile on culture. Renal toxicity is common with the use of amphotericin B, and bone marrow depression may be caused by 5-flucytosine therapy. Therefore twice-weekly leucocyte and platelet counts are advisable during treatment with these drugs. Fluconazole, a recently-introduced, orally-active antifungal agent, is proving to be an effective alternative to the above regime (dose 200 mg daily for a period of 4–6 weeks).

Prognosis: Relapses usually manifest within 12 months, but can occur up to 30 months after completion of treatment. Nearly 20% of patients cured of the infection will have positive CSF Indian ink smears but negative CSF cultures for *Cryptococcus neoformans*. The cure rate for cryptococcal meningitis with antifungal agents approaches 70%.

Parasitic infections

Cysticercosis

Cysticercosis is the most common parasitic disease affecting the CNS in children, and is endemic in Central and South America, South-East Asia, India, and the Caribbean. In southern Africa the highest incidence is recorded in black children from the Transkei and Ciskei.

The clinical features are extremely variable, necessitating a high index of suspicion, especially in children from endemic areas *(see Table 15.18).*

Table 15.18   Clinical features in 61 African children with cysticercosis

	%
Convulsions	82
Headache	38
Raised intracranial pressure	34
Focal neurological signs (hemiplegia, paraplegia)	34
Mental deterioration	13
Vomiting	10
Pain in limbs	3

(After Thompson *et al*, 'Cerebral cysticerosis in children in South Africa', in *Annals of Tropical Paediatrics* 1984: 4; 67-77)

Pathogenesis: Cysticercosis is caused by infection with the larval form of the porcine tapeworm *Taenia solium*, and humans are the only definitive host of the adult worm. Gravid proglottids are periodically passed in the stool of the host. In areas where sanitation is poor, the ova which contaminate the soil and vegetation are eaten by pigs, the intermediate host. The ova develop into oncospheres (larval form) in the pig's stomach, and penetrate the intestinal mucosa, gaining entrance to lymphatics and veins, leading to dissemination to muscle, brain, eye, and other tissues (larval or cysticercus stage of the life cycle). The cycle is completed when man eats undercooked 'measly' pork — the consumed cysticercus developing into

the adult tapeworm in the upper part of the small intestine.

Cysticercosis occurs when a human becomes the intermediate instead of the definitive host, i.e., he ingests food or water containing tapeworm ova or he auto-infests himself via the faecal-oral route. The ingested ova hatch into larval forms which penetrate the intestinal wall, and then lodge in various tissues of the body (viz. skin, muscle, liver, lungs, eyes, heart, etc.), with the CNS being the most important. In these tissues the oncospheres become mature cysticerci in about 10–12 weeks.

Symptoms, however, may take many months or even years to appear. The latent period is believed to be due to the fact that viable cysts incite little inflammatory response. Death of the larvae usually occurs about 2–5 years after infection, resulting in an increased inflammatory response, which produces the neurological signs and symptoms.

Clinico-pathological features: The signs and symptoms of cerebral cysticercosis are non-specific and varied. This diagnosis must therefore be considered in patients from endemic regions who present with neurological abnormalities.

The clinical presentation depends on three major pathological processes: the mass effect; the inflammatory response evoked by the parasite; and obstruction of the foramina and ventricular system of the brain, resulting in increased intracranial pressure.

For purposes of description the disease is classified into five types:

Parenchymal involvement is the most common variety in childhood, and may be acute or chronic. The lesions may be either focal or diffuse, with a predilection for the cerebral grey matter because of its elaborate capillary bed. The clinical manifestations of parenchymal cysticercosis are therefore variable, and may include seizures, focal neurological deficits, headaches, alterations in level of consciousness, mental retardation, and even dementia.

Meningeal involvement: When cysts are located on the surface of the brain, at its base, or in the subarachnoid space, they evoke an inflammatory response which results in chronic meningitis. Multiple cysts or 'racemose' cysts, which consist of grape-like clusters of proliferating larval membranes, tend to be localized to the base of the brain.

These cysts may obstruct the outlets of the 4th ventricle, producing obstructive hydrocephalus, while the host's inflammatory response causes basal adhesive arachnoiditis which obliterates the subarachnoid spaces and results in a communicating hydrocephalus. Basal arachnoiditis can also result in multiple cranial nerve palsies. Vasculitis with infarction of brain tissue is common in this form of the disease.

Ventricular involvement: If the larvae enter the choroid plexus the ventricles may be obstructed by the developing cysts or by racemose forms. Free-floating cysts may cause intermittent acute obstructive hydrocephalus, with resultant loss of consciousness and posture, brought on by sudden change in head position.

Mixed involvement occurs when there is a combination of parenchymal and meningeal forms of the disease.

Intraspinal involvement is rare, and may present as an intramedullary mass lesion with resultant paraplegia. Arachnoiditis and vasculitis may also be found.

Investigations: Blood eosinophilia (absolute count > 400/mm) may occur in some cases, but its value is reduced because black patients often have other parasitic infestations which may account for the eosinophilia.

The CSF changes are non-specific. CSF pleocytosis is usually present in patients with meningoencephalitis or the syndrome of raised intracranial pressure. The CSF protein may be raised and the glucose level may be lowered. The finding of eosinophilia in the CSF of a patient from an endemic area is highly suggestive of neurocysticercosis.

Two serological tests are presently available: haemagglutination (IHA) and ELISA tests, which are believed to be positive in over 80% of cases. A positive test on the CSF indicates past or present neurocysticercosis.

Soft tissue radiology may show calcific lesions of soft tissues. Skull X-ray is normal in many acute cases, but occasionally may show evidence of raised intracranial pressure or intracranial calcification.

The CT scan is one of the most useful tests, and is more sensitive and more specific than the serology tests. However, the scan appearance is very variable. It may show single or multiple cysts within the cerebral hemispheres, focal or diffuse low-density areas due to death and degeneration of cysts, patches of low density which enhance after administration of intravenous contrast media, single or multiple intraparenchymal calcified lesions, and occasionally hydrocephalus.

For the subarachnoid and intraventricular cysts which are difficult to detect with CT scan, ventriculography with addition of contrast media has been a useful investigation.

Biopsy of subcutaneous cysts is also helpful in the diagnosis of neurocysticercosis.

Treatment: Until the present decade, treatment of neurocysticercosis was largely limited to

---

Table 15.19   Aetiology of cerebral palsy

N.B. The aetiology of cerebral palsy is multifactorial; the most important causes are marked.

Congenital
  Prenatal causes
      *Infections
      *Toxaemia of pregnancy
      *Small-for-date baby
      Beeding during pregnancy
      Postmaturity
      Congenital hydrocephalus/microcephaly
  Perinatal Causes
      *Prematurity
      Prolonged labour with fetal distress
      Perinatal asphyxia (hypoxic ischaemic
          encephalopathy)
      Cerebral birth trauma
      Hyperbilirubinaemia (kernicterus)
      Metabolic complications, e.g., hypoglycaemia
      *Infections

Acquired
      *Head injury (motor vehicle accident)
      *Infections (meningitis, encephalitis, brain abscess, etc.)
      Metabolic- hypoglycaemia
              - hypocalcaemia
              - hypernatraemia
              - hyponatraemia
      Vascular- congenital AV malformations
              - sinus and cortical venous thrombosis from
                  gastroenteritis
              - embolic disease
      Toxins/drugs, etc.

treatment of the complications: anticonvulsants for seizure control, corticosteroids for raised intracranial pressure secondary to acute brain swelling, ventriculoperitoneal shunts for relief of hydrocephalus, and surgical removal of large cysts.

Recently praziquantel, an anthelminthic agent, has been hailed as a new hope for cysticercosis. It is given for a period of 14 days in a dosage of 50 mg/kg/day in four divided doses. Simultaneous steroids are used to prevent the Herxheimer reaction which may complicate praziquantel therapy. However, there is considerable debate as to the role of praziquantel in the treatment of neurocysticercosis. At King Edward VIII hospital praziquantel is presently not used, as our experience of intraparenchymal cysticercosis is that of a self-limiting disease which requires only symptomatic and supportive treatment (e.g., steroids for raised intracranial pressure, anticonvulsants for seizures, and occasionally surgical intervention for relief of hydrocephalus and removal of large cysts). Our experience is strengthened by recent reports of spontaneous resolution of clinical signs and CT scan appearances from other international centres.

The best intervention against neurocysticercosis is obviously one of prevention.

Cerebral palsy

Cerebral palsy refers to the motor deficit that results from a non-progressive lesion sustained during the developmental stage of the brain. Although the original brain damage is not progressive, the clinical picture will usually be modified with age. In the majority of cerebral palsied children there are varying degrees of associated disabilities besides the essential motor deficit.

Prevalence

The prevalence of cerebral palsy in South Africa is not known, but it is thought to be high, especially in socio-economically deprived communities and where maternal and child health care is suboptimal. In western countries the incidence ranges from less than 2% to 6%.

Aetiology

In a small percentage of patients the aetiology is obscure. However, in the majority of cases it is secondary to either a congenital or an acquired lesion *(see Table 15.19)*. In the past, perinatal causes, especially birth asphyxia, were overemphasized as causes of cerebral palsy.

It is now postulated that most of the congenital cases of cerebral palsy have a prenatal origin, with birth asphyxia playing only a minor role.

Types of cerebral palsy

The various clinical forms of cerebral palsy are based on the type of motor involvement, and this depends on the site of the main pathology *(see Table 15.20)*.

Diagnosis

Cerebral palsy must be considered in any infant with:
♦ delay in motor development, e.g., delayed development of head control, sitting, standing, and walking
♦ hypotonia or spasticity
♦ clumsiness
♦ abnormal movements
♦ persistent crying and feeding problems.

Clinical features

Useful clinical clues are persistent palmar thumbing, persistence of primitive reflexes, head retraction (due to increased extensor tone), 'scissoring' gait (adductor spasm), toe walking (increased gastrocnemius-soleus tone), and absent parachute response at 7–8 months (baby does not flex shoulder and extend arms when suspended supine in air and rapidly brought down to the floor or couch).

The tendon reflexes are brisk, and ankle clonus may be present. In children with severe cerebral palsy, feeding problems and drooling may be present because of pseudobulbar palsy. Constipation is common in severe cases.

Associated problems

The vast majority of children with cerebral palsy have one or more associated handicaps *(see Table 15.21)*. Often it is these handicaps which make cerebral palsy such a disabling condition.

More than 60% of cerebral palsied children in the UK are mentally retarded *(see Assessment, below)*. Children with hemiplegia, diplegia, and dyskinesia are more likely to be of normal

Table 15.20 Types of cerebral palsy

Type	Clinical features	Aetiology
1. Spastic (Most common type - 75% of cases)		
Diplegia	Spasticity mainly lower limbs	Perinatal hypoxia
		Intracranial haemorrhage — particularly periventricular haemorrhage in pre-term babies
		Pyramidal tract damage
Hemiplegia	Onset often silent, abnormal fisting may be an early sign	Vascular insult either prenatally or postnatally
	Arm affected more than leg	
	Elbow, wrist, and fingers are flexed, the forearm is pronated, and the foot acquires an equinus deformity	
	Limb asymmetry (progressive)	
	Epilepsy more common than in other types	
Quadriplegia	All four limbs and trunk affected, upper usually more than lower limbs	Perinatal hypoxic-ischaemic insult
	Initially hypotonic, followed in 2 – 5 years by severe spasticity	
	Microcephaly with severe mental retardation	
	Moderate to severe developmental delay	
	Feeding problems	
Monoplegia	Uncommon	
2. Dyskinetic	Involuntary movements often very marked	Hyperbilirubinaemia (kernicterus)
	Extensor spasm	Perinatal hypoxia
	Dysphagia	Basal ganglia damage from various causes
	Signs become progressively more marked and obvious by 1 – 2 years	
	Intelligence may be normal	
3. Ataxic	Limb and trunk ataxia, hypotonia	Cerebellar damage and/or hydrocephalus
4. Hypotonic	May precede other forms	
	Eventually become spastic, but rarely hypotonia is persistent	
5. Mixed	Combination of clinical signs, e.g., ataxia with hempilegia or diplegia	

intelligence. Recurrent seizures affect more than 30% of cases, and visual defects occur in about 25–30% of patients. As a result of the marked constraints placed on the child by the disease, social and emotional maladjustments are very common, particularly if the child is not handled correctly by the parents.

Management

Prevention: The prevalence of cerebral palsy is in inverse proportion to the availability of primary health care, in particular good prenatal and perinatal care; low birth weight and birth asphyxia are relatively common causes. Prompt attention to convulsive states from any cause is imperative.

Active management: This depends on:
- available facilities
- severity of handicap
- presence of associated disabilities.

Table 15.21   Associated problems of cerebral palsy

Intellectual impairment
Epilepsy
Speech/hearing/visual defect
Behavioural problems
Emotional problems
Social maladjustment

As with all handicapped children, ideally each child should be assessed by a team consisting of a physiotherapist, occupational therapist, speech therapist, social worker, psychologist, paediatrician, and possibly an orthopaedic surgeon.

Furthermore, special schooling is advisable where there are multiple or significant handicaps. Where such facilities are not available, health professionals are required to give advice. Suitable low-cost publications should be consulted to provide means for the child to receive maximal stimulation, particularly during the formative years. (For advice on such publications contact AHRTAG, 85 Marylebone High Street, London W1M 3DE.)

Physiotherapy should be commenced as soon as the diagnosis has been made. Both active and passive movements of joints should be encouraged, to avoid contractures. These should incorporate appropriate postures and movements which will inhibit abnormal reflex activity and facilitate the movement patterns found in normal older children. Treatment should be continued throughout childhood. Parents should be taught how to handle their children, and how to do simple exercises with them on a daily basis. They should be taught simple feeding techniques, and how to toilet-train their child.

Siblings of children with cerebral palsy should also be involved in the plan of care for a child with disabilities. Recent studies have shown that sibling participation increases ambulation, personal hygiene, dressing, and feeding abilities. This is so because sibling relationships include mental stimulation, interaction, competition, and approval or disapproval. Parents have noted that siblings are often more effective in motivating their disabled brothers and sisters than are parents themselves.

Either with or without a physiotherapist, an occupational therapist can be very helpful in improving the child's motor function and enabling the child to be as independent as possible.

Assessment: It may be difficult to assess the handicap, due to abnormal response.

Intellectual assessment of these children is difficult in the extreme, due to the multiplicity of physical and sensory handicaps, but it must be remembered that about 40% of children with cerebral palsy have normal to above-average intelligence. Furthermore, the facial expression and speech impairment frequently lead to an erroneous conclusion of mental retardation. However, where the child is clearly microcephalic, responds poorly to sensory stimuli, and has gross motor retardation, little can be offered.

Where hearing and visual deficits are thought to make a major contribution to the handicap, and facilities for testing and correcting these are available, referral is indicated.

Speech defects, which are particularly prominent in the choreoathetotic type, respond poorly to therapy.

Epilepsy, which occurs in over 30% of cases, is likely to cause further brain damage, and requires appropriate medication. Careful selection of suitable anticonvulsants is important, lest the side-effects increase the handicap.

Emotional and social maladjustments are more the rule than the exception. Much of this can be avoided by careful counselling of the parents and other members of the family. The likely cause and extent of the pathology and estimated potential must be explained. It is often necessary to do this in two or three sessions, with ample opportunity for questions. At the same time, counselling should aim to remove or avoid feelings of guilt, isolation, and stigmatization, and to replace this with active involvement in management. Community support groups can be of great benefit in this respect.

When the child is old enough, she should be told about her disability, as a well-balanced, well-motivated child will achieve much more than one who is not.

Medication: Diazepam (1–2 mg nocte) is useful in those children who display irritability and extensor spasms at night. Lioresal® (baclofen) is also a useful drug for decreasing flexor tone and spasms, but it seems to work better in cases of spasticity secondary to spinal rather than intracranial pathology. Recent studies on vigabatrin, a new anticonvulsant for relief of spasticity, have been encouraging. See below for anticonvulsants for associated epilepsy.

Surgery: Corrective orthopaedic procedures are particularly helpful in the spastic child with marked adductor spasms and contractures.

Selective posterior rhizotomy is used on a limited scale, but promises to be a major advance in skilled hands. It is of value only in the spastic form, and long-term physiotherapy is essential following surgery.

Convulsions

Convulsions are common in children. The cause and type of convulsion vary with age.

Neonate

See Chapter 5, Newborns.

Infancy

Convulsions in this age group are more readily recognized, but have features similar to those of the neonate. The most common causes are:

◆ intracranial infections
◆ structural abnormalities of the brain (including cerebral birth trauma)
◆ metabolic disturbance
◆ electrolyte disturbance.

Infantile spasms

A specific type of fit occurs in the age group 4–18 months, i.e., infantile spasms (West syndrome, 'salaam attacks'). These are sudden flexion (or rarely, extension) spasms of the head, trunk, and extremities, lasting a few seconds. They tend to occur in series, with intervening free periods of varying duration. In 80–90% of cases the attacks are in the first year, and in about 70% of cases within the first 6 months of life. Onset under 3 months of age is unusual. 'Salaam attacks' are idiopathic in over 50% of cases. In the remainder there is an association with perinatal asphyxia, birth trauma, infection, structural abnormalities of the brain, or metabolic disturbance, in which case there is often a history of poor development. Occasionally these attacks may be associated with tuberous sclerosis. These associated conditions must be excluded by appropriate diagnostic studies. Some patients who have infantile myoclonic spasms have a characteristic electro-encephalographic pattern (hypsarrhythmia). Absence of this typical pattern does not exclude the diagnosis, as these changes usually appear around 6 months and are rare before 3 months, with a tendency to disappear or become modified after 12 months of age. Furthermore, a hypsarrhythmic EEG may occur as a result of any early cerebral insult and is therefore not specific for West syndrome.

Management

An EEG and CT scan should be performed on all patients prior to initiation of therapy.

ACTH at a dose of 20 units per day is given for 2 weeks. At the end of this period an EEG is repeated. If the patient has responded, ACTH is tapered off and discontinued. If there has been no response, the dose of ACTH is increased to 30 units per day and is continued at this dose for an additional 4 weeks, after which it is tapered off and discontinued. A repeat EEG is performed at this stage. If there was a response, the patient is followed up in the routine clinical manner. However, if there was a relapse, the patient is given a repeat course of ACTH. If the patient does not respond to the repeat dose and has not had prior prednisone therapy, then the latter is given at a dose of 2–3 mg/kg/day after the patient has been off ACTH for 1 week. The protocol and follow-up is similar to that used for ACTH.

Throughout the course of therapy with ACTH or prednisone the patient's blood pressure should be monitored 12-hourly and serum electrolytes should be checked on a weekly basis. If severe hypertension, electrolyte imbalance, gastrointestinal bleeding, or ocular abnormalities result,

ACTH or corticosteroid therapy should be terminated.

It is advisable to start treatment with nitrazepam or clonazepam while the child is still on ACTH or prednisone, and to continue these when the latter are withdrawn. If the above therapy fails, valproic acid may be used.

The spasms usually cease spontaneously by 3–4 years of age, but approximately 50% will go on to other types of seizures after their spasms stop, and almost 80% subsequently have mental retardation.

Early childhood (1–5 years)
Febrile seizures
These are the most commonly encountered seizures in children. Three per cent of children under the age of 5 years will have at least one seizure with fever due to infection outside the central nervous system. Boys outnumber girls, and in more than one-third of cases a positive family history is elicited. Earlier studies have suggested a strong association between prolonged febrile seizures and subsequent complex partial seizures. Recent studies, however, suggest that this sequence, if it occurs at all, is rare.

Febrile seizures are either *simple* or *complex*. The following are features of **simple febrile seizures:**
◆ Occur in association with an extracranial febrile illness, usually viral, e.g., upper respiratory tract infection.
◆ Occur at onset of illness and often are the presenting symptom.
◆ Usually generalized, but may be focal.
◆ Occur once during the early phase of the illness.
◆ Usually last less than 15 minutes.
◆ On recovery there are no neurological abnormalities.
◆ Occur in age group 6 months to 5 years.

Febrile seizures are said to be **complex** if they last more than 30 minutes, occur several times during the same illness, are associated with postictal neurological deficits, or if there is a preceding history of neurological or neurodevelopmental disorder, or a family history of epilepsy.

Prognosis: About 40% of children will have a second febrile fit with a subsequent febrile illness. In spite of this the prognosis is excellent. There is no risk of intellectual impairment or subsequent epilepsy in simple fits. Complex seizures have a greater chance of resulting in subsequent mental retardation and epilepsy.

Management
Acute: Reduce temperature by removing clothing and exposing child to a fan, by tepid sponging, and by administering an antipyretic agent such as paracetamol. To terminate the fit, rectal diazepam (0.5 mg/kg/dose) is given by means of a narrow-bore syringe (e.g., Mantoux syringe), or a feeding tube inserted into the rectum. Absorption from this route is rapid. This can be repeated after 20–30 minutes if necessary. Intramuscular diazepam is not well absorbed.

Lumbar puncture and blood sugar estimates are essential in any young child (especially under the age of 18 months) with a febrile fit, even in the absence of clinical evidence of meningeal irritation.

Prophylaxis: The most important aspect of management of febrile seizures is counselling of parents. They should be reassured about the excellent prognosis of febrile convulsions, advised about treatment of recurrences, use of antipyretics, and risk of recurrence.

Prophylactic anticonvulsants are no longer prescribed, as there is no evidence that they have any long-term benefit in febrile convulsions. However, to prevent recurrent febrile convulsions, intermittent diazepam at a dose of 0.8 mg/kg/24 hours may be given 8-hourly for the first 24–48 hours after the onset of a febrile episode. Alternatively rectal diazepam (0.5 mg/kg/dose) can be given 8-hourly for up to 48 hours. Recent studies suggest that intermittent therapy should be reserved for children who have had a first convulsion lasting more than 20 minutes or before the age of 9 months, or for those who have had more than two previous convulsions.

Parents may be given a supply of rectal diazepam and syringes to use at the onset of seizures.

Childhood epilepsy (5–12 years)
Epilepsy refers to recurrent afebrile seizures occurring especially in those over the age of 5 years. The risk of recurrence after a single afebrile seizure in children is about 50%. The incidence of

epilepsy is highest in childhood, and it is estimated that approximately 3% will have at least one convulsion in their lifetime. In the vast majority of children epilepsy is idiopathic, but in a few cases it may be symptomatic of intracranial pathology, e.g., cerebral cysticercosis, tumour, or arteriovenous malformations.

Diagnosis

The diagnosis of epilepsy is clinical, and is based on a detailed description of events experienced by the patient before, during, and after a seizure, and relies heavily on an eyewitness account.

Because of the social and economic implications, the diagnosis of epilepsy should never be made without incontrovertible clinical evidence. A seizure should be suspected in any child who presents with a symptom that is episodic, involuntary, and involves any alteration in the level of consciousness or responsiveness, abnormal motor activity, or change in behaviour, sensation, or autonomic function.

Classification of epilepsy

(See Table 15.22.)
Accurate classification of the seizure type is important in confirming the diagnosis and for

Table 15.22   Classification of epilepsy

Partial seizure		Generalized seizures
Simple partial	(Consciousness not impaired)	*Absence* (petit mal)
Motor:	Focal, Jacksonian	
Sensory:	Tingling, light flashes, smell, vertigo	*Tonic-clonic* (grand mal)
Autonomic:	Pallor, flushing, pupillary dilation	*Tonic or clonic* *Myoclonic*
Psychic:	Déjà-vu	*Atonic* (akinetic)
Complex partial	(Consciousness impaired) Psychomotor or temporal lobe epilepsy	
Partial seizures evolving to generalized tonic-clonic seizures		

selection of the most appropriate choice of antiepileptic medication.

Epilepsy is classified into two major categories: partial and generalized. Partial seizures originate in a localized or focal area of the brain, and their clinical features depend on the area of the brain involved, e.g., motor, sensory, autonomic, or psychic. Generalized seizures result from simultaneous bilateral involvement of the cerebral hemispheres.

Grand mal is the most common, and has the characteristic aura, and tonic-clonic phases followed by loss of consciousness. Frothing, and incontinence of urine and faeces may occur.

Petit mal occurs especially in girls from 3–14 years of age. These attacks consist of sudden impairment of consciousness lasting a few seconds. The only motor component accompanying this may be a fluttering of the eyelids. Several of these can occur per day. They are often overlooked, and may interfere with school performance. Typical petit mal seizures may be brought on by hyperventilation.

Complex partial seizures have a motor and behaviour component. The motor component may be subtle (e.g., smacking of lips, twitching of hands, deviation of eyes), or a full-blown grand mal seizure. The behavioural components consist of hallucinations (especially auditory), epigastric discomfort, and sudden outbursts of laughter or anger.

Myoclonic seizures are sudden muscle jerks affecting individual muscle groups or the trunk, causing drop attacks. They may be benign, or symptomatic of some underlying degenerative disease, e.g., subacute sclerosing panencephalitis.

Differential diagnosis

In the pre-school child, breath-holding attacks, reflex anoxic seizures, rigors, and benign paroxysmal vertigo may be misdiagnosed as epilepsy. Syncope and conversion disorders may also be frequently mistaken for epilepsy *(see Table 15.23)*.

Investigation

Laboratory tests may be diagnostic or provide baseline data for monitoring antiepileptic medication therapy, but it must be remembered that

Table 15.23 Differential diagnosis of epilepsy

Syncope
Psychogenic attacks
  Pseudoseizures
  Panic attacks
  Hyperventilation
Migraine
Narcolepsy
Hypoglycaemia
Prolonged QT syndrome
Paroxysmal choreoathetosis
Kahn's syndrome
Tetanus
Temper tantrums

routine screening of haematological and biochemical indices provide an extremely low yield of clinically useful information.

In selected cases the following investigations may be indicated:

Newborns, infants, and children under 18 months of age: Lumbar puncture, blood sugar level, serum calcium, phosphate, and magnesium, and urinalysis. Rarely amino acid and organic acid determination is done to exclude inherited metabolic disorders.

Children from endemic areas: Tests for neurocysticercosis are indicated.

Skull X-rays provide no useful information, and if patients require neurological imaging they should undergo CT scanning, which is indicated for:

◆ focal neurological signs*
◆ focal EEG changes*
◆ raised intracranial pressure*
◆ progressive CNS disease
◆ cysticercosis
◆ intractable seizures.

(* When all three are present, CT scan abnormalities may be found in up to 80% of cases.)

Cranial ultrasound is a very useful investigation in infants with an open fontanelle.

An EEG study is important in the diagnosis and management of epilepsy, but it must be emphasized that an abnormal EEG does not establish a diagnosis of a seizure disorder unless the patient has a typical seizure during the recording; it only provides evidence that must be correlated with the clinical history.

An abnormal EEG characterized by epileptiform activity occurs in 3% of normal children aged 1–15 years. On the other hand, a normal EEG does not exclude the diagnosis of epilepsy.

In up to 20% of patients with epilepsy the EEG may be normal. An EEG is performed for the following indications:

◆ when there is doubt about the diagnosis (?hysteria, ?breath-holding attacks, ?syncope)
◆ petit mal or absence seizures (3 cps spike and wave pattern)
◆ complex partial seizures (temporal lobe focus) infantile spasms (typical hypsarrhythmia)
◆ herpes encephalitis (temporal spike and wave pattern)
◆ subacute sclerosing panencephalitis (typical periodic complexes)
◆ Lennox Gastaut (2 cps spike and wave pattern.)

N.B. EEG is of no value in febrile convulsions, and its value in determining when to stop anticonvulsant therapy is controversial. Combined video – EEG recording during a clinical seizure provides the most accurate means for the diagnosis of epilepsy. It is valuable when the diagnosis is in question (e.g., pseudoseizures), or when seizures are poorly controlled, as it may provide additional information to aid management of the seizure disorder.

Management of epilepsy

The aim of treatment is to integrate the child into society. This is done by controlling seizures, managing social and educational problems, counselling parents and the children themselves, and giving genetic advice.

Principles of treatment:

◆ Use a single drug wherever possible.
◆ Use the most effective drug for the specific seizure type (*see Table 15.24*).
◆ Initial dosage should be started at the lowest limit of the therapeutic range, with gradual increase after allowing an adequate time to achieve a steady-state plasma level.
◆ Ensure compliance before changing to another drug; this can be checked by measuring blood levels. If the first drug is not effective at maximal

Table 15.24   Seizure type and choice of anticonvulsant drugs

Seizure type		Drugs
Partial seizures		
Simple and complex	1st choice:	Carbamazepine
	2nd choice:	Phenytoin
		Phenobarbital
		Sod. valproate
		Clonazepam
		Vigabatrin
Partial seizures evolving to generalized tonic-clonic	1st choice:	As above
	2nd choice:	As above
Generalized seizures		
Absence (petit mal)	1st choice:	Ethosuximide
	2nd choice:	Sod. valproate
		Clonazepam
Tonic-clonic (grand mal)	1st choice:	Carbamazepine
	2nd choice:	Phenytoin
		Sod. valproate
		Phenobarbital
Myoclonic	1st choice:	Sod. valproate
	2nd choice:	Nitrazepam
		Clonazepam
Atonic/akinetic (drop attacks)	1st choice:	Sod. valproate
	2nd choice:	Phenytoin
Unclassified		
Infantile spasms	1st choice:	ACTH/prednisone
	2nd choice:	Sod. valproate
		Benzodiazepine
		Vigabatrin

N.B.

1. Benzodiazepines rarely for long-term treatment.
2. In the under 5s phenobarbitone is still the drug of choice for long-term control of seizures. Second choices would be phenytoin, carbamazepine, and sodium valproate.
3. Avoid phenytoin in girls, especially at puberty.
4. When using polypharmacy it is important to know about drug interactions. Carbamazepine, phenytoin, and phenobarbitone are inducers, while sodium valproate is a non-inducer. The inducers tend to reduce serum levels, while the non-inducers increase them.

therapeutic level, a second drug is added, and the first drug should be gradually tailed off after the second drug has reached a therapeutic plasma level.

◆ If the initial drug is partially effective, a second drug may be added, with the dosage being increased gradually to reach therapeutic plasma concentrations. On rare occasions a third drug may need to be added.

◆ Haematological and liver function tests should be performed at the onset of therapy, and thereafter at 6–12 month intervals to monitor for blood dyscrasias or liver dysfunction secondary to anti-convulsant therapy.

Monitor drug levels frequently with multi-drug regimens.

When to start anticonvulsants: Despite a recurrence risk of about 50% after a single afebrile seizure, most neurologists would commence anti-convulsant therapy only after two seizures have occurred. Anther consideration is the intervals between seizures: if the seizure-free interval is more than 12 months, anti-convulsant therapy is *not* recommended.

When to discontinue anticonvulsants: Continuous treatment is recommended until at least 2 years of freedom from seizures have elapsed. Thereafter it should be reduced gradually over a period of 6–12 months. A normal neurological examination and a normal EEG are good indications for stopping treatment after 2 years. Over 70% of children remain seizure-free if drugs are withdrawn after 2 years without seizures.

For seizures secondary to infective or metabolic abnormality, as in newborns, drug therapy is usually discontinued after 7–10 days. Maintenance anticonvulsant therapy is recommended if seizures recur on discontinuation.

Status epilepticus

Convulsive status epilepticus means a continuous state of epilepsy with major convulsions lasting longer than 30 minutes, and with no recovery of consciousness in between seizures. Any type of seizure disorder may become continuous. About 10–20% of epileptic patients will have at least one episode of generalized tonic-clonic status at some time. More than 80% of cases of status epilepticus occur in children under 5 years of age.

Management:

Status epilepticus is a medical emergency, as there is a risk of death and serious morbidity in up to a third of cases.

The aim of treatment is to stop the seizures within 30 minutes, but at the same time basic aspects of supportive management must not be neglected *(see Table 15.25).*

Supportive measures:

◆ Secure airway.

◆ Monitor vital signs (pulse, BP, respiratory rate).

◆ Supply facial/nasal O$_2$ with a high flow rate if cyanosis is present. Be prepared to intubate.

◆ Perform appropriate investigations:
— Metabolic: Dextrostix® (if < 45 mg per cent treat as hypoglycaemia) blood sugar; urea and electrolyte; calcium, phosphate, and mag-

nesium; and liver function tests and blood gases
— CSF
— CT scan.

◆ Start slow IV infusion with 5% dextrose in normal saline.

Table 15.26 lists the currently used anticonvulsant drugs, their dosage range, therapeutic range, and side-effects.

Coma

Consciousness is a state of being awake and appropriately responsive to stimulation. A normal level of consciouness is maintained by an interaction between the cerebral hemispheres and the reticular activating system located in the brain stem. Diseases affecting either of these will result in an altered level of consciousness.

Table 15.25   Management of status epilepticus

Drug	Route	Dose
Lorazepam	IV	0.05–0.10 mg/kg/dose, up to 4 mg max.
	Repeat after 10 minutes if seizures persist	
Diazepam	If lorazepam not available	
	IV	0.3 mg/kg/dose
	per rectum	0.5 mg/kg/dose, up to 10 mg/dose
	Repeat after 10 minutes if seizures persist	
	If status remains uncontrolled give:	
Paraldehyde	IM/rectal	0.1–0.3 ml/kg/dose, up to 5 ml max.
	If no response within 20 minutes to above, then give:	
Phenytoin	IV	15–20 mg/kg over 20 minutes (not exceeding 50 mg/min — may precipitate cardiac arrhythmias
	or	
Phenobarbitone	IV	20 mg/kg over 20 minutes
	If seizures are not controlled within 15 minutes of above therapy, refer to respiratory unit for IV thiopentone sodium and ventilatory support. Seizures usually controlled by 12–24 hours of phenobarbitone coma. Dose 5 mg/kg initially and maintain on 5 mg/kg/hour for 12–24 hours. Thereafter maintain on either phenobarbitone or phenytoin.	

Note: If seizures have not been controlled for 12 hours, give:
1. IV mannitol 0.5–1 mg/kg over 20 minutes. A repeat dose can be given 6 hours later.
2. Dexamethasone 2–4mg initially, followed by 1–2 mg 6-hourly x 48 hours.

Table 15.26   Anticonvulsant drugs

Drug	Dosage range	Therapeutic range	Side-effects
Phenytoin	3–8 mg/kg	5–20 µg/ml	Hirsutism, acne, gum hypertrophy, cerebellar disturbance
Phenobarbitone	3–5 mg/kg	10–40 µg/ml	Hyperactivity, restlessness, insomnia, learning difficulties
Carbamazepine	10–20 mg/kg	4–10 µg/ml	Skin reactions, fluid retention
Sodium valproate	20–50 mg/kg	50–100 µg/ml	Liver disturbance, bone marrow depression, alopecia, pancreatitis
Ethosuximide	20–40 mg/kg	40–100 mg/ml	GIT disturbance, skin rash, pancytopenia
Clonazepam	0.03–0.05 mg/kg (max. 0.2 mg/kg)		Hyperactivity, irritability, rarely thrombocytopenia
Nitrazepam	0.25–1 mg/kg		Drowsiness, hypersecretion of mucus and saliva

Note:

1. Phenobarbitone, phenytoin, and ethosuximide can be given as a total dose in the evening once the desired effect has been obtained. Carbamazepine and sod. valproate can be given thrice daily, and only rarely in two divided doses.
2. Although most anticonvulsants are excreted in breast milk, there is no contraindication to breast-feeding.

Evaluation of the child with coma

The comatose child is a major diagnostic and management challenge in paediatric practice. *Table 15.27* outlines the differential diagnosis of altered consciouness. A careful history is essential to elucidate one of these causes. The history preceding the onset of coma may give clues to the aetiology; for instance acute onset in a previously normal child is compatible with intoxications, drug effects, cerebrovascular accidents, trauma, and metabolic disease, whilst a gradual onset is often associated with an expanding intracranial mass lesion, infective process, or chronic intoxication.

Physical examination

The initial examination is performed to determine signs of systemic disease, trauma, and infection. The examination should include detection of airway patency, heart rate, pulse, blood pressure, respiratory rate and pattern.

The breathing pattern may give a clue to severity and level of brain dysfunction, e.g., Cheyne-Stokes respiration may occur with diffuse cerebral dysfunction; hyperventilation in the absence of metabolic acidosis indicates lesions of the midbrain or upper pons; ataxic (irregular, chaotic) respiration is associated with lesions of the medulla.

Table 15.27   Important causes of coma in childhood

Post-convulsive states	
Infections:	Meningitis
	Encephalitis
	Malaria
	Brain abscess
Trauma:	Oedema
	Haemorrhage
	Haematoma
Toxins/drugs:	Herbal medications
	Barbiturates, narcotics, tranquillizers
	Lead
	Alcohol
	Reye's syndrome
Circulatory/vascular disorders:	Hypertensive encephalopathy due to glomerulonephritis
	Stroke
	Basilar migraine
Raised intracranial pressure:	Oedema, tumour, hydrocephalus
Metabolic:	Hypoglycaemia/hyperglycaemia
	Hepatic encephalopathy
	Hypo- and hypernatraemia
	Hypoxia, hypercarbia
	Uraemia
	Inherited metabolic diseases

Blood pressure and pulse: A rising BP and bradycardia (Cushing's syndrome) indicate severe and increasing intracranial pressure. Occasionally hypertension may be the cause of the coma (hypertensive encephalopathy).

Temperature: An unstable temperature may indicate a brain stem lesion.

Neurological examination

The most important part of the neurological examination is the documentation of the level of consciousness. The Glasgow Coma Scale is a widely used method for the objective assessment of the degree of consciousness. Serial examinations of the Glasgow coma score have the added advantage of allowing one to assess the progress of the child. However, below the age of 5 years the verbal responses, and to a lesser extent the motor responses, are not easily graded. A paediatric modification of the Glasgow Coma Scale (Adelaide Scale) shown in *Table 15.28* provides a practical neurological coma scale for this age group and has proved useful in clinical practice.

Corneal reflexes: Loss of corneal reflex suggests brain stem damage.

Doll's eye manoeuvre: If the head is turned briskly to one side and the eyes turn in the opposite direction, the brain stem is intact. If this fails to occur, it may be due to brain stem lesion or infranuclear palsy.

Conjugate deviation of the eyes: In an irritative lesion of the hemisphere, the eyes are deviated away from the lesion, whereas with damage they are deviated towards the lesion. A hemiplegia on the side opposite to the deviation indicates a cortical lesion. Deviation of eyes to the same side as the hemiplegia indicates a pontine lesion. Failure of conjugate movement upward suggests a midbrain lesion (Parinaud's syndrome).

Roving eye movements, if full, suggest an intact brain stem.

Pupillary changes: The presence of normally reactive pupils makes a severe brain stem lesion unlikely. Small reactive pupils indicate hypothalamic or thalamic damage (loss of sympathetic input). Pin-point pupils (which may appear unreactive) suggest a pontine lesion. Fixed, dilated pupils indicate a midbrain lesion and are a poor prognostic sign. Mydriatics (atropine) will also cause dilated pupils. Small pupils may be seen in

Table 15.28 Objective assessment of coma

Adult Scale (Glasgow)		Paediatric scale (Adelaide)	
Eyes open			
spontaneously	4	As in adult scale	
to speech	3		
to pain	2		
none	1		
Best verbal response			
orientated	5	orientated	5
confused	4	words	4
inappropriate words	3	vocal sounds	3
incomprehensible sounds	2	cries	2
none	1	none	1
Best motor response			
obeys commands	5		
localize pain	4		
flexion to pain	3	As in adult scale	
extension to pain	2		
none	1		
Normal aggregate score	14	Birth–6 mths:	9
		6–12 mths:	11
		1–2 yrs:	12
		2–5 yrs:	13
		> 5yrs:	14

barbiturate and organophosphate poisoning. A unilateral dilated pupil indicates a 3rd nerve palsy and may be an early sign of transtentorial herniation.

Motor changes: Generalized hypotonia with depressed reflexes may be seen in the first 48–72 hours of 'cerebral shock', e.g., following head injury. Drug poisoning must also be considered.

Hemiplegia, decorticate posturing (upper limbs flexed and adducted, lower limbs extended and internally rotated) or decerebrate rigidity (upper limbs extended, adducted, and pronated, and lower limbs extended, internally rotated, and plantar flexed) may help to localize the lesion to the hemispheres or brain stem respectively.

Management

Principles:

◆ Ensure adequate ventilation.

◆ Ensure adequate blood sugar level.
◆ Arrive at aetiological diagnosis.
◆ General supportive measures.

Hypoxaemia and hypercarbia cause oedema of the brain, which frequently aggravates the pathology and further depresses the level of consciousness.

As the unconscious patient is not in a position to maintain a clear airway, this must receive priority. Secretions must be cleared and the child placed in the semi-prone position in order to prevent laryngeal obstruction. Occasionally endotracheal intubation is necessary.

Loss of consciousness of any duration renders maintenance of nutrition difficult, hence hypoglycaemia is often a consequence, and sometimes the cause, of loss of consciousness in children. Blood sugar estimation (by Dextrostix®) is essential in every case, with subsequent gavage feeding. Established hypoglycaemia requires intravenous glucose.

The history and general assessment of the patient may give an indication of the cause. A lumbar puncture is essential in any patient, provided there is no papilloedema. A pressure reading should be obtained and the Queckenstedt test performed. Lateral sinus thrombosis, complicating mastoiditis, will cause failure of a rise in pressure when the jugular vein on that side is compressed.

Other special investigations appropriate to the suspected diagnosis must be carried out as soon as possible, e.g., CT scan.

When cerebral oedema is suspected in septic meningitis and following trauma, fluid intake should be restricted and mannitol (7 ml/kg IV over 20 minutes) can be given.

Ensure adequate hydration and caloric intake. Regular monitoring of vital signs and level of consciousness is essential. Associated convulsions call for prompt and appropriate medication.

Headache

Headache is a common symptom in childhood. Its presence in the younger child must alert the clinician to the likelihood of organic disease.

Acute headache

Headache may be acute and associated with distinct signs that indicate its cause, such as in meningitis, encephalitis, brain abscess, intracranial haemorrhage, acute purulent sinusitis, viral infections, and systemic bacterial infections such as pyelonephritis and typhoid.

Acute headache with focal neurological signs and/or altered level of consciousness suggests meningitis, brain abscess, or intracranial haemorrhage. Headache may follow lumbar punctures in about 20–30% of cases, and may last for 2–3 days or longer.

Headache may be one of the signs of raised intracranial pressure. It may occur by day or night, but characteristically occurs in the morning and is made worse by coughing, sneezing, straining, or change in posture. A space-occupying lesion (tumour, abscess, haematoma) must be excluded by CT scanning. A lumbar puncture must not be done if a space-occupying lesion causing increased intracranial pressure is suspected.

Table 15.29   Types of recurrent headache in children

Tension headache
Vascular headache
   Migraine
   Hypertension
   Fever
Raised intracranial pressure
   Space-occupying lesions
   Hydrocephalus
   Benign raised intracranial pressure
Headache due to ocular muscle imbalance and refractive error
Headache from chronic sinusitis
Headache due to seizure equivalent

Chronic recurrent headache
See Table 15.29.

The majority of recurrent headaches in children are associated with migraine, muscle tension, or psychogenic factors. Some cases may be due to eye muscle strain or sinusitis, while a small percentage are secondary to serious neurological disease (space-occupying lesions or raised intracranial pressure).

Migraine

Migraine is a clinical diagnosis characterized by episodic attacks of throbbing headaches, often unilateral, and associated with nausea, vomiting, abdominal pain, and relief after sleep. The aetiology is thought to be a vascular instability due to a genetic defect. A positive family history is present in over 50% of cases.

Migraine headaches vary greatly in their intensity, frequency, and duration. There are several clinical variants of migraine:

Classic migraine consists of a prodromal phase of:

◆ Visual aberrations consisting of the perception of sparkling lights or coloured lines, scotomas, blurred vision, hemianopia, transitory blindness, and visual hallucinations.

◆ Sensory prodrome of paraesthesiae of the limbs and perioral region (due to vasoconstriction causing ischaemia), followed by typical unilateral headache with nausea and/or vomiting (due to vasodilation).

The headache is generally localized to one side of the head, contralateral to the visual symptoms, and most intense in the region of the eye, forehead, and temple. It usually lasts about a day, but it may be as short as a few hours or as long as 2 days.

Common migraine: The classic pattern is uncommon in children. More often prodromal symptoms are absent, or may consist of mood changes only, followed by unilateral or sometimes a diffuse throbbing headache, which may last for hours or several days.

Rarely, migraine may be associated with transient hemiplegia (**hemiplegic migraine**), or eye pain and oculomotor nerve palsy (**ophthalmoplegic migraine**).

Basilar migraine: In this rare type of migraine there are recurrent attacks of brain stem and cerebellar dysfunction. The peak incidence is in adolescence. An abrupt loss of consciousness lasting for a few minutes may develop. The neurological signs are usually followed by severe occipital headache and vomiting.

Migraine equivalents: These consist of episodic abdominal pain with nausea, vomiting, and diarrhoea (abdominal migraine), or benign paroxysmal vertigo. The attacks are brief in duration, lasting only minutes, and tend to be recurrent.

Cluster headaches

Cluster headaches are less common, and seem to occur predominantly in males, usually after the age of 10 years. Headache is the initial complaint;

the pain begins in the periorbital region and then spreads posteriorly to involve the entire hemicranium. The pain is intense and throbbing in nature; nausea and vomiting are absent, but rhinorrhoea, conjunctival injection with tears, sweating, and facial flushing develop ipsilateral to the headache. Cluster headaches may be caused by a systemic increase of histamine.

Seizure equivalents

Headache may be a feature of seizure equivalents. The distinguishing feature is that in classic migraine there is gradual onset of aura and headache (without loss of consciousness), whereas in the seizure equivalent it is of sudden onset, usually of short duration, and is often associated with loss of consciousness.

Psychogenic or tension headaches

These are the most common types of headache, especially in the older school-going child, and are due to anxiety, tension, and depression. Migraine may also be precipitated by anxiety, tension, and stress, but the characteristic features of the disease distinguish it from psychogenic headaches. Psychogenic or tension headaches are non-throbbing, bilateral, described as like a band, a heavy weight, or fullness, and is of varying severity.

Management of headache

A detailed history and complete physical examination are essential. Measurement of blood pressure, fundoscopy, and neurological examination are necessary. It is also essential to listen to the skull for a bruit and to examine the eyes for refractive error. Investigations may include:

◆ skull and sinus X-rays

◆ EEG

◆ CT scans if the clinical examination reveals signs of a mass lesion or raised intracranial pressure.

Drug treatment

For simple headaches analgesics are adequate, e.g., paracetamol.

In the case of a migraine, provocative factors should be avoided before drug treatment is contemplated.

Acute migraine attack: For mild headaches simple analgesics like paracetamol may be sufficient, especially if given in the prodromal phase. For the severe attack, ergot preparations may be given via the oral, sublingual, or rectal route. Sublingual administration is preferred, because it is less likely to produce gastric upset. The sublingual dose is 2 mg. It should be taken as early as possible, preferably before the headache is established. A second tablet may be taken 15–20 minutes later, during a single attack. Repeated administration is not advisable, as it may intensify nausea and vomiting. Intramuscular chlorpromazine 1 mg/kg is a safe alternative to ergotamine.

If the attacks occur more often than two per month, these drugs should be avoided.

Migraine prophylaxis: For the frequent recurrent attack (two or more attacks per month), prophylactic treatment is recommended. Propranolol and pizotifen (Sandomigran®) are the drugs of choice. In children propranolol is preferred. The dose is 2 mg/kg/day in three divided doses. Bradycardia, hypotension, and provocation of asthma may occur in some children. For this reason propranolol should be started at less than half the therapeutic dose and slowly increased as tolerated. Depression is a relatively common side-effect, and parents should be warned about this reaction when commencing treatment. The drug is usually given for about 6–12 months, and thereafter withdrawn gradually to prevent rebound headaches.

If propranolol is ineffective, calcium channel blockers may be tried. Cyproheptadine and nifedipine have been used in children with fairly good results. In adults, flunarizine (Sibelium®) has proved very effective as a prophylactic agent (5–10 mg nocte).

Prednisone in a dose of 1 mg/kg for 5 days and tapered over the next two weeks cures **cluster headaches** in more than 75% of cases.

Floppy infant and child

Introduction

A floppy infant is one who is hypotonic, whose legs abduct completely and hips and knees flex to give the so-called 'frog-like' posture, both in supine and prone position. When pulled from supine to sitting position, the head lags behind the trunk, and on reaching the sitting posture, the head flops forwards or backwards and the back is rounded. When suspended in air in the ventral position, the head, arms and legs hang down limply.

There is increased range of passive movements around joints, causing the knees to hyperextend, ankles to evert, and feet to flatten.

Once one has established that a child is floppy, the next step is to determine whether muscle weakness is present or not. In young children this is done by observing movement of the limbs against gravity: can the child lift her arms or legs off the couch, can she reach out for an object, stand, sit, hold up her head? In the older child, weakness of trunk and pelvic girdle muscles is assessed by making her get up from the supine position: if the child turns around and then 'climbs up her legs', using hands on knees for support (Gower's sign), then trunk and pelvic girdle muscles are weak.

Table 15.30   Features of spinal muscular atrophy (SMA) and Duchenne muscular dystrophy

	SMA (mild)	Duchenne muscular dystrophy
Motor milestones	Delayed	Normal or delayed
Marked hypotonia	+	–
Fasciculation	±	–
Tremor of hands	±	–
Calf hypertrophy	±	+++
Reflexes	–	Ankle jerk +
IQ	N or ↑	N or ↓
CK	N or mildly ↑	Gross ↑↑↑
EMG	Denervation	Myopathic

A floppy child who has muscle weakness is most likely to have a lesion in the lower motor neurone. The tendon reflexes will be depressed or absent, and there may be wasting of muscles. Predominantly proximal muscle weakness suggests either chronic anterior horn cell degeneration, myopathy, or polymyositis, whereas predominantly distal weakness suggests peripheral neuropathy (except for Guillain-Barré syndrome, which mainly affects proximal muscles). *Table 15.30* lists the features of two of the common causes of a lower motor neurone lesion in children. A common cause of muscle weakness and hypotonia of short duration is hypokalaemia,

Table 15.31 Differential diagnosis of paraplegia/paraparesis

A. With sensory level

i. Infective myelopathy

Viral (transverse myelitis)
Bacterial (suppurative myelopathy, TB myelitis)
Parasitic (cysticercosis, bilharziasis)

ii. Compressive myelopathy

Vertebral
   Trauma
   Pyogenic infections
   TB
   Malignancy 1°, 2° (leukemia, lymphoma, neuroblastoma)
Extradural
   Trauma (haematoma)
   Pyogenic infections (abscess)
   Malignancy (neurofibroma, meningioma)
Intradural
   Extramedullary
      Infections (arachnoiditis)
      Malignancy (neurofibroma, meningioma)
   Intramedullary
      Trauma (haematomyelia)
      Infections (tuberculoma, bilharzial granuloma)
      Malignancy (gliomas)
      Vascular malformations (AVM, haemangioblastoma, haemangioedothelioma)
      Congenital: syringomyelia or cord cyst

iii. Anterior spinal artery occlusion

B. Without sensory level

Guillain-Barré syndrome
Severe poliomyelitis
Parafalcine lesions
Superior sagittal sinus thrombosis
Recovering transverse myelopathy

commonly caused by prolonged diarrhoea *(see Chapter 20, Endocrine and Metabolic Disorders).*

Hypotonia without weakness may be due to cerebral palsy, chromosomal abnormality (e.g., trisomy 21), nutritional and emotional deprivation, hypothyroidism, rickets, infantile hypocalcaemia, and other rare inborn errors of metabolism (especially of connective tissue, resulting in laxity of ligaments and hyperextensibility of joints).

Hypotonia with muscle weakness

Poliomyelitis

See Chapter 8, Infectious Diseases.

Transverse myelitis

The hallmarks of this disease are acute onset of paraplegia, with loss of sensation up to a discrete level, bladder and rectal incontinence, areflexia which over days or weeks gives way to brisk reflexes and ankle clonus, and CSF lymphocytosis with normal CSF sugar. The causative organism is usually one of the neurotropic viruses, e.g., herpes, Coxsackie. Differential diagnosis includes spinal tuberculosis with extradural abscess, where the onset is usually insidious, kyphosis and tenderness of the spine may be present, and the Mantoux test is usually strongly positive. X-ray of the spine may show destruction of vertebrae. Other differential diagnoses are given in *Table 15.31.*

The disease is self-limiting and calls for supportive treatment.

Spinal muscular atrophy (SMA)

This is the most common chronic neuromuscular disorder seen in African children. It is more common than Duchenne muscular dystrophy, which occurs more frequently than SMA in white and Asian children. SMA is a degenerative disease of the anterior horn cell, of unknown aetiology. In European and Asian communities it is inherited as an autosomal recessive disorder, whereas most cases in the African population are of a sporadic nature. Modern techninques of clinical and laboratory investigation have been recently applied to SMA, culminating in the mapping of the genes responsible for this disease to chromosome 5. This means that DNA markers can now be used for prenatal diagnosis, and in the long term, the cloning of the actual genes will be a major step towards our understanding of the pathogenesis of this disease. The features of SMA are:

♦ floppy child with weakness
♦ symmetrical, proximal more than distal weakness
♦ lower limbs are affected more than upper limbs
♦ reflexes are absent or diminished
♦ fasciculation of tongue is diagnostic, but is not invariably present

◆ a coarse, irregular tremor of hands is diagnostic of the more benign forms of the disease

◆ mental function is normal, and often above average — the children are bright, alert, and responsive

◆ creatine kinase is normal or mildly elevated

◆ ECG shows a 'tremor', i.e., random spikes disturbing the baseline between the QRS complexes. These represent fasciculation potentials recorded from the limb muscles. They are found only in the mild form of the disease

◆ electromyography and muscle biopsy show denervation

◆ prognosis is determined by severity, especially respiratory and bulbar involvement.

The children fall into one of three groups, depending on severity:

Severe infantile form: The child is severely paralysed — unable to sit, hold up head, raise legs against gravity, or elevate arms. The only movements are of the elbow, wrist, ankle, and finger joints. Respiratory and bulbar involvement is invariable, and death ensues before the age of 2 years. Facial weakness is common in the African child.

The onset of the paralysis may be before, at, or within 3 months of birth.

Intermediate form: The child is able to sit, but unable to stand or walk. Respiratory weakness may or may not be present. Prognosis is good, with survival to adult life in a wheelchair.

Mild form: The child is able to stand and walk, but is weak. This form is most often confused with Duchenne muscular dystrophy. Prognosis is good.

Management of SMA is supportive. Particular attention is paid to prompt treatment of chest infection and prevention of contractures and scoliosis. Genetic counselling must be given where heredity is considered to be a factor *(see above)*.

Guillain-Barré syndrome (GBS)

This is the most common type of peripheral neuropathy seen in childhood. It is a demyelinating neuropathy induced by an autoimmune process, precipitated by a preceding viral or other infection. Coxsackie, echo, and herpes viruses, and *Mycoplasma pneumoniae* are known to cause the syndrome.

Clinical features:

◆ The onset is acute in a previously well child with normal motor development. A preceding upper respiratory tract infection is present 10–14 days prior to the onset of weakness. Occasionally the onset is insidious, the child presenting with frequent falls due to weakness.

◆ Proximal and distal weakness starts in the lower limbs and progresses in an ascending order, affecting the trunk, upper limbs, respiratory, bulbar, and facial muscles. The weakness tends to be symmetrical, and may take anything up to 3 weeks to reach a maximum, after which recovery occurs, usually in the same order (i.e., legs first). It may take anything up to 2 years for complete recovery to occur.

◆ Reflexes are depressed or absent, and sensory loss is minimal, but if present is of the 'glove and stocking' variety.

◆ Bladder and rectal paralyses are rarely present.

Table 15.32   Guillain-Barré syndrome diagnostic criteria

Essential criteria
> Progressive weakness of at least two limbs
> Areflexia
> Progression less than 4 weeks
> Absence of other causes of acute neuropathy

Helpful criteria
> Relatively symmetrical weakness
> Relatively mild sensory signs
> Facial weakness
> Autonomic dysfunction
> Absence of fever with neuropathic symptoms
> CSF (after first week) showing elevated protein and normal cell count (albumino-cytologic dissociation)
> Abnormally slow nerve conduction

Diagnostic criteria are given in *Table 15.32*.

Management is supportive. Respiratory care is important if intercostal and bulbar paralyses develop.

Any child in the early stages of Guillain-Barré syndrome must be carefully watched for development of respiratory and bulbar paralysis.

This usually occurs within 2 weeks of onset. Physiotherapy to prevent contractures and wasting is important. Plasma exchange is advocated for severe cases early in the course of the disease, but there is generally no place for steroids in the treatment of this disorder *(see Prognosis, below, for exception).*

Prognosis is good, with 80% showing complete recovery, although this may be slow. In 5% of cases there is subsequent relapse. Some may show residual weakness, and there is a small mortality in the acute phase from respiratory paralysis. In patients with the chronic relapsing forms of the disease, steroids are helpful.

The features of a poor prognosis in GBS are:
◆ an interval greater than 18 days from maximum deficit to onset of improvement
◆ areflexia from onset
◆ severe weakness in the distal muscles
◆ need for assisted ventilation
◆ electromyographic finding of profuse fibrillation indicating axonal degeneration
◆ marked reduction of mean compound muscle action potential (CMAP) amplitude (< 10% of lower limit of normal).

Other peripheral neuropathies
See Table 15.33.

Table 15.33 Causes of peripheral neuropathy

Autoimmune or idiopathic
Guillain-Barré syndrome
Miller-Fisher syndrome (ophthalmoplegia, ataxia, areflexia)
Chronic relapsing polyneuritis

Toxic neuropathies
Biological toxins — diphtheria
Chemical toxins — lead, thalium, mercury, gold, arsenic, benzine

Metabolic neuropathies
Acute intermittent porphyria
Diabetes mellitus
Uraemia

Hereditary neuropathies
Hereditary motor neuropathies
Hereditary sensory neuropathies

Miscellaneous
Collagen vascular disease
Sarcoidosis
Amyloidosis
Malignancies (lymphomas)

The other causes of peripheral neuropathy are rare in childhood. Hereditary peripheral neuropathies with autosomal dominant or recessive inheritance may ocassionally occur in childhood. A family history of peripheral neuropathy is therefore important in diagnosis. Toxins can cause peripheral neuropathy. The most common one in Natal is that resulting from benzine sniffing. Benzine (bought in corner stores for cleaning purposes) contains N-hexane, which is known to cause a neuropathy. The neuropathy is predominantly motor. Recovery is complete if sniffing is discontinued, but may take a year or more. Other conditions which cause a predominantly motor neuropathy include diphtheria, porphyria, and lead neuropathy.

Neuromuscular junction disorders
Disorders of the neuromuscular junctions are rare, and result from a lesion in the pre- or postsynaptic membrane. Such lesions may be hereditary or acquired, both of which may be present from birth or only manifest at a later stage.

Of the acquired disorders, **myasthenia gravis** is the best known, but is rare in childhood. It is caused by antibodies to acetylcholine receptors. Intermittent weakness which gets worse with exercise and improves with rest is characteristic. The weakness may be localized to the eye muscles or may be generalized. Respiratory or bulbar weakness may be life-threatening. The diagnosis is made by giving intravenous Tensilon® (1–2 mg). An immediate response is diagnostic. Treatment consists of anticholinesterase drugs, such as pyridostigmine, 15–60 mg 4-hourly except at night. Steroid therapy and thymectomy may occasionally be necessary.

Prognosis depends on the type. A transient neonatal form occurs as a result of maternal anti-acetylcholine receptor IgG antibodies crossing the placenta if the mother has myasthenia. Hypotonia, apnoeic attacks, and bulbar paralysis with pooling of secretions develop soon after birth and may be fatal if not treated. Complete recovery occurs by 3–4 weeks. Juvenile myasthenia occurs in older children, especially girls. Prognosis is excellent, particularly with modern therapy. Recently, rare inherited forms of myasthenia gravis have been described, in which defects of synthesis, storage, release, and degradation of acetylcholine have been implicated, as well as developmental defects of the postsynaptic membrane. These types may be refractory to treatment.

Botulism: In the United States and Britain botulism has been recognized as an important cause of acute, acquired hypotonia and weakness in infants between 3 and 18 weeks of age. Toxin is ingested from contaminated food (e.g., honey), and generalized weakness occurs. Total ophthalmoplegia, facial diplegia, and bulbar weakness may be present. The prognosis is good with supportive care. The diagnosis is made by identifying the toxin in stools or serum.

Organophosphorous poisoning: *See Chapter 27, Poisoning.*

Muscle disorders

Hypokalaemia is a common cause of hypotonia with weakness, especially in a malnourished child with diarrhoea.

There is marked head lag. The weakness may be asymmetrical and bulbar, and respiratory muscles may be involved. Hypokalaemia, normal CSF, and rapid recovery following potassium therapy distinguish it from poliomyelitis.

Congenital myopathies are much less common than Duchenne muscular dystrophy or spinal muscular atrophy, and cause the floppy infant syndrome with a variable degree of weakness. Contractures may or may not be present. Reflexes are depressed or absent, and muscles wasted. The creatine kinase (CK) is normal or mildly elevated, and the diagnosis can be made only by means of muscle biopsy. Centronuclear myopathy, though rare, is the commonest form of congenital myopathy seen in black children.

Muscular dystrophy: *(See Table 15.30.)* The common Duchenne type (DMD) affects boys and is X-linked. Females may be carriers. The disease is present from birth, but manifests between 2 and 5 years of age, with delayed motor milestones, frequent falls, difficulty in climbing hills or stairs, and difficulty in getting up from the floor. The weakness is progressive, so that by 10–12 years a wheelchair is needed. Pseudohypertrophy of calves and thighs is prominent. A tendency to walk on the toes is characteristic. Reflexes disappear from the arms early, but ankle jerks are preserved until late in the course of the disease. About 50% of the boys are mentally retarded. The ECG shows changes in R/S ratio and inverted T waves in almost all patients. A very high (100 times normal) serum CK is present from birth onwards. Muscle biopsy and electromyography will also help in making the diagnosis.

Management is supportive. Prevention of contractures (especially scoliosis and tight Achilles tendon) is important to prolong ambulation. Genetic counselling is also important. Female relatives who are carriers can be identified by doing three serial serum CK measurements. CK will, however, identify only 70% of definite carriers. Even with EMG and muscle biopsy, the carrier detection is not 100%. Fetal diagnosis using CK measurements of fetal blood is also not reliable. Recent advances in molecular genetics have led to the localization of the faulty gene in DMD to the short arm of the X chromosome (Xp21). Using the molecular approach, antenatal diagnosis by routine amniocentesis and the determination of the status of potential carrier females is possible in almost 95% of affected families.

Prognosis: The disease is invariably fatal, with death occurring from cardiac or respiratory failure in the late teens.

Polymyositis/dermatomyositis: Acute or insidious onset of muscle weakness in a previously well child (who becomes miserable, irritable, and weepy) must raise the possibility of polymyositis. In dermatomyositis skin lesions are present as well. These consist of an erythematous rash over the elbows, knees, and malar aspect of the face, with slight puffiness and purple tinge of upper eyelids (heliotrope sign). Muscle tenderness may be present. CK and ESR are usually markedly elevated, but may be normal. Muscle biopsy shows degeneration with an inflammatory cell infiltrate around vessels.

Treatment is with prednisone, 1 mg/kg/day until clinical improvement starts, and then slowly tailing off. Methotrexate may occasionally be used in addition.

The prognosis is generally good, but death in the acute phase from respiratory failure may occur. Contractures and muscle calcification and ulceration are late complications.

Hypotonia without weakness

Cerebral palsy
See above.

Chromosome disorders
See Chapter 3, Genetics and Congenital Disorders.

Hypothyroidism
See Chapter 20, Endocrine and Metabolic Disorders.

Rickets
See Chapter 21, Metabolic Bone Disorders.

Learning disabilities
See Chapter 30, Psychological and Behavioural Disorders.

Hyperactivity
See Chapter 30, Psychological and Behavioural Disorders.

Intracranial tumours

Introduction
Intracranial tumours are the second most common type of malignant neoplasm in children under the age of 15 years. Studies done in Durban have shown that primary brain tumours are the most common form of solid neoplasm in this age group, and second only to leukaemia if all malignant diseases are included. However, the prevalence of primary intracranial tumours among black children in Africa is lower than that reported for white children.

Whereas CNS tumours in adults are mostly supratentorial, those of childhood are predominantly infratentorial. In adults most CNS tumours are malignant astrocytomas and metastatic carcinomas, while in childhood most are either low-grade astrocytomas or embryonic neoplasms, e.g., medulloblastomas, ependymomas, or germ cell tumours. In contrast to other childhood malignancies, CNS tumours have responded less dramatically to modern multimodal forms of treatment, particularly chemotherapy.

The peak age of occurrence in Durban was 6 years, and the major histological types were astrocytoma (47%), medulloblastoma (22%), and craniopharyngioma (16%). The high incidence of craniopharyngiomas in black children has also been documented in other African series. There was an overall male predominance, which was especially striking in craniopharyngiomas.

Classification
CNS tumours are classified as *primary* or *metastatic*. The primary tumours have been further classified on the basis of:
- *Location:* Infratentorial (posterior fossa), or supratentorial (cerebral hemisphere lesions or lesions of midline structures). *(See Table 15.34.)*
- *Tissue of origin:* Neuroectodermal tumours are those of other structures. *(See Table 15.35.)*

Table 15.34   Primary intracranial tumours according to location

Supratentorial
Cerebral hemispheres and meninges
   Astrocytoma
   Ependymoma
   Meningioma
Midline structures
   Pituitary adenoma
   Craniopharyngioma
   Colloid cyst
   Pineal parenchymal tumour
   Germ cell tumour
   Astrocytoma
   Optic nerve glioma
Infratentorial
Cerebellum and 4th ventricle
   Astrocytoma
   Medulloblastoma
   Ependymoma
Brain stem
   Astrocytoma

Clinical features
Symptoms: The early recognition of CNS tumours in children is difficult because of the non-specific nature of symptoms. In infancy the easily separable sutures delay detection, as raised intracranial pressure develops slowly. In Durban many patients present at a late stage with signs of severe raised intracranial pressure and/or focal neurological deficits.

Early morning headache is often the first symptom, followed by nausea and vomiting. Other symptoms may include dizziness, and blurred vision may follow, with personality changes and poor school performance. In our experience the major presenting features were as listed in *Table 15.36.*

Table 15.35   Primary brain tumours according to tissue of origin

Neuroectodermal/neuroepithelial tissue
  Glial tissue
    Astrocytoma
    Oligodendrogliomas
    Optic nerve gliomas
  Ependymal cells
    Ependymoma
  Embryonal cells
    Medulloblastomas
  Choroid plexus
    Choroid plexus papillomas
  Pineal body
    Pineocytoma
    Pineoblastoma
Never sheath cells
  Neurilemmoma (Schwannoma, neurinoma)
  Neurofibroma
Meninges
  Meningioma
  Meningeal sarcoma
Pituitary
  Adenoma
  Craniopharyngioma
Blood vessels
  Haemangioblastoma
Miscellaneous
  Malignant lymphoma
  Colloid cyst of 3rd ventricle

Table 15.36   Symptoms in 100 patients with primary brain tumours in Natal

	Percentage of all tumours
Ataxia	50
Headache	44
Vomiting	43
Visual disturbance	28
Convulsions	14
Mental changes	8

Visual disturbances were more common in supratentorial tumours, while ataxia occurred more frequently in infratentorial lesions. Convulsions and mental changes were less frequent.

Signs: Presenting signs of intracranial tumours among black children in Natal are given in *Table 15.37.*

Table 15.37   Signs in 100 patients with primary brain tumours in Natal

	Percentage of all tumours
Raised intracranial pressure	66
Cranial nerve palsies	54
Focal signs	49
Gait disturbance	33
Meningeal irritation	25
Mental changes	13

Raised intracranial pressure occurred more frequently in supratentorial tumours, while gait disturbances and cranial nerve palsies were more prominent in infratentorial lesions.

The late presentation of these patients is the most likely reason for the high incidence of signs of raised intracranial pressure and focal neurological deficits.

Raised intracranial pressure is caused by the tumour mass, the associated cerebral oedema, or obstructive hydrocephalus. In older children the predominant symptom is headache. Symptoms requiring urgent attention are failing vision, deteriorating level of consciousness, and neck stiffness. Papilloedema is present in less than 50% of patients. Bulging fontanelle, separation of sutures, and a 'cracked-pot' note are useful indicators of raised intracranial pressure.

Diagnostic evaluation
See Table 15.38.

Plain skull X-rays may show:
◆ signs of raised intracranial pressure, displacement of the pineal body, or hyperostosis adjacent to a meningioma
◆ calcification: craniopharyngioma, malignant glioma, oligodendroglioma, pineal tumour, and, rarely, ependymoma.

CT scan with contrast enhancement: This allows rapid and non-invasive delineation of CNS tumours. CT scans are excellent for delineating supratentorial and posterior fossa lesions, but are less accurate in evaluating brain stem lesions.

Where there are no facilities for CT scans, radio isotope brain scans may be helpful.

Table 15.38   Focal neurological deficit: a clue to site of lesion

Likely site of lesion	Deficit
Cerebral hemisphere lesions	
Frontal	Mental and personality changes
Post-frontal	Hemiparesis
Parietal lobe	Hemianopia, astereognosis, sensory inattention, etc.
Temporal	Memory and mood disturbance
Dominant hemisphere	Speech disorder
	Focal convulsions
Optic nerves and optic chiasma	Visual failure
Cerebellar lesions	Ataxia
Cerebello-pontine angle tumours	Ataxia, multiple cranial nerve palsies, e.g., V, VIII, IX, and X
Pineal tumours	Pupillary paralysis and defective vertical conjugate gaze (Parinaud's syndrome)
Brain stem tumours	Progressive cranial nerve palsies and long tract signs in the absence of raised intracranial pressure until a late stage

Magnetic resonance imaging: By virtue of abolishing bone images it is useful in evaluating tumours near the base of the skull.

Cerebral angiography: is useful in distinguishing between tumour and vascular malformation. It can also assist in planning surgery.

Management

Deteriorating level of consciousness, failing vision, and neck stiffness indicate a marked elevation of intracranial pressure, and require urgent attention. Mannitol may be given to reduce cerebral oedema, prior to urgent transfer to a neurosurgical unit for decompression and immediate surgery if indicated. Radiotherapy and chemotherapy are adjuncts in treatment.

M. Moodley

16

Renal disorders

This chapter will present disorders of the kidney and urinary system by two different methods:

◆ a clinical problem-orientated, practical approach

◆ a theoretical outline of specific diseases.

Clinical problem-orientated approach

A consistent approach to solving the clinical disorders given below is to uncover the *site* of the lesion and then the *nature* (aetiology) of the lesion. The following are problems arising from disturbances of this system which should be drawn to the attention of health professionals.

Oedema

Swelling of the body which pits on pressure may be due to renal, nutritional, cardiac, hepatic, gastrointestinal, and allergic diseases. Non-pitting oedema reflects disordered lymphatics.

A **renal cause** for the oedema is suggested by urine abnormalities (especially proteinuria), hypertension (and its neurological consequences), and oedema which begins around the eyelids.

Nutritional oedema is easily recognized by the features of kwashiorkor; ascites is uncommon.

Congestive cardiac failure presents with dyspnoea, tachycardia, raised jugular venous pressure, tender hepatomegaly, crackles at lung bases, and an abnormal heart (enlarged, murmurs, gallop rhythm, etc.).

Oedema of **hepatic origin** invariably starts as ascites. The liver is enlarged, and may be firm-to-hard, with an irregular edge; there are other signs of chronic liver disease, such as hypoglycaemia, bleeding tendency, rickets, clubbing of fingernails, palmar erythema, spider-naevi, pruritus, pale stools, deficiencies of fat-soluble vitamins, and portal hypertension.

Malabsorption leads to oedema. Stools are fatty and may be foul-smelling; and there may be deficiencies of other nutrients (fat-soluble vitamins, iron, folate, etc.).

Allergic reactions give rise to sudden swelling around the eyes, mouth, or upper respiratory tract, and to urticaria. These signs are localized, and rarely confused with the causes of generalized oedema.

Urine abnormalities

See Table 16.1.

These are noticed by the patient or parents, or detected during routine examination.

Haematuria

Haemoglobinuria and myoglobinuria give a red colour and a positive reagent strip test, but will not show RBC'c on microscopy. It is essential to determine the *site* from which blood is leaking into the urine.

◆ Clinical features *(see below)* often suggest glomerular or tubular disease.

◆ Bright red blood at the end of micturition suggests lower urinary tract disease, e.g., *S. haematobium*, adenovirus cystitis. Tea-like discoloration throughout the urinary stream indicates kidney disease, e.g., glomerulonephritis.

Urine collection in three glasses is simple and can be informative: blood in the first glass suggests urethral disease, blood in the third glass suggests bladder problems, and blood in all three glasses indicates kidney disease.

◆ Asymptomatic, gross haematuria, sometimes with clots, often arises from the bladder (foreign body, tumour), although renal parenchymal diseases may occasionally present in this manner.

◆ Small, crenated red cells of varying sizes point to the glomerulus as the site of disease, while round, smooth-walled red cells of similar size arise outside the glomerulus.

◆ Accompanying proteinuria (> 2+) and casts indicate renal parenchymal disease.

Table 16.1 Urine examination

Test	Normal				Abnormal
Colour	Pale yellow				- red stain on napkin = decomposition of urates - red = RBCs, haemoglobin, myoglobin - colourless = dilute - food/drugs can alter colour
Odour	Ammonia-like				- acetone smell = ketonuria - faecal odour = coliform infection

Quantity		ml/day	GFR	ml/min	- acute renal failure = urine output < 300 ml/m²/day
	Birth	30–60	(corrected to 1.73 m²	26 ± 2*	
	2nd wk	100–300		54 ± 8	
	0.5–1 yr	400–500		77 ± 14	- clinical problems in chronic renal failure = when GFR < 20 ml/m²/min
	1–3 yrs	500–600		96 ± 22	
	4–12 yrs	700–1 400		118 + 18	
	*mean± SE				

Osmotic capacity		mOs/kg	- after 12 hr fluid restriction = > 850 mOs/kg
	2nd week:	600–1 250	↓ = hypokalaemia, hypercalcaemia, chronic renal failure, pyelonephritis, sickle-cell anaemia, hydronephrosis, diabetes insipidus
	> 0.5 yrs	870–1 310	↑ = pre-renal failure
	(N.B. 900 mOs/kg = specific gravity 1.025)		

pH	Serum HCO₃	Urine pH	> 6.0 = distal renal tubular acidosis, metabolic alkalosis
	17 mmols/l	5.0	< 5.0 = metabolic acidosis, hypokalaemia
	30 mmols/l	8.0	*see text*

Protein	< 150 mg daily. Dipstick® = + or -ve	
Cells	- White cells 10/mm³ or < 5/HPF	- pus cells + > 10⁵ bacteria/ml + single organism = infection *see text*
	- RBC 0/mm³ or < 5/HPF	

Casts	- 1/mm³ or 1–2/HPF	cellular = parenchymal renal disease red cell = glomerulonephritis white cell = pyelonephritis hyaline = nephrotic syndrome epithelial = acute tubular necrosis broad casts = renal failure all casts = glomerular + tubular disease

		Gluc	↑ = low renal threshold. Diabetes mellitus, transient hyperglycaemia
Glucose	Not detectable	*Na*	↑ = chronic renal failure
Na	1.6–4 mEq/kg/day	*K*	↑ = diuretics, metabolic acidosis
K	0.4–1.2 mEq/kg/day	*Ca*	↑ = distal renal tubular acidosis, hyperparathyroidism ↓ = rickets, hypoparathyroidism
Ca	1–5 mg/kg/day		
P	15–20 mg/kg/day	*P*	↑ = resistant rickets, hyperparathyroidism

♦ Petechiae, ecchymoses, and mucosal haemorrhages suggest a systemic bleeding disorder.

♦ Renal parenchymal diseases which should be considered when there is haematuria without heavy or significant proteinuria are Alport's syndrome, IgA nephropathy, recovering post-streptococcal glomerulonephritis, benign familial nephritis, and idiopathic haematuria/nephritis.

♦ Hypercalcinuria can cause haematuria. Calcium oxalate crystals may be seen on urine microscopy.

♦ Investigations should be undertaken only after detailed history, clinical examination, and careful urine analysis. Invasive procedures, in particular, should be done only when other investigations (ultrasound, abdominal radiograph, etc.) are non-contributory.

Proteinuria

It is important to rule out proteinuria which is not clinically significant, such as that due to fever, posture, surgery, and trauma. This type of proteinuria is usually transient and mild (< 0.5 $gm/m^2/24$ hrs; < 100 mg/day; early morning urine protein/creatinine ratio < 20 mg/mmol^{-1}).

Investigation can uncover the source of the proteins and convey some idea of the type and severity of disease. Haematuria co-existent with proteinuria indicates renal parenchymal diseases. If the proteinuria comprises mainly albumen or high molecular weight proteins, the lesion is likely to be in the glomeruli; low-molecular-weight proteinuria is from the tubules (Fanconi syndrome, cystinosis, etc.).

Heavy proteinuria (> 2 $gm/m^2/24$ hrs) is characteristic of nephrotic syndrome, but can also occur with constrictive pericarditis. Moderate proteinuria (0.5–2.0 $gm/m^2/24$ hrs; 100 mg/day) is a feature of acute glomerulonephritis, while mild proteinuria may be caused by interstitial nephritis and acute glomerulonephritis. Mild to moderate proteinuria may also be caused by chronic renal failure and congenital abnormalities of the kidneys. When the majority of protein in the urine in nephrotic syndrome is of low molecular weight (e.g., transferrin), the histological lesion is likely to be 'minimal change'. In such cases steroids are effective and prognosis excellent. The loss of high molecular weight proteins in urine in nephrotic syndrome is suggestive of steroid-unresponsive disease.

Further investigations are influenced by the clinical and biochemical findings. Ultrasound is especially helpful in identifying congenital lesions, obstructive uropathy, and shrunken kidneys.

Little or no urine passed (oligo-anuria)

This should always be regarded as an emergency, as it may be a sign of kidney failure. It is critical to determine the anatomical site of the disease process leading to oligo-anuria, as replacement of fluids, which is life-saving for shock, is dangerous for renal or post-renal diseases. Dehydration, blood loss, and shock (cold peripheries, impalpable or thready pulse, hypotension, diminished consciousness) are the key events leading to pre-renal failure. Fluid or blood should be infused urgently. Strangury or palpable bladder and ureters suggest obstructive uropathy. Catheterization is necessary to bypass urethral and bladder-neck obstruction. Features of renal parenchymal causes of oliguria or anuria are given below. Plasma electrolytes and urine examination are essential to identify the pre-renal, renal, or post-renal location of the disease. An ultrasonogram of the abdomen is extremely useful: information is sought on size and shape of the kidneys, echogenicity of renal parenchyma, size of ureters, and calculi.

Change in behaviour, fits, coma or other neurological signs

These may be related to high blood pressure or renal failure (*see appropriate sections for management*). Neurological complications require immediate investigation and treatment; for the many causes of these problems, and management, *see Chapter 15, Neurological Disorders.*

Fever of unknown origin

Always exclude an urinary tract infection (UTI). The clinical features which sometimes accompany UTI are discussed below.

Growth retardation, rickets, acidosis, anaemia (alone or in combination)

These often signify <u>chronic renal disease</u>. All such children should be referred for detailed investigation unless the cause is obvious and easily remedied, e.g., <u>protein-energy malnutrition</u>, <u>nutritional rickets, diarrhoeal acidosis, iron-deficiency anaemia</u>.

Renal masses

These may be <u>hydronephrosis</u>, <u>renal cystic disorders</u> (e.g., dysplastic kidney, polycystic disease, medullary cystic diseases, etc.), ectopic kidney, renal vein thrombosis, or nephroblastoma. Evaluation requires detailed <u>nephro-urological tests, of which ultrasonography is the simplest</u>.

Specific diseases

Glomerulonephritis

Definition

This is an all-embracing term which refers to diseases of glomeruli. In the main, these diseases are recognized by a combination of certain clinical features, histopathological changes in the kidney, biochemical abnormalities, immunological findings, and alterations to the electrical charge in the glomerular basement membrane.

Introduction

The **clinical syndromes** of glomerulonephritis are:
- acute nephritis
- nephrotic syndrome
- persistent or recurrent haematuria and/or proteinuria
- acute renal failure (urine output < 180 ml/m^2/day; < 0.5 ml/kg/hr in infants)
- chronic renal failure.

In some of these syndromes the cause is identifiable, e.g., post-streptococcal nephritis and malarial nephrotic syndrome, but in many it is not. These problems may arise in the setting of a systemic illness, e.g., Systemic lupus erythematosus, and Schönlein-Henoch purpura.

Histology: The changes seen on light microscopy may be obvious, with thickening of the glomerular basement membrane *(membranous)* or proliferation of the cellular components *(proliferative);* or the changes may be hard to discern, with virtually normal glomeruli *(minimal change).* (*Figs 16.1–16.3* demonstrate these features on electron microscopy.)

Abnormal function: Altered glomerular function results in a pattern of biochemical changes, primarily of protein and lipid metabolism, which is characteristic of some of the clinical syndromes indicated above. Diminished function leads to increased serum creatinine and urea.

Pathogenesis: The pathogenesis of these glomerulonephritides is unclear, but in many it is

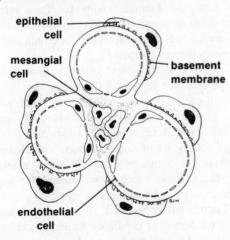

Fig. 16.1 Normal glomerulus on electron microscopy

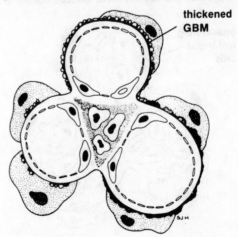

Fig. 16.2 Membranous glomerulonephritis on electron microscopy

on an immunological basis. Disturbances of immune factors in plasma and deposits of immunoglobulin and complement in renal tissue can therefore assist in more precise diagnosis. For example, serum C3 is markedly diminished in post-streptococcal glomerulonephritis; there is an absence of deposits of immunoglobulin or complement in minimal change nephrosis; and linear deposits of IgG are found on the glomerular basement membrane in Goodpasture's syndrome.

In some cases the damaging processes are not immune-related, but linked to vascular, coagulation, toxic, or congenital factors. Alteration of the anionic electrical charge in the basement membrane, which presents a barrier to the escape of serum proteins, has also been implicated.

Correlations: The difficulty with the above classification of glomerulonephritis is that there is considerable overlap among the different parameters given. There may be little correlation between histology, clinical features, and biochemical and immunological changes. A single histological group, for example, can occur with any of these clinical syndromes, and include a range of biochemical and immunological abnormalities.

Post-streptococcal glomerulonephritis (PSGN)

Although glomerulonephritis may be caused by a number of different organisms and agents *(see Table 16.2),* the streptococcal-induced disease is

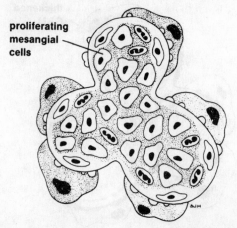

Fig. 16.3 *Acute proliferative glomerulonephritis on electron microscopy*

proliferating mesangial cells

the most common. The nephritic syndrome is recognized by the presence of abnormalities in quality (haematuria, proteinuria, casts) and quantity (oliogo-anuria) of urine, oedema, and hypertension.

Table 16.2 Some causes of acute glomerulonephritis

Infections:	
Bacteria:	Streptococci, staphylococci, *S. typhi*, *T. pallidum*, pneumococci
Viruses:	HBs, echovirus, E.B. virus, varicella, HIV
Protozoa:	Malaria
Collagen-vascular disease:	Schönlein-Henoch purpura, SLE, progressive systemic sclerosis, polyarteritis nodosa
Genetic:	Alport's syndrome
Drugs:	Methicillin
Miscellaneous:	Sickle-cell disease, sarcoid, irradiation

Pathogenesis: The triggering event is a streptococcal infection of the skin or the throat. In African children, the skin is the more frequent site, and bacterial infection is often superimposed on preceding scabies. Roughly one out of every six or seven infections with nephritogenic streptococci results in glomerulonephritis. The risk is higher after skin than throat infections. Infection at either site elicits an immune response to the streptococcus, and the consequent combination of streptococcal antigens with specific antibodies results in the formation of immune complexes. These enter the circulation and are largely deposited in the glomeruli, which have receptors for certain components in these complexes.

The precise component of the streptococcus responsible for glomerular damage has not been identified. Antigen and antibody may also reach the glomeruli separately and combine to form immune complexes at this site. Glomerular damage occurs when these immune complexes activate the complement cascade, which in turn produces factors which cause inflammation and attract polymorphonuclear leucocytes.

Endothelial cells swell, fibrin is deposited, and the lumen of capillaries thereby occluded. Release of proteolytic enzymes from polymorphs disrupts the integrity of the glomerular basement membrane and allows the excessive escape of blood cells and plasma constituents in the urine. Evidence of these immunopathogenic responses is the presence in serum of detectable antibodies (e.g., ASOT, anti-NADase, anti-DNase B, anti-hyaluronidase) to the corresponding streptococcal antigens, and reduction of complement globulins, especially C3. These changes are very useful in diagnosis.

Pathology: The imprint of these immunological processes on the histology of the kidney is a diffuse *proliferative* nephritis, with a striking *exudation* of polymorphs in the glomeruli. Proliferation is caused by an increase in endothelial and mesangial cells. Deposits in the shape of humps, possibly representing immune complexes, are detected by electron microscopy on the subepithelial aspect of the basement membrane.

Incidence: As PSGN can occur with minimal symptoms and physical discomfort, the true incidence of this disease among African children in South Africa cannot be estimated. In other studies, the ratio of subclinical to overt disease is usually four or five to one. It may be as high as nineteen or as low as less than one. The incidence of acute glomerulonephritis has declined in most richer countries in recent years, together with a decrease in the number of cases following streptococcal sore throat, although epidemics have reappeared with streptococcal outbreaks. In South Africa the disease is common among underprivileged African and Indian children, and infrequent among privileged children. It may occur in epidemic form in poorer communities. In Durban, PSGN is the most common renal problem seen in the King Edward VIII Hospital, and accounts for about 2% of all admissions to the children's wards. Chronic overcrowding among urbanized black families in South Africa is an important factor responsible for the predominance of post-streptococcal diseases, including rheumatic fever.

Clinical features: Unlike rheumatic fever, only certain nephritogenic strains of Group A β-haemolytic streptococci, identified by specific M or T antigens, can cause PSGN. Inexplicably, the disease usually occurs in adequately-nourished children. It is possible that a vigorous immune response to streptococci is necessary to produce glomerular injury, and that this response is blunted

by protein-energy malnutrition. There is an increased familial susceptibility to PSGN.

Table 16.3 Glomerulonephritis according to infected site

	Skin	Throat
Country	Tropical, subtropical	Temperate
Season	Summer	Winter/spring
Age of onset	Pre-school and school children	Mainly school children
Sex distribution	M = F	M > F
Streptococcal M serotype S	49, 55, 57, 60	12
Risk of developing nephritis	High	Low
Period from infection to nephritis	21 days	10 days
Antibodies	Anti-DNase B Anti-hyaluronidase	Anti-NADase ASOT

There are a few differences in PSGN secondary to skin or throat infection *(see Table 16.3)*.

The onset of symptoms is usually abrupt. Those children who seek medical advice always have haematuria, proteinuria, casts in the urine, and oedema. Milder cases with fewer signs, however, go undetected in the community. In addition, most of the hospitalized cases of PSGN have hypertension, impetigo, and oliguria *(see Fig 16.4)*.

Haematuria is rarely gross. It is most often microscopic, and persists for a few months after onset. Proteinuria is usually mild, and its disappearance parallels that of red cells in the urine. The urine contains varying numbers and types of casts, and of these, red cell casts are pathognomonic of glomerulonephritis *(see Urine Examination, Table 16.1)*.

Hypertension occurs in about three-quarters of the children with PSGN; and is directly related to encephalopathy. There is no correlation between encephalopathy and fluid retention. This complication is suggested by headache, restlessness, drowsiness, vomiting, blurring of vision, and convulsions. Papilloedema and fundal haemorrhages are exceedingly rare in hypertensive encephalopathy. The high blood pressure usually settles in a week, but in a small minority of cases it may persist for longer periods.

Oedema is usually periorbital, and occasionally extensive. Circulatory congestion is present in about

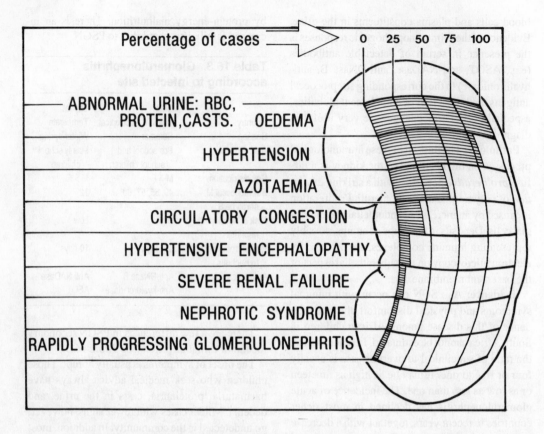

Fig. 16.4 Frequency of signs and complications in post-streptococcal glomerulonephritis

20% of cases *(see Table 16.4)*, and mimics signs of left- and right-sided heart failure. These features, however, are not due to myocardial damage and 'cardiac failure', because the important indices of cardiac function are normal in this disease.

Useful clinical distinctions from failure due to primary cardiac disease (e.g., rheumatic fever),

Table 16.4 Serious complications of acute glomerulonephritis in African children

Total number of children studied	2 765
Volume overload (CCF)	20%
Hypertensive encephalopathy	2.9%
Severe renal failure (i.e. requiring peritoneal dialysis)	1.2%
Deaths	1.84%

are the absence in PSGN of a hyperdynamic, thrusting apex beat and a relatively slower pulse. In the majority of children, the oedema and congestion clear as diuresis appears, i.e., within a week to ten days.

A decreased urinary output is frequent, and in severe cases leads to anuria. It is a complication which can easily be monitored, but is frequently overlooked. The management of oligo-anuria depends on careful observation (increasing oedema, weight gain) and good nursing. There is an improvement in urine output by the end of the first week in most cases, and by a fortnight in nearly all. This diuresis is accompanied by amelioration of oedema and circulatory congestion.

Prolongation of oligo-anuria beyond this period is an ominous sign, and suggests either a rare complication of PSGN or another diagnosis.

Important investigations:
- Urine — *see Urine Examination, Table 16.1*
- blood urea, serum creatinine and electrolytes (especially K), acid-base indices
- chest X-ray may show cardiomegaly, congestion of lungs, and small bilateral pleural effusions
- full blood count — mild leucocytosis
- ECG to monitor effects of hyperkalaemia
- streptococcal antibodies — usually positive
- skin or throat culture for streptococci is frequently negative
- C3 — markedly reduced in vast majority.

Differential diagnosis: *See Table 16.2.* Special efforts must be made to exclude typhoid; *Table 16.5* gives features which are useful in distinguishing PSGN from typhoid nephritis.

Prevention:
- Improvement of socio-economic status, in particular housing.
- treatment for pyoderma and pharyngitis
- treatment of contacts.

Table 16.5 Features helpful in recognizing typhoid nephritis

	PSGN	Typhoid
Oedema	Brief (± 7 days)	Prolonged (± 30 days)
Fever and splenomegaly		✓
Antibodies to streptococci	✓	
Blood culture		✓
C3	Markedly diminished	Moderate diminution
Recovery	Within 30 days	Longer than 30 days
Renal failure	Rare	Frequent
Mortality	2%	20%

Management: In developing countries, a rough guide to the requirement for hospital admission would be: (i) hypertension; (ii) oliguria.

Fluid and food intake: In the presence of marked oliguria (< 300 ml/m^2/day) the fluid intake should be restricted to 300–400 ml/m^2/day plus the volume of previous day's urine output. Aim at a high calorie intake (400 kcals/m^2/day). Lactose is more palatable than glucose/dextrose. This can be supplemented by sweets and high-calorie formulas. Avoid proteins and electrolytes. As renal function returns to normal, proteins and electrolytes can be reintroduced.

Regular monitoring: Daily fluid intake and output, weighing, urine testing (albuminuria, appearance, volume, specific gravity), 3-hourly blood pressure monitoring.

Drugs: If possible avoid drugs excreted by the kidney. Remember that during renal failure, these drugs accumulate rapidly and very small maintenance doses are required. Digoxin is best avoided.

Furosemide (1 mg/kg per dose IV; maximum 400 mg in 24 hours). A diuresis may be induced when given intravenously, especially for pulmonary oedema and circulatory congestion. Penicillin should be given for 10 days, after a throat and/or skin swab has been taken. *See Table 16.16 for details of anti-hypertensive medications.* Diazepam is given for convulsions.

Uraemia: Protein should be restricted or absent from the diet while the blood urea is elevated. *See below for indications for peritoneal dialysis.*

Hyperkalaemia: May cause bradycardia, fibrillation, heart block, and death. Typical ECG changes are prolonged QRS, depressed ST segment, and high T wave.

Treatment is urgent when these changes are present and/or serum potassium is more than 7.0 mEq/l.

a. Calcium gluconate (10%) 0.5 ml/kg is given over 2–4 minutes with an ECG monitor. Sodium bicarbonate 2.5 mEq/kg counteracts the arrhythmia, but must not be repeated. Glucose (50%) 1 ml/kg is given as a bolus, and then 30% glucose infusion is commenced as for fluid requirements. This is usually effective within 1–2 hours, but if hyperkalaemia persists, insulin 1 u/kg is given IV with blood sugar monitoring and glucose infusion.

b. If serum potassium is < 6.0 mEq/l with normal ECG, omit (a). Use an ion exchange resin orally, or by retention enema.

c. Repeat (a) once if not below 6.0 mEq/l after 2–3 hours, and plan for peritoneal dialysis.

Circulatory congestion and pulmonary oedema call for the following steps:
- furosemide IV
- peritoneal dialysis
- O$_2$
- morphine
- rotating tourniquets
- venesection

◆ artificial ventilation.

Acidosis is corrected with sodium bicarbonate given IV.

Peritoneal dialysis (or haemodialysis in special units only) is implemented for the indications listed below:

◆ deterioration in the clinical condition

◆ blood urea rising above 50 mmol/l (preferably it should be kept below 35 mmol/l)

◆ hyperkalaemia (> 7.0 mEq/l)

◆ severe metabolic acidosis, unresponsive to alkali therapy

◆ acute water and salt overload manifesting as severe circulatory congestion.

Unusual complications: *(See Fig. 16.4.)* In the vast majority of children with PSGN, the tendency is towards quick resolution and rapid recovery. However, a small minority develop complications in the short term. These are:

Rapidly-progressive glomerulonephritis: This occurs in less than 1% of children with PSGN. The clinical picture is dominated by prolonged oligoanuria, progressing relentlessly to chronic renal failure or death, and histology shows crescent formation of glomeruli. There is no satisfactory treatment, although quadruple therapy with cyclophosphamide, steroids, anticoagulants, and antiplatelet agents may be useful.

Nephrotic syndrome: This occurs in less than 0.5% of children with PSGN. No specific therapy is indicated, and the disease usually resolves in a few months *(see below)*.

Long-term sequelae of PSGN: There is conflicting evidence about the long-term effects of PSGN. The vast majority of children with PSGN suffer no permanent sequelae, but a small minority (probably less than 1%) may develop chronic nephritis and hypertension. This minority proportion probably increases in older patients.

Nephrotic syndrome

General features

The term nephrotic syndrome, refers to a heterogeneous group of glomerular disorders which are the end result of heavy proteinuria (> 40 mg/m^2/hr, or > 3 gm/1.73m^2/day, or 4+ on reagent strip).

Massive loss of proteins in the urine leads to hypoalbuminaemia and oedema.

In addition, the serum lipids and α_2 globulin levels are often raised. The presentation is usually insidious, with oedema of the eyelids which is usually worse in the morning. Oedema is often severe in African children, and can spread to become anasarca. This may be due to a combination of factors which, in addition to massive proteinuria, include dietary and infective causes of low serum albumin. Except for a swollen body, the patient often does not have many other signs of renal disease, and does not appear to be seriously ill. Hypertension, hypertensive encephalopathy, volume overload, and renal failure are rare. Complications include a predisposition to infection (especially pneumococcal peritonitis), vascular thrombosis (affecting any vessel), haemolytic uraemic syndrome, and circulatory failure.

The last-mentioned is caused by excessive loss of fluids from the intravascular compartment, and presents with cold peripheries, cyanosis of extremities, pallor, hypotension, and a thready pulse.

Investigations should aim at confirming the biochemical abnormalities characteristic of this syndrome and determining the aetiology.

In most patients the cause of nephrotic syndrome is unidentified. Some known causes are given in *Table 16.6.*

Table 16.6 Some causes of nephrotic syndrome

Infections	*P. malariae, S. mansoni, T. pallidum,* streptococci, hepatitis B, infective endocarditis, hydatid disease
Toxic causes	Heavy metals (Hg, Pb), drugs (trimethadione, penicillamine, captopril)
Allergy	Bee stings, pollen
Vasculitis	SLE, Schönlein-Henoch purpura, polyarteritis nodosa, dermatomyositis
Malignancies	Lymphoma
Miscellaneous	Renal vein thrombosis, constrictive pericarditis, diabetes, amyloidosis, Alport's syndrome, haemolytic-uraemic syndrome

Plasmodium malariae is an important cause of nephrosis in endemic areas in Nigeria, Uganda, and Kenya; as is the hepatitis B virus in Namibia, Zimbabwe, South Africa, and West Africa.

Schistosoma mansoni and *haematobium* are implicated in Egypt and Sudan, and group B haemolytic streptococci in Zimbabwe. Other infections such as *Salmonella typhi, Treponema pallidum, Streptococcus viridans* and *Mycobacterium leprae* are less frequently identified as aetiological agents. Onchocerca have been pin-pointed as a cause in the Cameroons. Autoimmune disorders, vascular diseases, malignancies, and idiopathic factors are much less common causes of the disease in Africans than in non-African people. Histological classification of the disease, based on tissue obtained at renal biopsy, aids management and prognosis.

The closest identity between histological lesions and micro-organisms has been between membranous nephropathy and hepatitis B surface (HBs) antigen in countries where HBs incidence is high. There is also a close correlation between diffuse proliferative exudative glomerulonephritis and group B haemolytic streptococci in South Africa, Zimbabwe, and North Africa. Specific histological changes have been attributed to quartan malaria in childhood nephrosis in Nigeria. In South Africa (among whites and Indians), Ghana, and Libya, the renal biopsy picture is similar to that seen among children in the rest of the world: in most cases minimal change. Elsewhere minimal change is uncommon.

The pattern of this syndrome is not uniform throughout the world, but is strongly influenced by geographical location and by environmental and possibly other factors acting on particular communities. These differences have been kept in mind in the discussion below.

Nephrotic syndrome among children in continents other than Africa
(See Table 16.6 and Fig. 16.5.)
In the vast majority of non-African children nephrotic syndrome is not a serious disease, and when properly managed has an excellent prognosis, allowing a full and active life. Nephrotic syndrome is less common in temperate countries than in tropical and sub-tropical Africa. The disease is dominated by **minimal change** lesions, which account for roughly 80% of all children with nephrosis. Most children with minimal change disease are male, younger than 5, have a less insidious onset of symptoms and signs, have less uraemia, haematuria, and hypertension, have selective proteinuria, i.e., excrete small (e.g., transferrin) rather than large (e.g., IgG) molecular weight proteins, and 90% respond to steroid therapy *(see Table 16.7).* The major clinical problem in these children

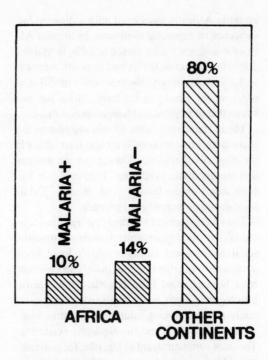

Fig. 16.5 Frequency of minimal change nephrotic syndrome

is that of frequent relapses (i.e., two relapses within 6 months of onset of disease), which occur in just under half the patients. The child with frequent relapses is usually managed on cyclophosphamide, chlorambucil, or levamisole, which prolong remission periods.

Nephrotic syndrome in Africa
Malaria-endemic areas: *(See Table 16.8.)* In the African environment, where malaria is endemic, the incidence of nephrotic syndrome (assessed by estimates of hospital admissions) is higher than in temperate countries. This is supported by the fact that the transition from malarial to non-malarial

Table 16.7 Steroids in minimal change nephrotic syndrome

Initial attack	Prednisone 2 mg/kg/day (max. 80 mg/day) x 6 wks; then 1/4 of this dose every 48 hours x 6 wks
Relapse	Prednisone (2 mg/kg/day) until urine protein-free; then 1/4 of this dose every 48 hrs x 4 wks

zones in Africa is associated with a diminishing incidence of nephrotic syndrome. In tropical Africa for instance, the incidence is 2.4%, in Malawi 1.4%, in Zimbabwe 0.7%, and in South Africa it is 0.2%. Accordingly, the frequency of this disorder among blacks in southern Africa lies between that of tropical and temperate countries.

The outstanding feature of this disorder in the malaria-endemic areas of West and East Africa is the compelling evidence linking quartan malaria and the nephrotic syndrome. This evidence has been based on epidemiological, clinical, pathological, and immunological grounds.

The vast majority of affected children have 'obvious' structural glomerular lesions. Distinctive renal histological changes which have been attributed to quartan malaria, mainly in children, have been reported from Nigeria. This specific histological pattern, however, has not been consistently detected among adults and children elsewhere with malaria and the nephrotic syndrome. The most common lesion in Uganda, for example, was diffuse proliferative glomerulonephritis.

The peak age of incidence of nephrosis in tropical Africa is between 5 and 8 years, and the sexes are equally represented. These children usually have poorly selective proteinuria, and an overall unsatisfactory response to therapy with antimalarials, steroids, and immunosuppressives. Death from progressive renal failure is common in those

Table 16.8 Features of childhood nephrotic syndrome in malaria-endemic zones of Africa

Incidence	High
Peak age	5–8 years
Sex incidence	M = F
Aetiology	*P. malariae* in majority
Histological groups	Dominated by changes attributed to malaria. Minimal change in 8–10%
Immunofluorescence	Deposits in most
Response to therapy (steroids, cyclophosphamide)	Poor in majority. Frequent and alarming complications. Steroids and cyclophosphamide produce a favourable response in minority with selective proteinuria and/or minimal change
Prognosis	Poor

with poorly selective proteinuria, supervening in about 50% at 5 years. Between 8 and 10% of children have minimal change nephrotic syndrome. These children usually have a short history of disease, selective proteinuria, and a favourable response to steroid therapy.

Non-malarial zones: *(See Table 16.9.)* Despite the absence of the damaging effects of malaria on the kidney, there still remains in African children in southern Africa an unusual distribution of histopathological types of nephrosis, which distinguishes them from children in tropical Africa and on other continents. The disease clearly behaves differently in African children generally, compared to most non-Africans. The nephrotic syndrome in Indian and white South African children is similar to that in other countries.

The majority of African children (86%) have 'obvious' structural glomerular lesions, while only a minority (14%) have minimal change. Even this small group with minimal change does not always show a close identity with the classical features of minimal change alluded to and seen among Indian children, and may in fact have focal glomerular sclerosis. *Membranous nephropathy* is the most common lesion among African children, followed by the different subgroups of proliferative glomerulonephritis. The cause of the disease in the vast majority of these patients is not known, although HBs is very closely linked with membranous lesion.

Indeed, if an African child with nephrotic syndrome is HBs-positive, there is no need for a renal biopsy, as the patient has a very high probability of having membranous nephropathy. The disease is seen most frequently in either pre-school or late-primary school children, and is more common among males. Haematuria and hypertension occur frequently, and are detected in almost all the histological groups, but renal failure is uncommon at initial presentation. Prognosis depends on the histological group.

There is no firm evidence that African children with nephrosis disease (including many, though not all, of those with minimal change) respond to drugs used conventionally for this disease (i.e., steroids and cyclophosphamide). As these drugs can have serious side-effects, their use is best avoided in the vast majority of African children, except the small group with minimal change who

Table 16.9 Features of nephrotic syndrome in South African children

	African	Indian
Incidence	Midway between temperate and tropical countries	–
Peak age	2 peaks: 4 years and 8 – 11 years	Pre-school
Sex incidence	M > F	M > F
Aetiology	Unknown in many; HBS in nearly all with membranous disease	Unknown in majority
Histological groups	Dominated by 'obvious' structural glomerular lesions (86%); especially membranous. Minimal change in 14%	Dominated by minimal change (75%)
Immunofluorescence	Deposits in majority	No deposits in majority
Response to therapy (steroids, cyclophosphamide)	Do not respond	Majority respond
Children who relapse frequently	As in temperate countries	± 30%
Prognosis	Related to histological group	Excellent

are steroid-responsive. Management is supportive, with recommendations of a high protein diet and use of diuretics. The former is of some benefit, as a few children who do badly in their deprived home environments lose oedema rapidly when treated in hospital. Intravenous 20% albumin combined with diuretics is useful for alleviation of severe oedema.

Haemolytic-uraemic syndrome (HUS)

This is not a distinct and single clinicopathological entity, but a complex syndrome of which the essential features are:

◆ haemolytic anaemia, with fragmented cells on the peripheral blood smear

◆ thrombocytopenia

◆ acute renal damage manifesting as azotaemia (uraemia).

It is a disease primarily of infancy and childhood, and is seen in both developed and develop-

ing countries. In the former, HUS is an important cause of renal failure, requiring dialysis and transplantation. While the syndrome is rare in African children in Zimbabwe and South Africa, it is frequently seen among white children in Johannesburg. It is eight times more frequent in whites than in blacks. It affects both boys and girls equally, and there is considerable variation in the mean age of onset (from under 1 year to over 4 years).

There is no satisfactory unifying hypothesis to explain the nature of the disease. The observed effects on blood factors and the kidney may be the end result of haematological, metabolic, or immunological derangements.

The central event in pathogenesis is injury to endothelial cells in the glomeruli by the agents or processes listed in *Table 16.10*. Shiga-like toxins are especially important as triggering agents. Damaged endothelial cells become swollen and partially dislodged from the underlying basement membrane; exposure of collagen and other constituents in this sub-endothelial space activates platelets. Intravascular clumping of platelets is initiated by vasoactive substances released by endothelial cells and platelets: there is decrease in anti-aggregating factors (such as prostacyclin) and increase in aggregating agents (such as thromboxane, high molecular weight von Willebrand factor). The sub-endothelial space becomes filled with the debris of platelets, fibrin, and lipids. Polymorphs increase damage by releasing proteases. Swollen endothelial cells, and debris-filled subendothelial space and thrombi, reduce the diameter of the capillary lumen. These changes

Table 16.10 Aetiology of haemolytic-uraemic syndrome

Idiopathic*	
Infections	*E. coli* 0157: H7#
	Shigella dysenteriae#
	S. pneumoniae#
	Other bacteria and viruses
Inherited	Autosomal recessive*
	Autosomal dominant*
Drug-induced	
Miscellaneous	Glomerulonephritis, post-transplant*, pregnancy, malignancy

*recurrent   # produce Shiga-like toxins

[handwritten: Damage to endoth. cells of glomeruli; Collagen → Platelet act. → I.V. clumping]

[handwritten at bottom: ① Fragmented cells → Blood smear. ② Thrombocytopaenia ③ Uraemia]

cause a reduction in glomerular filtration rate (GFR).

The exact reasons for the fragmentation of red cells and destruction of platelets unclear; these effects may be the result of passage through tiny renal capillaries webbed by strands of fibrin.

Pathology

This is a glomerular disease in which the endothelial cells are swollen and changes occur in the subendothelial region. A heterogeneous material comprised of cellular (platelets) and non-cellular (fibrin, lipids) components is interposed between the endothelial cells and glomerular basement membrane. This can lead to narrowing of the capillary lumen, which may be further occluded by microthrombi. This combination of lesions may occur dominantly in glomeruli, or in renal arteries and arterioles. In some cases there is cortical necrosis.

Clinical features

Preceding the more dramatic features of renal failure are episodes of afebrile bloody diarrhoea, vomiting, and upper respiratory tract infection. There is an unexpected deterioration, with symptoms and signs of acute renal failure *(see below)* with pallor, oliguria, and convulsions.

Gastrointestinal signs may be severe in some cases. The clinical presentation will indicate mild, moderate, or severe renal damage. Prognostic indices are given in *Table 16.11*. Recurrences of HUS have been indicated in *Table 16.10*.

The complications include bleeding, encephalopathy, cardiac failure, infection, and the metabolic disturbances characteristic of renal failure. Sequelae are neurological problems and chronic renal failure.

Management   *Early dialysis*

Management is primarily that of renal failure. Mild cases are treated by conventional methods, and usually recover in 10 days. One of the most important aspects of treatment is early institution of peritoneal dialysis (within 24 hours) for severe cases. This determines survival. Careful management reduces mortality to less than 5%. Particular attention must be paid to control of convulsions, hypertension, and of fluid, electrolyte, and calorie requirements. Blood transfusions must be re-

Table 16.11   Features suggesting poor outcome in haemolytic-uraemic syndrome

Clinical deterioration
Older age
Concomitant problems: pneumococcal and shigella infections, intestinal gangrene
Inherited disease
Recurrences

stricted to those with haemoglobin below 6 g/dl, as they aggravate or induce hypertension. Infusions of fresh frozen plasma can prove useful in some cases.

The evidence at present does not support the use of anticoagulants, aspirin, streptokinase, urokinase and dipyridamole.

Recurrent haematuria due to glomerular disease

In such cases macroscopic haematuria occurs during a mild upper respiratory tract infection or after exercise. The usual causes are:

♦ Berger's disease (IgA nephropathy)
♦ benign familial haematuria
♦ glomerulonephritis (minimal change, mesangial proliferative, etc.)
♦ Alport's syndrome (family history, male, eye signs, deafness, progressive renal impairment).

Inherited and congenital renal disorders

These usually present with renal masses or signs of advancing renal failure. Those seen in Durban include obstructive uropathy (e.g., pelvi-ureteric stricture, urethral valves), ureteric abnormalities, renal agenesis, renal cysts, dysplastic kidney, polycystic kidneys, primary oxalosis, Alport's syndrome, and ectopic kidneys.

Urinary tract infection (UTI)

One of the most important considerations of this disease in poor communities is that it may be overlooked because of the silent nature of the infection, which may be completely obscured by the overwhelming burden of other problems. The clinical features of UTI are often inconspicuous, especially in the younger child, and pyelonephritis is not infrequently diagnosed for the first time at post-mortem. As UTI can cause much morbidity, and in a minority result in chronic renal destruction and death, it must be actively excluded in any unexplained illness in childhood, and adequate treatment provided.

Definition
◆ More than 10^5 organisms/ml of fresh urine, *or any growth* in suprapubic aspirate or in catheter specimens
◆ pure culture
◆ pus cells often found.

Aseptic precautions *(see Chapter 31, Procedures)* in collection are a minimum condition for interpreting these urine findings.

If facilities for culture are not available, the following fact can prove useful for diagnosis: pus cells in the urine are present in more than 90% of patients with positive cultures, and absent in more than 90% of patients with negative cultures. Commercial kits for diagnosis of UTI may also be helpful; these include medium-impregnated slides for immediate plating, and reagent strips which detect pus cells and bacteria. These techniques may be especially useful in poor countries. Pyuria without significant bacteriuria indicates partially-treated infection, or delay in culture of urine sample.

Organisms: Predominantly *E. coli*; although other bacteria such as klebsiella, proteus, enterococci, pseudomonas, and staphylococci also cause UTI. The source of infection is usually bowel flora, but may be blood-borne in infants *(see Fig. 16.6)*. Virulence has been correlated with fimbria on *E. Coli* which adhere to specific receptors on mucosal cells.

The incidence is similar in male and female infants, whilst among older children females predominate.

In the West, among apparently healthy school-girls who are usually asymptomatic, about 2% have UTI. Fewer boys (0.3%) have such infection. Widespread screening for covert bacteriuria is not a cost-effective measure given the relatively low return and uncertainty of success of treatment. Covert bacteriuria has been detected in up to 0.8% of male and 3.6% of female children in India.

Studies in Africa have suggested that UTI is a common problem in apparently healthy as well as obviously ill children. It has been detected in a significant proportion of children in the community and in hospital. UTI may often be present in children with protein-energy malnutrition and *Schistosoma haematobium* infestations.

Clinical features
The majority of infants have no symptoms referable to the urinary tract, and many older children

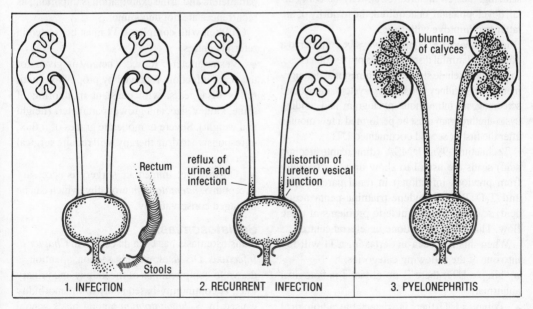

Fig. 16.6 Pathogenesis of pyelonephritis

are asymptomatic. This fact underlines the absolute necessity for a proper urine examination in order to establish a diagnosis.

◆ In **infancy,** lethargy, failure to feed, unstable temperature, poor colour, apnoea, jaundice, anaemia, purpura, and hepatosplenomegaly are the common features.

◆ **Children** may have some urgency as an isolated feature but be otherwise asymptomatic. Frequency, dysuria, fever, abdominal and flank pain, and enlarged tender kidney do occur infrequently.

Associated abnormalities

One of the major concerns is to prevent the progressive destruction of renal tissue by infection of the urinary tract. A factor underlying this is the high frequency with which abnormalities of the urinary tract have been detected in children with UTI. The most frequent abnormality is reflux of urine. The downward flow of urine constantly clears bacteria originating in the bowel which regularly traverse the urethra near the external meatus. If this flow of urine is interrupted, infection is more easily established. Reflux of urine from the bladder into the ureters (vesico-ureteric reflux) or from calyces into the renal parenchyma (intrarenal reflux) during micturition predisposes to persistent infection, pyelonephritis, and renal scarring. Vesico-ureteric reflux may be congenital, developmental, or acquired; the majority of the latter two improve with time.

In other words, UTI must always be considered a potentially harmful disease unless proved otherwise. In order to exclude structural or functional derangements of the kidney and urinary system, ultrasound screening, an intravenous pyelogram and voiding cysto-urethrogram must be performed a few months after the first or second documented UTI.

Technetium-99m DMSA (dimercaptosuccinic acid) scans are useful to show up scars (usually from previous infections) in renal parenchyma, and T$_c$DTPA (diethylene-triamine-penta acetic acid) scans provide a guide to problems of urine flow. This can only be done in referral centres.

When this has been undertaken, UTI will fall into one of the following categories:

◆ simple UTI: there is no obvious radiological abnormality

◆ complex UTI: there is a detectable radiological defect, which may be:

— vesico-ureteric reflux:, during voiding, urine refluxes into the ureter. This predisposes to stasis and infection, leading to pyelonephritis.

— obstruction: this may be congenital or acquired (e.g., stones).

Management

Treatment of acute infection: Sulphonamides, given over 5–7 days, are effective. The use of other agents will depend on culture of urine and sensitivity of the organism. Useful chemotherapeutic agents and antibiotics for UTI are: co-trimoxazole, synthetic penicillins, nitrofurantoin, and nalidixic acid.

Sulphonamides still have a place in poor countries. In very ill children, gentamicin should be given IM.

Recurrent infections: Treatment in the acute phase depends on the sensitivity of the infecting agent. Prophylactic therapy may have to be administered for several years if recurrences are frequent. The drugs used prophylatically at half or a third of the usual dosage are: co-trimoxazole, nitrofurantoin, ampicillin, nalidixic acid, or sulphonamides.

Simple UTI: Treatment is simply that of the acute infection *(as above).* Follow-up of growth parameters and urine examination is important, as recurrences are not uncommon.

Children with **complex UTI** must be treated in referral centres.

◆ Vesico-ureteric reflux: Therapy is given for the acute infection, followed by prophylaxis until reflux disappears, with constant monitoring of urine, kidney size, and growth parameters (height and weight). Severe or moderate grades of reflux, unresponsive to drug therapy, will require surgical intervention.

◆ Obstruction: Immediate surgery is necessary except in *S. haematobium* uropathy, which can be managed conservatively.

Schistosomiasis

Schistosomiasis has been discussed in *Chapter 8, Infectious Diseases;* in this section attention is drawn to complications of the kidney and urinary tract. A community-based study of the morbidity caused by *S. haematobium* among black school children in an endemic area of Natal gives an accurate impression of the problem at this level.

Up to 98% of children in some areas were infected. Both sexes were equally affected by *S. haematobium,* and 93% of these were under 15 years of age. The intensity of infection, as estimated from the egg load in the urine, was moderate to heavy in 80% of children studied, especially in those between 6 and 10 years of age. The children with a heavy burden of parasites were more likely to have symptoms, proteinuria, haematuria, and rectal granuloma. The infected children could be classified into three clinical categories *(see Table 16.12).* It can be seen that three-quarters of children with *S. haematobium* had infection of the rectum.

Children who had contact with river water were likely to have more serious disease than those who used water from taps or tanks.

Excretory urography showed pathological features in 42% of the infected children; these radiological changes revealed polypoid lesions, bladder calcification, ureteric dilatation and hydronephrosis. Most of the children with urographic abnormalities had severe changes; ureteric involvement was often bilateral.

A most important finding was that despite these clinical and radiological abnormalities, the renal function assessed by blood urea, serum creatinine, and glomerular filtration rate was normal. The natural history of the untreated cases is not clear, as symptoms generally disappear; anatomic abnormalities of the urinary tract resolve, remain static, or deteriorate. Treatment with the appropriate drug leads to resolution of hydronephrosis in a few months.

In hospital practice the following uncommon and extreme forms of the disease are seen:

- iron deficiency anaemia
- strangury
- acute retention of urine

Table 16.12 Clinical presentation of *S. haematobium*-infected children

Presentation	Proportion
Asymptomatic	12%
Dysuria/haematuria	12%
Dysuria/haematuria/rectal mucosal lesions	76%

- renal failure secondary to obstructive uropathy
- an 'acute nephritic' presentation.

The last-mentioned does not appear to be a 'true' nephritis; it is rare, and the pathogenesis not understood. Clinically, the presentation is similar to that of post-streptococcal glomerulonephritis, with one essential difference: there are no casts in a fresh sample of urine which contains ova of *S. haematobium.* Evidence of streptococcal infection is obviously negative. Clinical improvement occurs rapidly on specific therapy.

Studies in Brazil and Africa show that *S. mansoni* can cause nephrotic syndrome.

Renal tubular diseases

Renal tubular disorders may be caused by congenital defects or by acquired damage from drugs, toxins, etc.

Tubular necrosis presents as renal failure *(see below and Table 16.13).*

Proximal tubular diseases

Proximal tubular diseases may be asymptomatic, or may present with growth retardation, somatic abnormalities, rickets, stones, and metabolic abnormalities (acidosis, hypokalaemia). Examples are Fanconi syndrome, glycosuria, renal tubular acidosis, and vitamin D-dependent rickets.

Distal tubular diseases

Distal tubular diseases manifest as growth retardation, acidosis, rickets, and diabetes insipidus. Examples are renal tubular acidosis and nephrogenic diabetes insipidus.

An approach to hypertension in childhood

Introduction

Long-standing hypertension is uncommon in childhood. Among Third World doctors the marginalization of hypertension has been accentuated by the overwhelming dominance of nutritional and infectious diseases. During the past 20 years, however, there has been increasing support for the recognition of apparently normal children in the uppermost range of blood pressure levels as being potential, if not actual, hypertensives. This pattern of being on a relatively fixed higher centile is set as early as 1–4 years of age. There is direct evidence to suggest that these children are at high risk for essential hypertension in adult life.

Hypertension can only be diagnosed if the blood pressure (BP) is properly taken and sensibly interpreted.

Measurement of blood pressure

In children above the age of 2–3 years, BP can be taken by auscultation. The cuff size of the baumanometer should cover two-thirds of the upper arm,

and the inflatable bladder within it must encircle the arm girth. The child should be sitting and relaxed. Systolic pressure is at the appearance of sound during release from occlusion of the artery, and diastolic pressure is at the level of muffling (phases 1 and 4 respectively). Alternative techniques such as Doppler ultrasound and flush method are used to estimate BP in infancy. Mistakes in recording BP arise due to inaccurate cuff size, poor equipment, observer error, and an uncomfortable or anxious child.

Interpretation of blood pressure levels

In the absence of local data, BP percentile charts based on American studies are useful for ascertaining normal and abnormal values.

A single BP recording is sufficient if it confirms obvious symptoms and signs of hypertension (e.g., in nephritis or Cushing's syndrome). However,

Table 16.13 Some tubular disorders

Defect/disease	Clinical features	Helpful tests
Multiple defects:		
Fanconi syndrome	Rickets,	Proteinuria
	Growth retardation	Glycosuria
	Polyuria	Hyperaminoaciduria
	Polydipsia	Phosphaturia
	Dehydration acidosis	Proximal RTA
		Uricosuria
		Reduced serum
		PO4, K, uric
		acid, HCO3
Amino acids:		
Cystinuria	Urinary stones	Cystine
		Ornithine
		Arginine
		Lysine in urine
Glucose:		
Glycosuria	Diabetes	Glucose in urine
	Low renal threshold	
	Fanconi syndrome	
	Renal failure	
Electrolytes:		
Hypercalciuria	Haematuria	Urinary Ca:
Hypophosphataemic	Stones	Creatinine
rickets		(mmols) ratio
		> 0.7
Concentration:		
Nephrogenic	Polyuria	
diabetes insipidus	Polydipsia	Dilute urine
	Hypernatraemic	(< 100 m Os/kg)
	dehydration	Unresponsive to
	Vomiting	vasopressin
Acid-base:		
Renal tubular	Like Fanconi	Failure to acidify
acidosis (types I,	syndrome	urine
II, III, IV)		Low bicarbonate
		threshold in
		tubules
		Nephrocalcinosis

Table 16.14 Definition of hypertension in children

> 95th percentile

Newborn	1st 12 hours	Premature 65/45
	1st week	Full term 80/50
		Premature 80*/50*
		Full term 100/70

	SYSTOLIC RULE OF 5s	mmHg	DIASTOLIC RULE OF 2s
6 weeks to			
6 years		115/80	
8 years		120/82	
9 years		125/84	
10 years		130/86	
12 years		135/88	
14 years		140/90**	
16 years		#145/92	
18 years		#150/94	

Kilopascals (kPa) = mm Hg x 0.133

* Arbitrary figures

\# Systolic 3–5 mm Hg less in girls

**Take >140/90 in adolescents 14 years and older as hypertension. Repeat measurements recommended in all children and adolescents. (At least three readings at weekly/monthly intervals, unless child is symptomatic or has an obvious cause.)

three measurements on separate occasions must be taken if the BP is borderline.

Any value outside the normal range (97th percentile) is clearly hypertension. Some workers define hypertension (diastolic and systolic) as values of BP beyond the 95th percentile, while P.D. Thomson and S.E. Levin from Witwatersrand University have collected data from a number of studies and proposed criteria as outlined in *Table 16.14*.

Causes of hypertension

Essential hypertension is a diagnosis arrived at by exclusion of other causes. Renal diseases account for more than 80% of those cases where the aetiology is identifiable. Some of these causes are given in *Table 16.15*.

Table 16.15   Causes of hypertension

Renal diseases
    Glomerulonephritis (due to infections, autoimmune
        processes, or radiation)
    Interstitial nephritis
    Reflux nephropathy (pyelonephritis)
    Obstructive uropathy
    Congenital abnormalities (dysplasias, polycystic disease)
    Renin-secreting tumours
Vascular diseases
    Coarctation of the aorta
    Renal artery stenosis or thrombosis
    Non-specific arteritis (Takayasu's)
Endocrine disorders
    Adrenal disorders (adrenogenital syndrome, Cushing's
        syndrome, primary hyperaldosteronism,
        phaeochromocytoma)
    Hyperthyroidism
    Hyperparathyroidism
    Diabetes mellitus
Miscellaneous causes
    Poliomyelitis, Guillain-Barré syndrome, neuroblastoma,
        neurofibromatosis, hypercalcaemia, mercury poisoning,
        leg traction, raised intracranial pressure, administration of
        corticosteroids and other drugs. Excessive intake of
        liquorice should always be borne in mind as being
        responsible for hypertension.

Clinical features

Symptoms include headaches, vomiting, blurred vision, and fits. Neurological complications can be varied; there may be signs and symptoms of heart failure, with an enlarged heart and a left ventricular apex beat. Retinal blood vessel changes can be detected.

Diagnostic evaluation

A logical approach to obtaining a relevant history, performing a problem-orientated physical examination, and requesting appropriate investigations, is to remember common causes of hypertension (*see Table 16.15*) and systematically seek evidence of these. Having defined the problem (hypertension), one should attempt to identify the organ involved (site of the lesion) and then the exact disease causing the problem (nature of lesion).

Family history may indicate familial tendencies to hypertension, a clear genetically-transmitted disorder, or the effects of high BP (i.e., myocardial infarctions, cerebrovascular accidents, uraemia). Information should be sought on other family members with renal disease, (e.g., hereditary nephritis, polycystic disease), endocrine disorders (e.g., diabetes, adrenal hyperplasia), autoimmune disease (e.g., SLE), and blood disorders (e.g., sickle-cell anaemia). Essential hypertension and obesity in the family will suggest essential hypertension in the patient.

A past history of growth retardation may mean a chronic renal disorder. The patient should be questioned on previous episodes of renal problems (especially urinary tract infections), and symptoms and signs of vascular, endocrine, or neurological disease.

The present history of illness ought to reveal the effects of hypertension and its causes. Once again, enquiry should be directed to the recognizable clinical expression of common disease, given in *Table 16.15*.

Physical examination can be most rewarding, particularly in children from poor communities, where histories are often inadequate or misleading. First of all BP and pulse must be measured in all limbs. Absence at any one site suggests a vascular cause. Long-standing hypertension results in growth retardation, left ventricular hypertrophy, and occasionally retinopathy. Even severe acute elevations in blood pressure do not produce these effects.

Kidney disease must be carefully excluded by looking for fever, oedema, abdominal masses and bruits, and the specific signs of SLE (such as arthritis, rash, lymphadenopathy, and alopecia).

Table 16.16 Drugs used in hypertension

A. HYPERTENSIVE EMERGENCY

Drug	Initial dose	Further treatment
Hydralazine	1.7–3.5 mg/kg/24 hrs IM or IV; qid, 0.15 mg/kg IV when given with reserpine	Acts in 0–20 minutes
Reserpine	0.02 mg/kg IM	Double dose if BP high in 4–6 hours; double 2nd dose again if BP still high in 4-6 hours. Acts in 1–2 hours.
Furosemide	5–40 mg IV or 5.6 mg/kg day	Repeat to maximum of 400 mg/24 hours
Labetalol	1 mg/kg/hr IV	Can increase to 3 mg/kg/hr; use alone
Sodium nitroprusside	0.5 μg/kg/minute IV in a 0.01% solution	Maximum dose 8 μg/kg/minute IV; use under close supervision; stop if no response in 10 minutes

Other drugs

Clonidine	2–6 kg	2nd line drug
Verapamil	1–10 mg/kg/hr	2nd line drug
Captopril	0.1–0.3 mg/kg/dose orally	2nd line drug
Minoxidil	0.1–0.2 mg/kg/dose orally	2nd line drug

Peritoneal dialysis for patients with azotaemia and severe hypertension due to sodium and water retention.

B. PERSISTENT HYPERTENSION

Drug	Daily dose Initial – maximum (mg/kg)
Diuretics	
Hydrochlorothiazide	1–2
Chlorothiazide	10–20
Furosemide	1–3
Spironolactone	1–2
Triamterene	2–6
Drugs acting on adrenergic system	
Propranolol	1–15
Alphamethyldopa	10–60
Reserpine	0.1–0.5 mg/day
Clonidine	25–100 μg/tid
Prazosin	0.05–0.4
Vasodilators	
Hydralazine	1–8
Minoxidil	0.1–2
Calcium channel inhibitor	
Nifedipine	0.25–1
Enzyme blocker	
Captopril	0.3–6

Hearing should be tested for hereditary nephritis. Chronic renal disease results in multiple problems, such as severe wasting, muscle weakness, tetany, rickets, and acidosis.

Cushing's syndrome, hyperthyroidism, adrenogenital syndrome, and diabetes mellitus present with characteristic features which are not difficult to identify. The CNS must be carefully examined.

It must be reiterated that essential hypertension is a diagnosis of exclusion, and is supported by a positive family history and the presence of obesity. This diagnosis may be especially insecure in the pre-pubertal child, and therefore such children should be fully investigated.

Investigations

Simple, inexpensive, and non-invasive investigations are done first, usually on an outpatient basis. Complicated and invasive techniques are performed last, and in hospital. Urine analysis, full blood count, and blood chemistry (urea, creatinine, sodium, potassium, chloride, bicarbonate, anion gap, glucose, calcium, phosphorus, alkaline phosphatase, uric acid) are the first-line tests.

Careful interpretation of these will in many cases convey some idea of the underlying cause.

Next a chest radiograph and plain X-ray of the abdomen are undertaken. These may show up an enlarged heart and nephrocalcinosis or calculi, or possibly indicate hydronephrosis. Ultrasound of the kidneys is essential, as it can reveal size and configuration of renal outlines.

A rapid sequence intravenous urogram and voiding cysto-urethrogram are necessary to dia-

gnose intrinsic and extrinsic disease and reflux respectively.

In most instances of hypertension no further investigations will be required. In a minority, radionuclide studies, DMSA (for renal cortical function) and DTPA (for renal excretory function) scans, renogram, computed tomography scan, or angiography may have to be done. Specialized tests on plasma and urine need to be undertaken for Cushing's syndrome, aldosteronism, phaeochromocytoma, neuroblastoma, and thyrotoxicosis.

In children with hypertension of obscure aetiology, a percutaneous renal biopsy is sometimes necessary.

Treatment

There is no strict uniformity in the sequence of drugs used in treatment of hypertension. The most commonly used drugs, in order of priority, are the

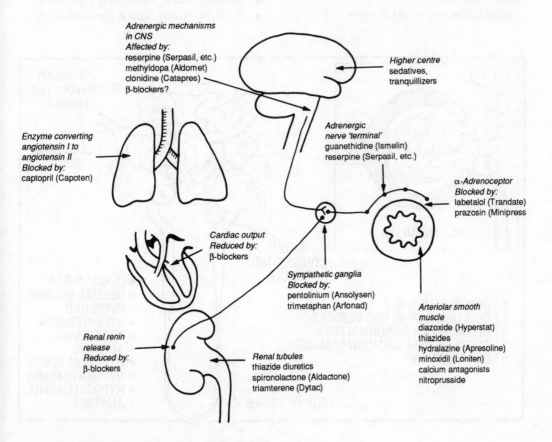

Higher centre
sedatives,
tranquillizers

Adrenergic mechanisms in CNS
Affected by:
reserpine (Serpasil, etc.)
methyldopa (Aldomet)
clonidine (Catapres)
β-blockers?

Enzyme converting angiotensin I to angiotensin II
Blocked by:
captopril (Capoten)

Adrenergic nerve 'terminal'
guanethidine (Ismelin)
reserpine (Serpasil, etc.)

α-Adrenoceptor
Blocked by:
labetalol (Trandate)
prazosin (Minipress)

Cardiac output
Reduced by:
β-blockers

Sympathetic ganglia
Blocked by:
pentolinium (Ansolysen)
trimetaphan (Arfonad)

Arteriolar smooth muscle
diazoxide (Hyperstat)
thiazides
hydralazine (Apresoline)
minoxidil (Loniten)
calcium antagonists
nitroprusside

Renal renin release
Reduced by:
β-blockers

Renal tubules
thiazide diuretics
spironolactone (Aldactone)
triamterene (Dytac)

Fig. 16.8 Antihypertensives and their sites of action

371

thiazide diuretics, beta blockers, and vasodilators *(see Table 16.16).* Treatment is begun at a low dose and then increased to maximum. If single-drug therapy at maximum tolerated doses is ineffective, drugs from the three groups are given in combination. Some of the antihypertensive agents and their sites of action are given in *Fig. 16.8.* An alternative approach to treatment, especially in the adolescent, is to promote dietary salt restriction, weight reduction, physical exercise, and relaxation. Emergency treatment for accelerated hypertension requires intravenous administration of hydrallazine, labetalol, or sodium nitrusside.

Acute renal failure

(See Fig. 16.9.)
This is a serious and infrequent problem which requires care in specialized units and must be considered in any child who stops passing urine at normal frequency.

Renal failure may be of two types:

♦ acute: usually sudden in onset, potentially reversible
♦ chronic-insidious onset, irreversible, leads to death if no dialysis or kidney transplant available.

Definition

The function of the kidneys is to excrete waste materials and maintain homeostasis of fluid and electrolytes in the body. Renal failure occurs when the kidneys are unable to discharge this function. This is nearly always accompanied by oligo-anuria. Therefore, renal failure is present when urinary output falls below 300 ml/m^2/day, and this usually causes the serum creatinine to rise to twice the normal value, and the blood urea to be above 16 mmol/l.

Causes

These may be:
♦ pre-renal: due to impaired renal perfusion
♦ renal: when there is renal disease or injury

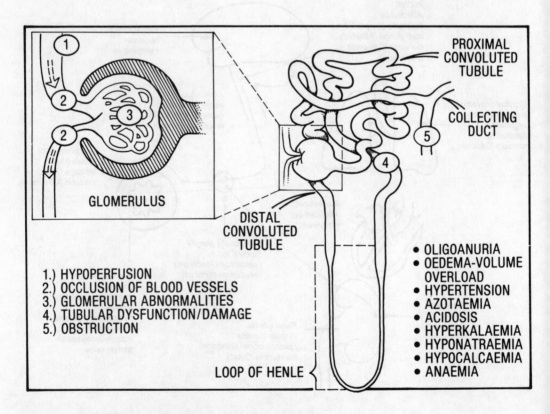

PROXIMAL CONVOLUTED TUBULE

COLLECTING DUCT

GLOMERULUS

DISTAL CONVOLUTED TUBULE

1.) HYPOPERFUSION
2.) OCCLUSION OF BLOOD VESSELS
3.) GLOMERULAR ABNORMALITIES
4.) TUBULAR DYSFUNCTION/DAMAGE
5.) OBSTRUCTION

LOOP OF HENLE

• OLIGOANURIA
• OEDEMA-VOLUME OVERLOAD
• HYPERTENSION
• AZOTAEMIA
• ACIDOSIS
• HYPERKALAEMIA
• HYPONATRAEMIA
• HYPOCALCAEMIA
• ANAEMIA

Fig. 16.9   Renal failure: Site of lesion and abnormal features

♦ post-renal: due to obstruction of outflow of urine.

History, physical examination, and urine analysis will reveal the cause in most instances.

The most common cause of renal failure in childhood is dehydration, leading to pre-renal hypoperfusion. This is eminently preventable by oral rehydration, and easily treated by intravenous fluids. Delay in treatment can lead to parenchymal kidney damage.

On the other hand, injudicious use of intravenous fluids in the presence of renal parenchymal damage can be extremely dangerous, leading to volume overload and peripheral, pulmonary, and cerebral oedema. Therefore it is crucial to know whether oligo-anuria is caused by pre-renal or renal parenchymal disease. *Table 16.17* gives simple tests to make this distinction.

Acute post-streptococcal glomerulonephritis is the most frequent renal cause of kidney failure in developing countries, and responds satisfactorily to simple management procedures. Haemolytic-uraemic syndrome is an important cause in developed countries. A list of the causes of renal failure is given in *Table 16.18*.

Abnormal features

These may be dominated by the antecedent illness. For example, the features may be those of post-streptococcal glomerulonephritis or haemolytic uraemic syndrome. In tubular necrosis, the picture

is most often the result of acidosis, azotaemia, and oliguria. The abnormalities are:
♦ oliguria/anuria
♦ oedema, 'volume overload', and hypertension — if fluid intake has been uncontrolled
♦ hypertension
♦ azotaemia — serum creatinine and blood urea rise
♦ acidosis — hyperventilation
♦ hyperkalaemia — cardiac toxicity: ECG changes, arrhythmias and cardiac arrest. Serum potassium levels > 7.0 mEq/l require urgent intervention (*see above*)
♦ hyponatraemia — this is usually dilutional and asymptomatic

Table 16.18   Causes of renal failure

Pre-renal	Dehydration:	Gastroenteritis
	Shock:	Gastroenteritis, haemorrhage, burns, septicaemia
	Hypoproteinaemia:	Nephrotic syndrome
	Vascular occlusion:	Renal artery occlusion
Renal	Acute glomerulonephritis	Post-streptococcal, non-streptococcal (e.g., typhoid, staphylococcal, vasculitic diseases)
	Haemolytic-uraemic syndrome	
	Tubular necrosis:	Dehydration, shock, nephrotoxins
	Cortical necrosis:	Septicaemia, ischaemia, intravascular coagulation, dehydration
	Pyelonephritis	
	Interstitial nephritis	Drugs (sulphonamides, methicillin)
	Congenital renal anomalies:	Polycystic kidneys, dysplasia
Post-renal	Obstructive uropathy:	Congenital (urethral valves)
		Acquired (e.g. *S. haematobium*, sulphonamides, uric acid nephropathy in acute leukaemia therapy)
	Vesico-ureteric reflux	

Table 16.17   Test to distinguish pre-renal from renal failure

	Pre-renal	Renal
Fractitional excretion of sodium		
$\dfrac{UNa}{PNa} \times \dfrac{PCr}{UCr} \times 100$	< 1%	> 3%
Urine sodium (mmol/l)	< 25	> 25
Urine/plasma ratios of		
osmolality	> 1.2	< 1.1
urea	> 8	< 8

UNa = urine sodium
PCr = plasma creatine
PNa = plasma sodium
UCr = urine creatinine

373

◆ hypocalcaemia — usually asymptomatic; tetany if alkali therapy given

◆ anaemia — normocytic, normochromic; usually no therapy indicated; severe in haemolytic uraemic syndrome *(see Fig. 16.9)*.

Management

In pre-renal failure the overriding consideration is replacement of body fluids. Once this is achieved, urine will be passed in a few hours and renal failure will resolve. The type of fluid used depends on the nature of the insult. If this is gastroenteritis, then electrolyte solutions such as half Darrow's may be given intravenously. If urine is not passed after intravenous fluids, the problem may be:

◆ incomplete fluid replacement

◆ renal parenchymal damage (e.g., tubular necrosis), or

◆ obstructive uropathy.

For management of renal parenchymal damage *see above*.

Post-renal failure due to *S. haematobium* requires bladder catheterization, antibiotic cover, and antischistosomal therapy. Other surgical obstructions must always be excluded by appropriate investigations (e.g., ultrasonography).

Important investigations are listed in *Table 16.19*.

Table 16.19   Investigations for post-renal failure

Full blood count with smear
Blood urea, creatinine, electrolytes
Urine examination
Coagulation studies
Blood culture
Ultrasound and X-ray abdomen

Chronic renal failure (CRF)

This is a rare condition in children, and refers to a state in which irreversible renal disease leads to insufficient functional kidney tissue, with a glomerular filtration rate below a third or quarter of what is necessary to maintain normal body homeostasis. The causes are often not known, but the disease may be due to glomerulonephritis (although post-streptococcal nephritis has not convincingly been shown to result in chronic failure), pyelonephritis, and congenital renal abnormalities *(see Table 16.20)*.

Table 16.20   Causes of chronic renal failure

Glomerulonephritis
Pyelonephritis + obstructive uropathy
Congenital anomalies
Hereditary diseases
Kidney stones

The proportions of the various diseases causing CRF varies in rich and poor communities. Reflux nephropathy and congenital anomalies are prominent causes in rich countries.

The **manifestations** of chronic renal failure, are: vomiting, polydipsia, polyuria, anorexia, growth retardation, wasting, hypertension, anaemia, bleeding disorders, hypotonia, muscle weakness, neurological disturbances, tetany, rickets, acidosis, hyperkalaemia, hyponatraemia, hyposthenuria, and susceptibility to infection. Oedema and oligo-anuria occur late in the disease.

Management

Management must be carried out by experienced personnel, with special care being given to diet, acidosis, rickets, hyperphosphataemia, hyperkalaemia, anaemia, hypertension, intercurrent infections, etc. *(see Chapter 20, Endocrine and Metabolic Disorders)*.

Dialysis and transplantation, whenever available, are the treatments of choice; these are indicated when signs and symptoms become unmanageable, or when complications are severe. Dialysis is used prior to transplantation, or if the latter is contraindicated. Dialysis at home, with continuous ambulatory peritoneal dialysis or haemodialysis, is being widely employed. The vast majority of patients are alive more than five years after a renal transplant from a living donor or a cadaver.

H.M. Coovadia

17
Cardiac disorders

Introduction

Cardiac disorders in children may be considered under two broad categories: congenital or acquired. Congenital heart abnormalities occur with equal frequency among black and white children. On the other hand, rheumatic heart disease has a prevalence among black school children at least equal to that of congenital heart anomalies, but is rare in white children. These two entities account for the majority of cardiac problems. Other important causes that may be encountered are idiopathic congestive cardiomyopathy (more common among blacks), infective endocarditis (either on a previous rheumatic valvular lesion or complicating a congenital heart abnormality), and cor pulmonale consequent upon upper airways obstruction — the result of enlarged adenoids and tonsils (very common in black infants and children). An arrhythmia is less likely to occur in children than is the case with adults. If it does so, it will almost certainly be a supraventricular tachyarrhythmia. *(See Chapter 1 for examination of the cardiovascular system.)*

The top five cardiac disorders

Congenital heart abnormality (++)
Rheumatic heart disease (++)
Idiopathic congestive cardiomyopathy
Cor pulmonale (due to upper airways obstruction)
Infective endocarditis

Congenital heart disease (CHD)

Incidence and aetiology

Congenital heart malformations occur in at least 7 per 1 000 live births. If follow-up of every newborn were complete, it is probable that the figure would increase to 10 per 1 000 live births (i.e., 1%).

In the majority of instances (85–90%) the cause is not known. It is thought to be due to an interaction between environmental factors and a degree of genetic predisposition. Known teratogenic agents include maternal alcohol and phenytoin ingestion during pregnancy, and exposure to rubella in the first trimester. Single gene abnormalities, e.g., Marfan's syndrome, may have associated congenital heart malformations. Similarly, congenital heart abnormalities may be found in children with chromosomal aberrations (e.g., 40% chance in trisomy 21 or 45X0; 90% chance in trisomy 13 or trisomy 18).

A positive family history of congenital heart disease may be found in at least 10% of first degree relatives. The six abnormalities listed below account for 80% of all congenital heart disease.

The top six cardiac abnormalities

Ventricular septal defect	38%
Patent ductus arteriosus	20%
Coarctation of aorta	10%
Tetralogy of Fallot	6%
Atrial septal defect	3%
Isolated pulmonic stenosis	3%
TOTAL	80%

Clinical features of heart disease

Infants

◆ **Central cyanosis** which does not respond to oxygen therapy is indicative of cyanotic CHD.

◆ **Heart failure** presents with rapid breathing, sweating, inability to complete feeds, failure to gain weight or sudden increase in weight (due to oedema), puffy eyes (early sign of oedema), hepatomegaly, and a palpable spleen.

◆ **Heart murmurs:** Careful, repeated auscultation of infants will reveal transient systolic murmurs in most normal infants.

375

▶ Systolic murmurs which *persist*, or are *loud*, or are associated with *other signs of cardiac disorder* should be considered significant. Serious heart malformations may not have a murmur.

Diastolic murmurs are always significant, but are found in very few infants with congenital heart defects.

◆ All neonates should be examined soon after birth for possible congenital heart disease, and again at 6 weeks of age. This is because a significant murmur arising from a ventricular septal defect (VSD) may only become audible some time after birth, after the fall in pulmonary artery pressure and vascular resistance.

Children

◆ **Central cyanosis** and clubbing are cardinal features.

◆ **Heart murmurs:** Fifty per cent of all children will have a functional murmur when febrile, excited, or after exercise. Significant systolic murmurs are usually loud, often associated with a thrill, and heard maximally at one of the main auscultatory areas, i.e., the lower left sternal edge. Diastolic murmurs are always significant.

◆ **Cardiac failure** at this age presents with tachypnoea, moist sounds at the bases of the lungs, elevated jugular venous pressure, hepatomegaly and dependent oedema.

Functional murmurs

Functional systolic murmurs at the fourth left interspace (vibratory ejection) or at the second left interspace (blowing ejection) must be differentiated from organic murmurs. They are very common in schoolchildren (60–70%). The common features are:

◆ usually grade 3/6 or less, occurring in midsystole

◆ louder during fever

◆ louder in supine, softer in erect position

◆ second sound splits normally, i.e., widens on inspiration

◆ commonly a dull 3rd sound at the apex

◆ there may be associated venous hums (continuous) below both clavicles. These disappear with alteration of neck position or pressure over the external jugular veins at the root of the neck.

Dynamics

The clinical identification of congenital heart defects requires a basic knowledge of the dynamics of the CVS. The normal heart consists of two pumps working simultaneously alongside each other *(see Fig. 17.1)*. The right side has a low-pressure atrium receiving desaturated blood from the systemic circulation, and a muscular pumping ventricle which propels the blood into the pulmonary circulation. The pressure which the right

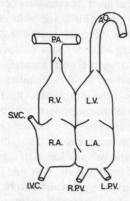

Fig. 17.1 A normal heart

ventricle (RV) must generate depends on the resistance to flow in the sponge-like pulmonary vascular bed. This is normally low, therefore the RV pressure does not need to be more than 15–25 mmHg in systole.

In the right atrium (RA) pressure is determined by the compliance of the RV, which is normally good, and RA pressure does not rise above 5 mmHg.

On the left side of the heart the left atrium (LA) receives saturated blood from the pulmonary veins, and the left ventricle (LV) has to generate enough pressure to ensure that the blood will circulate throughout the body. The systemic resistance is much higher than pulmonary resistance, so LV pressure needs to be 60 mmHg systolic in an infant, rising to 120 mmHg in the normal adult. The LV is a thick, muscled chamber, which makes it relatively non-compliant, and LA pressure therefore needs to be greater than RA pressure to fill the LV (normal LA mean pressure is 5–10 mmHg).

In the normal situation, the mean pressure in the LA is always higher than RA pressure, and the LV

Table 17.1 Distinguishing features of acyanotic defects

Defect	Pulse	Systolic murmur	Diastolic murmur	2nd heart sound	Chest X-ray	ECG
Coarctation	Branchials bounding. Femorals absent (or delayed)	Ejection at back	Mid (33%)	Normal	Large proximal aorta. 3 sign (in older children)	Normal or LVH
Aortic stenosis	Small volume	Ejection at 2RS radiates to neck. Ejection systolic click if valvar. Thrill = severe	Early (20–25%)	Normal	Large proximal aorta	Normal axis. LVH if severe
Ventricular septal defect	Normal	Pan at 4LS Grade 3–5/6 (Maybe thrill)	Mid at apex = high flow	Loud P2 = pulm. hypertension	Cardiomegaly. Pulm. plethora	Biventricular enlargement
Endocardial cushion defect (ASD + MI)	Normal	Pan at apex. Ejection at 2LS	Mid at 4LS	Fixed split. Loud P2 = pulm. hypertension	Cardiomegaly. Pulm. plethora	QRS axis – 60°. RsR in V1
Atrial septal defect (ostium secundum)	Normal	Ejection at 2LS	Mid at 4LS	Fixed split	RA and RV enlarged. Pulm. plethora	Rt. axis RsR in V1
Patent ductus arteriosus	Collapsing	Ejection at 2LS in infants. Continuous machinery		Loud P2	Cardiomegaly. Pulm. plethora. (Normal in asymptomatic)	Normal or biventricular enlargement
Pulmonary stenosis	Normal	Ejection at 2LS. Ejection systolic click. Thrill severe	Nil	Soft P2. Wide split	Large MPA, RV enlargement. Normal lung vascularity	Rt. axis, RVH

ASD = Atrial septal defect   RA = Right atrium   LS = Left intercostal space   MPA = Main pulmonary artery   LVH = Left ventricular hypertrophy   P2 = 2nd pulmonic sound
MI = Mitral incompetence   RVH = Right ventricular hypertrophy   RS = Right intercostal space   RV = Right ventricle

systolic pressure is always about four times greater than the RV pressure. In the same way, the pulmonary artery systolic pressure, being that generated by the RV, is always lower than the aortic pressure generated by the LV.

It is obvious, therefore, that if there is a simple defect connecting the two sides of the heart at any level, from the atrium to the great vessels, blood will only flow across the defect from left to right. Patients with these defects are not cyanosed.

Congenital heart defects are classified into those which cause cyanosis, and those which are acyanotic.

Acyanotic conditions are divided into two groups:
◆ Obstructive defects which affect either the left or right side of the heart, and cause hypertrophy of the chamber which is obstructed, e.g., aortic or pulmonary stenosis.
◆ Defects connecting the two circulations, allowing left-to-right shunting of blood to occur, e.g., VSD, atrial septal defect (ASD), and patent ductus arteriosus (PDA) *(see Dynamics, above)*.

Acyanotic congenital heart defects

Table 17.1 should be consulted for the distinguishing features of conditions discussed below.

These either present with symptoms and signs of cardiac failure, or are discovered due to a cardiac murmur being found at examination.

Defects presenting with heart failure in infants

Coarctation of the aorta *(see Fig. 17.2)*: This is a constriction in the thoracic aorta in the region of the ductus arteriosus (i.e., juxtaductal). If severe, this causes left heart and, soon thereafter, right heart failure, usually in the second week of life. Diagnosis is made by palpating the pulses in the arms and legs. The arm pulses are easily felt, whereas the femoral pulses are impalpable. The difference in blood pressure by means of the flush technique is more than 20 mmHg. A systolic murmur is usually heard at the back between the left scapula and the spine. An apical mid-diastolic murmur is audible in about one-third of infants, and is due to mild mitral valve deformity. Two-thirds of these symptomatic babies have an associated major cardiac defect, e.g., VSD and/or PDA.

Patent ductus arteriosus (PDA) *(see Fig. 17.3)*:

In infants born pre-term, particularly those with respiratory distress, the ductus arteriosus often remains patent, and a significant left-to-right shunt develops through it towards the end of the first week of life. These infants develop tachypnoea again, and a systolic murmur becomes audible on the left just below the clavicle. The pulse pressure is large and the dorsalis pedis is easily palpable. PDA may also occur in full-term infants. This is characterized by a continuous (machinery) murmur just below the left clavicle.

If there is a large flow through the PDA, a mid-diastolic murmur will be heard at the apex.

PDA in term infants very rarely closes spontaneously and always requires surgical removal before six months of age, even if it is asymptomatic.

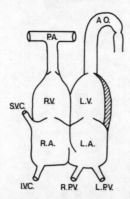

Fig. 17.2   Coarctation
Cross-hatching = hypertrophy

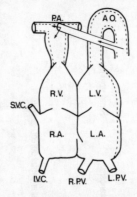

Fig. 17.3   Patent ductus arteriosus
Broken line = dilation

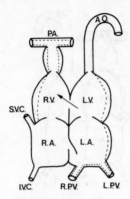

Fig. 17.4 Ventricular septal defect (VSD)

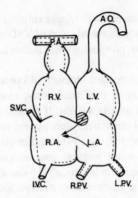

Fig. 17.5 Endocardial cushion defect (ECD)

Ventricular septal defect (VSD) *(See Fig. 17.4)*

Large defects present between 2 and 6 weeks of life (later at higher altitudes), when the pulmonary vascular resistance has decreased from the high fetal level. These infants become breathless on feeding and, as a result, fail to gain weight adequately, due to the large left-to-right shunt causing overloading and failure of the left ventricle. The typical loud pansystolic murmur is heard at the left lower sternal edge, below a line drawn through the nipples. If the left-to-right shunt is large, a mid-diastolic murmur will be heard at the apex. If there is pulmonary hypertension, the pulmonary component of the second sound (P2) will be loud.

Note: Small VSDs are asymptomatic. They have the typical pansystolic murmur, but will have neither symptoms nor the loud P2, nor diastolic murmur. The majority will close spontaneously before adult life, particularly within the first 2 years.

Endocardial cushion defect (ECD) *(see Fig. 17.5):* Atrio-ventricular septal defect (AVSD), a common form of this abnormality, is an ostium primum ASD, associated with a cleft in the mitral valve which allows a left-to-right shunt between the left ventricle and the right atrium. Such a shunt may be very large and cause cardiac failure early in life. Half of the infants with this defect have Down's syndrome *(see Chapter 3, Genetics and Congenital Disorders)*. On auscultation, a pansystolic murmur is heard at the apex, due to mitral incompetence, and an ejection systolic murmur is heard at the left sternal border due to increased flow through the pulmonary valve.

The ECG usually shows left anterior hemiblock, with a QRS axis between -60° and -90°, and an RsR pattern in lead V1, indicating right ventricular hypertrophy due to the volume overload.

Aortic valve stenosis (rare) *(see Fig. 17.6):* If severe, these present in infancy with left heart failure. An ejection systolic murmur is heard at the second right intercostal space, and the pulse pressure is small, with poor volume pulses.

Other conditions which cause left heart failure in infancy, without cyanosis, which must be considered in the *differential diagnosis*, are myocarditis and tachyarrhythmias.

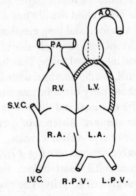

Fig. 17.6 Aortic valve stenosis

Immediate treatment

For all infants presenting with heart failure, treatment is digoxin and diuretics, regardless of the diagnosis. Coarctation of the aorta and severe

379

aortic valve stenosis will require surgical management in infancy, but most cases of VSD will close spontaneously, provided cardiac failure is controlled.

The most important measure of control is the infant's ability to feed adequately, assessed by checking the gain in weight. If a child with the signs of a VSD fails to respond, a coexistent defect must be suspected, e.g., PDA and/or coarctation of the aorta, when surgical intervention will be required. In pre-term infants, a PDA usually closes by the time the infant reaches its expected term. If it does not close, surgical removal of the PDA will be necessary.

Defects presenting with cardiac murmurs

Aortic stenosis, valvar (rarely subvalvar or supravalvar) *(see Fig. 17.6)*: Aortic stenosis accounts for 4% of congenital heart defects, with males predominating 4:1.

Isolated aortic stenosis presenting in childhood is almost always congenital in origin. Rheumatic fever invariably causes incompetence as well as stenosis of the aortic valve, and is rare before the age of 10 years.

Aortic stenosis is usually asymptomatic in infancy, as it commonly develops later in an aortic valve which is often bicuspid. Significant aortic stenosis in the older child usually has a palpable thrill, as well as a loud and long ejection systolic murmur which radiates to the right side of the neck from the second intercostal space. The chest X-ray may look normal, but the proximal aorta is usually enlarged. A short, early diastolic murmur is audible in 20–25% of cases, and there is an ejection click in valvar stenosis. Absence of a click suggests subvalvar or supravalvar stenosis.

Pulmonary valve stenosis *(see Fig. 17.7)*: This is a common congenital heart defect, but varies widely in its degree of severity. The majority of cases are mild and asymptomatic. The most severe cases may develop right heart failure. More often they present with cyanosis due to right-to-left shunting through a patent foramen ovale, because the right atrial pressure exceeds the left atrial pressure. An ejection systolic murmur is heard at the second left intercostal space, and is often preceded by an ejection systolic click. In severe cases

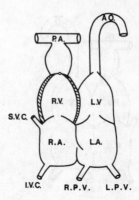

Fig. 17.7 Pulmonary valve stenosis

the murmur will be long, obscuring the aortic component of the second heart sound, and a thrill will be palpable. The pulmonary component of the second heart sound is soft and delayed. Severe cases, i.e., those with a thrill, should undergo cardiac catheterization during which a balloon valvuloplasty is performed. If this is not possible, then surgical treatment is indicated.

Coarctation of the aorta: In older children and adults, coarctation may be symptomatic, or may present as hypertension with symptoms of headache, chest pain, or cerebrovascular accidents. Some patients complain of claudication in their legs. The diagnosis is made by palpating the discrepancy between the pulses in the arms and legs. Because of the development of collateral circulation, the femoral pulses will be palpable, but weaker and delayed compared to the arm pulses. Recording the blood pressure in the arms and legs will confirm the discrepancy, with hypertension in the arms and relatively low pressure in the legs.

The right arm must always be used for blood pressure recordings, as the left subclavian artery may occasionally be involved in the coarctation.

A systolic thrill may be felt in the suprasternal notch, and the typical harsh systolic murmur may be heard at the back, at the angle of the left scapula — but often there is only a soft systolic murmur over the precordium. The chest X-ray in infants presenting with severe coarctation shows generalized cardiomegaly and congestion of the lungfields. In older children and adults, there is slight enlargement of the left ventricle due to concentric hypertrophy. The proximal aorta is enlarged, and an indentation may be seen in the descending aorta to the left of the vertebral column, making a figure '3' sign. A radiological feature of children of school-going age and older is notching of the inferior edges of the 3rd to 8th ribs, caused by enlarged collateral intercostal arteries. The ECG is usually normal in children, but may show left ventricular hypertrophy in older patients.

Older asymptomatic infants and children require elective surgical repair to prevent the development of permanent hypertension (recommended age: 2 years).

If a child older than a year presents with signs of coarctation and is in congestive cardiac failure (CCF), aortic arteritis (Takayasu's disease) should be suspected.

Atrial septal defect: (Ostium secundum and solitary ostium primum) *(See Fig. 17.8.)* Children with these defects are usually asymptomatic, although they are not athletic, and may suffer frequently from chest infections because of a large left-to-right shunt into the pulmonary circulation.

They show clinical signs of right ventricular hypertrophy, with a palpable lift over the pulmonary outflow tract. A grade 2/6 ejection systolic murmur is heard at the 2nd left intercostal space, and there is fixed splitting of the second heart sound. A tricuspid diastolic murmur may be heard at the lower left sternal edge. The chest X-ray is typical, showing a large main pulmonary artery and plethoric lung fields.

The ECG differentiates secundum from primum defects, there being right axis deviation in the former and left axis deviation in the latter. Both show RsR' in Vl. Most patients with secundum defects require surgical closure of the defect during childhood, preferably prior to school attendance. Only large primum defects require closure.

Asymptomatic VSD: These children have a loud pansystolic murmur at the 4th left interspace due to a high-velocity but low-volume shunt from the LV to the low-pressure RV. They do not have either a loud P2 or apical mid-diastolic murmur. The ECG and chest X-ray are usually within normal limits. The prognosis is good for spontaneous closure of the defect, and they should be allowed unrestricted physical activity.

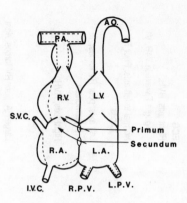

Fig. 17.8   Atrial septal defect (ASD)

Prophylactic amoxicillin must always be given 1 hour before the extraction of teeth, to prevent infective endocarditis occurring in the right ventricle opposite the defect.

Asymptomatic PDA: These patients have a typical, continuous machinery murmur, heard just below the left clavicle, and may have a wide pulse pressure. The ECG and chest X-ray are usually within normal limits.

Even an asymptomatic PDA must be removed surgically, because there is a high risk of bacterial endocarditis occurring.

Cyanotic congenital heart defects

Congenital heart defects which cause central cyanosis can be divided into two groups:

◆ those in which desaturated, systemic, venous blood cannot reach the pulmonary circulation to pick up oxygen, and

◆ those in which there is mixing of saturated and desaturated blood, i.e., common mixing situations.

Table 17.2 should be consulted for the distinguishing features discussed below.

Systemic venous blood unable to reach the pulmonary circulation

Transposition of the great vessels (with intact ventricular septum) *(see Fig. 17.9):* The aorta arises from the right ventricle and the pulmonary artery from the left ventricle.

Table 17.2 Distinguishing features of cyanotic conditions

Cardiac anomaly	Cyanosis	Pulse	Auscultation	Chest X-ray	ECG
Transposition	Within the first week of life. Increasing	Normal	Usually without murmur. May be precordial systolic murmur.	Plethora	Right axis, RVH. Upright T wave in V4R, V1
Pulmonary atresia	From birth	Poor/Normal	Pansystolic xiphisternum. Single HS2	Oligaemia	Normal to left axis. Poor RV forces
Tricuspid atresia	From birth	Poor/Normal	No murmur or soft systolic over precordium. Single HS2	Oligaemia	Left axis, poor RV forces, P pulmonale
Tetralogy	Variable. Often acyanotic in infancy, increases gradually. May have spells	Normal	Long systolic at left sternal border. Single HS2	Oligaemia	Right axis, RVH
Ebstein	From birth. Tends to improve	Normal	Pansystolic murmur and diastolic scratch at xiphisternum	Oligaemia	Large RA, poor RV forces, right bundle branch block
Eisenmenger	Initially not cyanosed. Progressive	Normal	Ejection systolic click at left sternal border. Soft ejection systolic murmur. Very loud pulmonary HS2	Oligaemia	Right axis, RVH
Critical pulmonary stenosis	Mild to moderate	Small	Ejection systolic murmur at 2nd right interspace. Soft pulmonary HS2	Oligaemia	Right axis, RVH, P pulmonale
Truncus arteriosus	Mild to moderate	Collapsing	Systolic ejection click and long systolic murmur at left sternal border. May be early diastolic murmur as well	Plethora	Normal to right axis, biventricular hypertrophy
Total anomalous pulmonary venous connection	Moderate	Small	Ejection systolic murmur at 2nd right space. Wide split of HS2. Mid-diastolic murmur at xiphisternum	Plethora	Right axis, RVH
AVCC	Mild to moderate. Variable	Normal	Precordial systolic murmur	Plethora	Left axis, biventricular hypertrophy. Prolonged PR
Hypoplastic left heart syndrome	Mild to moderate	Very poor	Precordial systolic murmur. Ejection systolic click. Gallop	Plethora	Right axis, RVH. Poor LV forces

AVCC = Atrio-ventricular communis canal
HS2 = 2nd heartsound
RV = Right ventricle
RVH = Right ventricular hypertrophy
LV = Left ventricle
RA = Right atrium

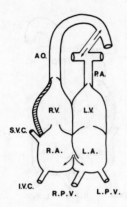

Fig. 17.9   Cyanotic: transposition of the great vessels with intact ventricular septum

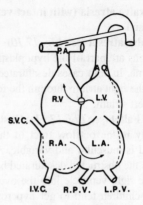

Fig. 17.10   Cyanotic: tricuspid valve atresia

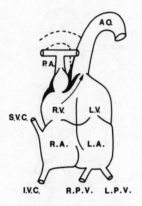

Fig. 17.11   Cyanotic: tetralogy of Fallot

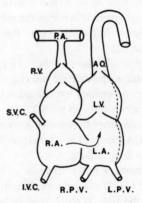

Fig. 17.12   Cyanotic: Ebstein's anomaly of the tricuspid valve

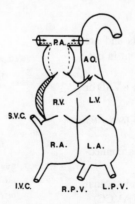

Fig. 17.13   Cyanotic: Eisenmenger syndrome

Pulmonary valve atresia (with intact ventricular septum) and
Tricuspid valve atresia *(see Fig. 17.10)*
Both conditions are part of the hypoplastic right heart syndrome. In both cases desaturated blood passes from the right atrium through the foramen ovale to the left atrium.
Tetralogy of Fallot *(see Fig. 17.11):* Obstruction occurs mainly in the outflow tract of the right ventricle, and is muscular and variable. A large VSD permits the obstructed desaturated blood to pass from the right ventricle into the overriding aorta. These children tend to get hypercyanotic attacks due to infundibular spasm. Emergency treatment for this is given below.
Ebstein's anomaly of the tricuspid valve *(see Fig. 17.12):* The tricuspid valve is displaced into the body of the right ventricle and is incompetent. Part of the right ventricle is above the valve (atrialized). A right-to-left shunt occurs through the foramen ovale.
Eisenmenger syndrome *(see Fig. 17.13):* Obstruction is due to pulmonary arteriolar disease causing severe pulmonary hypertension. A right-to-left shunt occurs through a VSD.

   If severe pulmonary hypertension complicates an ASD or PDA there will also be a reversal of the shunt through these defects.
Critical pulmonary valve stenosis — (trilogy) *(see Fig. 17.14):* If the stenosis is critical, the pressures in the right ventricle and right atrium may be greater than on the left, and a right-to-left shunt will occur through the foramen ovale, or sometimes across a coexistent ASD.

Common mixing situations

All of these have plethoric lung fields and are moderately cyanosed. They often present in cardiac failure:

◆ transposition of great vessels (TGV) + VSD or PDA

◆ persistent truncus arteriosus (PTA) *(see Fig. 17.15)*

◆ total anomalous pulmonary venous connection (TAPVC) *(see Fig. 17.16)*

◆ persistent atrioventricular communis canal (complete endocardial cushion defect) (AVCC)

◆ single ventricle: this is usually associated with transposition of the great vessels

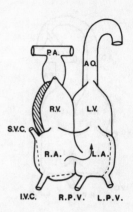

Fig. 17.14 Cyanotic: critical pulmonary valve stenosis

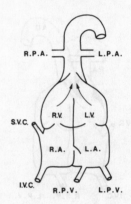

Fig. 17.15 Cyanotic: persistent truncus arteriosus

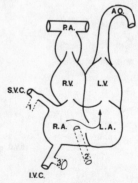

1. **Supracardiac into S.V.C.**
2. **Intracardiac into R.A. (coronary sinus)**
3. **Infracardiac into I.V.C.**

Fig 17.16 Cyanotic: total anomalous pulmonary venous connection (TAPVC)

◆ hypoplastic left heart (LH) syndrome: this usually comprises aortic valve atresia, mitral atresia or hypoplasia, hypoplastic ascending aorta, and a diminutive left ventricle.

Approach to cyanotic congenital heart disease in the young baby

Other causes of cyanosis must first be excluded, viz., pulmonary conditions, central nervous system problems, and metabolic causes (hypoglycaemia, hypocalcaemia).

The respiratory pattern of the child must be observed, while physical examination should particularly include the signs of CCF. Thereafter, a chest radiograph is taken (antero-posterior and lateral), and an ECG performed *(see Table 17.2)*.

While most infants with cyanotic congenital heart defects need referral to a specialized cardiac unit, and many require prompt surgical intervention or atrial septostomy to survive, some do not require, or are not suitable for, immediate treatment. All these, as well as those who have had palliative procedures, remain cyanosed.

Patients with complicated and multiple defects, e.g., transposition of the great vessels with single ventricle and subpulmonary stenosis, are cyanosed, but may be haemodynamically balanced so that their lives and well-being are not immediately threatened. Patients with other conditions, e.g., Ebstein's anomaly, continue through to adult life without any surgical intervention being indicated or suitable.

The **long-term management** of these cyanosed children requires regular examination, with particular reference to the following points:

◆ Serial measurements of height, weight, and skull circumference: their growth may be stunted, especially if they are in cardiac failure; otherwise they should maintain a steady gain. If cyanosis is severe, there is a delay in closure of the anterior fontanelle.

◆ Estimation of the haemoglobin level and haematocrit: anaemic children do not look cyanosed. A raised haematocrit indicates severe cyanosis. Iron deficiency is common, and must be corrected. If not, this may lead to cerebral thrombosis, especially in children below the age of 2 years.

◆ Septic skin lesions and dental caries should be avoided, and must be treated promptly. The greatest danger to children with cyanotic heart defects is paradoxical embolization and the development of cerebral abscesses.

A brain abscess should always be suspected in cyanosed children who develop intractable headache, unexplained fever, or neurological signs. This is more likely to occur above the age of 2 years.

◆ Early detection and management of cardiac failure is vital. If complications occur, appropriate action must be taken, including referral for reappraisal.

Children with cyanotic heart defects are not athletic, but should be allowed to exercise within their own limits. They should be encouraged to take an interest in non-athletic pursuits, and require the support and encouragement of the whole family to enable them to develop their personalities and achieve intellectual satisfaction. Many have the ability to attain the highest intellectual levels. Children with tetralogy of Fallot, who may develop syncopal attacks from infundibular spasm, should not be allowed to overexert themselves or become too excited. Generally, gentle exercise should be encouraged and competitive exercise excluded.

Rheumatic fever

In Africa, Asia, and South America, rheumatic fever remains a common disease and is associated with significant morbidity and mortality rates, both in the acute phase of the disease and as a result of chronic cardiac valvular sequelae. It remains the most common cause of acquired heart disease in children.

In most European and North American countries, the incidence of rheumatic fever declined in the 50 years preceding 1980. The reduction, both in incidence and severity, commenced before the advent of antibiotics and appears to have been related mainly to improvements in the general health and socio-economic standards of the populations in these countries.

However, since the mid 1980s there has been an unexpected resurgence of rheumatic fever in the United States. This has occurred in middle-class families with ready access to medical care. The exact reasons are still unclear, but there has been the re-appearance of 'rheumatogenic' strains of Group A haemolytic streptococci (M-types 1,3,5,6, and in particular 18) in the affected areas *(see below)*.

Aetiology

In susceptible individuals (possibly with a specific class II HLA antigen) rheumatic fever is a sequel to a pharyngeal infection with one of the Group A ß-haemolytic streptococci. Specific 'rheumatogenic' strains of streptococci can now be identified, and it is significant that these strains are rarely found today in populations where rheumatic fever has virtually disappeared.

Clinical features of acute rheumatic fever

In children between the ages of 5 and 15 years, the signs and symptoms of rheumatic fever occur 2–3 weeks after a pharyngeal infection. Very rarely it occurs in children as young as 18 months.

A fairly wide spectrum of presenting features exists, from the unequivocal signs of fever associated with flitting polyarthritis, and obvious carditis causing signs of cardiac failure, to milder, almost insignificant symptoms, where the diagnosis must be made on the evidence of a combination of factors. In 1944, Jones *(see Select Bibliography)* enumerated major and minor criteria which, with modifications in 1965 by a committee of the American Heart Association, have been accepted as indicators of probability in making the important diagnosis of acute rheumatic fever. The need to make an *accurate diagnosis* in all cases is emphasized, because serious involvement of heart valves may follow a relatively mild first attack, and prevention of further attacks is imperative if the grave long-term cardiac complications are to be avoided.

Major criteria

(See Table 17.3.)

Carditis: In the author's experience, 70% of black children in hospital presenting with rheumatic

Table 17.3. Diagnostic criteria of rheumatic fever

Major	Minor
1. Carditis	1. Prolonged PR interval on ECG.
2. Polyarthritis	2. Arthralgia
3. Chorea	3. Previous history or evidence of rheumatic fever
4. Fever	4. Fever
5. Nodules	5. Acute phase reactants

Note: Use 1 and 2 as either minor or major criteria, but not as both.

fever have evidence of carditis on their first admission (world figures vary from 40–75%). The diagnosis of carditis is made if one or more of the following signs is present:

♦ *Cardiac murmurs* indicating endocarditis. The most common of these is a high-pitched, blowing, pansystolic murmur heard at the apex, and is due to mitral valve incompetence caused by distortion of the mitral valve cusps. Sometimes this is associated with a short mid-diastolic murmur at the apex, which disappears as the acute process resolves. Involvement of the aortic valve causes incompetence, which is recognized by an early diastolic murmur, heard best at the aortic area and down the left sternal edge when the patient is sitting up and leaning forward. A wide pulse pressure and collapsing pulses will also be present.

♦ *Cardiac enlargement*, most easily detected by X-ray examination of the chest. When this is associated with soft heart sounds, a diffuse apical impulse, and tachycardia (out of keeping with the degree of fever), myocarditis must be suspected even if murmurs are absent. When the patient is asleep, a record of the pulse will reveal a fast rate if the myocardium is involved. A rapid 'sleeping' pulse may be the only indication of carditis.

♦ *A friction rub*, usually heard early in the illness if there is pericarditis. This often disappears, or may be absent if a pericardial effusion occurs. A large pericardial effusion may cause tamponade, distended neck veins, hepatomegaly, and pulsus paradoxus, or may be suspected if there is a globular enlargement of the cardiac shadow on the chest X-ray and S–T elevation on the electrocardiogram. Pain in the chest or abdomen is often a presenting feature of rheumatic fever, with or without pericarditis. Careful repeated auscultation for a rub should be done if pain is a symptom.

◆ *Pancarditis*, with involvement of the endocardium, myocardium, and pericardium, which often presents with congestive cardiac failure.

Polyarthritis: The typical presentation is a flitting arthritis with red, hot, swollen, tender, large joints, which become involved sequentially: as a new joint is involved, the arthritis in the previously-affected joint subsides.

It is important to consider rheumatic fever in the differential diagnosis of monoarthritis in children.

Once the acute inflammation has settled, the joints recover completely.

Chorea: This occurs most often in girls between 7 and 14 years of age. There is a long latent period of weeks or months between the streptococcal infection and the onset of symptoms. In some cases, chorea may develop some weeks after joint symptoms, but often it occurs without any recognized symptoms or signs of rheumatic fever. Between 20 and 30% of patients with chorea either have or develop cardiac valvular disease. The onset is gradual over 1 or 2 weeks, during which the child is scolded for being clumsy, spilling drinks, or dropping articles. Involuntary grimacing is accompanied by purposeless, uncoordinated, asymmetrical, jerky movements, which may be bilateral or unilateral and make writing impossible, and managing buttons and shoelaces difficult. Emotional lability is striking: crying alternating with laughing. Speech may be affected. When asked to perform tasks, the involuntary movements become exaggerated, and the hand grip cannot be sustained. When asked to extend their arms forward, their hands and wrists form a typical 'eating-fork' configuration. In the most severe cases, patients cannot even remain lying on a bed because of violent, involuntary movements. Chorea often runs a prolonged and relapsing course over weeks and months.

◆ **Erythema marginatum:** This is a transient erythematous rash. When it fades, it leaves irregular thin lines which make circular patterns on the trunk and occasionally the limbs, but never on the face. It is easily seen on light-skinned patients, but neither easily nor often seen on darkly-pigmented skin.

◆ **Nodules:** Subcutaneous, non-tender, small, mobile nodules are found over the extensor surfaces (around the elbows, wrists, knuckles, knees, ankles), over the spinous processes of the vertebrae, the occiput, and sometimes on the scalp and ears of patients, who usually have or develop severe cardiac involvement.

Minor criteria
(See Table 17.3)

◆ **Previous history** of rheumatic fever.

◆ **Arthralgia:** It is important to exclude vague limb pains due to myalgia. This should not be used as a criterion if arthritis is a major manifestation.

◆ **Fever:** Temperature recordings are usually 38 °C or more in acute rheumatic fever.

◆ **Prolonged P–R interval** on the electrocardiogram to greater than 0.18 seconds. This should not be used where carditis is a major criterion.

◆ **Acute phase reactants:** These are not specific for rheumatic fever:

— leucocytosis. This is usually between 12 and 15 x 10^9/l

— erythrocyte sedimentation rate (ESR). This is raised, but the level does not correlate with severity

— C-reactive protein (CRP). This is invariably found in the serum of almost all cases.

◆ Evidence of a *previous episode* of rheumatic fever. Use this or previous history, not both.

The presence of two major criteria, or one major and two minor criteria, together with evidence of a preceding streptococcal infection, make the diagnosis of rheumatic fever probable.

Invariably, the acute pharyngitis has resolved before the symptoms of rheumatic fever commence, but a throat swab should always be done, as it may reveal streptococci. Indirect evidence of a preceding streptococcal infection may be obtained from an elevated antistreptolysin 0 titre (ASOT), or the finding of other streptococcal antibodies (anti-DNAase B or anti-hyaluronidase) in high titre in the blood. These findings by themselves are not diagnostic of rheumatic fever, and all streptococci do not cause elevation of the ASOT.

Treatment of rheumatic fever

Prevention

Rheumatic fever is rare where standards of living are good. A high incidence is associated with poor housing, overcrowding, and lack of primary health care facilities. Treatment of streptococcal throat infections with penicillin within one week of the onset of symptoms prevents the development of rheumatic fever, provided the treatment is adequate. The recommended dosages are:

◆ one IM injection of benzathine penicillin G 600 000 units (below 30 kg body weight) or 1 200 000 units (over 30 kg), or

◆ oral penicillin V, 50 mg/kg/day, given 3 times a day for 10 days. It is important that oral penicillin is given before meals, and the course completed.

◆ in patients sensitive to penicillin, treatment is with erythromycin 125–250 mg, 4 times daily for 10 days; or cephaloridine IM 30–50 mg/kg/day in divided doses, 8-hourly; or oral cephalexin, 25–100 mg/kg/day in divided doses, 8-hourly.

Ideally all children complaining of a sore throat should have a throat swab cultured, and if group A ß-haemolytic streptococci are found, the patient should be given penicillin treatment (or erythromycin, if they are penicillin-sensitive). As this is frequently not possible, the decision to give antibiotics depends on the likelihood of the pharyngitis being streptococcal. This, in turn, can be extremely difficult to determine.

Acute rheumatic fever

Antibiotics: Once a throat swab has been taken, treatment with penicillin (or a substitute) must be started immediately. The first dose should be intramuscular, and is followed by intramuscular or oral administration for 10 days.

Rest: Children with painful joints and acute carditis invariably lie still. As they recover, they may be allowed to move around in bed, but should not be allowed to walk until joint involvement has subsided, cardiac enlargement decreased, and the 'sleeping' pulse rate diminished. Thereafter they should be allowed progressively more activity; most children on adequate treatment should be back to normal, non-strenuous activity within 3 weeks. If there has been cardiac failure, convalescence may be prolonged, and activity should be restricted until evidence of rheumatic activity has been absent for 2 weeks.

Anti-inflammatory treatment:

◆ *Salicylates* are particularly useful in alleviating the pain of arthritis and the discomfort of fever. The ESR returns to normal more quickly, but salicylates do not have any effect on valvular damage.

Dosage: Sodium salicylate 40–60 mg/kg/day, or acetylsalicylic acid (aspirin), 80–120 mg/kg/day.

Treatment should continue until all signs of activity have subsided, and then be gradually withdrawn over a 2-week period. Recurrence of symptoms will require increasing the dosage until control is achieved.

Side-effects: Symptoms of salicylate toxicity (tinnitus, dizziness, nausea, and vomiting), are rarely seen at the recommended dosage. If they occur, treatment must be stopped for 48 hours and recommenced at a lower dosage. Gastric irritation with bleeding from the mucosa may occur, therefore stools should be examined regularly for occult blood while the patient is on treatment. Giving extra milk or using buffered aspirin may overcome this problem.

Contraindications: Salicylates may precipitate pulmonary oedema in patients with acute carditis, and are therefore best avoided in patients with obvious cardiac embarrassment.

◆ The value of *corticosteroids* in the treatment of children with carditis is controversial. They may possibly be lifesaving in cases of pancarditis. Signs of acute rheumatic fever (e.g., fever, raised ESR, and arthritis) may respond rapidly to corticosteroid therapy, but there is no effect on long-term valvular damage.

A recent double-blind, placebo-controlled trial of prednisone failed to show any benefit either in the short-term clinical response or in the long-term follow-up of patients with active rheumatic carditis.

Dosage: Prednisone, 2 mg/kg/day in 4 divided doses.

Treatment should be continued at full dosage until the patient is symptomatically well and the acute phase reactants have been normal for a week. This usually takes 2–3 weeks. Thereafter the dosage should be reduced by 10% every second day, until the daily dose is one-third of the initial dose.

Thereafter the reduction should be by 5% every second day. Regular assessment of the acute phase reactants should show a decline to normal levels. Should these become elevated again during the withdrawal period, the dosage should be increased to the previous level and maintained at that until signs of activity have subsided, before gradual withdrawal is recommenced.

Congestive cardiac failure: Slow digitalization with digoxin, 0.04–0.06 mg/kg total in 4 equal doses at 6-hourly intervals is recommended. Maintenance dose is 0.01 mg/kg/day in 2 divided doses. Large doses of digoxin are dangerous in children with myocarditis. Diuretics are indicated if there is pulmonary oedema or severe congestive failure. Hypokalaemia is particularly dangerous in children with myocarditis during digitalization, and potassium supplements must be given if a diuretic which eliminates potassium is used.

Hydrochlorothiazide, 0.5–2.0 mg/kg/day in 2–3 divided doses, is a safe diuretic. Furosemide, 1 mg/kg/dose IV, is used for pulmonary oedema. This can be repeated until improvement occurs. Potassium supplementation is essential when using furosemide.

Spironolactone (Aldactone®), 2–3 mg/kg/day, divided in 2–3 doses may be required when oedema is chronic and does not respond to the above-mentioned drugs. Captopril (a vasodilator) in a dose of 0.5–6.0 mg/kg/day, in 4 divided doses may be added to the anti-failure therapy, especially if there is significant mitral regurgitation.

Emergency surgery may be indicated in the acute phase of carditis, particularly with the rapid onset of pulmonary oedema. This indicates haemodynamic deterioration in the degree of mitral regurgitation.

Chorea: If involuntary movements are severe, haloperidol (Serenace®) 0.025–0.05mg/kg/day, in divided doses can be given orally. In milder cases, phenobarbitone 3–5 mg/kg/day may be used.

Chronic rheumatic heart disease

The symptoms and signs of acute rheumatic fever subside, the joints recover completely, and in those who have not had carditis, there is a return to complete normality. Once rheumatic fever has occurred, however, there is always a danger of recurrence. If there had been carditis during the first attack, subsequent attacks will again involve the heart, causing increasing damage to the valves. These become progressively more distorted and incompetent, and/or adherent and stenotic.

Mitral valve disease

The mitral valve is the one most commonly affected by rheumatic fever, either alone or in combination with the aortic valve and, occasionally, with the tricuspid valve.

By far the most common lesion is **mitral incompetence.** The apical pansystolic murmur radiating to the axilla, heard during the acute attack, may disappear within a few months, only to reappear and become harsher and louder as the valves contract. The haemodynamic effect of mitral incompetence depends on the amount of blood which regurgitates into the left atrium through the damaged valve during ventricular systole. A small amount has little effect, but large amounts of blood result in distension and increased pressure in the left atrium and pulmonary vein. The left ventricle becomes enlarged and hypertrophied and, if the load becomes too great, left heart failure and pulmonary oedema will occur.

In severe mitral incompetence there is displacement of the apex, which is thrusting in character, and the pansystolic murmur will be loud and may be heard not only in the left axilla, but at the back as well. A mid-diastolic rumbling murmur is heard at the apex due to the large amount of blood passing across the damaged mitral valve in diastole. If a third heart sound is heard before the diastolic murmur, it indicates critical overloading of the left ventricle. Such patients are symptomatic, with poor effort tolerance, orthopnoea, and paroxysmal nocturnal dyspnoea, and require treatment with digoxin to prevent cardiac failure. In these cases a chest X-ray shows enlargement of both the left atrium and left ventricle. Only severe cases show ECG changes of left atrial and left ventricular hypertrophy.

Mitral stenosis usually takes some years to develop, as the cusps of the damaged valve fuse together along their commissures. The author has, however, seen children as young as 8 years old with tight mitral stenosis. When rheumatic fever occurs at a young age in impoverished Third

World children, the progression of the valvular disease to incompetence and/or stenosis appears to be more rapid. The obstruction of flow into the left ventricle causes enlargement and increased pressure in the left atrium and pulmonary veins, which leads to pulmonary arteriolar hypertension. When the overloading of the left atrium becomes critical, pulmonary oedema will occur.

Children with mitral stenosis have poor effort tolerance, dyspnoea, and coughing, but haemoptysis is rare in childhood. Examination reveals a tapping apex, and a rumbling diastolic murmur which increases in intensity just before a loud first heart sound. An opening snap may be heard if the valve cusps are mobile. A chest X-ray shows left atrial enlargement and increased pulmonary vascular markings. Right ventricular enlargement is demonstrated on the ECG, which will also show wide bifid P waves, indicative of left atrial enlargement.

Aortic valve disease

Involvement of the aortic valve may occur alone following rheumatic fever, but it is more often associated with mitral valve disease. Pure aortic stenosis is usually due to a congenital defect. Incompetence invariably occurs if the aortic valve is damaged by rheumatic fever, and this may be associated with some degree of stenosis if the distorted cusps fuse together. The progression of aortic valve damage is much slower than mitral valve disease, and rarely causes severe disability or symptoms during childhood unless there is gross incompetence. In most cases of isolated aortic valve disease, left ventricular failure occurs only after many years.

There may be evidence of left ventricular enlargement, clinically detectable as a thrusting apical impulse. Significant aortic incompetence always causes a large pulse pressure with collapsing pulses. A 'pistol shot' is heard over the femoral arteries. In addition, there may be a positive Durosiez sign, i.e., both systolic and diastolic bruits will be heard with the stethoscope proximal to the site of gradual compression of the femoral pulse. The soft, early diastolic murmur, heard during the acute attack, often persists for many years before becoming longer and louder, with wider radiation as the degree of incompetence increases. It often

sounds like the cooing of a dove, but may be harsh and associated with a thrill. An ejection systolic murmur, which may be soft or loud, with a thrill if there is significant stenosis, is often heard at the aortic area as well.

In severe aortic incompetence, a mid-diastolic murmur is frequently heard at the apex (Austin–Flint murmur). This is caused by the regurgitant flow in diastole striking open the anterior mitral leaflet which then shudders, thus setting up turbulence. This may lead to a mistaken diagnosis of coexistent mitral stenosis.

Tricuspid valve disease

Occasionally the tricuspid valve may be damaged by rheumatic fever. This usually causes incompetence, with or without some degree of stenosis. Usually the mitral valve, but occasionally the aortic valve, is involved.

More often, tricuspid valve incompetence occurs as a functional complication of severe pulmonary hypertension associated with mitral valve disease, particularly tight mitral stenosis. The features of tricuspid incompetence are a pansystolic murmur (heard best at the xiphisternum and becoming louder during inspiration), systolic pulsation in the neck veins, and pulsation of the liver. A mid-diastolic murmur is heard over the xiphisternum on inspiration if the regurgitant flow is great, or if there is stenosis of the valve.

Management

Prevention of recurrent attacks: Once rheumatic fever has occurred, the most important aspect of treatment is to prevent recurrences, particularly if there has been any evidence of carditis, as each subsequent attack causes increasingly severe damage to the heart valves. This is achieved by preventing streptococcal infection, using continuous prophylactic treatment with penicillin or, in those few patients who are allergic to penicillin, by sulphonamide or erythromycin therapy.

Whilst it is rare for a patient to develop a recurrence of rheumatic fever after the age of 10 years, adolescents and young adults in close communities such as boarding-schools, army camps, or mine compounds are at risk of developing streptococcal pharyngitis with rheumatogenic strains, and recurrence of rheumatic fever. Prophylactic treatment should, therefore, be continued into adulthood in patients who are in these situations. When prophylactic treatment is uninterrupted, incompetent lesions have been found to improve in some patients. The most effective prophylactic regime is achieved with an injection of long-acting benzathine penicillin (Bicillin LA®), 600 000 units IM for those under 30 kg, and 1 200 000 units for bigger children and adults, administered every 3 weeks.

Oral penicillin V, 250 mg twice daily, may be used, but is less successful in achieving complete protection. Patients forget to take their pills before meals, and absorption can be disturbed by enteral illness.

Oral suphonamide 0.5–1 g twice daily, or erythromycin 250 mg daily, may be used as alternatives, but patient compliance must be ensured.

Surgical correction of valve defects: Patients who are incapacitated by damaged valves should be referred for detailed echocardiographic and catheterization studies so that surgical intervention or mitral balloon valvuloplasty can be planned.

Tight pliable mitral stenosis can be relieved either by balloon valvuloplasty (at catheterization), or by surgical commissurotomy with or without cardiopulmonary bypass support. Mitral stenosis, with significant subvalvar thickening, or incompetent valves can be repaired or replaced by prosthetic, homograft, or heterograft valves at open heart operations.

Occasionally, a child with established mitral incompetence and acute carditis who fails to respond to anti-failure therapy will require surgical correction of the mechanical defect. Occasionally ruptured chordae are also in need of repair. Despite the presence of active carditis, such patients recover well in the short term.

Unfortunately, no child who undergoes a surgical procedure for valves damaged by rheumatic fever ceases to be a patient, and most require repeated operations.

In Africa, acute rheumatic fever still has a mortality of 2–3%, and there is a considerable morbidity. The life-span in those who have established heart disease has been prolonged by surgical intervention, but it is still limited, and the quality of life is poor, with affected individuals being unable to undertake occupations requiring physical exertion.

Only through well-organized health programmes aimed at improved living standards (especially housing), early treatment for streptococcal infections, and persistent prophylaxis of affected individuals, can a reduction in this common and eminently-preventable cause of serious cardiac disease be achieved.

Cardiomyopathy

The term cardiomyopathy is used to describe a variety of non-inflammatory conditions causing myocardial dysfunction and resulting in cardiac failure. These may present acutely, but all have the characteristic feature of chronic myocardial failure with a tendency to form intracardiac thromboses.

When faced with the problem of a child in cardiac failure, it is important to look first for signs of a remediable cause:
◆ rheumatic fever
◆ congenital heart defects
◆ anaemia
◆ acute glomerulonephritis
◆ thyrotoxicosis.

The diagnosis of cardiomyopathy is made only after treatment for failure and exclusion of all other causes. The definition of the type of cardiomyopathy usually requires investigation in a specialist cardiac unit.

Cardiomyopathy is a common disease in Africans; it is one of the most frequent causes of heart failure. In most cases an aetiological factor cannot be identified, and prognosis is generally poor. The most common variety is congestive cardiomyopathy.

Clinical features of congestive cardiomyopathy

Most patients present with congestive cardiac failure and a history of effort dyspnoea, fatigue, and orthopnoea. Occasionally children present with syncope, and sometimes with signs of systemic embolization from intracardiac mural thrombosis. Hemiplegia, loss of consciousness, or sudden death from cardiac arrhythmia or cerebral embolus occur.

Examination reveals distended neck veins (often with a large 'A' wave followed by a sharp 'Y' descent), peripheral oedema, hepatomegaly, and in long-standing cases, ascites and pleural effusions.

The pulse pressure is often reduced due to peripheral vasoconstriction raising the diastolic pressure. Pulsus alternans may be present, indicating a severely compromised myocardium, or there may be atrial fibrillation. The apex is usually displaced towards the axilla, and is left ventricular in type, but not overactive. The heart sounds are usually soft, and a triple rhythm due to a third heart sound is common.

Cardiac murmurs are usually absent, but in grossly enlarged hearts there may be dilatation of the mitral and/or tricuspid rings, causing incompetence of the valves. Accordingly, pansystolic murmurs may be heard, which, with treatment for failure, diminish or disappear.

The ECG, although not specific, is always abnormal. There may be left axis deviation. T wave inversion on the left-sided leads is common, and there may be evidence of left ventricular hypertrophy. Large, wide, P waves indicate biatrial enlargement. Arrhythmias may occur; atrial or ventricular ectopics and atrial fibrillation are not uncommon. Occasionally there may be evidence of the Wolff-Parkinson-White (W-P-W) syndrome, i.e., a short PR interval with a prolonged QRS complex due to a 'delta' wave.

The chest X-ray usually shows a grossly enlarged heart with pulmonary congestion. Occasionally the heart is not markedly enlarged, and the term 'restrictive cardiomyopathy' has been used to describe these cases.

Treatment

See under Rheumatic Heart Disease: Congestive Cardiac Failure.

Differential diagnosis

Acute myocarditis, pericarditis, and rheumatic fever can usually be excluded on clinical, ECG, and X-ray features, but echocardiography may be necessary to differentiate pericarditis from cardiomyopathy. Pericardial paracentesis to confirm an effusion should not be undertaken without ECG control.

Cardiac failure due to severe anaemia or acute glomerulonephritis must also be excluded by appropriate investigations. An aberrant left coronary artery arising from the pulmonary artery causes left ventricular hypoxaemia and ischaemia, leading to heart failure. Characteristic ECG changes assist in the diagnosis.

Specific types of cardiomyopathy

Familial and congenital cardiomyopathy

Familial cardiomegaly: A family history of cardiomyopathy or sudden death identifies this rare condition. Bundle branch block is an ECG feature.

Hypertrophic obstructive cardiomyopathy (HOCM): A family history of heart disease and sudden death is usual. There is symmetrical or asymmetrical hypertrophy of the myocardium, affecting particularly the ventricular septum and papillary muscles, causing obstruction of the outflow tract and distortion of valves, especially on the left side. Systolic murmurs may be present. The ECG shows septal hypertrophy, left axis deviation, and bundle branch block patterns.

Treatment with a beta-blocking agent (propranolol) together with a calcium channel blocker (verapamil) is often successful, but surgical removal of the obstructing muscle is sometimes necessary. Digoxin should not be used, as it increases myocardial contractility.

Asymmetrical septal hypertrophy (ASH) can occur in infants born to diabetic mothers, particularly if control of the diabetes has been poor. If the baby is symptomatic, treatment is the same as for HOCM. ASH usually resolves in about 6 months.

Cardiomyopathy may be associated with **inherited disorders of the muscles and nerves,** e.g., Duchenne muscular dystrophy, myotonia atrophica, and Friedreich's ataxia, in all of which it is often the cause of death. It also occurs in **disorders with deposition of abnormal substances,** e.g., mucopolysaccharides in Hurler's syndrome and Hunter disease, and glycogen in Pompé's Type 2 glycogen storage disease.

Primary endocardial fibroelastosis (EFE) presents within the first 2 years of life with congestive cardiac failure. The disorder is confined to a greatly thickened endocardium, particularly in the left ventricle, which restricts contraction of the heart. Left ventricular hypertrophy is striking on the ECG, and the heart size does not diminish with treatment, even though failure may be controlled. If the mitral valve is involved, the characteristic pansystolic murmur of mitral incompetence will be heard. The cause of EFE has not been identified, but it is probably the result of fetal myocarditis.

Acquired cardiomyopathy

Cardiomyopathy of unknown origin is the most usual variety found in children and adults in southern Africa. The clinical features are those of congestive cardiomyopathy, and the course is one of repeated episodes of cardiac failure and multiple embolic episodes, resulting in early death. Post mortem examination of the heart shows dilatation and hypertrophy without fibrosis. Adherent thrombus may be present on the endocardium of the left ventricle.

Endomyocardial fibrosis is a common cause of heart failure in central Africa, and sporadic cases have been described from other parts of the world. Incompetence of the mitral and tricuspid valves is more common in this type of cardiomyopathy, but emboli are rare. Fibrosis of the endocardium of both ventricles, with involvement of the valves, is the outstanding pathological feature. In some cases the cavity of the right ventricle is almost completely obliterated.

Beriberi due to thiamine deficiency causes a high-output cardiac failure, with tachycardia, a large pulse pressure, dilated pulsating forearm veins, and warm extremities. (Low-output failure with orthopnoea and oliguria has also been described). Neurological signs of thiamine deficiency, peripheral neuropathy, nystagmus, encephalopathy, and malnutrition will also be present Beriberi is found in children fed exclusively on a diet of polished rice, and the cardiac dysfunction is dramatically corrected by treatment with thiamine 50–100 mg IM daily, together with digoxin and a diuretic.

Chagas' disease occurs in South and Central America, where it is caused by the parasite *Trypanosoma cruzi*. Infestation of children, particularly in the first year of life, may cause an acute interstitial myocarditis which heals by fibrosis, causing chronic myocardial dysfunction associated with hypertrophy and arrhythmias. Effective treatment is not available, and the prognosis in children is poor *(see Chapter 8, Infectious Disorders)*.

Cardiomyopathy in AIDS can present in various ways, most commonly as a congestive cardiomyopathy. This may be evident clinically, or only discovered at autopsy. Damage to the cardiac conduction system has been reported, as well as the presence of pericardial effusions. An arteriopathy involving small and medium-sized arteries (heart, lungs, kidneys, spleen, intestine, brain) has also been documented.

Infective endocarditis

This is a serious infection of the endocardium, usually caused by organisms lodging on previously-abnormal valves. It is an uncommon disease in both rich and poor communities, and is seen in about 1 out of 4 600 hospital in-patients in both groups.

Changing pattern of the disease

Since the classic accounts by Osler and Horder at the turn of the century, the pattern of this disease has altered among children in the West. The spectrum has been shifting from the subacute to the acute form. This has been attributed to the more frequent use of antibiotics. Whereas *Strep. viridans* used to be the cause in the vast majority of cases, its importance has decreased. Despite this, it is still the most frequently-isolated organism in this disease. Congenital heart disease has replaced rheumatic fever as the main cause of susceptibility to endocarditis. Children who have undergone open-heart surgery are particularly at risk.

Aetiology

Staphylococci and streptococci account for more than 90% of cases in most parts of the world. In South Africa, *Staph. aureus* is the most common cause of infective endocarditis in black children. The source of staphylococci is probably the skin, but may occasionally be other sites, such as bones. *Strep. viridans* infection follows dental extractions or other oropharyngeal surgery.

Underlying cardiac disease

In Africa this infection occurs predominantly in valves damaged by rheumatic fever. This is not unexpected, as rheumatic heart disease is widely prevalent, is severe, and requires cardiac surgery at a young age. Occasionally there is no pre-existing heart lesion.

Clinical features

The cardinal features are due to infection, cardiac abnormalities, and immune complex/embolism. The full-blown picture, which is rarely seen, includes fever, anaemia, clubbing, murmurs, cardiac failure, splenomegaly, petechiae, purpura, Roth spots (haemorrhagic areas with white centre in retina), absent pulses, splinter haemorrhages under the nails, Osler's nodes (tender red nodules in finger pulp), Janeway's lesions (painless haemorrhagic areas in palms and soles), haematuria, and proteinuria. Fever and anaemia occur early in the disease, while splinter haemorrhages, Osler's nodes and Janeway lesions are late features.

Affected African children are usually 7–10 years old, and the frequent features are:

◆ fever
◆ murmurs, and
◆ anaemia.

The late features are not seen at all among black South African children, while the remaining signs described above are uncommon. Glomerulonephritis is sometimes a serious problem in *Staph. aureus* endocarditis. Neurological complications can be severe.

Diagnosis

A high index of suspicion must be maintained in those with pyrexia of unknown origin, and in patients with rheumatic heart disease who have fever and anaemia. Positive blood cultures confirm the diagnosis, but often these can be negative. If in doubt, treat!

Prognosis

The mortality rate is lowest for *Strep. viridans*, and greatest for *Staph. aureus*. Depending on which organism predominates, the average mortality is between 17% and 60%.

Treatment

Preventive measures include attention to skin sepsis and antibiotic cover (penicillin) during surgery (especially to the oropharynx, ears, and nose) in children with any heart lesion. *(See Table 17.4 for details.)*

Choice of antibiotics for cure depends on sensitivity of the organism. Useful combinations (intravenous) are penicillin and gentamicin or amikacin (for *Strep.viridans*), and cloxacillin together with gentamicin or amikacin (for *Staph. aureus*). Minimum duration of treatment is 6 weeks.

Table 17.4 Recommended endocarditis prophylaxis for dental, oral, or upper respiratory tract procedures

Drug	Dose
Standard regimen	
Amoxicillin	50 mg/kg orally 1 hour before the procedure; then 25 mg/kg 6 hours later
	or
	Initial dose: < 15 kg, 750 mg; 15–30 kg, 1 500 mg; and > 30 kg, 3 000 mg, then half the dose 6 hours later
Amoxicillin/penicillin-allergic patients	
Erythromycin (ethylsuccinate or stearate)	20 mg/kg orally 2 hours before the procedure, then half the dose 6 hours later
	or
Clindamycin	10 mg/kg orally, 1 hour before the procedure, then half the dose 6 hours later

Miscellaneous

Myocarditis

Myocarditis can occur at any age and is caused by a variety of viral infections. A newborn infant may be infected if the mother has pleurodynia due to a Coxsackie B virus, and epidemics have occurred in nurseries when the infection has spread to other infants.

Infants present with cardiac failure; tachypnoea and tachycardia are the earliest features. Older children may complain of precordial pain. A loud third heart sound is heard at the apex, there is generalized cardiomegaly on the chest X-ray, with pulmonary congestion, and the ECG shows inversion of T waves in leads 1, V5, and V6. Treatment aims at control of cardiac failure with digoxin and a diuretic.

Pericarditis

Three types of pericarditis are recognized, both pathologically and clinically, in children.

Dry pericarditis
Here a fibrinous exudate involves both layers of the pericardium. This type often presents with pain in the epigastrium or over the lower chest. A squeaky friction rub is heard in about half the cases. This is best heard at the left sternal border when the child is sitting, and is accentuated by pressing on the chest with the stethoscope.

Pericardial effusion
This may be serous, haemorrhagic or purulent. There may be epigastric pain, and dyspnoea is common. A friction rub may be heard, and the heart sounds are muffled. The area of cardiac dullness is increased. Cardiac tamponade occurs if an effusion collects rapidly, compressing the heart and obstructing diastolic filling. The pulse is rapid, and there is a small pulse pressure with pulsus paradoxus. The jugular venous pressure is greatly elevated, and the liver is distended and tender. Pleural effusions are commonly found in children with pericarditis.

Constrictive pericarditis
This usually follows an effusion with the heart shadow becoming smaller. There is distension of the neck veins and liver, often with ascites. A diastolic 'beat' is felt medial to the apex due to rapid filling of the constricted ventricle, and there is pulsus paradoxus.

Causes of pericarditis
Rheumatic fever may cause either dry pericarditis or with effusion, when it is most often associated with a pancarditis. Other features of rheumatic fever will usually suggest the diagnosis. It does not cause constrictive pericarditis.

Tuberculosis is the most common cause of pericardial effusion in endemic areas, but it may

cause a dry pericarditis and become constrictive. The effusion may be straw-coloured or blood-stained. Diagnosis is made by aspiration of the fluid and tuberculin testing *(see Chapter 9, Tuberculosis).*

Viral infections may be associated with any type of pericarditis. The onset is abrupt, usually following an upper respiratory infection. There may be precordial or epigastric pain.

Bacterial infections with staphylococci, streptococci, pneumococci, or *H. influenzae* can cause a purulent pericarditis. These, particularly staphylococci, are often associated with other sites of infection, e.g., osteitis or trauma.

Amoebic pericarditis results from rupture of a liver abscess into the pericardial sac.

Malignant lymphomas in the mediastinum may cause both pericardial and pleural effusions.

Treatment
Treatment depends on the cause. Pericarditis due to rheumatic fever responds dramatically to treatment with prednisone, and does not require aspiration. Effusions should be aspirated once to establish the diagnosis, and tamponade must always be relieved by aspiration. Tuberculous pericarditis calls for treatment with isoniazid, ethionamide, and/or rifampicin. Purulent pericarditis requires repeated aspiration or surgical drainage, as well as appropriate antibiotic treatment. Constrictive pericarditis may complicate tuberculous and amoebic pericarditis. In these cases surgical stripping of the pericardium is required.

Arteritis

Takayasu's disease (or pulseless disease)
(Also see Chapter 23, Juvenile Chronic Arthritis and Vasculitides.)
Congenital coarctation of the aorta is relatively uncommon in African children and will be symptomatic within the first month of life. Thus aortic arteritis should be suspected in older infants and children presenting with upper limb hypertension and poor leg pulses, especially if they are in CCF.

Kawasaki disease

(Also see Chapter 23, Juvenile Chronic Arthritis and Vasculitides.)

Aneurysms of the proximal portions of the coronary arteries may occur in 20–25% of cases. Deaths, in 2% of patients, are due to myocardial infarction or myocarditis.

Pulmonary hypertension

(Not due to congenital heart disease)

Chronic upper airway obstruction

Severe upper airway obstruction may be caused by very large tonsils and adenoids, resulting in chronic hypoxaemia which causes reflex constriction of the pulmonary arterioles. These children present with right heart failure and are recognized by their noisy breathing. They also snore loudly when asleep.

Attention to cardiac failure with digoxin, diuretics, and oxygen, followed by removal of the tonsils and adenoids, results in complete cure.

Bilharzia

(Also see Chapter 8, Infectious Disorders.)

Schistosomal infestation of the bladder and/or bowel may be complicated by embolization of ova to the lungs, causing both obstructive and reactive pulmonary arteriolitis which proceeds to fibrosis. This cause of pulmonary hypertension produces unremitting right heart failure and death. The diagnosis is presumptive in a child with schistosomiasis, but can be confirmed by lung biopsy.

Cor pulmonale

(Also see Chapter 13, Respiratory Disorders.)

This can occur following lung damage secondary to measles and adenovirus infections. It has also been recently described in children with AIDS, who present with progressive nodular and interstitial pulmonary disease.

Persistent pulmonary hypertension of the newborn (persistent fetal circulation syndrome)

(Also see Chapter 5, Newborns.)

This problem usually occurs in full-term or post-date neonates appropriate for gestational age. There may be a history of meconium staining and/or birth asphyxia, as well as maternal risk factors such as increased maternal age, pre-eclampsia, Caesarian section, precipitous delivery, polyhydramnios, or diabetes. The baby usually has signs of respiratory distress and is cyanosed soon after birth. The blood pressure may be normal or decreased. There is a right ventricular heave, and on auscultation there is a pansystolic murmur of tricuspid incompetence, best heard at the 4th left interspace. There may even be signs of congestive cardiac failure. The ECG may display evidence of right ventricular and/or right atrial hypertrophy with ischaemic changes. A chest radiograph will show cardiomegaly.

These infants are often difficult to distinguish from those with cyanotic congenital heart disease. They should be referred to a specialist centre, where echocardiography will resolve the problem. Treatment includes hyperventilation with the aid of a ventilator, additional oxygen, and correction of metabolic acidosis, to induce pulmonary arteriolar vasodilatation.

Arrhythmias

Paroxysmal supraventricular tachycardia

This is the most common arrhythmia. Infants present with pallor, diminished activity, and difficulty in finishing their feeds. Often there is a precipitating febrile illness, e.g., urinary tract infection. Older children complain of suddenly feeling their heart beat faster, together with weakness. Examination reveals a heart rate in excess of 240/minute. Attacks may stop as abruptly as they start, without treatment. ECG will show tachycardia with P waves followed by normal QRS complexes.

Infants require digitalization, and treatment for any precipitating causative illness.

In older children the tachycardia may be stopped as abruptly as it started by pressing on the right carotid artery or the eyeball, or by getting the child to perform the Valsalva manoeuvre. These manoeuvres are rarely successful in infants, and eyeball pressure must never be used, as it may result in detachment of the retina. A cold (ice) pack to the face can be tried in these babies.

If medical treatment fails, electrical (DC) conversion is recommended — 2–4 joules/kg.

Atrial flutter

Atrial flutter may be present at birth, causing congestive cardiac failure. It has been diagnosed *in utero* by the finding of fetal tachycardia before labour commences. The ECG shows typical flutter waves instead of P waves. Treatment is with digoxin. If the flutter is resistant to medical therapy, electrical conversion is indicated — 2–4 joules/kg.

Congenital heart block

This presents at birth, and is suspected if an otherwise-normal infant has bradycardia, i.e., less than 100/minute. The diagnosis is confirmed by the ECG, which shows an atrial rate faster than the ventricular rate. The QRS complexes are usually of normal duration (< 0.10 seconds). If Stokes-Adams attacks occur, an artificial pacemaker is required.

There is a frequent association between congenital heart block and maternal systemic lupus erythematosus. The mothers of affected infants should therefore be routinely checked for specific antibodies (Anti-Rho and Anti-La).

Management of paediatric cardiac emergencies

Cyanosis of newborn infants

◆ Administer oxygen. If there is no immediate improvement, and there are no other signs of respiratory disease or cerebral depression, the cause is probably cardiac-related.

If the cyanosis is of cardiac origin *do not* continue to give oxygen, which may aggravate the situation by provoking closure of the ductus arteriosus.

◆ Maintain the infant's temperature.

◆ Give 5% glucose solution IV.

◆ Give sodium bicarbonate IV to correct acidosis.

◆ Give oral prostaglandin E_2, 30–60 μg/kg hourly. (Dissolve 500 μg tablet in 10 ml sterile water. Each 1 ml = 50 μg.)

All cyanotic infants should be referred to a specialist unit as soon as possible.

Cyanotic spells in tetralogy of Fallot

◆ Place infant in knee–chest or squatting position.

◆ Administer morphine 0.1–0.2 mg/kg SC or IM.

◆ Administer propranolol 0.1 mg/kg IM and continue on propranolol by mouth 1–5 mg/kg/day in divided doses.

◆ Check for anaemia and treat accordingly.

Cardiac failure

◆ Nurse the baby propped up at 60°.

◆ Administer oxygen by mask or funnel.

◆ Restrict fluid intake (60 ml/kg/day in neonates); preferably breast milk or low-sodium milk.

◆ Digoxin (elixir 0.05 mg/ml, tablets 0.125 and 0.0625 mg, or injection 0.25 mg/ml) *(see Table 17.5)*. Oral digoxin acts almost as quickly as an intramuscular injection, and is preferred for infants who are not vomiting. Intravenous digoxin is rarely indicated, and must be given with care at 3/4 of the oral or IM dosage, under ECG control.

Furosemide (Lasix®) is the most effective diuretic for acute cardiac failure. It is best given IV initially and then by mouth for maintenance (1–6 mg/kg/day; 0.5–1.0 mg/kg/dose).

Potassium supplementation is required to provide 1–2 mmol/kg/day in divided doses if a diuretic which causes potassium loss is used.

An intravenous infusion of either isoprenaline at a rate of 0.05–0.10 μg/kg/min or dopamine at a rate of 3–10 μg/kg/min. can be used in severe cardiac failure.

Spironolactone (Aldactone®) can be used as a potassium-sparing diuretic in a dose of 2–3 mg/kg/day in 2–3 divided doses, given orally. This can be combined with furosemide.

Vasodilators will reduce the left ventricular after-load, and are particularly useful in cases of dilated cardiomyopathy. Captopril is used in a dose of 0.5–6 mg/kg/day divided into 3–4 doses.

Table 17.5 Digitalizing schedule for infants

Age of Infant	Total digitalizing dose (TDD) divided into 4 doses, 6-hourly	Daily maintenance given in 1 or 2 doses
Pre-term	0.04–0.05 mg/kg	¼ of TDD
2 mths–2 yrs	0.06–0.08 mg/kg	¼ of TDD
Over 2 years	0.04–0.06 mg/kg	0.01 mg/kg/day

Cardiac arrest

Asystole accounts for 90% of cases, the other 10% being caused by ventricular fibrillation. The only way to differentiate is by ECG.

Management

◆ Establish a clear airway and give artificial ventilation, 20–30 breaths a minute, with 100% oxygen from a bag via a face mask, or by endotracheal intubation. Use mouth-to-mouth ventilation if equipment is not available.

◆ Give external cardiac massage simultaneously. For infants, the operator's hands should be placed on either side of the chest and the infant's sternum compressed by both thumbs at a rate of 80–100/minute.

◆ Give sodium bicarbonate, 2 mEq/kg body weight IV, to counteract metabolic acidosis.

◆ Check serum electrolytes and correct hypokalaemia and/or hypocalcaemia.

◆ If ECG reveals ventricular fibrillation, electrical defibrillation is necessary.

S.E. Levin

18

Blood disorders

Anaemia

Anaemia is defined as a decrease in haemoglobin (Hb) or haematrocrit (HCT) below the normal value for age and sex. The main pathogenic mechanisms are:

◆ impaired or ineffective blood production
◆ haemorrhage
◆ haemolysis — increased red cell destruction.

Anaemia is not a disease in itself, but a manifestation of an underlying disorder. In the developing world there may be multifactorial causes, e.g,. nutritional, infective, or parasites causing blood loss in the same patient. The prevalence of low-birth-weight infants contributes to the high incidence of nutritional anaemias. The cause must therefore always be established before treatment is given.

Normal values

The diagnosis of anaemia in infancy and childhood is based upon knowledge of the changes in Hb, HCT, and red cell characteristics which occur during growth and development (*see Fig. 18.1 and*

Table 18.1). The high Hb level (*physiological polycythaemia*) at birth reflects recent exposure to the relatively hypoxic intrauterine environment.

Delay in clamping the cord can increase the blood volume by 60%. The Hb level of capillary blood may be 2 g/dl more than that of venous

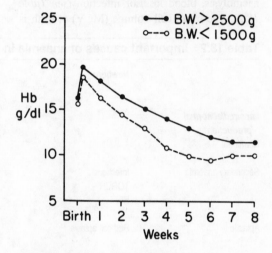

Fig. 18.1 Changes in haemoglobin levels in early infancy

Table 18.1 Normal blood values in infancy and childhood

Age	Hb g/dl	HCT %	MCV fl	MCH pg	Retics %
Cord	16.5	52	108	36	5
1 day	19.6	61	107	37	5
1 week	18.2	58	98	33	1
1 month	14.5	44	96	32	1
2 months	11.5	35	94	30	1
6 months	11.6	35	90	30	1
1 year	11.5	35	78	27	1.5
2–5 years	12.5	37	80	27	1.5
6–12 years	13.5	40	85	29	1.5
Adolescent					
Male	15–17	46–52	78–98	26–32	0.5–2
Female	13–15	40–46	78–98	26–32	0.5–2

Hb = haemoglobin   HCT = haematocrit   MCV = mean cell volume   MCH = mean cell haemoglobin   Retics = reticulocytes

blood. A further increase on day one is due to postnatal reduction in plasma volume. The progressive postnatal decrease in Hb, which reaches a nadir between 6 and 12 weeks *(physiological anaemia)*, is a physiological adjustment, more marked in pre-term infants. It is not due to iron deficiency; nor is it corrected by iron therapy.

Anaemia in the newborn
Also see Chapter 5, Newborns.
This is defined as a Hb less than 14 g/dl in the full-term infant, and is most commonly due to haemolysis, blood loss, or infection *(see Table 18.2)*. The mean cell volume (MCV) at birth is

higher *(physiological macrocytosis)* and may fall to lower than adult levels by about 3 months. The red cells tend to be microcytic from 3 months to approximately 6 years, which could be mistaken for iron deficiency anaemia or thalassaemia minor. (As a rough guide, the MCV = 70 + 1 for each year of age up to 6 years.) The reticulocyte count is approximately 5% at birth and returns to adult levels at 1 week. Hypoplastic anaemia is rare. Evaluation of the aetiology includes a detailed history of pregnancy and delivery, with particular reference to infections, blood loss, and drug ingestion. The family ethnic background, and history of previously anaemic or jaundiced infants,

Table 18.2   Important causes of anaemia in infancy and childhood

	Newborn	Infancy and pre-school	Later childhood
Impaired/abnormal production Nutritional	–	Iron deficiency PEM Folate deficiency	Iron deficiency Folate deficiency Vit. B_{12} deficiency
Secondary anaemia	Infections TORCH HIV	Infection	Infection Systemic disease
Aplastic	Red cell aplasia	Acquired (infection, idiopathic, drugs) Fanconi's anaemia	Acquired (infection, idiopathic, drugs) Fanconi's anaemia
Neoplastic	Congenital leukaemia	Acute leukaemia Solid tumours	Acute leukaemia Lymphoma Solid tumours
Blood loss	Feto-maternal Twin-twin Cord Cephalhaematoma Haemorrhagic disease Blood sampling	Gastrointestinal (malformations, polyps parasites) Platelet/ coagulation abnormalities	Gastrointestinal (malformations, ulcer, parasites) Urogenital (bilharzia) Platelet coagulation abnormalities
Haemolysis	Rh/ABO Infection Hereditary — spherocytosis — G6PD	Infection N.B. malaria Autoimmune Hereditary — spherocytosis — Hb–pathies — thalassaemia — G6PD	Infection N.B. malaria Autoimmune Hereditary — spherocytosis — Hb–pathies — thalassaemia — G6PD

miscarriages, or blood transfusions are particularly important in relationship to hereditary haemolytic anaemias, and Rh and ABO incompatibility. Jaundice and hepatosplenomegaly suggest haemolysis or infection, whereas pallor, shock, or overt bleeding indicate blood loss anaemia *(see Table 18.2)*. Cephalhaematoma and bleeding into organs (e.g., spleen) should be excluded. The placenta should always be examined as a possible source of the haemorrhage. In twin births, twin-to-twin haemorrhage may occur, resulting in anaemia in one and polycythaemia in the other. Feto-maternal transfusions may cause chronic anaemia in the neonate.

As the profoundly anaemic, jaundiced, or sick neonate requires immediate intervention, it is important to have a logical approach to the differential diagnosis *(see Fig. 18.2)*. The results of appropriate investigations should be available before any form of treatment is commenced.

The reticulocyte count is the most useful test to differentiate hypoplastic anaemia from anaemia due to haemolysis or blood loss. A direct Coombs' test will differentiate the immune (Rh/ABO) from non-immune haemolytic anaemias (hereditary or infective) and blood loss. *(For further details see Chapter 5, Newborns.)*

Infection must be considered in the first instance when a jaundiced and anaemic infant with hepatosplenomegaly shows no evidence of blood group incompatibility. Hereditary haemolytic anaemia should be suspected if there are specific red cell morphological abnormalities: spherocytes (hereditary spherocytosis), elliptocytes (hereditary elliptocytosis),

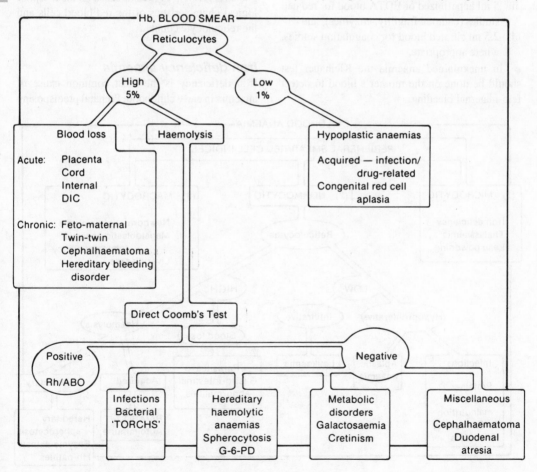

Fig. 18.2 Approach to anaemia in the newborn

pyknocytes (glucose-6-phosphate dehydrogenase or pyruvate kinase deficiency). The more common haemoglobinopathies (Hb S, Hb C) and thalassaemia are asymptomatic at birth. Anaemia develops only at 3–6 months, as fetal Hb F is replaced by adult Hb A, which contains the defective globin chains *(see Haemoglobinopathies, below).*

If an emergency blood transfusion has to be given before a definitive diagnosis has been made, certain rules should be followed:

◆ The transfused blood must be compatible with both mother and baby in case there are maternal antibodies present in the infant's circulation.

◆ Diagnostic blood samples must be taken before transfusion and should include:

i. 10 ml clotted blood for serological studies (e.g., red cell antibodies, TORCHS, HIV)
ii. 5 ml heparinized or EDTA blood for red cell studies (osmotic fragility, enzymes), and
iii. 2.5 ml citrated blood for coagulation studies, where appropriate.

◆ In unexplained anaemia the Kleihauer test should be done on the mother's blood to detect feto-maternal bleeding.

Haemolytic disease of the newborn (erythroblastosis fetalis)
See Chapter 5, Newborns.

Anaemia in infancy and later childhood
The most common causes of childhood anaemia are outlined in *Table 18.2.* In Third World countries, nutritional deficiencies and anaemias secondary to infection, systemic disease, and parasites predominate. However, the cause of the anaemia is often multifactorial. *At all ages blood loss must be excluded.* Hereditary haemolytic anaemias are less common, but cause significant morbidity and mortality in certain well-defined population groups. A schematic approach to differential diagnosis is given in *Fig. 18.3,* based on the morphological characteristics of the red blood cells and the reticulocyte count.

Iron deficiency anaemia
Iron deficiency is the most common cause of anaemia in early childhood. Prenatal predisposing

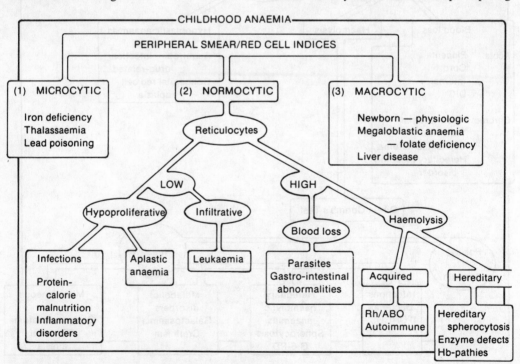

Fig. 18.3 Approach to anaemia in infancy and childhood

factors include maternal multiparity, twin births, low birth weight (LBW), and blood loss, all of which result in depleted iron stores at birth. As the total body iron stores at birth are directly related to birth weight, all LBW infants start life with deficient stores. The single most important post-natal cause of iron deficiency is inadequate dietary intake relative to rapid growth. LBW infants, even if breast-fed, will become iron deficient unless they are given supplementary iron from the age of 2 months. Additional contributory factors include bacterial, viral, and parasitic infections, which impair iron uptake and utilization, or cause chronic blood loss. The age groups at greatest risk are 6 months to 3 years, and then in adolescence.

The incidence of iron deficiency varies inversely with socio-economic status, ranging from less than 5% in affluent western societies to more than 50% in developing countries.

Clinical manifestations

Initial symptoms and signs are vague and non-specific e.g., tiredness and lethargy. Irritability, anorexia, and pica are common. Frequently the child presents with an intercurrent infection, with anaemia as an incidental finding. As the development of anaemia is a gradual process, children may adapt to haemoglobin levels below 5 g/dl with minimal systemic upset. Varying degrees of pallor, koilonychia, moderate splenomegaly, and a soft ejection systolic murmur, may be the only abnormal physical findings. Parietal bossing of the skull may be present in patients with iron deficiency due to chronic blood loss. Other signs of suboptimal nutrition may be present.

Haematological findings

The characteristic blood findings in iron deficiency are microcytosis (MCV < 70 fl), hypochromia (MCH < 26 pg), reduced serum iron (< 40 µg/dl), increased iron-binding capacity (> 450 µg/dl), decreased transferrin saturation (< 16%), and decreased serum ferritin (< 10 ng/ml). The free erythrocyte protoporphyrin level (FEP) and red cell distribution width (RDW) is increased. These changes precede the development of anaemia. The reticulocyte count is increased where blood loss is the cause.

Differential diagnosis

A hypochromic, microcytic blood picture occurring in a child aged 6 months to 3 years with a poor dietary history or low birth weight is usually accepted as sufficient evidence for a diagnosis of nutritional iron deficiency. Biochemical tests need not be done routinely. The diagnosis can be confirmed with a therapeutic trial of oral ferrous sulphate. In areas where intestinal parasites are common, proctoscopy should be done and stools should be examined for occult blood and ova. A source of blood loss should always be sought in children with recurrent episodes of hypochromic anaemia, and in older children with a good dietary history who present with an iron-deficient blood picture. Raw cows' milk may cause chronic subclinical intestinal blood loss: heating or boiling the milk denatures the protein and hence obviates this problem. Pulmonary haemosiderosis should be suspected in infants fed on cows' milk, or in older children with repeated respiratory problems and associated iron deficiency. Lead poisoning is often found with iron deficiency in certain urban populations, and can be confirmed by blood lead level estimation.

Other disorders giving a hypochromic, microcytic anaemia are the thalassaemia syndromes and long-standing chronic infections or inflammatory disorders (*see later in this chapter*).

Treatment

Oral ferrous sulphate (citrate, gluconate, or fumarate), in a dose of 5 mg Fe^{++}/kg/day, will correct nutritional iron deficiency anaemia within 4 weeks in over 90% of cases. Symptoms of lethargy and irritability improve within days of commencing treatment — a feature which is confirmatory of the diagnosis. The minimum acceptable response is a rise in haemoglobin of 2 g/dl in 3 weeks. Lack of response is most often due to poor drug compliance or incorrect diagnosis. Slow or incomplete response may be due to intercurrent infection, impaired absorption, continuing blood loss, occult folate deficiency, or inadequate dosage.

Parenteral iron therapy is rarely indicated for medical reasons, but may be necessary in cases of poor compliance with oral therapy or in malabsorptive states. It should not be given to patients with active infections or underlying systemic disease.

Blood transfusion is not recommended for chronic iron deficiency anaemia unless it is very severe (Hb ≤ 4 g/dl) and there are cardio-pulmonary symptoms, continuing blood loss, or severe infection is present. Packed red cells 10 mg/kg should be transfused slowly, with a diuretic given simultaneously.

Dietary factors: Milk is a poor source of iron, but the iron in breast milk is more readily absorbed than that in cows' milk, and fully breast-fed infants rarely develop iron deficiency. The haem iron present in meat is more easily absorbed than the inorganic iron in cereals and vegetables. The availability of iron from iron-fortified foods varies widely. Rice is a poor source. Egg iron is very poorly absorbed, and the addition of eggs to a mixed meal will retard the absorption of iron from other foods. Citrus fruits or medicinal vitamin C significantly enhance the availability of dietary iron.

Iron requirements and prevention of iron deficiency: A minimum daily intake of 1 mg Fe^{++}/kg/day (maximum 15 mg/day) is recommended for full-term infants, and 2 mg/kg/day for premature babies. Promotion of breast-feeding, the introduction of mixed feeding by 4 months of age, and appropriate advice regarding iron-rich foods are the most important factors in prevention of iron deficiency. LBW infants, however, require additional iron supplementation by 6–8 weeks of age. This can be given as medicinal iron, or as iron-fortified formula in infants who are not breast-fed. Supplementation from birth is not indicated, and may be harmful. Term infants who are fed on cows' milk formula from birth and who receive mainly cereals and vegetables as weaning foods require iron supplements from the age of 3 months if iron deficiency is to be prevented.

Megaloblastic anaemias

These are uncommon in children, but more prevalent in Third World countries than in developed communities. The main cause is dietary folate deficiency. This is most often due to decreased intake or absorption associated with general malnutrition, chronic diarrhoeal disorders, and intercurrent infection. Other aetiological factors are chronic haemolytic anaemias, where there is an increased requirement due to rapid red cell turnover, and to anti-convulsant therapy which impairs folate absorption. LBW infants who grow rapidly have an increased demand for folate and are therefore at risk.

Clinical features
The age group at greatest risk is 6 months to 3 years, and in particular malnourished (kwashiorkor) or LBW infants. Presenting signs include pallor, occasionally mild icterus, and in severe cases a petechial rash. Children with megaloblastic anaemia are usually more ill than those with iron deficiency and a comparable degree of anaemia.

Haematological findings
Anaemia is often severe, with Hb levels below 7 g/dl. The MCV is usually more than 100 fl, but may be misleadingly low due to marked variation in cell size and shape or concomitant iron deficiency. The peripheral smear frequently shows a combination of oval macrocytes, normochromic, normocytic cells, and microcytes. Leucopenia and thrombocytopenia are common, and hypersegmentation of neutrophils is characteristic. Serum folate is below 3 ng/ml, red cell folate below 160 ng/ml, and serum iron elevated. Bone marrow examination confirms the presence of megaloblastic changes in both red and white cell precursors.

Prevention and treatment
The minimum daily requirement of folic acid is 50 µg. Good dietary sources are liver, eggs, fresh green vegetables, yeast, and nuts. Breast milk and cows' milk have small but adequate amounts of folate for young infants. Goats' milk is markedly deficient. Folate is heat-labile and thus destroyed by cooking.

Treatment with folic acid, 1 mg daily for 10–14 days, will correct the anaemia. Further supplementation for approximately a month is recommended to replenish stores. The diet should contain adequate protein, and iron and vitamin C supplements may be necessary.

Vitamin B$_{12}$ deficiency occurs rarely in children. The most common causes are chronic ileal disease, resection of the lower ileum, and deficient or abnormal intrinsic gastric factors. It is not uncommon to find megaloblastic anaemia due to Vitamin B_{12} deficiency in older black children in Durban. Preliminary investigations suggest malabsorption due to giardia infestations. Juvenile pernicious anaemia and inherited disorders of B_{12} metabolism are extremely rare.

Confirmatory diagnostic tests include determination of serum vitamin B_{12}, the Schilling test of B_{12} absorption, and investigation for gastrointestinal pathology.

Long-term replacement therapy with parenteral vitamin B_{12} 50–100 µg monthly, is usually required.

Protein-energy malnutrition (PEM)
(Also see Chapter 7, Nutritional Disorders.)
Anaemia is a regular feature of PEM. Numerous factors contribute to the aetiology, varying in different geographical areas. Protein deficiency *per se* causes anaemia. Iron deficiency is uncommon at presentation, but develops in most cases during recovery as growth requirements increase. Folate deficiency is less common than iron deficiency, but frank megaloblastic anaemia can occur. Other contributing factors are bacterial and parasitic infections, dilutional effects due to blood volume changes, and variable vitamin and trace element deficiencies.

Haematological features
The anaemia of protein deficiency is moderate — Hb 8–10 g/dl — normocytic, and normochromic. Reticulocytosis develops within 7–10 days of dietary rehabilitation. A transient decrease in Hb coincides with loss of oedema and plasma volume expansion. Bone marrow iron stores are frequently increased on admission, but decrease rapidly during dietary rehabilitation. Overt iron deficiency with hypochromia and microcytosis commonly develops within four weeks. The WBC varies with the presence or absence of infection. Thrombocytopenia may occur in severely ill, infected patients.

The presence of severe anaemia suggests coincidental folate or iron deficiency or infection.

Treatment
Treatment is directed towards nutritional rehabilitation and control of intercurrent infection. Folic acid supplementation, 1–5 mg daily for 10 days, is advisable early in the therapeutic regimen. Iron supplementation should be deferred until infections are controlled and until the initiation of transferrin regeneration within 2–3 weeks. Transfusion of packed red cells may be required in severely anaemic patients, or if infection is present.

Anaemia of infection
Anaemia associated with acute infection is usually haemolytic in type *(see Haemolytic Anaemias, below)*. Transient red cell aplasia can also occur *(see Red Cell Aplasia, below)*. Chronic infections are a common cause of low-grade anaemia in children, particularly chronic respiratory, urinary, and parasitic infections.

An underlying infection should always be excluded in an anaemic child. ◄

Chronic systemic diseases
Rheumatoid arthritis, renal, hepatic, and endocrine disorders are also associated with chronic anaemia. Such anaemia varies with the activity of the underlying disease.

The characteristic features are a moderate normocytic, normochromic anaemia (Hb 8–10 g/dl) with evidence of subclinical haemolysis, impaired marrow response to anaemia, and impaired iron utilization. In long-standing cases, microcytosis and hypochromia may develop. Serum iron and transferrin are both decreased. The RDW is normal. Serum ferritin and bone marrow iron are increased. These features distinguish this type of anaemia from iron deficiency, with which it is often confused *(see Fig. 18.4)*.

As both absorption and utilization of iron are impaired, iron therapy is ineffective and contraindicated. The treatment is that of the underlying disease. Once this is controlled, the anaemia will also resolve.

Aplastic anaemia
Bone marrow failure may be either hereditary or acquired, and can affect all haemopoeitic elements (pancytopenia), or be restricted to a single cell line

(erythroid, myeloid, or megakaryocytic), in which case it is referred to as hypoplastic anaemia.

Acquired aplastic anaemia

The most common causes of acquired aplastic anaemia are listed in *Table 18.3*. In the majority of cases no precipitating factor can be identified. There is increasing evidence that immunological factors may play an important aetiological role.

Clinical and haematological features: The onset is usually insidious, with pallor, lethargy, easy bruising, and petechiae progressing to overt haemorrhage and serious intercurrent infection.

Hepatosplenomegaly is rarely seen in acquired aplastic anaemia, and hence is a useful differentiating feature from acute leukaemia, which may otherwise have a similar clinical presentation.

The blood picture is one of peripheral pancytopenia. Diagnosis is confirmed by bone marrow aspirate and trephine biopsy.

Treatment: The treatment of choice in severe aplasia is bone marrow transplantation from a histocompatible sibling. Where this is not feasible, immunosuppressive therapy (antithymocyte globulin, cyclosporin-A, corticosteroids) and/or androgens are indicated. Supportive transfusions of blood granulocytes and platelets should be reserved for life-threatening situations, as bone marrow transplantation is most successful in those who have had the least transfusions.

The **prognosis** is generally poor. Approximately 50% of patients die within 5 months, and less than 15% make a complete haematological recovery. With bone marrow transplantation, over 55% survive in full haematological remission for longer than 2 years. The major complication is the development of graft-versus-host reaction.

Fanconi's anaemia

This familial hypoplastic anaemia is inherited as an autosomal-recessive trait. A high prevalance has been recorded in some geographical areas in South Africa amongst certain population groups, white and black. Associated physical abnormalities in

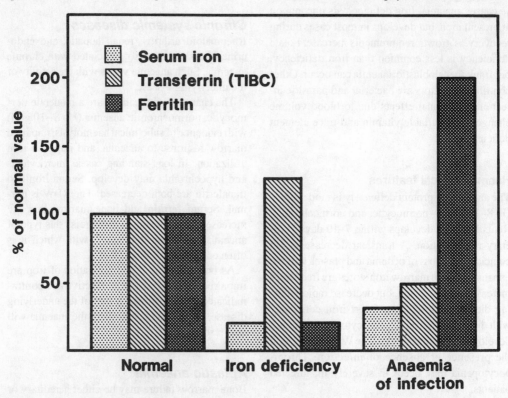

Fig. 18.4 The haematological features of anaemia due to iron deficiency and infection

Table 18.3 Causes of acquired aplastic anaemia

Idiopathic
Antibiotics:
  Chloramphenicol, sulphonamides
Anticonvulsants:
  Phenobarbitone, phenytoin
Antimalarials:
  Quinine, amodiaquine
Cancer chemotherapeutic agents
Chemicals:
  Benzine, carbon tetrachloride, glue
Insecticides:
  DDT, chlordane, parathione, lindane
Infections:
  Hepatitis A, HIV, EBV, rubella, measles, mumps, influenza
Protein-energy malnutrition (PEM)
Irradiation
Pre-leukaemic conditions

order of frequency are pigmentary skin changes (76%), LBW, short stature, thumb anomalies, microcephaly, hypogenitalia, renal anomalies, other skeletal anomalies, strabismus, hyperreflexia, microphthalmia, mental retardation, deafness, and congenital heart disease. The bone marrow is hypercellular, and chromosomal analysis typically reveals chromosomal breakages and structural abnormalities.

Pancytopenia rarely develops before 4 years of age, and often responds to androgens and steroids. Bone marrow transplants have been performed with limited success. Patients have a high risk of developing myeloid leukaemia and cancer. Repeated transfusions are associated with iron overload. The life expectancy is markedly shortened.

Acquired red cell aplasia

Transient erythroblastopenia of childhood (TEC) occurs as a complication of viral infections. The aplasia usually lasts no more than 7–10 days, and in children with no pre-existing haematological abnormality it rarely causes significant anaemia. However, in patients with pre-existing chronic haemolytic anaemias, a similar transient aplastic episode may result in sudden severe anaemia, requiring blood transfusion. A decrease in reticulocyte count is usually the first sign of impending

crisis in these patients. It may be precipitated by a viral infection, e.g., parvovirus.

Congenital pure red cell aplasia (Blackfan-Diamond syndrome)

This is a rare disorder in which a selective aplasia of erythroid precursors is present at birth. Treatment with corticosteroids is effective, and long-term maintenance therapy is required.

Haemolytic anaemias

Haemolytic anaemias are characterized by evidence of increased red cell destruction (anaemia, jaundice, urobilinuria or haemoglobinuria) and a compensatory increase in bone marrow erythropoeisis (reticulocytosis). In long-standing haemolytic anaemia, extramedullary haemopoeisis in liver and spleen may contribute to hepatosplenomegaly, and expanded bone marrow cavities from erythroid hyperplasia will cause skull bossing and thinning of the cortices of long bones.

When red cell destruction occurs mainly extravascularly in spleen and reticulo-endothelial system, the predominant clinical feature is jaundice. When destruction is mainly intravascular, the main features are pallor and haemoglobinuria.

Aetiology

Haemolytic anaemias may be due either to hereditary intrinsic defects of the red cell membrane, enzymes, or haemoglobin, or to acquired extrinsic factors such as infections, antibodies, and mechanical trauma. The most common causes are listed in *Table 18.4.*

Hereditary spherocytosis (HS)

This is the most common inherited haemolytic anaemia in people of north European extraction. In South Africa it is seen in all ethnic groups, and is the most common inherited haemolytic anaemia seen in blacks. The inheritance pattern is autosomal-dominant. In 25% of cases it is due to a new mutation with no family history.

The red cells are spherocytic in shape. The basic defect is in the red cell membrane, which is deficient in spectin and is associated with increased permeability to sodium. The degree of spectin deficiency correlates closely with the severity of disease and the degree of spherocytosis. The

Paediatrics and child health

Table 18.4   Classification of haemolytic anaemia

Hereditary
Membrane defect
    Hereditary spherocytosis
Enzyme deficiencies
    Glucose-6-phosphate dehydrogenase (G6PD)
Haemoglobin abnormalities
    Sickle-cell anaemia
    Thalassaemia
Acquired
Isoimmune
    Haemolytic disease of newborn
Autoimmune
    Viral infection
    Bacterial septicaemia, protozoa, e.g., malaria
    Penicillin, sulphonamide, cephalosporin, rifampicin
Nonimmune
    Malaria
    Burns
    Hypersplenism

spherocytes are trapped and destroyed in the venous sinuses of the spleen; hence splenectomy will cure the anaemia.

Clinical features

These are very variable, ranging from an asymptomatic, compensated haemolytic process to severe recurrent anaemia requiring transfusion. Most cases exhibit jaundice in the newborn period. Differentiation from ABO haemolytic disease may be difficult. In HS the persistence of spherocytes beyond the neonatal period, together with evidence of increased osmotic fragility in the infant and one parent, confirms the diagnosis.

In later childhood, episodic jaundice precipitated by infection is a common presentation, frequently associated with splenomegaly. Complications include transient aplastic crises, which are usually precipitated by infection (e.g., parvovirus) and resolve spontaneously with a brisk reticulocytosis. Gallstones and leg ulcers are uncommon complications in young children, but become increasingly prevalent from adolescence onwards.

Haematological features

Anaemia is moderate (Hb 8–10 g/dl), but may become severe (Hb 3–5 g/dl) during aplastic or hyperhaemolytic crises. Reticulocytes range from 5–15%. Diagnosis is based on the finding of spherocytes, increased red cell osmotic fragility, and increased autohaemolysis corrected (*in vitro*) by glucose. In most instances one parent will show similar abnormalities. Autoimmune haemolytic anaemia, which also has spherocytes, can be excluded by a negative Coombs' test.

Treatment

Splenectomy effectively controls haemolysis by removing the main site of red cell destruction. The intrinsic abnormality of the red cell is unchanged. The most severe post-splenectomy complication is overwhelming pneumococcal septicaemia. Risk of this complication is minimized by deferring operation until 5 years of age, giving preoperative pneumococcal vaccine, and prophylactic penicillin postoperatively.

Hereditary elliptocytosis

This is characterized by oval-shaped red cells, and is due to abnormality of the red cell membrane. In the majority of patients (85–90%), inheritance is autosomal-dominant and the disease is asymptomatic. In the remainder it appears to be autosomal-recessive, and characterized by moderate to severe haemolysis. Splenectomy is effective in ameliorating haemolysis in severe cases.

Enzyme deficiencies

The most common red cell enzyme deficiencies causing clinical haemolysis are, in order of frequency, glucose-6-phosphate dehydrogenase (G6PD), pyruvate kinase (PK), glucose-phosphate-isomerase (GPI), and hexokinase (HX) deficiency.

G6PD deficiency is distributed world-wide, with particular prevalence in people originating from areas where falciparum malaria is endemic. The deficiency provides a limited protective effect against the development of falciparum malaria. There are numerous genetic mutants of the G6PD enzyme throughout the world. The enzyme deficiency is always associated with a reduction in the red cell life-span. The magnitude of this effect depends on the particular gene mutation and the enzyme levels. In Caucasians the incidence ranges from approximately 3% in Greeks to more than

50% in Sephardic Jews. In American blacks the incidence is 10% and in South African blacks 3–5%, depending on the tribal group. The gene for G6PD is carried on the X-chromosome and transmitted as a sex-linked recessive. Female heterozygotes (XX) are asymptomatic carriers. Affected males (XY) and homozygous females (XX) show full expression of the disease.

Clinical and haematological features

Expression varies, and neonatal jaundice is often the presenting feature.

In Caucasians, enzyme levels are usually lower than in blacks, and Caucasians exhibit a low-grade, compensated haemolytic anaemia with increased reticulocytes and occasional splenomegaly. Blacks usually show no clinical or haematological abnormalities until exposed to oxidant stress. The typical acute haemolytic episode develops 3–4 days after ingestion of oxidant drugs or the development of infection (*see Table 18.5*). Jaundice and haemoglobinuria are followed by a sharp drop in Hb. Brisk reticulocytosis develops within 3–7 days, and Hb returns to normal over 1–2 weeks. Neonates may develop haemolysis from substances excreted in the breast milk. Diagnosis is confirmed by G6PD screening tests or quantitative assay in red cells.

Treatment: This involves avoidance of oxidant drugs, and the use of blood transfusion during acute haemolytic episodes. Splenectomy is not helpful.

Pyruvate kinase (PK) deficiency is a rare autosomal-recessive disorder occurring mainly in people of northern European stock. Diagnosis is confirmed by an enzyme screening test or red cell assay.

Glucose-6-phosphate isomerase (GPI) deficiency and **hexokinase (HX) deficiency** are rare disorders, transmitted as autosomal recessives and not restricted to any specific ethnic group. Diagnosis is confirmed by red cell enzyme assay.

Haemoglobinopathies and thalassaemia syndrome

Abnormalities of haemoglobin causing clinical disease are due either to substitutions or depletions of amino acids in the globin chains, or to impaired rates of globin chain synthesis.

Table 18.5 Causes of haemolysis in G6PD deficiency

Drugs:	Antimalarials
	Sulphonamides
	Chloramphenicol
	Nitrofurantoin
	Nalidixic acid
	Aspirin/phenacetin compounds
	Vitamin K (large doses)
Chemicals:	Naphthalene moth balls
	Benzine
Food:	Fava beans
Infections:	Bacterial
	Viral
Metabolic:	Diabetic acidosis

Normal haemoglobins

(*See Table 18.6.*)

Normal adult haemoglobin has three components: Hb A, Hb A2 and Hb F, with Hb A comprising more than 95% of the total. Hb F is the major component at birth, and decreases by 3–4% per week to reach adult levels by approximately 6 months of age.

The alpha globin chains are common to all the normal haemoglobins. Defect of alpha chains will therefore be manifest from birth, whereas defects of beta chains will not manifest clinically until 3–6 months of age, when beta chain synthesis predominates.

Haemoglobinopathies

The most common haemoglobinopathy, sickle-cell disease (HbSS), is the result of the substitution of valine for glutamic acid in the 6th position of the beta chain. This renders the Hb less soluble on deoxygenation. Tactoids form within the red cell, distorting its shape, impeding passage through small capillaries, and causing vaso-occlusive crises and haemolytic anaemia. Other beta chain defects causing less severe haemolysis are Hbs C, D, and E.

Table 18.6 Haemoglobin composition and concentration related to age

Haemo-globin	Globin chains	Birth %	6 months %	Adult %
HbA	$\alpha_2\beta_2$	10–35	92	> 95
HbA$_2$	$\alpha_2\delta_2$	0–1.8	1–3	2–3
HbF	$\alpha_2\gamma_2$	65–90	< 5	< 1

Sickle-cell disease

This condition represents the homozygous state for the sickle-cell gene (Hb SS). Heterozygote carriers have sickle-cell trait (Hb AS). The disease is inherited as an autosomal co-dominant.

It is the most common severe inherited disease in Africa generally, except in South Africa. Approximately 10% of American blacks have the sickle-cell trait. In Africa the incidence is highest in West Africa (30 – 40%) and lowest in South Africa (1%). The gene is also prevalent in certain peoples of Mediterranean, Saudi Arabian, and Asiatic origin. The geographical distribution tends to parallel that of falciparum malaria.

Clinical and haematological features: The characteristic features of sickle-cell disease are those of a chronic haemolytic anaemia, punctuated by painful crises due to vaso-occlusive episodes. The clinical picture varies with age and environmental factors. In infancy, painful swelling of hands and feet (so-called 'hand and foot syndrome') may be the presenting feature. Varying degrees of pallor, jaundice, and hepatosplenomegaly will also be noted.

Intravascular sickling — with or without infarctive episodes involving mesenteric. renal, cerebral, skeletal, or pulmonary capillaries — gives rise to a wide variety of clinical signs, ranging from acute abdominal pain, haematuria, and hemiplegia, to bone pains and haemoptysis. Repeated infarcts in the spleen result in progressive splenic hypofunction and atrophy by about 5 years of age. Intravascular sickling crises may be precipitated by acute infections, hypoxia, shock, dehydration, acidosis, or exposure to cold. In addition, patients may develop aplastic crises or hyperhaemolytic crises associated with worsening of the anaemia. Acute exacerbation of anaemia with a rapid increase in the size of the spleen occurs in sequestration crises, and requires an urgent blood

transfusion. Patients with sickle-cell disease are also particularly prone to pneumococcal and *H. influenzae* infections, and to salmonella osteomyelitis, which simulate infarction of the bone.

In the steady state the anaemia may be moderate or severe (Hb 5–9 g/dl), but tends to be relatively constant for each individual. Reticulocytes are increased. Sickle-cells are usually demonstrable on the blood smear. The diagnosis is confirmed by Hb electrophoresis. Hb S constitutes over 80% of the total haemoglobin, and the remainder is Hb F. Both parents will show sickle-cell trait (Hb AS), and are usually asymptomatic, but sickling crises can be provoked by anaesthesia or anoxic stress.

Treatment: There is no curative treatment for sickle-cell disease. Treatment of sickling crises is supportive, and aimed at restoring dehydration, correcting acidosis, relieving pain, and controlling underlying infection. Blood transfusion may be required in aplastic or hyperhaemolytic crises, but is not indicated on a regular basis for anaemia. Folic acid in a dose of 5 mg/day has been shown to improve growth and the Hb level.

Thalassaemia syndromes

The thalassaemia syndromes are a heterogeneous group of hereditary disorders characterized by imbalanced globin chain synthesis and abnormalities of haem synthesis, resulting in ineffective microcytic, hypochromic erythropoeisis and, in severe cases, chronic haemolytic anaemia and progressive haemosiderosis. Defective production or translation of mRNA-controlling globin chains results in decreased synthesis of either α, β, σ or γ chains. The most common form is thalassaemia. In the most severe type, no chains are sythesized at all (β-type). Hb A is absent, and the predominant haemoglobin is Hb F.

The α thalassaemias are characterized by decreased chain synthesis. Homozygous thalassaemia is incompatible with life. The predominant haemoglobin is Hb Barts (γ 4). Heterozygotes may exhibit transient Hb Barts at birth, or Hb H (β 4) in later life.

β-thalassaemia is most prevalent in people of Mediterranean, Middle Eastern, and Asiatic origin. Clusters of patients with thalassaemia are seen in the Indian community in Natal and in the Transvaal provinces of South Africa, but it is rare in blacks. **Thalassaemia major** (Cooley's anaemia) is the term used for individuals homozygous for the β-thalassaemia gene, with severe clinical disease. **Thalassaemia minor** indicates the heterozygous state, and is usually asymptomatic.

Individuals who are doubly heterozygous for two different thalassaemia genes have clinical manifestations of variable severity, and are classified as **thalassaemia intermedia.**

Clinical and haematological features: Signs of β-thalassaemia major are usually evident within the first year of life, with most patients presenting in the first 4–6 months. The disease is characterized by pallor, mild jaundice, fever, failure to thrive, abdominal distension, and hepatosplenomegaly. It progresses to a severe transfusion-dependent haemolytic anaemia. Skull bossing and maxillary hypertrophy develop within the first 2 years, resulting in the so-called 'mongoloid facies'. Progressive haemosiderosis results in hepatic, cardiac, and endocrine dysfunction. Growth is stunted, and intercurrent infections are common. Few patients survive beyond the second decade without treatment.

Anaemia is severe (Hb 4–7 g/dl). The red cells are microcytic and hypochromic, with bizarre poikilocytes, target cells, stippled cells, normoblasts, and increased reticulocytes. Serum iron, transferrin saturation, serum ferritin, and bone marrow iron are all increased.

Hb F is markedly increased (60–100%), Hb A decreased or absent, and Hb A2 variable. Both parents will show features of thalassaemia trait *(see Table 18.7).*

Treatment: All new patients with Hb greater than 7 g/dl should be observed to make sure that they do not have thalassaemia intermedia. If the child is asymptomatic and growing well, regular blood transfusions should not be given. Severe forms of thalassaemia require regular transfusions designed to maintain the Hb at 11–14 g/dl. On this regimen, skull bossing, skeletal deformities, and growth retardation are minimized. Patients feel and look well, and can participate in normal activities. Iron-chelating agents such as desferrioxamine, given by continuous overnight subcutaneous infusion, promote urinary iron excretion and delay the progression of haemosiderosis. Splenectomy may be required in patients with

gross splenomegaly and increasing transfusion requirements.

Prevention: Screening for thalassaemia trait should be encouraged in high-risk population groups. Appropriate premarital counselling of affected couples is recommended, and consanguineous marriages should be discouraged. Prenatal diagnosis can be made either from direct fetal blood sampling or from skin fibroblasts obtained by amniocentesis.

β-thalassaemia minor (trait) is associated with mild anaemia, and rarely causes clinical symptoms. It is frequently misdiagnosed as iron deficiency. In communities where both conditions are common, it is important to be able to distinguish between the two *(see Table 18.7).*

Table 18.7 Features of thalassaemia trait and iron deficiency anaemia

	β-Thalassaemia minor	Iron deficiency
Anaemia	Mild or absent	Mild to severe
Hb g/dl	Rarely < 10 g	Frequently < 10 g
MCV/RBC ratio	< 11	> 12
RDW	Normal	Increased
Serum iron	Normal	Decreased
Serum ferritin	Normal	Decreased
FEP*	Normal	Increased
HB A2	Increased	Decreased
Hb F	Usually increased	Normal

* FEP – Free erythrocyte protoporphyrin

Iron therapy is ineffective in thalassaemia ◀ minor, and is contraindicated.

If both parents have thalassaemia minor there is a 25% chance of transmitting thalassaemia major and a 50% chance of thalassaemia minor in any children *(see Chapter 3, Genetics and Congenital Disorders).*

Acquired haemolytic anaemias

Infections

In developing countries, where severe bacterial and parasitic infections are common, acquired haemolytic anaemia may complicate septicaemia due to *E. coli*, *H. influenzae*, staphylococci, or streptococci, particularly in infants and young children. Haemolysis is a regular feature of malarial infection, and may be the presenting feature. It is important to remember that infections or drug therapy may also precipitate or exaggerate haemolysis in children with hereditary haemolytic anaemia, such as G6PD deficiency. Therapy consists of treatment of the child for the underlying disease, and supportive transfusion of packed red cells as necessary .

Autoimmune haemolytic anaemia

This is uncommon in children, but may occur as a very acute self-limiting episode in association with viral or mycoplasma infections. Steroid therapy is the treatment of choice. Chronic autoimmune haemolytic anaemia is usually a manifestation of underlying lymphoma, generalized autoimmune disease, or an immune deficiency disorder.

Leucocyte disorders

Quantitative or qualitative changes in the white blood cells accompany a wide variety of childhood illnesses. The significance must be interpreted in relationship to the normal variations in white cells which occur during growth and development (see Table 18.8).

Neutrophil leucocytosis is a physiological finding at birth, and persists for 24 – 72 hours. Thereafter there is a progressive decrease in total white cell count and neutrophils. Lymphocytes are the predominant cells from 1 month to 3 years of age. By 4 years of age, equal proportions of granulocytes and lymphocytes are present, and thereafter granulocytes predominate.

The total granulocyte mass is distributed between:
  i. the bone marrow reserve pool
  ii. the marginating granulocyte pool lining blood vessel walls
  iii. the circulating granulocytes, and
  iv. tissue granulocytes.

Changes in the peripheral white cell count may therefore result from an absolute increase or decrease in bone marrow production, or from shifts in a redistribution of cells between the four sites mentioned above.

Table 18.8 Normal white blood cell counts in infancy and childhood

	WBCx10^9/l Birth weight		N%	L%
	> 2.5 kg	< 2.5 kg		
Cord blood	16.0 *	9.3	70	30
1 day (capillary)	20.5	14.9	75	25
1 week	15.6		60	40
1 month	10.6		40	60
1 year	10.0		40	60
2–5 years	5.0–15.0**		50	50
6–14 years	5.0–10.0**		65	35

* Mean value   ** Range   N = neutrophils   L = lymphocytes

Leucocytosis

Infection is the most common cause of an increased white blood cell count (WBC) in children. The predominant cell-type frequently indicates the type of infection. Neutrophils predominate in bacterial infections, lymphocytes in viral infections and whooping cough, monocytes in tuberculosis, and eosinophils in parasitic and allergic disorders.

Other causes of leucocytosis are summarized in Table 18.9.

Leukaemoid and leuco-erythroblastic reactions are relatively common in Third World countries where severe and recurrent infections are prevalent in children. Myeloid leukaemoid reactions (WBC > 50.0 x 10^9/1 and/or > 5% immature cells in the peripheral blood) are most often associated with overwhelming bacterial infections (E. coli, staphylococcus, shigella) and congenital syphilis; less commonly with tuberculosis, haemolytic anaemias, and neoplastic disorders. Lymphocytic leukaemoid reactions are usually due to whooping cough. Leukaemia and neoplastic disorders are discussed in Chapter 19, Common Neoplastic Disorders.

Leucopenia

A reduction in total WBC usually reflects neutropenia and occurs in typhoid fever, brucellosis, and severe or prolonged bacterial infections which deplete both peripheral granulocytes and the marrow storage pool. These patients are usually febrile, sick, and toxic. Leucopenia in the newborn

(WBC $< 5.0 \times 10^9$/l) is often a manifestation of septicaemia. Immune neutropenia, due to anti-bodies derived from the mother, is a cause of transient neutropenia in the newborn period, caus-ing minimal systemic upset. Acquired bone marrow aplasia due to drug therapy, either alone or in conjunction with infection, may cause severe neutropenia. Hereditary aplasia and neutropenia are rare conditions, characterized by severe, recur-rent bacterial infections. Copper deficiency is often an unrecognized but correctable cause of neutropenia in malnourished, infected infants and those receiving hyperalimentation. Approxi-mately 20% of blacks exhibit leucopenia (WBC $< 4.0 \times 10^9$/1) due to neutropenia, which appears to be genetic in origin and is not associated with an increased susceptibility to infection.

Functional disorders of neutrophils

The ability of neutrophils to eradicate infection by destruction of bacteria involves four major func-tions: chemotaxis, opsonization, phagocytosis, and bacterial killing. Hereditary or acquired de-fects of any of these functions result in increased susceptibility to bacterial and/or fungal infections.

Treatment

The management of the child with leucocytosis is essentially that of addressing the underlying dis-ease. Neutropenia and functional neutrophil disor-ders call for eradication of bacterial infections by appropriate antibiotic therapy. Granulocyte trans-fusions may be indicated in overwhelming infec-tions. Children with hereditary neutropenic

Table 18.9 Causes of leucocytosis

	Neutrophils	Monocytes	Lymphocytes	Eosinophils
Physiological	Newborns Stress, anxiety Exercise	Recovery phase of acute infections	Early childhood (1 mth–4 yrs)	Recovery from shock/infection
Infections	Bacterial Fungal Syphilitic Endotoxin	Tuberculosis SBE Congenital syphilis	Viral: Infectious mononucleosis, cytomegalovirus Whooping cough Acute infectious lymphocytosis	Parasitic: Ascariasis Strongyloidiasis Ankylostomiasis Toxocariasis Trichinosis
Drugs	Steroids Epinephrine	—	—	Penicillin and others (hypersensitivity reaction)
Haematological/ neoplastic	Haemorrhage Haemolytic anaemias Transfusion reactions Metastatic tumours Myeloblastic leukaemias (immature cells)	Hodgkin's lymphoma Histiocytosis Monoblastic leukaemia Neutropenic states	Lymphoblastic leukaemia Lymphomas Aplastic anaemia Neutropenias	Histiocytosis Hodgkin's lymphoma Metastatic tumours
Miscellaneous	Connective tissue disease Diabetic acidosis Chronic inflammatory disorders Post-splenectomy	Connective tissue disease Sprue Regional ileitis	Thyrotoxicosis	Allergic disorders Pulmonary eosinophilia Idiopathic hyper- eosinophilic syndrome

disorders, or those on long-term cancer chemotherapy should be protected from exposure to infections. Oral hygiene and the use of oral antiseptic and antifungal agents are particularly important. Oral antibiotics such as neomycin, which cannot be absorbed, may be indicated. Biological substances such as erythropoietin, granulocyte monocytic colony stimulating factor (GMCSF), and interleukin III, which influence growth and function of haematopoeitic cells, are being used in clinical practice for cytopenias, but the cost is exorbitant.

Bleeding disorders

These disorders often present as emergencies. Prompt diagnosis and treatment can modify a life-threatening haemorrhage to a moderate one. The problem is characterized by persistent or excessive bleeding following minor trauma, dental extractions, or surgical operations; or by spontaneous bleeding into the skin or joints.

The basic mechanism of haemostasis depends on three major components:

◆ the integrity of the vessel wall resulting in vasoconstriction

◆ the platelets forming the primary haemostatic plug, and

◆ the coagulation factors which form the fibrin clot.

The abnormality may be quantitative or qualitative, and the cause can be inherited or acquired. The diagnosis is based on the history, clinical findings, and four basic laboratory tests.

History

A recent history of trauma and the severity of the injury should be elicited. One needs to enquire about symptoms of infections, drug ingestion (such as aspirin), and possible inadequate intake of vitamins C and K. The site of the bleeding must be established, viz., joints, muscles, mucous membrane, and/or skin.

When taking the history, age of onset and details of any prolonged bleeding following minor trauma or surgery are important. Conversely, a negative response excludes an abnormality unless the missing factor(s) had been inadvertently replaced. Recurrent bleeding from a single orifice such as the nose or rectum may be due to a bleeding disorder, but a local cause should always be excluded.

A recent past history of a viral infection is important for the diagnosis of idiopathic thrombocytopenic purpura (ITP). A family history of abnormal bleeding suggests an inherited cause. If only male siblings and maternal uncles are involved, haemophilia A or B should be suspected. A negative history. however, does not rule out haemophilia, as 30% of cases are due to spontaneous mutation.

Clinical signs

On examination, every attempt should be made to make a clinical diagnosis *(see Table 18.10)*. Anaemia or signs of shock may be present with severe bleeding. An acquired cause is likely if the child looks ill, whereas a child with an inherited cause usually looks well. Other signs suggestive of an acquired disorder are fever, jaundice, bone tenderness, lymphadenopathy, hepatosplenomegaly, and arthritis.

The type and site of bleeding and the sex of the patient may throw further light on the possible cause.

Purpura means bleeding into the skin ('dry purpura') or mucous membranes ('wet purpura'). It may be superficial, as in platelet or small vessel defects, or deep, as in coagulation defects. Petechiae, or pinhead-sized purpuric lesions which tend to occur over pressure sites, are highly suggestive of the former, and are rare in coagulation disorders. Ecchymotic lesions alone suggest a coagulation disorder. Coexisting petechiae and ecchymoses occur in severe platelet deficiency. Palpable purpura is characteristic of hypersensitivity vasculitis, e.g., Schönlein-Henoch purpura.

Multiple bleeding sites are common in acquired causes, as in disseminated intravascular coagulation (DIC). Bleeding into joints and/or muscles is the hallmark of haemophilia. Gastrointestinal bleeding occurs frequently in vitamin K deficiency, severe liver disease, and platelet abnormalities.

If the patient is male, haemophilia is likely.

Haemophilia must always be considered as a possible cause in a boy with a bleeding disorder.

The four basic screening tests outlined in *Table 18.11* are needed to localize the defect in the

Table 18.10   The clinical diagnostic approach to bleeding disorders

Physical findings	Level of disorder	Disease
Petechiae, superficial ecchymoses, mucous membrane bleeding	Platelets	Platelets: – quantitative defect, e.g., ITP – qualitative defect e.g., drugs
	Blood vessels	Scurvy, vasculitis, etc.
Palpable purpura	Blood vessels	Hypersensitivity, vasculitis, Schönlein-Henoch purpura
Haemarthrosis deep ecchymosis + mucous membrane bleeding	Coagulation factors (VIII, IX)	Haemophilia A & B, von Willebrand's disease
Other signs, e.g., fever, jaundice, hepatosplenomegaly, etc.	Combination of above	Leukaemia, liver disease, portal hypertension, DIC, SLE, etc.

Table 18.11   Four basic screening tests

Test	Evaluates
Platelet count (part of FBC)	Platelet numbers and size
Bleeding time	Quantative and qualitative platelet defect Vessel wall
Prothrombin time (PT)	Coagulation factors— extrinsic pathway— factors I, II, V, VII, X
Partial thromboplastin time (PTT)	Intrinsic pathway: factors I, II, V, VIII, IX, X, XI, XII

haemostatic mechanism. As a guide, if a single coagulation test is abnormal, an inherited cause is most likely, e.g., prolonged PTT in haemophilia. Conversely, multiple abnormal tests suggest an acquired cause.

The full blood count and smear will detect the severity of the anaemia, thrombocytopenia, and red cell and leucocyte abnormalities, e.g., leukaemia. Megathrombocytes in the peripheral smear are indicative of increased platelet production due to destruction, consumption, or sequestration, as in idiopathic thrombocytopenic purpura (ITP), DIC, or hypersplenism. Bone marrow aspiration is necessary if thrombocytopenia, pancytopenia, macrocytosis, or blasts are present, in order to elucidate the cause or confirm diagnosis.

Determination of the bleeding time is contra-indicated in the presence of severe thrombo-cytopenia.

In the absence of suitable laboratory facilities, a provisional diagnosis can be based on the bleeding time, Hess test, and clotting time.

Blood vessel disorders

These are discussed in detail in other chapters: Schönlein-Henoch purpura and SLE in *Chapter 23, Juvenile Chronic Arthritis and Vasculitides*; infections in *Chapter 8*; and scurvy in *Chapter 7, Nutritional Disorders*.

A diagnosis of a vascular defect is suspected when bleeding is confined to the skin (palpable purpura) and mucous membranes and the basic laboratory tests are normal. The bleeding time may be prolonged, and the Hess test is usually positive. In Durban the most common forms are those due to infection and drugs causing a vasculitis. Schönlein-Henoch purpura is uncommon in black children. Purpura fulminans is seen occasionally, with severe extensive vasculitis usually involving the skin of the buttocks and lower extremities. It may follow measles, other viral infections, or bacterial infections, but the cause is unknown. It is often fatal, and probably represents a severe immunological reaction involving the vessel walls.

Quantitative platelet disorders — thrombocytopenia

Thrombocytopenia is defined as a platelet count below $100 \times 10^9/l$. This may be the result of diminished bone marrow production, excessive destruction or consumption, excessive pooling (as in an enlarged spleen), or ineffective thrombopoiesis (as in folate and vitamin B_{12} deficiency). Bleeding occurs if the platelet count falls below $50 \times 10^9/l$. Bone marrow aspiration is usually performed to establish whether or not the megakaryocytes are decreased, normal, or increased, and to exclude abnormalities of the red and white cell series.

The cause of defective production of megakaryocytes is occasionally congenital, as in Fanconi's anaemia and congenital megakaryocytic aplasia. More commonly it is acquired due to marrow damage by infections, drugs, chemicals, or irradiation. It may also be due to marrow infiltration, as in leukaemia or neuroblastoma.

The most common cause of thrombocytopenia is probably infection resulting in marrow damage, immunological destruction, or consumption (DIC). It is postulated, however, that bacteria and their endotoxic products may cause direct injury to the platelets, or alter the vascular endothelium, resulting in adhesion of platelets.

Drugs may also induce immune thrombocytopenia, with recovery on withdrawal of the offending drug. Falciparum malaria is associated with IgG and IgM platelet antibodies and thrombocytopenia in the acute phase. The platelet count recovers when an appropriate therapy is followed.

A rare immunological process is involved when maternal isoimmune antibodies are formed in response to fetal platelet antigens, as in blood group incompatibilities. On the other hand, autoimmune antibodies may be transferred across the placenta from a mother with idiopathic thrombocytopenic purpura or systemic lupus erythematosus (SLE). Intrauterine infections are a common cause of neonatal thrombocytopenia, so the mother's FBC, platelet count, and infection screen are called for.

Idiopathic thrombocytopenic purpura (ITP)

ITP is the commonest cause of thrombocytopenia in children aged between 2 and 6 years in western countries, but appears less common in the South African black population. This may either be genetic or due to under-diagnosis. A history of a viral infection in the preceding 3 weeks is present in the majority of children. The following diagnostic criteria must be met:

- presence of spontaneous purpura
- a platelet count of less than $100 \times 10^9/l$
- normal white and red cells
- absence of pathological cells in peripheral blood or marrow
- normal clotting and prothrombin times
- no history of drug ingestion or disease which may produce thrombocytopenia, and
- no enlargement of the spleen or lymph nodes.

ITP can be acute or chronic: in both instances it is on an immunological basis. In childhood the acute self-limiting disease usually occurs following viral infections. In this condition platelets are destroyed as 'innocent bystanders' in an interaction of antigen–antibody complexes related to the infective agent. There is an inverse relation between the decline in level of platelet-associated IgG antibodies and the recovery in the platelet count. In chronic ITP, however, platelet antibodies are formed, resulting in an insidious onset of purpura and a protracted course. An underlying cause, such as SLE, should always be excluded.

Clinical picture

There is an acute onset of spontaneous bruising, petechial mucous membrane bleeding from the gums and nose, and sometimes bleeding in the urinary or gastrointestinal tract. Pressure areas and the palate should be inspected for petechiae. Cerebral haemorrhage occurs in less than 1% of children. Blood loss is seldom severe enough to warrant a blood transfusion. The child is apyrexial and otherwise well. Petechiae and ecchymoses are easily missed in dark-skinned patients. Black patients may also present with anaemia or shock, due to delay in presentation.

Laboratory investigations

The platelet count is normally below $50 \times 10^9/l$, with megathrombocytes in the peripheral blood. The bone marrow aspirate demonstrates normal or increased numbers of active megakaryocytes, with decreased platelet budding and normal white cell and red cell precursors. Platelet antibody determinations are of no use in patient management. Children over 10 years, especially girls, should be investigated for autoimmune disorders such as SLE. HIV infection may be associated with immune thrombocytopenia, and should be excluded.

Course and treatment

Eighty per cent of children recover within a month without specific therapy. Patients should be observed, preferably in hospital, until spontaneous or treatment-induced recovery occurs. Treatment is indicated only if significant mucous membrane haemorrhage is present. Epistaxis can be controlled effectively with a nasal plug. Prednisolone 2 mg/kg/day is given for 14 days. Intravenous high dose immunoglobulin will effect a transient rise in platelet count in the majority of patients, but general use is limited due to the high cost. A splenectomy is indicated in patients who remain both symptomatic and thrombocytopenic after a year. Cytostatics and immune-regulating drugs are not routinely indicated. Platelet transfusions are not helpful because of the extremely short platelet survival due to platelet antibodies.

Neonates of mothers with ITP have a 33% chance of transient thrombocytopenia at birth, because maternal platelet antibodies may cross the placenta.

Onyalai

This immune thrombocytopenia occurs only in certain black population groups of southern Africa, and was responsible for 1% of all admissions to the Kavango Regional Hospital in Namibia during the past decade. The disease is also common among the Ovambo people of Namibia, Simbundu people of Angola, and is known to occur in Zambia, Botswana, and Zimbabwe. The clinical hallmark is the sudden appearance of haemorrhagic bullae on the buccal mucosa and skin of a previously healthy person, and severe loss of blood. The mortality from haemorrhagic shock

and/or cerebral haemorrhage may reach 10% if active support with blood and intravenous fluid is not provided. Corticosteroids are not effective. Intravenous vincristine sulphate, high dose immunoglobulin, and a splenectomy may cause a rise in the platelet count.

Hypersplenism

This is the term used for a lowered platelet red cell and white cell count, single or in any combination, which results from pooling or increased destruction of blood cells in an enlarged spleen. Production of the various elements by the bone marrow is normal or increased, and the peripheral cell count reverts to normal after a splenectomy.

Qualitative platelet disorders

These disorders may be congenital or acquired. The former variety is very rare (e.g., Glanzmann's thrombasthenia, storage pool disease). Acquired platelet function defects occur following drug ingestion (e.g., aspirin), and in patients with uraemia. Characteristically the bleeding time is prolonged but the platelet count, PT, and PTT are normal. Platelet function tests are abnormal.

Coagulation disorders

Defective coagulation occurs as a result of inherited clotting defects, such as haemophilia, or due to an acquired problem, as in DIC or vitamin K deficiency.

Haemophilia

Haemophilia is said to be uncommon in blacks, but there is increasing evidence to the contrary. There are more than 200 known cases in the province of Natal. Haemophilia A is caused by the production of an abnormal factor VIII with reduced clotting activity. Haemophilia B (Christmas disease) is due to deficiency of factor IX. The former is four to five times more frequent, and both have sex-linked recessive inheritance. Haemophilia C (factor XI deficiency) is an autosomal-recessive disease with a high frequency in the Jewish population. Characteristically the PTT is prolonged. About 30% of cases of haemophilia A occur sporadically, either because the disease was previously unrecognized in the family or because of a mutation. Carrier females can often be detected, as they may possess an excess of immuno-reactive factor VIII.

Severity is inversely proportional to factor levels in haemophilia A and B: mild bleeding occurs when levels are between 30 and 5%; moderate bleeding with levels of 5–1%; and severe symptoms or spontaneous bleeds when the level is less than 1%.

Haemorrhage may develop during the neonatal period, but nearly always during the first few years of life, when the child begins to crawl and walk. Whilst bleeding can occur from any site, the hallmarks of haemophilia are haemarthrosis and intramuscular haematoma. During the first year of life, bleeding occurs mainly into muscles and subcutaneous tissue. The most serious bleeding is intracranial, which may be spontaneous and lethal. Bleeding into the forearm may cause neurovascular occlusion and result in Volkmann's ischaemic contracture. Paralytic ileus may result from retroperitoneal bleeding; compression of the femoral nerve may occur if blood tracks down behind the inguinal ligament. Respiratory obstruction and dysphagia are the result of bleeding into the posterior pharyngeal wall. Haematuria can be a problem.

Haemophilia B has similar clinical problems; severity corresponds to factor IX levels. Haemophilia C is a milder disease.

Management

The parents and the child must be fully informed about the disease. Genetic counselling is clearly very important after investigation of family members. The child should wear an identity disc which displays the diagnosis of the disease.

The following must be strictly avoided before factor replacement: jugular or femoral vein puncture, lumbar puncture, intramuscular injections, and any form of surgery. Aspirin should never be given. Local pressure must be applied whenever feasible.

Inhibitors to factor VIII should be excluded before surgery or any invasive procedure. A multidisciplinary approach is desirable, involving a paediatrician, haematologist, physiotherapist, orthopaedic surgeon, and psychologist.

Replacement therapy aims at raising the factor VIII level in haemophilia A to between 30 and 60% of normal. As the half life of factor VIII is

8–12 hours, treatment should be repeated at 12-hourly intervals. Fresh frozen plasma, 15–20 ml/kg given every 12 hours, raises the level to about 30%. Factor VIII concentrates, 15–40 units/kg, raise the level to 30–100% respectively. Treatment usually has to be continued for 3 days or more, but can be discontinued if there is no further evidence of haemorrhage or continuing pain.

Acute knee arthrosis requires additional attention. The patient should be admitted to hospital and weight-bearing avoided. A plaster of Paris back-slab must be applied to immobilize the joint in slight flexion. Aspiration is indicated if the joint is tense and very painful. The procedure must be performed with strict aseptic precautions, and cryoprecipitate must be administered immediately prior to the aspiration. A short course of steroids (prednisone 2 mg/kg/day for 3 days) accelerates the reduction of pain and swelling.

Surgical procedures and dental extractions should be preceded by administration of 20–40 factor units/kg. Antifibrinolytic agents (e.g., epsilon-amino-caproic acid) should be given before and after dental extraction. The presence of inhibitors must always be excluded preoperatively, and replacement therapy must continue for 5 days postoperatively .

As a therapeutic or prophylactic measure, factor VIII can be given by the family at home, or in a clinic, on a regular basis. Fresh frozen plasma, 15–20 ml/kg is used for haemophilia B and C. Prothrombin complex concentrates 20–40 units/kg can be used for haemophilia B.

Mild cases of haemophilia and von Willebrand's disease can be treated prophylactically with desmopressin (DDAVP®), which raises the level of factor VIII.

Von Willebrand's disease

This is an autosomal-dominant disorder in which there is a combined quantitative factor VIII deficiency and a qualitative defect of platelets (decreased adhesiveness due to lack of von Willebrand factor). The bleeding time is therefore increased and the PTT is prolonged. The most frequent presentation is mucosal bleeding and epistaxis. Treatment is similar to that for haemophilia A.

Vitamin K deficiency

This vitamin is required by the liver for synthesis of factors II, VII, IX and X. The natural K vitamins are synthesized by intestinal flora. Being fat-soluble, they require bile for absorption, and are not stored in the body. In vitamin K deficiency the liver synthesizes abnormal proteins known as PIVKAs, which are inactive and may cause inhibition of coagulation. The PT and PTT are characteristically prolonged.

Haemorrhagic disease of the newborn *(see Chapter 5, Newborns)* is due to functional immaturity of the liver and poor stores of vitamin K, because the infant's gut flora have not been established and breast milk contains very little vitamin K. Bleeding occurs on the second or third day of life, or later in breast-fed babies, due to a deficiency of factors II, VII, IX and X. Melaena, haematemesis, and umbilical cord bleeding may occur. This can be prevented by giving 1 mg of vitamin K IM or IV to the baby at birth, or to the mother before delivery. In overt bleeding, 1–5 mg of vitamin K stops the blood loss within 2–4 hours. Should bleeding continue, 10–15 ml/kg of fresh plasma and/or blood should be given, and DIC must be excluded.

Other causes of vitamin K deficiency are obstructive jaundice, malabsorption syndromes, prolonged use of broad spectrum antibiotics, oral anticoagulants, and a diet deficient in vitamin K.

Liver disease

All coagulation factors except factor VIII are synthesized in the liver; blood levels of factor VIII are therefore normal or even raised in liver failure. Coagulation factor deficiencies may occur in both acute or chronic liver disease.

The liver also degrades activated clotting factors and fibrinolytic enzymes. Failure of this procedure may trigger DIC and cause excessive fibrinolysis. The levels of vitamin K-dependent factors are the first to fall, followed by factor V and fibrinogen. The PT, PTT, and possibly thrombin time are prolonged. Thrombocytopenia may also occur secondary to cirrhosis and portal hypertension. Bleeding may also be due to a local cause, e.g., varices in portal hypertension.

Treatment is with fresh frozen plasma. Prothrombin complex should be avoided.

Disseminated intravascular coagulation (DIC)

This is the most common acquired cause of severe life-threatening bleeding. It complicates a number of conditions, such as septicaemia, viraemia, shock, hypoxia, burns, malignancy (e.g., promyelocytic leukaemia), and postoperative states. The newborn is particularly susceptible *(see Chapter 5, Newborns)*.

Episodes of DIC result from intravascular activation of the coagulation system, with consequent widespread deposition of platelets and altered fibrinogen in the microcirculation. If it is severe, this results in generalized haemorrhage and/or end-organ failure due to blockage of the microvessels by thrombi. The kidneys are particularly susceptible to this ischaemic damage, as are the brain, heart, and adrenals, resulting in renal failure and microangiopathic haemolytic anaemia.

All four basic screening tests may be abnormal, due to consumption of clotting factors and platelets, which are the first to fall. In addition, the thrombin time is prolonged, the fibrinogen is low, and there are increased fibrin degradation products (FDPs). As this is a dynamic process of consumption and regeneration, these parameters may not always be abnormal. Factor assays are not always necessary, but in contrast to liver disease, factor VIII is low.

In severe DIC the FDPs are not elevated, due to inhibition of the fibrinolytic response. This indicates a poor outcome, with irreversible organ failure.

Management

The management is controversial, but the first step is to treat for the underlying cause. If the bleeding is severe, platelet concentrates, fresh frozen plasma, and cryoprecipitate should be given. Heparin may be used if replacement therapy has failed to alleviate severe bleeding and purpura fulminans, and in acute promyelocytic leukaemia to prevent DIC.

J.A. Naidoo
P. Hesseling

19

Common neoplastic disorders

Introduction

Malignant disease is infrequent in childhood, but despite this, in western countries it is the second most frequent cause of death, after trauma. In Third World countries on the other hand, trauma and malignancy rank fourth or fifth. In South Africa there is an affluent society living alongside a Third World society, which provides an opportunity to compare these groups and identify differences.

Tables 19.1 and *19.2* illustrate some of these differences, e.g., acute myeloid leukaemia occurs in black children more frequently than in Caucasians, and nephroblastoma is more common in black children than neuroblastoma.

The aetiology of malignancy in childhood is becoming clearer. Genetic factors, chromosomal abnormalities, mutations in tumour suppressor genes, immunological deficiency, virus infections (e.g., EB virus in Burkitt's lymphoma), and environmental factors have been implicated.

The organs which are involved in neoplastic disorders in children differ from those in adults. The bronchus, gastrointestinal tract, and breast are predominantly involved in adults, whereas nephroblastoma, neuroblastoma, and retinoblastoma are exclusive to childhood. Acute leukaemia is the most common malignancy in children, with brain tumours coming second.

Tremendous advances have been made in management of malignancies, and with multimodal therapy complete cure is becoming increasingly feasible in developed countries. New diagnostic aids such as magnetic resonance imaging and electron microscopy of biopsy material have improved diagnostic accuracy considerably. However, as the costs involved are very high, these benefits have not been realized in developing countries. Poor socio-economic conditions and inadequate infrastructure result in delay in diagnosis and initiation of therapy, inadequate therapy, and poor compliance and follow-up, all of which have an adverse effect on the prognosis. The data in *Table 19.3* illustrate how these factors affect black children and those of mixed racial origin from disadvantaged communities. The variation in survival due to late presentation is particularly notable in neuroblastoma, where delay in diagnosis has a marked effect on the prognosis. Ethnic differences probably determine the disease behaviour, and hence the outcome, of acute lymphoblastic leukaemia. Successful modern therapy may carry a risk of permanent damage to various organs as well as of a second cancer years later.

All children with cancer should be referred to a paediatric oncology unit for assessment.

Table 19.1 Haemotological malignancies, Durban, 1988–90*

	African	Indian	White	Mixed	Total
Acute lymphoblastic leukaemia	38	24	15	–	77
Acute myeloid leukaemia	25	5	–	1	31
Chronic myeloid leukaemia	5	–	–	–	5
Hodgkin's disease	12	1	–	1	14
Non-Hodgkin's lymphoma	17	4	2	–	23
Burkitt's lymphoma	10	–	–	1	11
Langerhans cell histiocytosis	2	–	–	–	2
Miscellaneous	4	1	–	–	5

* Includes patients < 12 years

Table 19.2 Solid tumours in children, Durban, 1988–90*

	83	4	1	33
Brain tumours	47	2	–	19
Nephroblastoma	18	–	1	3
Neuroblastoma	33	1	–	3
Retinoblastoma	17	–	–	17
Rhabdomyosarcoma	3	2	1	5
Osteosarcoma	1	2	–	14
Ewing sarcoma	14	1	1	
Germ cell tumours	4	2	**Total**	
Liver tumours	11	**White**	94	
Miscellaneous	**Indian**	3	54	
African	8	3	21	

* < 12 years of age

Table 19.3 Percentage survival at Tygerberg Hospital (Cape Town) 1974–88

Ethnic group	Acute lymphoblastic leukaemia	Wilms' tumour	Hodgkin's disease	Neuro-blastoma
Black	21	77	71	25
White	60	78	75	85
Mixed	25	68	85	29

▶ Personnel at primary and secondary level health care facilities should be acutely aware of the urgency of referring these patients for further management. For example, a child with an abdominal mass is very likely to have a malignant tumuor and should be referred without delay.

Leukaemia

The acute leukaemias are characterized by uncontrolled proliferation or defective maturation of white blood cells, and account for 30–35% of neoplastic disorders in children. The aetiology is unknown. Most childhood leukaemias are acute, and 85–90% are lymphocytic. Acute non-lymphocytic leukaemias (myelocytic, promyelocytic, myelomonocytic, monocytic, etc.) account for 10–15% of cases, except among black children in central, eastern, and southern Africa and among children in Turkey, where non-lymphocytic leukaemias may account for up to 50% of cases. Chronic myelocytic leukaemia is rare in children, and occurs in two forms: a chronic adult variety, and a more fulminant juvenile form. Chronic lymphocytic leukaemia does not occur in children.

Clinical features

Acute lymphocytic leukaemia (ALL) has a peak age incidence at 3–4 years, but may occur at any age. Acute non-lymphocytic leukaemia (ANLL) has no comparable age peak. The incidence is slightly higher in males than females for both ALL and ANLL. Common presenting features include malaise, pallor, lymphadenopathy, petechiae, bruising, hepatosplenomegaly, and signs of infection.

Symptoms and signs are due to:

1 Bone marrow replacement resulting in:
◆ anaemia, causing pallor, fatigue, and oedema
◆ thrombocytopenia, causing a bleeding tendency, manifesting as purpura, epistaxis, bleeding gums, fundal haemorrhages
◆ neutrophilia (abnormal cells) or neutropenia, predisposing to infection.

2 Invasion of organs resulting in enlargement and dysfunction:
◆ hepatosplenomegaly
◆ lymphadenopathy (in ALL)
◆ gum hypertrophy (mainly in monocytic leukaemia)
◆ bone and joint pain (can mimic rheumatic fever or osteitis)
◆ neurological signs, including fundal changes, e.g., haemorrhages, leukaemic deposits, papilloedema
◆ ulceration of gums, tonsils, palate.

3 Immunological malfunction: delayed hypersensitivity.

The early signs may be indistinguishable from
common viral infections. Bone and joint pains are
often a feature of ALL and may be mistaken for
rheumatic fever. Pain in the bones may be mistaken for 'growing pains'. Gingival hypertrophy
and ulcerative oropharyngeal lesions occur more
commonly in ANLL. Orbital chloromata may be
a feature of ANLL in black children, but are rarely
seen in whites. Infection at presentation is more
common in ANLL than ALL.

In developing countries, where children may
present late with advanced disease, the clinical
picture of fever, adenopathy, hepatosplenomegaly, and wasting, in conjunction with pulmonary or abdominal symptoms, may mimic
disseminated tuberculosis, or chronic bacterial or
parasitic infections. Patients with lytic bone lesions and periosteal reactions, which occur chiefly
in ALL, may be misdiagnosed as having osteomyelitis or neuroblastoma.

Haematological features

Anaemia (haemoglobin < 10 g/dl) is common, and
usually normocytic, normochromic in type. The
white blood cell count can be low (< $5.0 \times 10^9/1$),
normal, or increased ($20-100 \times 10^9/1$).

Leukaemic blast cells are usually present in the
peripheral blood, particularly in patients with
increased total white blood counts. Severe thrombocytopenia (platelet count < $50 \times 10^9/1$) is
common.

Bone marrow examination confirms the diagnosis, and is essential for accurate classification of the leukaemia. Identification of the
morphologic, cytochemical, immunological (surface marker), and cytogenetic characteristics of
the blast cells is necessary for correct classification into subtypes of ALL and ANLL (*see Tables
19.4 and 19.5*). Improved techniques have demonstrated that both ALL and ANLL are heterogeneous. Furthermore, there is an increasing number
of mixed lineage and even biclonal leukaemias
being described. These findings have important
therapeutic and prognostic implications, and
account for the varied response to therapy.

Most childhood ALLs are PAS-positive and
exhibit the C ALL antigen, i.e., 'common' ALL.

A minority show T- or B-cell characteristics.
The ANLLs are PAS-negative, Sudan black-
and/or peroxidase-positive. Esterase stains help to
differentiate myelocytic from monocytic leukaemias. Chromosomal translocations (8:21,15:17),
deletions (monosomy 7), and trisomies 7, 8, or 9
occur in approximately 50% of ANLL cases. ALL

Table 19.4 French–American–British (FAB) classification of acute leukaemia

1. Acute nonlymphocytic leukaemia
M1 Acute myeloblastic without maturation
M2 Acute myeloblastic with maturation
M3 Acute promyelocytic
M4 Acute myelomonocytic
M5 Acute monocytic
M6 Erythroleukaemic
M7 Acute megakaryoblastic

2. Acute lymphoblastic leukaemia
L1 Paediatric type
L2 Adult type
L3 Burkitt type

Table 19.5 Immunological classification of childhood acute lymphoblastic leukaemia (ALL)

ALL variant	Tdt	T	CALLA	Sig	Incidence %
Common	+	-	+	-	70
T cell	+	+	-	-	15
B cell	-	-	-	+	1.5
Null	+	-	-	-	10

TdT = Terminal deoxynucleotidyl transferase
T = T antigen
CALLA = common acute lymphocytic leukaemia antigen
Sig = surface immunoglobulin

B-cell leukaemia is associated with karyotype t(8:14), t(2:8) or t(8:22). The t(1:19) translocation is specific for pre B-cell ALL. The t(14:11) translocation is associated with T-cell ALL.

Other investigations

Before commencing therapy the following investigations should be done:

◆ urea and electrolyte
◆ uric acid estimation
◆ liver function tests
◆ LDH
◆ immunoglobulin levels
◆ screen for disseminated intravascular coagulopathy (essential in promyelocytic leukaemia)
◆ chest radiograph to exclude tuberculosis or mediastinal masses
◆ radiograph of long bones
◆ culture of nose and throat swabs, and blood, stool, and urine
◆ tuberculin test.

Complications

The most serious complications of leukaemia include CNS and testicular involvement, haemorrhage, infections with Gram-negative organisms (pseudomonas, klebsiella), fungi (candida), viruses (chickenpox, cytomegalovirus), and *Pneumocystis carinii*.

Complications of drug therapy include bone marrow suppression, hair loss (vincristine, alkylating agents), mouth ulcers (methotrexate), cardiomyopathy (adriamycin, duanomycin) and leukoencephalopathy (intrathecal methotrexate).

Management

Management of childhood leukaemia comprises not only medical treatment of the disease itself, but provision of constant guidance, encouragement, and support for the child and family.

Specific therapy

(see Table 19.6.)

These patients should be treated in a tertiary centre. Chemotherapy is designed to provide a combination of drugs which interfere with different phases of DNA synthesis or cell metabolism and have their greatest effect on immature or dividing cells.

Table 19.6 Chemotherapy in acute leukaemia

	ALL	ANLL
Remission induction (3 – 6 wks)	Vincristine + Prednisone + L'asparaginase or Duanomycin	Cytosine arabinoside + Thioguanine + Duanomycin
CNS prophylaxis (2–3 wks)	Intrathecal methotrexate + Cranial irradiation	Intrathecal methotrexate/ cytosine arabinoside Cranial irradiation
Maintenance	6 Mercaptopurine + Methotrexate + Periodic vincristine/ prednisone + Intrathecal methotrexate	Cytosine arabinoside + Thioguanine or BCNU/ cyclophosphamide

In ALL, induction with a combination of vincristine and prednisone will effect remission in approximately 90% of cases within 3–6 weeks. Addition of a third drug — l'asparaginase or an anthracycline (duanomycin, adriamycin) — increases both the remission rate and length of survival.

The second phase of therapy involves CNS prophylaxis, using a combination of intrathecal methotrexate and cranial irradiation. This is followed by maintenance therapy with oral 6-mercaptopurine and methotrexate, with or without periodic reinforcement with vincristine and prednisone.

After 2–3 years of sustained haematological remission without evidence of extramedullary disease, maintenance therapy is discontinued. The subsequent relapse rate is approximately 20% and usually occurs within 18 months of stopping treatment. Apart from bone marrow relapse, the common sites are the CNS and the testes.

In ANLL the most effective chemotherapeutic agents for induction of remission include duanomycin (or adriamycin), cytosine arabi-noside and 6-thioguanine. The current remission rate is between 50 and 70%. Subsequently CNS prophylaxis with intrathecal methotrexate and/or cytosine arabinoside and cranial irradiation is ad-visable for those who achieve remission. Main-tenance chemotherapy in ANLL is at present unsatisfactory, and sustained remissions are diffi-cult to achieve. Periodic courses of combination chemotherapy at 4- to 6-week intervals appear to be more effective than daily oral maintenance therapy.

Bone marrow transplantation has a place in childhood leukaemia. Promising results have been obtained in ANLL, and in patients with ALL who have relapsed on conventional chemotherapeutic regimens.

Supportive treatment

To prevent infection, isolation facilities should be provided and careful attention should be paid to washing of hands before handling a patient.

If severe neutropenia is present, prophylactic

antibiotics may be necessary. Prophylactic INH, zoster, and measles immune globulins should be given. The haemoglobin level should be kept above 10 g/dl by giving packed red cell transfusions, and platelet infusions are necessary if there is bleeding or if the platelet count is below $20 \times 10^9/l$.

Allopurinol is necessary to prevent uric acid nephropathy. Careful attention should be paid to hydration, to alkalinization of the urine by giving bicarbonate, and to monitoring of the electrolytes and uric acid levels to prevent the tumour lysis syndrome. This is a complication of hyperleuco-cytosis and/or massive organomegaly.

Family support

There is an appreciably high prevalence of marital and family discord, psychiatric and emotional problems, school difficulties and sibling rivalries in families of leukaemic children. Prolonged therapy and numerous hospital visits are a tremen-dous financial and practical burden for most fami-lies. A supportive team of medical and nursing personnel, social workers, religious and psychiat-

---

Table 19.7 Prognostic factors in acute leukaemia

Prognostic factor	ALL Good	ALL Poor	ANLL Good	ANLL Poor
Age (yrs)	3–8	< 2, > 10	5–10	< 5, > 10
Race	White	Black	White	Black
Sex	Female	Male	?	?
Clinical				
Hepatosplenomegaly	Moderate	Massive	N/A	N/A
Mediastinal mass	Absent	Present	N/A	N/A
Large node mass(es)	Absent	Present	N/A	N/A
CNS disease	Absent	Present	Absent	Present
Gingival hypertrophy	N/A	N/A	Absent	Present
DIC	Absent	Present	Absent	Present
Remission at 2 wks	Present	Absent	–	–
Laboratory findings				
WBCx 10^9/l	< 10	> 20	< 100	> 100
Hb g/dl	> 7	< 7	?	?
Platelets 10^9/l	> 100	< 50	> 100	< 50
Morphology*	L1	L2, L3	M1, M2	M3–M7
Surface markers	Common ALL	B	?	?
Chromosome abnormalities	Absent	Present	Absent	Present

* French–American–British (FAB) classification
N/A — Not applicable

---

ric advisors is therefore an essential part of total patient and family care.

Every patient should be discussed by the whole team on a weekly basis.

Prognosis

(See Table 19.7.)

The average survival in untreated patients with acute leukaemia is 8 –12 weeks. With chemotherapy, life expectancy has improved greatly. In ALL approximately 60% of children receiving combination chemotherapy will be alive and free of disease 3–5 years after diagnosis. In ANLL, the outlook is much less favourable. The median survival with most current therapeutic regimens is less than 1 year, and fewer than 20% of patients survive for 2 years or longer. However, with bone marrow transplantation the prognosis has improved.

Apart from the morphologic type of leukaemia, other factors which influence the prognosis significantly include age, sex, ethnic origin, 'tumour load', extramedullary disease, blast cell subtype, and chromosomal abnormalities. The prognosis is less favourable for children under 2 years or over 10 years, for males, blacks, patients with marked hepatosplenomegaly, WBC in excess of 20.0 x $10^9/1$, or CNS involvement. Subtypes of ALL with B-cell characteristics, or ANLL with promyelocytic, erythroleukaemic or megakaryocytic features carry a poor prognosis. In ALL a poor response to two weeks of therapy is also a bad prognostic sign. As stated above, certain chromosomal abnormalities have a predictive value.

The most important prognostic factor is the height of the white cell count at presentation.

Lymphomas

The malignant lymphomas have a wide range of cell types and histological patterns involving lympho-reticular tissue. These neoplasms may arise from the stem cell, the lymphocyte, or the histiocyte, and accurate morphological identification and classification can be difficult. Non-Hodgkin's lymphoma and Hodgkin's disease are unrelated disorders. In childhood they behave differently from the adult versions.

Non-Hodgkin's lymphoma (NHL)

This is a highly malignant disorder. It is not common in Durban, where approximately six cases are seen annually. In contrast, in Uganda and central Africa, the incidence of Burkitt's lymphoma is high. Childhood NHL differs from adult NHL in that extranodal presentation is predominant. Widespread dissemination and leukaemic transformation are common initially, making the distinction between NHL and ALL difficult. Tumour growth is rapid, hence the relapse and mortality rates are high. Follicular lymphoma — differentiated and mixed types as seen in the adult — are rare, and the main histological pattern in childhood is essentially limited to one of three diffuse types: lymphoblastic, undifferentiated, or so-called 'histiocytic' or large lymphoid cell type, with a small number being unclassifiable. Immunological markers are used for further classification .

Age and sex incidence: The disease occurs in children over the age of 2 years, with a peak incidence between 3 and 5 years, and a male predominance. There is an increased incidence in children with HIV infection.

Main clinical presentations

Abdominal swelling (40 –50%)**:** The malignant cells are B lymphoblasts. This includes Burkitt's lymphoma (the 'American type'). Leukaemic transformation and nodal involvement are uncommon. Intussusception of the small bowel occurs with an easily removable tumour, or with massive intra-abdominal disease.

Mediastinal mass/pleural effusion (35%)**:** This is T lymphoblastic in most cases. Leukaemic transformation is common, usually with a very high white cell count and CNS and/or gonadal infiltration. Bony swellings may be present. Abdominal involvement is rare. Superior vena caval obstruction may occur, and calls for urgent treatment. Refractory tonsillitis is not uncommon, and has a poor prognosis. Peripheral lymphadenopathy (usually cervical) may be present. The nodes are painless, and stony-hard, discrete and mobile.

Involving several sites (15%)**:** This may affect the lymph nodes, abdomen, and bones, with prominent swellings. Histologically this is a heterogeneous group and is termed large cell lymphoma, histiocytic or immunoblastic. B-cell markers may be present.

Staging of the disease is based on Murphy's system *(see Table 19.8)*. As this is usually a diffuse disease in childhood, clinical staging is used. More accurate information is obtained by radiological studies: chest X-ray, ultrasonography, CT scanning, IV pyelography, bone marrow aspiration, and CSF examination.

Table 19.8 Murphy modified staging system for non-Hodgkin's lymphoma

Stage I	Single nodal or extranodal site (not mediastinal or abdominal)
Stage II	One or more extranodal site plus regional nodes, or two extranodal sites on the same side of diaphragm
Stage III	Two or more sites on both sides of diaphragm, inlcuding all primary intrathoracic and extensive abdominal tumours
Stage IV	Stage I-III plus bone marrow involvement (< 25% infiltration) and/or CNS disease

Treatment

Chemotherapy, using a combination of vincristine, prednisone, cyclophosphamide, and anthracyclines, is given together with CNS prophylaxis. Radiotherapy is not used primarily, as this is never a localized disease. Surgery is limited to biopsy and to removal or debulking of abdominal nodes.

Prognosis

The prognosis varies from 20 to 70% long-term survival. The prognostic factors are similar to ALL, and include the histological type and stage of the disease.

Burkitt's lymphoma

This is an undifferentiated lymphoma of B-cell origin which has a predilection for the jaw and facial bones ('African type') and abdominal nodes and viscera ('American type'). Nodal and mediastinal involvement and leukaemic transformation is uncommon. Involvement of the CNS is a frequent complication, especially in the 'African type'. It is highly malignant, and the fastest growing of all tumours. Histologically the characteristic 'starry sky' appearance is seen. It is endemic in central Africa and Uganda, is associated with the prevalence of malaria, and is aetiologically linked to the Epstein-Barr virus. The two types have different chromosomal abnormalities. Both the 'African' and 'American' types occur sporadically in South Africa.

Treatment

The mainstay of treatment is cyclophosphamide in combination with methotrexate (parenteral and intrathecal) and vincristine. However, more aggressive treatment protocols have achieved an improved cure rate. The prevention of metabolic death by the tumour lysis syndrome, which is precipitated by treatment, has also improved survival. This requires an adequate fluid intake, and alkalinization of the urine with allapurinol.

Whilst there are reports of good prognosis for this tumour from Uganda, local experience has been to the contrary. Remission is achieved, but relapses are common.

Hodgkin's disease

This is a less malignant lymphoma. It is rare in childhood, and occurs more commonly in the second decade. However, the disease has been seen in children as young as 2 years. Approximately four cases are seen per year at King Edward VIII Hospital, Durban. Males predominate.

The **common presentation** is painless enlargement of a group of lymph nodes, usually cervical. Generalized lymphadenopathy occurs less often. The nodes are firm, rubbery, non-tender, and mobile, in contrast to tuberculosis *(see Chapter 9, Tuberculosis)*. Primary extranodal presentation is rare in childhood.

Hepatosplenomegaly and extranodal disease may occur in any organ, with or without systemic symptoms (B symptoms) such as fever, sweating, weight loss, and pruritus. Pruritus has no prognostic significance and is uncommon in childhood.

The **diagnosis** is established on excision lymph node biopsy (after excluding TB by tuberculin tests, etc.). The histology is graded according to the Rye modification of the Lukes/Butler classification, i.e.,

◆ lymphocyte predominance (LP)
◆ nodular sclerosis (NS)
◆ mixed cellularity (MC)

◆ lymphocyte depleted (LD).

In the Caucasian and Indian child, LP and NS predominate and have a better prognosis. By contrast, in 70% of black children the common histological patterns are MC and LD, which have a poorer prognosis .

Table 19.9 Ann Arbor clinical staging of Hodgkin's disease

Stage I	Involvement of a single lymph node region, or of a single extra-lymphatic organ or site	(I)
Stage II	Involvement of two or more lymph node regions on the same side of the diaphragm,	(IE)
	or localized involvement of extra-lymphatic organ or site and one or more lymph node regions on same side of the diaphragm	(IIE)
Stage III	Involvement of lymph node regions on both sides of the diaphragm	(III)
	+ involvement of the spleen	(IIIS)
	or localized extra-lymphatic organ or site	(IIIE)
Stage IV	Diffuse or disseminated involvement of one or more organs or tissues, e.g., liver, marrow, pleura, lung, bone, and skin	

N.B. If systematic symptoms absent = Stage IA, IIA, etc.
If systemic symptoms present = IB, IIB, etc.

Determining the **extent of the disease** is based on the Ann Arbor Classification of clinical staging *(see Table 19.9)*. To determine the extent and stage of the disease, detailed investigations have to be undertaken, e.g., chest X-ray, ultrasonography of abdomen, and trephine biopsy of the bone marrow. However, laparotomy and splenectomy to stage the tumours are not being done in children. Currently CT scanning is being used as an adjunct.

Chemotherapy is the mainstay of **treatment** except for children in stage I. Six cycles of mustine or chlorambucil with vincristine, prednisolone and procarbazine are used. Radiotherapy is used for stage I, and if life-threatening pressure symptoms are present.

Prognosis depends on the histology and stage of the disease, but is generally relatively good.

Malignant solid tumours

Nephroblastoma

Nephroblastoma (Wilm's tumour) is a malignant renal tumour derived from embryonic cells. It may grow rapidly in size, and commonly invades the renal vein. Minor trauma may dislodge haematogenous tumour emboli which metastasize to the lungs, liver, and bones. The tumour spreads locally into adjacent organs and along the ureter, and lymphatic spread occurs to the para-aortic nodes. There are various histological patterns which have a direct bearing on the prognosis.

Nephroblastoma is the third most common malignant solid tumour encountered in young children in Natal; at King Edward VIII Hospital (Durban) an average of 17 new patients are admitted each year. Approximately 5% of patients have bilateral tumours.

Most patients present between 2 and 4 years of age with an abdominal mass – usually a large, firm, irregular, non-tender tumour arising from the flank. Often the underprivileged child is severely malnourished, with a massive abdominal tumour. Other presenting features include abdominal pain, haematuria, hypertension (due to increased renin production), varicocele (due to left renal vein occlusion), pyrexia, and symptoms due to metastases. These may occur in lungs, liver, opposite kidney, other intra-abdominal sites, bones, and brain (depending on the histological type). Rupture of a large tumour causes acute abdominal signs due to haemoperitoneum. Certain congenital abnormalities, notably aniridia, hemihypertrophy, genito-urinary anomalies and Beckwith's syndrome, may occur in association with nephroblastoma. The differential diagnosis includes neuroblastoma, hydronephrosis, and polycystic kidneys.

Investigations

These include full blood count, urea and electrolyte estimation, and liver function tests to assess the patient's general status.

Straight X-rays of the abdomen and chest (for metastases), ultrasound, and CT scan show a solid renal tumour containing cystic areas. Hydronephrosis and multicystic renal disease can usually be excluded with certainty. The opposite kidney is assessed. Inferior vena caval involvement can also be excluded. Intravenous pyelography (done if CT scanning is not available) shows distortion of the kidney by an intrinsic tumour. Less commonly, the abnormal kidney fails to opacify, indicating invasion with obstruction of the ureter.

Staging and classification

The staging used internationally for nephroblastoma may be summarized as follows:

Stage I: Tumour limited to the kidney and completely resected

Stage II: Tumour extends beyond the kidney, but is completely resected

Stage III: Residual non-haematogenous tumour confined to the abdomen

Stage IV: Haematogenous metastasis

Stage V: Bilateral renal involvement at diagnosis.

Tumours are further classified histologically into 'favourable and 'unfavourable' groups.

Management

The child with nephroblastoma is treated with a combination of surgery, chemotherapy, and radiotherapy. Treatment is regarded as urgent because of the risk of embolization along the renal vein. When the tumour is very large, a course of chemotherapy is given to reduce the size of the tumour before operation. If there is no residual disease after resection, actinomycin-D and vincristine are administered at regular intervals for 6 months. When resection has not been complete, or if there is metastasis, adriamycin and radiotherapy are added.

Prognosis

With modern treatment regimes, the 2-year survival rate for stage I tumours is over 95%. Even in the presence of metastasis at the time of presentation (stage IV), a 2-year survival rate in excess of 40% has been reported. The prognosis is least favourable when the histology shows sarcomatous or anaplastic features.

Children under 2 years of age have a significantly better survival rate than older children .

Neuroblastoma

Neuroblastoma is a malignant tumour of the sympathetic nervous system, arising from primitive cells of the dorsal neural crest of the embryo. The tumour may originate in any part of the sympathetic nervous system, most occurring in or near the adrenal gland. Spread occurs early by local extension into neighbouring tissues along the lymphatics.

Neuroblastoma may differentiate into ganglioneuroblastoma or ganglioneuroma, which are more mature, benign tumours. This maturation may occur spontaneously or in response to treatment. Complete spontaneous remission and cure have been reliably documented.

Neuroblastoma produces catecholamines, and metabolites of adrenaline and noradrenaline, notably vinylmandelic acid and homomandelic acid, may be identified and measured in the urine.

In Europe and North America it is the most common solid malignant tumour of childhood, but in Natal the tumour is considerably less common than nephroblastoma. In Durban about six new cases are seen each year *(also see Table 19.3 for the incidence in Cape Town)*. Neuroblastoma occurs early in life, and metastasis may be present at birth. Most tumours present between 18 months and 5 years of age.

Clinical features

The clinical features depend on the site of the tumour. The usual presentation is with a large, irregular abdominal mass, which consists of the primary lesion plus locally invasive tumour and infiltrated lymph nodes. Dissemination occurs early, to the cortex of long and flat bones, regional lymph nodes, liver, bone marrow, and subcutaneous tissue. Pulmonary involvement is rare. It is not uncommon for patients to present with rapidly progressive metastases and a small primary lesion which is not detectable clinically. Such patients may have prominent swellings on the skull, proptosis with periorbital blue discoloration, disseminated skin metastases, painful skeletal lesions, or gross and irregular hepatomegaly. Fever, anaemia, and bone pain are common. In developing countries these children are often emaciated and ill with advanced disease. If the abdominal mass is missed, a mistaken diagnosis of leukaemia may be made. Occasionally there is chronic diarrhoea, opsimyoclonus, and ataxia.

Diagnosis

Plain abdominal X-rays may show calcification of the tumour, and metastatic lesions may be identified on chest and skeletal X-rays. The ultrasound

Table 19.10 Clinical staging of neuroblastoma

Stage I	Tumour confined to the organ or structure of origin
Stage II	Tumour extends beyond the organs or structure of origin but does not cross the midline. Regional ipsilateral lymph nodes may be involved
Stage III	Tumour beyond the midline with or without bilateral lymph node enlargement
Stage IV	Remote disease – skeleton, parenchyma, or distant lymph nodes
Stage V	Classified as Stage I and Stage II, but with remote disease confined to liver, skin, or bone marrow. Usually 1 year old

scan shows downward renal displacement by a suprarenal tumour. CT scans of the chest and abdomen are useful to determine the extent of the disease and lymph node involvement. A radio-labelled guanethine analogue, iodine-131 meta-iodo-benzyl guanidine (131 I-M IBG), which has a strong affinity for adrenergic nerve tissue, is useful for locating the primary tumour and detecting metastases.

The diagnosis is confirmed by elevated urine catecholamine levels, the presence of tumour cells with rosette formation on bone marrow aspiration, or direct biopsy. The histology may be very difficult to distinguish from other 'small round cell' tumours such as lymphoma, and various sarcomas.

The staging system used is that of Evans *et al.* (*see Table 19.10*).

Treatment
Surgical removal of the primary lesion is undertaken whenever possible, as this frequently increases the response of metastases to chemotherapy, possibly by reducing tumour bulk. The response to chemotherapy is dramatic, but relapse is common.

Prognosis
The prognosis depends on the age and stage of the disease, ranging from more than 80% for stage I to less than 20% for stage IV disease. Tumours orginating in the abdomen have a worse prognosis

than thoracic tumours. Children under 1 year of age have the best chance of cure, even when there are metastases to skin, liver, and bone marrow (but not bone), i.e., stage IV-S disease. Expert evaluation is thus essential before deciding to withhold treatment in this age group.

Rhabdomyosarcoma
Rhabdomyosarcoma, arising from the embryonic rhabdomyoblasts, is the most frequently occurring soft tissue sarcoma in childhood. Tumours may occur in any part of the body, the common regions being the genitourinary system, the trunk, and extremities. Local invasion is usual, and spread may occur along lymphatics to the regional nodes, or in the blood stream to the lungs and liver.

At least 25% of cases will have metastases at diagnosis.

Most tumours present as a polypoid lesion in the ear, nose, bladder, or vagina (sarcoma botryoides). Early signs include obstruction or a blood-stained or offensive discharge. On the trunk and extremities the tumour presents as a soft tissue mass, which may be tender and is easily confused with an acute abscess. Orbital swelling may be mistaken for a retinoblastoma, neuroblastoma, or Burkitt's lymphoma. There are four histological types: embryonal (sarcoma botryoides), alveolar, pleomorphic, and mixed types.

The **diagnosis** is established by biopsy of the lesion and regional lymph nodes. The CSF should be examined carefully for malignant cells if the tumour involves the head, neck, or parameningeal sites.

Treatment includes surgery, chemotherapy, and radiotherapy. Primary total resection offers the best chance of cure; extensive mutilating surgery may be minimized by first shrinking the lesion with chemotherapy and/or radiotherapy.

Hepatomas
There are two morphological types, with clinical and prognostic differences. They present as abdominal swelling, weight loss, and/or anaemia. The enlarged liver may or may not be tender. The **hepatoblastoma** predominates in males and generally occurs before the age of 3 years. The right lobe of the liver is usually involved. Other anomalies, e.g., hemihypertrophy and virilization, may

be present. Serum alpha-fetoprotein is elevated in most children. Some secrete human chorionic gonadotrophin.

Hepatocellular carcinoma is rare, but there is a high incidence in parts of Africa, e.g., Mozambique, which may be causally linked to hepatitis B-associated cirrhosis.

It occurs after the age of 3 years, and rarely before 6 years.

Treatment consists of partial hepatectomy where possible, followed by chemotherapy. If the disease is limited this may be curative. Preoperative intensive chemotherapy may convert an inoperable lesion to an operable one.

Prognosis is good if the tumour is completely removed, but if unresectable, or if metastases are present, the outlook is poor.

Germ cell tumours

These are rare tumours which develop from primordial germ cells of the embryo, normally destined to produce sperm or ova. The signs and symptoms depend on the site of orgin. They may present as an ovarian or testicular tumour, or in an extragonadal site. The sacrococcygeal region is the commonest extragonadal site. Other sites are the retroperitoneum, vagina, mediastinum, and the pineal region. Tumours arising from the ovary may be associated with chromosomal or endocrine abnormalities. The malignant histological types are:

- germinoma:
  - dysgerminoma of ovary
  - seminoma of testis
- immature teratoma
- embryonal carcinoma
- endodermal sinus tumour (yolk sac tumour)
- choriocarcinoma.

Most of these tumours secrete the tumour marker alpha-fetoprotein (the highest level is seen in yolk sac tumours). Human chorionic gonadotrophin is another marker which is high in choriocarcinoma. These markers are useful for clinical evaluation, for assessing response to treatment, and for monitoring for recurrence.

Treatment: Total excision is performed if possible, followed by radiotherapy and/or chemotherapy.

Prognosis varies with age, histology, surgical resectability, and response to radiotherapy and adjuvant chemotherapy.

Retinoblastoma

(Also see Chapter 25, Disorders of the Eye.)
Retinoblastoma is a relatively rare malignant tumour of the eye, but a high frequency has been found in parts of Africa and India. At King Edward VIII Hospital, Durban, about ten new cases are seen each year in black children. There is a familial tendency with autosomal dominant inheritance, which is particularly pronounced in bilateral disease. It is associated with an abnormality of chromosome 13. Spread is either into the orbit or along the optic nerve, with intracranial extension being the usual cause of death. Blood spread with bone marrow involvement is a late manifestation. Most present before the age of 3 years, with the mother having noticed a white spot in the pupil (leukocoria or 'cat's eye reflex'), a squint, or proptosis. Gross proptosis or a large orbital mass is not uncommon at presentation in Third World countries. The differential diagnosis should include rhabdomyosarcoma, neuroblastoma, Burkitt's lymphoma, and visceral larva migrans.

Investigations
These include ophthalmological examination under anaesthesia, radiography of the local area, and skeletal survey, CT scan, CSF cytology, and bone marrow aspiration.

Treatment
Treatment involves enucleation of the eye in the early stages (and if unilateral), followed by radiotherapy and chemotherapy. If both eyes are affected, the more severely involved eye is removed, followed by radiotherapy and chemotherapy. Cryotherapy and photocoagulation may be used.

Prognosis
Early stage disease has a good prognosis. Regular ophthalmological examination of the normal eye should be performed. Any siblings should be examined regularly because of the familial tendency.

Late stage disease: The prognosis varies, but there is hope.

Brain tumours

See Chapter 15, Neurological Disorders.

Bone tumours

The two important primary malignant tumours of childhood are osteogenic sarcoma and Ewing's sarcoma. They tend to occur in the older child, where pain and swelling as the usual presenting complaints may mimic osteomyelitis. A pathological fracture may be the initial feature. Most osteogenic sarcomas arise in the lower femur or upper tibia, producing a limp. Ewing's sarcoma is said to be rare in blacks, and locally only one or two cases are seen per year. It involves the long bones of the lower extremities, the pelvis, vertebrae, and ribs. Metastases occur early. Biopsy is necessary to confirm the diagnosis. Chest X-ray, isotope bone scan, and CT lung scan are done for accurate staging.

Treatment

Chemotherapy is the mainstay of treatment. High-dose methotrexate with folinic acid rescue is the treatment of choice for osteogenic sarcoma. The cost is exorbitant.

Combination therapy with vincristine, actino-mycin-D, cyclophosphamide, and adriamycin is used for Ewing's sarcoma.

Radiotherapy is given to achieve local control. The tendency today is for limb preservation using *en bloc* resection of the tumour rather than amputation.

Prognosis

This has improved from 5–10% to 50–60% disease-free survival.

Langerhans cell histiocytosis (histiocytosis X)

This term is used to describe a spectrum of diseases of the reticulo-endothelial system where there is an abnormal proliferation of histiocytes associated with varying degrees of eosinophilic and lymphocytic infiltration. The diagnostic cell is the Langerhans cell, which resembles the epidermal Langerhans cell and is characterized by a lobulated, grooved nucleus, a delicate nuclear membrane, a small nucleolus, and eosinophilic cytoplasm. On electron microscopy these cells have unique cytoplasmic organelles called Birkbeck granules or X bodies, which are racket-shaped structures. They have a specific Langerhans cell marker which is the S-100 neurotropin.

It is debatable whether this is an inflammatory or neoplastic condition, and whether it represents a single disease entity or not. The aetiology is unknown. It may be an abnormal response to an infectious agent or a disorder of immune regulation. Recent work suggests that it is not a malignancy, but rather a form of immunodeficiency, possibly involving a soluble thymic or T-lymphocyte product.

It is essentially a disease of childhood and is rare in black children, with only one case a year seen in Durban.

There are three clinical syndromes with overlapping features.

Eosinophilic granuloma of bone

This is the most benign form. It presents in children over the age of 8 years, either with single or multiple lesions, predominantly in membranous bones. It manifests with pain, swelling, spinal cord signs, or pathological fractures.

On X-ray the characteristic finding is a single, well-demarcated, lytic lesion. A full skeletal survey should be done to exclude other lesions. Dissemination occurs in about 5% of cases.

The **diagnosis** is confirmed by biopsy.

Treatment: If possible, the lesion is curetted at the time of biopsy; otherwise radiotherapy is applied.

Hand-Schüller-Christian disease

This is a disseminated form which tends to be subacute and occurs between 2 and 8 years of age. It often presents with chronic otorrhoea, a seborrhoeic rash, exophthalmos, hepatosplenomegaly, diabetes insipidus, and lytic lesions in the skull and mastoids.

Investigations should be directed at detecting organ involvement and dysfunction.

Diagnosis is confirmed on biopsy of the skin lesions.

Treatment: *See under Letterer-Siwe disease, below.*

Letterer-Siwe disease

This is the most severe form, and a malignant expression of the disease. It presents in infancy with failure to thrive, fever, haemorrhagic seborrhoeic rash, lymphadenopathy, hepatosplenomegaly, pulmonary involvement, lytic lesions in bones, and haematological manifestations (e.g., pancytopenia). Loose teeth may be present. The condition may be mistaken for Burkitt's lymphoma.

Diagnosis is confirmed by biopsy of skin or lymph nodes.

For **treatment** of the latter two forms of the disease, the decision to treat with cytotoxic drugs is based on the severity of the disease and level of organ dysfunction. If not severe, and if there is no organ dysfunction, the child can be observed. If the child is ill and vital organs are threatened, cytotoxic drugs — with or without prednisone — should be used with caution because of the danger of further immunosuppression. The drugs used are chlorambucil, vincristine, methotrexate, VP-16,

and cyclophosphamide — individually or in combination. A humoral factor from calf thymus has been found to bring about dramatic clinical improvement in some cases. Radiotherapy should preferably be avoided, and used in small doses if necessary.

Prognosis

In single-system disease the prognosis is good. The recurrence rate is 25%, but systemic spread is unusual. In multi-system disease the prognosis must be guarded: cure occurs in less than 50%; 30–50% show transient or no response, with high mortality despite chemotherapy. Surviving patients have a high morbidity, with growth failure, growth hormone deficiency, diabetes insipidus, orthopaedic sequelae, and pituitary insufficiency.

J.A. Naidoo
P. Hesseling

20

Endocrine and metabolic disorders

Endocrine disorders

The endocrine system plays an important part in the progressive biological change taking place during the period of intrauterine development and through childhood and adolescence. The growth of the endocrine glands is followed by the establishment of hormonal feedback mechanisms. The sexual differentiation of the fetus has a very important endocrine component. The endocrine status of the mother, placental function, and exogenous hormone administration may profoundly affect the baby *(see Table 20.1)*. Postnatally, the sleep-wake cycle gradually assumes a vital role in the determination of normal circadian rhythms, but stresses such as trauma, exercise, emotions, or hypoglycaemia operate through the central nervous system to overcome the circadian rhythms of various hormones. Puberty depends on a series of integrated endocrine events operating through the hypothalamus to increase gonadal sex hormone output. The cellular responses to hormone actions are modulated through their binding to specific receptors and intracellular second-messenger mechanisms. Thus, normal homeostasis is maintained by integrated autonomic, endocrine, immune, and metabolic responses.

Endocrine disorders may be congenital or acquired. Congenital disorders arise because of absence or maldevelopment of an endocrine organ. This is usually a sporadic occurrence, or because of inherited enzymatic defects in hormone production or cellular receptor insensitivity.

There are differences in the incidence of endocrine disorders in different societes. These conditions seem to be rare in Third World countries. However, the preponderance of nutritional and infective diseases, the lack of diagnostic experience and sophisticated laboratories, and the scarce availability of life-saving treatment may make these differences more apparent than real.

Endocrine disorders may present with classical clinical features, but more often their early non-specific signs and symptoms are easily overlooked or misdiagnosed. They should be considered in the following clinical situations:

In the newborn:
- sexual ambiguity
- persistent vomiting
- goitre
- convulsions.

In the older child:
- slow development
- abnormally slow or fast growth in stature
- polydipsia, polyuria, weight loss
- unexplained drowsiness, coma
- sexual precocity
- recurrent convulsions
- delayed puberty
- obesity in a short child
- persistent unexplained biochemical abnormality
- in the context of disorders known to affect endocrine glands, e.g., tuberculous meningitis, craniopharyngioma, following cranial irradiation.

Occasionally, the treatment of a suspected endocrine disorder cannot wait for laboratory confirmation. In such cases, obtaining a random sample of frozen separated serum is often all that it is necessary before a therapeutic trial is started. Care must be taken in transporting the frozen samples to a distant main laboratory for confirmation of the

Table 20.1 Congenital disorders associated with maternal endocrine factors

Maternal	Infant
Thyrotoxicosis	Thyrotoxicosis or hypothyroidism
Hyperparathyroidism	Hypocalcaemia
Diabetes mellitus	Hypoglycaemia, hypocalcaemia
Androgen treatment	Virilization
Antithyroid drugs and iodine	Goitrous hypothyroidism

diagnosis, which usually involves a radioimmuno-assay procedure.

Disorders of growth

Growth *in utero* depends on maternal nutrition and an intact placenta, and is largely independent of fetal hormone output. In infancy, somatic growth is mainly regulated by adequate nutrition. Thereafter it depends on an interaction of the endocrine and skeletal systems in the absence of chronic disease.

The assessment of growth depends on repeated, accurate measurements of stature *(see Chapter 2 for details of the procedure)*. This is a more sensitive index of long-term health and nutrition than weight, which is subject to wide fluctuations from intercurrent illness. Although many children in underdeveloped countries fall under the third centile for height, growth charts from the western world are representative of many diverse populations under conditions of optimal growth, and are applicable to all ethnic groups.

The **growth velocity** is the rate of growth in centimetres per year *(see Chapter 2, Growth and Development)*, and is derived from two consecutive height measurements at least 6 months to a year apart. Growth rates vary with age, and an abnormality should be suspected if the yearly rate is less than 7 cm under 4 years of age, less than 6 cm under age 6, and less than 4.5 cm from 6 years until the onset of puberty. Girls' pubertal growth spurt occurs earlier than that of boys and is of shorter duration.

The **radiological bone age** is obtained by comparing X-rays of the left hand and wrist with those of a standard atlas, or more conveniently with simple line diagrams highlighting the critical epiphyses *(see Fig. 20.1)*. In genetic short stature, the bone age corresponds to the chronological age. In malnutrition and chronic disease, the bone age is usually less retarded than the physical growth. In constitutional delay and isolated growth hormone deficiency, the bone age and physical growth are equally retarded. When retardation of the bone age far exceeds physical stunting, it suggests hypothyroidism or long-standing malnutrition. An advanced bone age indicates excess sex hormone or thyroid activity. In congenital adrenal hyperplasia or true precocious puberty, this results in early cessation of growth and reduced final height, even if the child appears tall for age at the time.

Failure to grow normally is an important symptom in childhood. It may be overlooked for many years if height records are not commonly kept, as endocrine causes of poor growth are relatively uncommon. Amongst poorly-growing children in

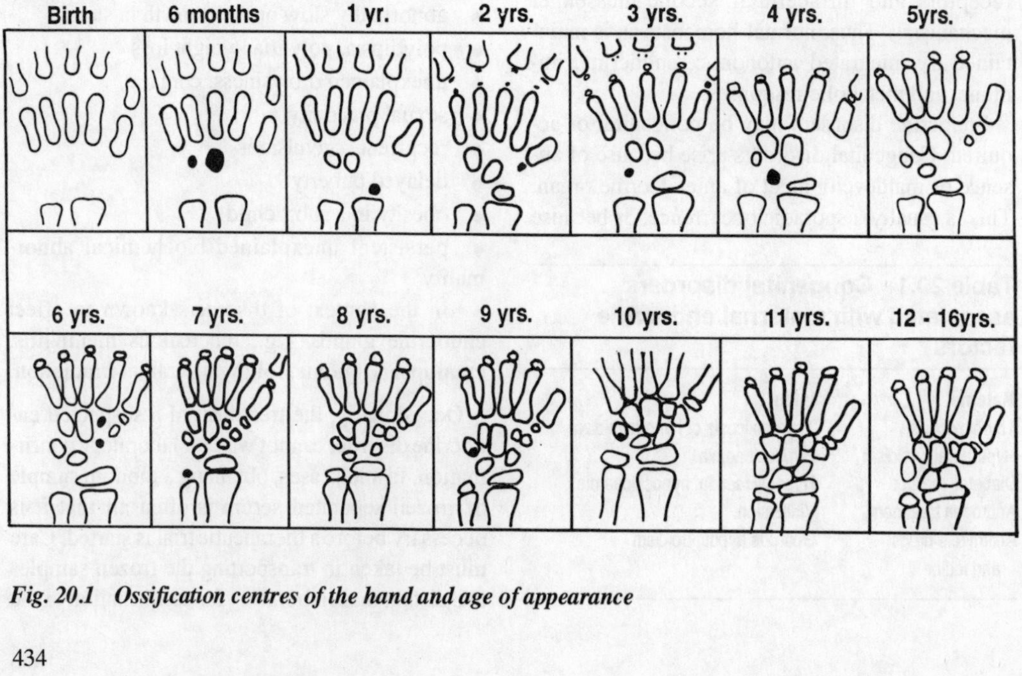

Fig. 20.1   Ossification centres of the hand and age of appearance

the Third World, the following conditions must first be excluded:
- small for gestational age
- inadequate nutrition
- anaemia
- parasitic infestation, and
- chronic infection.

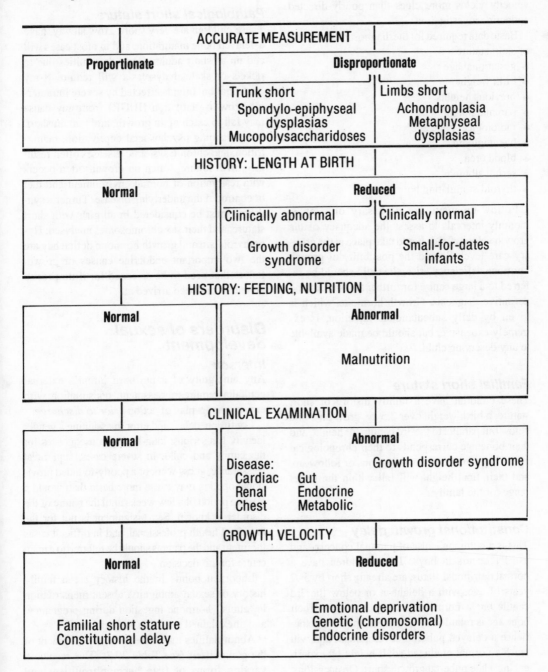

Fig. 20.2 Short stature: clinical approach

ACCURATE MEASUREMENT

Proportionate	Disproportionate	
	Trunk short	Limbs short
	Spondylo-epiphyseal dysplasias	Achondroplasia
	Mucopolysaccharidoses	Metaphyseal dysplasias

HISTORY: LENGTH AT BIRTH

Normal	Reduced	
	Clinically abnormal	Clinically normal
	Growth disorder syndrome	Small-for-dates infants

HISTORY: FEEDING, NUTRITION

Normal	Abnormal
	Malnutrition

CLINICAL EXAMINATION

Normal	Abnormal
	Disease: Growth disorder syndrome
	Cardiac Gut
	Renal Endocrine
	Chest Metabolic

GROWTH VELOCITY

Normal	Reduced
Familial short stature Constitutional delay	Emotional deprivation Genetic (chromosomal) Endocrine disorders

The approach to a child with short stature *(see Fig. 20.2)* demands a careful systematic history and examination and accurate measurements. This information taken in conjunction with the growth velocity yields more clues than poorly-directed endocrine investigation.

Basic data required for the diagnostic evaluation of short stature:

◆ gestational age
◆ birth weight
◆ previous heights
◆ parental height
◆ radiological bone age
◆ haemoglobin
◆ blood urea
◆ serum albumin
◆ thyroid-stimulating hormone.

Follow-up visits are necessary only at 3-monthly intervals to assess the adequacy of the growth velocity, and should take place at the primary care level. Should the possibility of growth hormone deficiency arise, the child should be referred to a large centre for further assessment and definitive diagnosis. Growth hormone, which is given by daily subcutaneous injection, is extremely expensive, but should be made available to any deserving child.

Familial short stature

These children have a family history of short stature, a birth weight over 2.5 kg, grow on a line below but parallel to the 3rd centile for height, and their bone age corresponds to their chronological age. They require no investigations or follow-up, and their final height will fall within the target range for the family.

Constitutional growth delay

This is a common cause of parental concern, and usually occurs in boys. These children have a normal nutritional status, are already short by 5–7 years of age, with a height at or below the 3rd centile but a normal annual growth rate. Their bone age is retarded by 2–4 years, they will experience a delayed pubertal development, and will reach a normal predicted adult height by experiencing a late pubertal growth spurt. On occasions, causes of pathological growth disorders such as acquired hypothyroidism need to be excluded in

these children. Treatment with anabolic steroids or testosterone may be indicated for psychological reasons near the time of puberty.

Pathological short stature

These children are very short, grow slowly, have a delayed bone maturation, and in most cases will end up as short adults. Bony deformities due to rickets or skeletal dysplasia will require X-ray confirmation. Infants affected by severe intrauterine growth retardation (IUGR) from any cause may fail to catch up in growth, and remain short. Long-standing psychosocial deprivation, malnutrition, and chronic systemic diseases often result in growth failure. Catch-up growth often occurs with restoration of normal environment and diet or control of the underlying disease. Turner's syndrome must be considered in all girls with short stature, and their sex chromosomes analysed. Hypothyroidism and growth hormone deficiency are the two important endocrine causes of growth failure that need to be screened for if no precise diagnosis has been arrived at.

Disorders of sexual development

Intersex

Any ambiguity of a newborn infant's external genitalia requires assessment, consultation with experts, and a plan of action *prior to discharge*.

Confusion, delay, and error in assigning a gender identity has serious, long-lasting consequences for the family and child. In severe cases, superficial reassurance, guess-work or a poorly-founded provisional opinion may cause more harm than would a waiting period of a few weeks until the nature of the disorder is known. Sex assignment is not for the untrained health professional, and in difficult cases the infant and the parents should be referred to a main centre for this decision.

Important points in the history are a family history of sexual ambiguity, absent menstruation in 'aunts', hormone ingestion during pregnancy, and unexplained deaths in early infancy.

Abnormalities may arise in the development of the gonad itself *(see Table 20.2)*. This results in varying forms of **true hermaphroditism** and mixed gonadal dysgenesis. The former condition, in which both functioning ovarian and testicular

Table 20.2   Abnormal sexual differentiation

Abnormal development of gonads. Sex chromosome abnormalities
a. True hermaphroditism
b . Mixed gonadal dysgenesis

Abnormal genitalia in presence of XY karyotype and testes (male pseudohermaphroditism)
a. Deficiency in testosterone biosynthesis
b. Disorder of function at androgen-dependent target areas
    - complete androgen resistance
    - incomplete androgen resistance

Abnormal genitalia in presence of XX karyotype and ovaries (female pseudohermaphroditism)
a. Congenital adrenal hyperplasia
    - with salt-losing syndrome
    - without salt-losing syndrome
b. Exogenous androgens in pregnancy

Table 20.3   Approach to ambiguous genitalia

What is the phenotypic sex and functional anatomy?
Clinical examination (presence of gonads?)
Ultrasound
Exploratory laparotomy

What is the aetiological diagnosis?
Chromosome analysis
Sodium and potassium balance
Plasma 17-OH-progesterone
Gonadal biopsy

tissue are present, appears to be the most common intersexual disorder amongst Africans.

Pseudohermaphroditism refers to abnormal genital development despite the presence of concordant chromosomes and gonads. In the XY fetus it is due to insufficient testosterone secretion or action; in the XX fetus it is the result of exposure to male hormones *in utero*.

The approach to a child with ambiguous genitalia *(see Table 20.3)* entails a careful clinical assessment of the external genitalia: length and width of the phallic structure, degree of hypospadias, whether the urethra is separate from the vaginal opening, whether posterior fusion of the labio-scrotal folds exists, as well as the presence or absence of gonads in the labia or bifid scrotum. A rectal examination is rarely helpful. Intersexed newborns without palpable gonads need to have the potentially fatal disorder of congenital adrenal hyperplasia (CAH) excluded before being sent home.

In general, the patient will fall into one of two broad groups: those who have a reasonable phallus with perineal hypospadias, and those in whom gender assignment is difficult because the genitalia are truly ambiguous. The sex of rearing, except in genetic female infants with virilization due to CAH, is usually determined by practical considerations and the ability to achieve functional sexual

activity rather than by the sex chromosome pattern. Particularly in true hermaphrodites, strong preference of the parents or late presentation with well-established gender identity may override other factors in helping to make the decision.

Premature thelarche

This refers to isolated breast development without other signs of puberty. It is not rare, and may be found quite incidentally during physical examination. It usually presents below the age of 2 years, often as an extension of the breast enlargement in the newborn period, and with a tendency to wax and wane over intervals of 1–2 months. Provided the child's growth rate is appropriate for age, and there is no pubic or axillary hair development, the condition is not serious, and is usually due to small amounts of oestrogens secreted by a few isolated, small ovarian cysts. No referral is necessary, but follow-up is important at 3-monthly intervals. The parents can be reassured that the condition will subside, but they need to be cautioned against the use of any locally-applied treatment.

Premature adrenarche

Early development of pubic and axillary hair, associated with adult body odour, may develop in some children around the age of 4–7 years. Growth in stature may be slightly advanced, but genital development and testicular size remain at prepubertal level. It is necessary to exclude exogenous androgen administration, late-onset congenital adrenal hyperplasia, and adrenal tumours. Once this has been done, the parents can be reassured of the benign nature of the condition.

True precocious puberty

The rate of normal pubertal development is outlined in *Chapter 2, Growth and Development*.

True precocious puberty refers to premature activation of the hypothalamo-pituitary-gonadal axis. It frequently starts in the first few years of life, and is much more common in girls than in boys. Overall body growth and full-blown sexual development (in boys pubertal-sized testes longer than 2.5 cm in the longitudinal axis) proceed at an alarming rate. Physical aggressiveness may be a problem in boys. In 80% of girls with true precocious puberty no organic cause is found, whereas approximately 50% of boys have evidence of tumours or hamartomas near the hypothalamus. Precocious puberty may be a sequel to tuberculous meningitis, encephalitis or hydrocephalus.

All children should be referred as early as possible for investigation and initiation of suppressive therapy, either with cyproterone acetate (100 mg/m^2/day) or preferably with monthly injections of long-acting gonadotrophin-releasing hormone analogues.

Precocious pseudopuberty

Precocious pseudopuberty refers to the development of secondary sex characteristics as a result of increased sex steroid activity without normal activation of the hypothalamo-pituitary-gonadal axis. It may be isosexual or heterosexual, and may be due to exogenous administration of sex hormones, or to autonomous overproduction as a result of an ovarian, testicular, or adrenal tumour, or congenital adrenal hyperplasia. In view of the possible gravity of the diagnosis and the necessity of sophisticated tests and therapy, urgent referral is indicated.

Pubertal gynaecomastia

Transient breast enlargement occurs commonly in boys at the mid-pubertal stage of development. It may be asymmetrical and tender, and can last for 1–2 years before regression occurs. Occasionally it is associated with primary hypogonadism (Klinefelter's syndrome), and in extremely rare instances with testicular or adrenal tumours.

If physical examination is normal and puberty is unequivocally under way, no investigation is necessary, but reassurance and psychological support should be offered. Medical suppressive treatment is rarely successful, and surgical excision is reserved for very large breasts or for cases with severe adjustment problems.

Delayed puberty

Delay of growth and puberty is much more common in boys than girls. Investigations should be undertaken when breast development has not started by age 13–14 in girls, or testicular growth by age 14–15 in boys. It must be remembered that long-standing undernutrition and chronic systemic disease of any kind may lead to pubertal delay.

In boys, simple physiological delay is much more common than testicular failure due to Klinefelter's syndrome or permanent lack of pituitary gonadotrophins. Treatment with long-acting testosterone 50–100 mg IM monthly for 3–4 months may be sufficient to produce a rapid sustained advance in pubertal development.

In girls, delayed puberty often has an organic basis, such as ovarian dysgenesis (Turner's syndrome), androgen-insensitivity disorders (in genetic 46XY males), or gonadotrophin deficiency. Referral for further investigations is appropriate.

Disorders of water balance

Syndrome of inappropriate antidiuretic hormone secretion (SIADH)

This is associated with a variety of intracranial and extracranial conditions, but is most commonly seen in severe meningitis (mainly tuberculous), head injury, pulmonary disorders, and with vincristine therapy. Increased renal tubular water reabsorption results in diminished output of a highly concentrated urine in the face of plasma hypo-osmolality and dilutional hyponatraemia without dehydration. The clinical features are those of water intoxication: nausea, vomiting, muscle weakness, neurological irritability, convulsions, and coma.

In conditions known to predispose to SIADH, excessive oral and intravenous fluids should be avoided. The mainstay of treatment consists of severe restriction of water intake until a steady rise in serum sodium and a loss of body weight occur. In emergency situations, the slow intravenous administration of 3% saline (5 ml/kg) combined with furosemide therapy (0.5–1 mg/kg) may help for a while.

Diabetes insipidus

The symptoms of this disorder include polyuria, thirst, chronic dehydration, and growth failure. The passage of large amounts of dilute, glucose-free, pale-coloured urine may be due to a deficiency of ADH or to a lack of its effect on the kidney. The diagnosis is confirmed when inappropriately dilute urine is excreted in the presence of serum hypertonicity. Overnight water deprivation tests may be dangerous in children suspected of having diabetes insipidus (DI). The test is best done in the morning, when fluids can be totally withheld under supervision, preferably in a secondary or tertiary institution. In DI, the test leads to rapid dehydration with a rise in plasma osmolality and sodium, but with little change in urine output, urine osmolality, or specific gravity. If the defect can be corrected with vasopressin administration, a central nervous system cause is implicated.

Central diabetes insipidus

The lack of ADH secretion by the posterior pituitary may be partial or complete. Rarely, this is inherited or idiopathic, but it is more commonly acquired as a result of organic lesions of the hypothalamo-pituitary area such as trauma, craniopharyngioma and other tumours, histiocytosis, and following neurosurgery. On occasions, the ADH deficiency may precede the symptoms of the underlying pathology, hence a CT scan is essential if no obvious cause is found. Older children are not dehydrated unless the thirst centre is also involved. When plasma osmolality or sodium are normal, the condition must be distinguished from compulsive water-drinking.

The treatment consists of hormone replacement, either with lysine vasopressin or desamino-D-arginine vasopressin (DDAVP), given as intranasal spray. DDAVP needs refrigeration to ensure stability, has a long duration of action (12–24) hours and excessive administration carries a risk of water intoxication.

Nephrogenic diabetes insipidus

ADH insensitivity at the renal tubular level is a familial condition and occurs mainly in boys as an X-linked dominant trait. Occasionally heterozygous girls may also be affected clinically. Soon after birth, the infants present with vomiting, constipation, failure to thrive, and recurrent hypertonic dehydration. Very rarely, the condition may be mimicked by chronic hypokalaemia due to kwashiorkor or long-standing diarrhoea.

There is no response to vasopressin administration. Treatment is difficult, and must always include a high water intake with frequent feeding, even during the night. A low-salt diet, and hydrochlorothiazide (3 mg/kg/day) with indomethacin (1.5–3 mg/kg/day) reduce the urine losses only partially, but help prevent recurrent admissions for rehydration, and promote weight gain.

Disorders of the thyroid

Hypothyroidism

Endemic cretinism is still found in areas where iodine deficiency has not been corrected by iodination of salt or water supplies. These infants are born to mothers with goitres and significant iodine deficiency throughout pregnancy.

Primary congenital hypothyroidism due to aplasia or dysgenesis of the thyroid seems to be rare among African children. It is very difficult to diagnose early because the symptoms and signs are non-specific. Thyroxine is essential for normal brain development, but treatment within the first few months of life will prevent significant mental deficit. If untreated, the infant shows retarded linear growth and is slow in achieving developmental milestones.

Only 10–15% of hypothyroid newborns present with a suspicious clinical picture. The most reliable signs are an open posterior fontanelle (greater than 1 cm), an umbilical hernia, coarse facial features, and poor sucking. In the absence of systematic screening programmes, a high index of awareness may be maintained by the use of a Congenital Hypothyroidism Score *(see Table 20.4)*, where a total score greater than 5 suggests hypothyroidism. Although jaundice is not highly weighted in the scoring system — being a common occurrence in the first week of life — *prolonged unconjugated hyperbilirubinaemia* lasting

Table 20.4   Congenital hypothyroidism score

Symptom	Score
Hernia, umbilical	2
Hypothermia	1
Coarse facial features	2
Enlarged tongue	1
Hypotonia	1
Jaundice (> 3 days)	1
Dry skin	1
Wide posterior fontanelle	1
Constipation	2
Duration of gestation > 40 wk	1
Birth weight > 3.5 kg	1
Female sex	1
Total	15

Score > 5 suggests hypothyroidism

Table 20.5   Causes of hypothyroidism

Dysgenesis
  Aplasia
  Maldescent
Iodine deficiency
Familial enzyme defect
Ingestion of goitrogens
  Antenatal
      Iodide-containing cough mixtures
      Antithyroid drugs
      Para-aminosalicylic acid
  Postnatal
      Iodide-containing cough mixtures
Autoimmune thyroiditis
Secondary hypothyroidism
  Hypothalamic or pituitary disease

a few weeks should raise suspicion of congenital hypothyroidism. The laboratory diagnosis is not difficult. Serum T_4 is low to low–normal, and the thyroid-stimulating hormone (TSH) value is always significantly elevated (except in the rare instance of secondary pituitary hypothyroidism).

The causes of hypothyroidism are shown in *Table 20.5*. Patients with dysgenesis and secondary hypothyroidism have no goitre. Delayed skeletal maturation, as assessed by the size of the distal femoral epiphysis on an X-ray of the knee, can provide an added argument in favour of therapeutic trial, if no reliable laboratory is available.

Treatment can always be stopped in the second year of life, when brain development is no longer vulnerable, to allow for retesting. When hypothyroidism occurs after infancy, there is much less severe brain damage, but these children are sluggish, puffy, and grow slowly. Treatment consists of L-thyroxine in a dose ranging between 25 and 50 µg daily in the first year. Growth, bone age, and measurement of T_4 and TSH may be used to monitor the adequacy of the dosage.

Hyperthyroidism

Thyroid hyperfunction is rare in children but may occur at all ages, including the neonatal period, when it is caused by the transplacental passage of thyroid-stimulating immunoglobulins from a mother with Graves' disease. The main presenting features in children are emotional lability, nervousness, behavioural disturbances, sweating, and nocturnal enuresis, but a large goitre and severe ophthalmopathy are rare. The diagnosis is confirmed by an elevated serum T_4 and a suppressed TSH. The various methods available for treatment are antithyroid drugs, subtotal thyroidectomy, and radioactive iodine.

Disorders of the adrenal cortex

Acute adrenal insufficiency

An adrenal crisis may be the presenting feature of any of the conditions listed in *Table 20.6*, or it may occur in treated patients as a result of acute stress. Inadequate secretion of glucocorticoids and mineralocorticoids results in salt loss, hypoglycaemia, and circulatory collapse. The serum potassium is high, the sodium low to low–normal, and there is a poorly compensated metabolic acidosis.

This is an acute medical emergency requiring immediate treatment before any transfer.

If there is any suspicion of acute adrenal insufficiency, treatment must be commenced before a confirmatory diagnosis, as a short therapeutic trial could be life-saving.

Acute management

◆   Take blood samples for electrolytes, acid base, urea, glucose, and freeze extra serum for plasma cortisol assay.

◆ Fluid and electrolyte replacement to re-expand the blood volume and elevate the blood pressure must be infused intravenously: plasma or Haemaccel® for severe shock, otherwise 0.9% sodium chloride in 5% dextrose at the rate of 10–20 ml/kg over the first hour, thereafter at a maintenance rate to deliver 60 ml/kg over the following 24 hours.

◆ Hydrocortisone sodium succinate (Solu-Cortef®) is given as an IV bolus (50 mg for small children and 100 mg for larger children), followed by 50–100 mg/24 hours added to the IV maintenance solution.

◆ Fludrocortisone (Florinef®) 0.05– 0.1 mg/day orally.

◆ Monitor circulation, electrolytes, and glucose levels.

Table 20.6 Adrenocortical insufficiency

Aplasia/hypoplasia
Enzyme defect
   Congenital adrenal hyperplasia
Destruction
   Haemorrhage
   Infection
   Waterhouse-Friedrichsen syndrome
   Autoimmune disease
   X-linked adrenoleucodystrophy
Suppression of pituitary-adrenal axis
   Iatrogenic steroid therapy
ACTH deficiency
   Hypothalamic/pituitary damage
Congenital unresponsiveness to ACTH

Congenital adrenal hyperplasia

This is an autosomal-recessive condition due to a partial or severe deficiency of an enzyme in the biosynthetic pathway of cortisol, and in 50% of cases also of aldosterone. It is now being more frequently recognized in African babies. Cortisol deficiency is present early on in fetal life, resulting in stimulation of excessive ACTH release, which causes hyperplasia of the adrenal cortex and virilization of the external genitalia. The most common type is due to 21-hydroxylase deficiency. The diagnosis should be suspected in any newborn with intersexuality in whom gonads are not palpable, or in any male infant who presents with a salt-wasting syndrome soon after birth. The electrolytes will be abnormal (high potassium, low sodium, low bicarbonate and glucose) only if salt-loss is present. Pre-treatment serum has to be stored in the deep-freeze for later confirmation of the diagnosis, which will rest on finding increased levels of 17 OH progesterone and adrenal androgens. After acute management as for adrenal crisis, life-long maintenance is started with oral hydrocortisone or cortisone acetate (20–25 mg/m^2/day in divided doses) in all infants, and fludrocortisone (0.05–0.1 mg once daily) with added dietary salt if necessary for the salt-losers.

The child is issued with an identity disc with the diagnosis engraved on it. When stable, the infant should be referred to a tertiary centre for a review of the diagnosis, assessment of the need for surgical repair of the intersexed genitalia in female patients, and for genetic counselling. With good follow-up care and constant availability of medication, long-term survival may be ensured.

Addison's disease

The adrenal cortex may atrophy as part of an autoimmune or metabolic disorder, or be destroyed by tuberculous infection. Patients with Addison's disease are weak, anoretic, and may present with vomiting, diarrhoea, dehydration, and hypotension. There is an increase in pigmentation of the skin, buccal mucosa, and nails. The biochemical features of hypoadrenalism are present and, although basal cortisol may be low– normal, there is a poor response to an ACTH stimulation test. Life-long maintenance treatment is similar to that of congenital adrenal hyperplasia. With intercurrent illness or stress, the hydrocortisone dose should be doubled or tripled until the illness has resolved.

Hyperadrenocorticism

Hyperfunction of the adrenal cortex may present clinically with Cushing's syndrome or with marked virilization, depending on the specific steroid secretion.

Cushing's syndrome is caused by:

◆ excess steroid therapy (most common)

◆ adrenal tumour (onset of symptoms occurs before 8 years of age, usually in early childhood, and is associated with virilization; often malignant)

◆ ectopic ACTH-secreting microadenoma (more frequent in adolescence)

◆ ectopic ACTH-secreting tumours (very rare).

The moon face, truncal obesity, and 'buffalo hump' are characteristic. Growth failure with retarded bone age is an important point in differentiation from nutritional obesity, unless androgens are also excessively secreted. Muscle wasting and weakness, thinning of the skin with purple striae, personality changes, hypertension, and virilization may be present.

Florid cases should be referred to a tertiary care centre without delay. In a doubtful case, there may be a place for attempting to confirm or exclude the presence of an elevated cortisol secretion. Useful screening laboratory tests are the estimation of a 24-hour urinary free cortisol excretion, and the overnight dexamethasone adrenal suppression test (dexamethasone 0.3 mg/m^2 is given orally at 11 p.m. and plasma cortisol is measured the next morning at 8 a.m.). Adrenal tumour localization may be made by ultrasonography, IVP, or CT scan.

The predominantly virilizing adrenal tumours have to be differentiated from congenital adrenal hyperplasia by radiological localization and by the fact that their elevated androgens cannot be suppressed by dexamethasone.

Surgical resection, either by unilateral adrenalectomy or trans-sphenoidal microadenodectomy, should only be attempted in a very specialized centre with experienced surgeons and endocrinologists.

Disorders of the parathyroid glands

Parathyroid hormone (PTH) is intimately linked to the maintenance of normal serum calcium and is therefore an important factor in the development of metabolic bone disease (see Chapter 21).

Primary hyperparathyroidism

Hypercalcaemia caused by hyperfunctioning parathyroid glands is uncommon in children. Familial parathyroid hyperplasia may occur on its own or as part of dominantly inherited multiple endocrine adenomatosis. Solitary adenomas are even rarer; they present in later childhood or adolescence, usually with longstanding symptoms, representing a poor awareness of the disorder and the lack of routine biochemical screening in children. Malaise, gastrointestinal symptoms, abdominal pains, nephrolithiasis, bone pain, and fractures are the most common presenting symptoms. An elevated serum calcium and a lowered serum phosphorus level in the presence of a normal urea strongly suggest the diagnosis, which can be confirmed by finding raised PTH levels. Surgical removal is curative, but only an experienced surgeon should attempt the neck exploration.

Hypercalcaemia may also be due to vitamin D intoxication, malignant secondary bone deposits, and leukaemia.

Secondary hyperparathyroidism

This is much more common than primary hyperparathyroidism in children, and is due to chronically decreased serum calcium, which leads to parathyroid hyperplasia. This is well demonstrated in vitamin D deficiency and chronic renal failure. Excessive bony resorption with deformities and fractures may ensue. The serum calcium is at low–normal levels, the serum phosphorus is decreased in patients with normal renal function, and the alkaline phosphatase is elevated. Treatment consists of vitamin D or its active metabolites in order to maintain serum calcium levels as close to normal as possible.

Hypoparathyroidism

Transient neonatal hypoparathyroidism may occur in association with maternal hyperparathyroidism or diabetes. It presents with hypocalcaemic convulsions and apnoeic spells. The treatment is intravenous calcium for convulsions.

Congenital hypoparathyroidism

◆ *Sex-linked recessive type:* Onset with hypocalcaemia occurs at a few days to a few months of age.

◆ *Hypoplasia:* Associated with heart and thymus defect, e.g., Di George syndrome.

Idiopathic acquired hypoparathyroidism presents after one year of age and may be associated with other autoimmune conditions (Addison's disease, thyroiditis) presenting later in life. Patients present with tetany, convulsions, intellectual impairment, dental enamel hypoplasia, cataracts, and may have mucocutaneous candidiasis. Another form is secondary to hypomagnesaemia.

The diagnosis is suspected on the findings of a low serum calcium, a high serum phosphorus, a normal alkaline phosphatase and urea, together with X-ray evidence of metaphyseal density and intracranial basal ganglia calcification.

Vitamin D or its active metabolites, extra calcium, and aluminium hydroxide as phosphate binder are the prescribed treatment, with regular monitoring of serum calcium levels to avoid hypercalcaemia.

Parathyroid resistance syndrome
This comprises a group of disorders with the clinical and biochemical pictures of hypoparathyroidism but with normal or raised PTH levels. Not all patients have the typical features of Albright's hereditary osteodystrophy, which are short stature, mental retardation, and skeletal changes. Treatment is as for hypoparathyroidism.

Insulin-dependent diabetes mellitus
The incidence of diabetes in children is fairly low in the Third World, with the result that health care systems have limited experience in the diagnosis and treatment of the disorder.

Thus the clinical presentation of diabetes is still very often an acute metabolic emergency with frequent unwarranted deaths.

In patients who have inherited specific genes linked to the HLA locus, environmental factors such as viruses or toxins may trigger repeated autoimmune attacks on the pancreatic beta cell, leading to insulin deficiency. Polydipsia, polyuria, weight loss, and fatigue are usually evident for a period of less than a month, during which time the diagnosis is rarely entertained. The clinical presentation is often more abrupt, and occasionally fulminating, with severe **diabetic ketoacidotic coma (DKA)** occurring even before the diagnosis is established.

Rapid breathing, vomiting with abdominal guarding, and alteration in the sensorium may lead to an initial erroneous diagnosis of pneumonia, gastroenteritis, acute abdomen, meningoencephalitis, acute salicylate intoxication, or cerebral malaria. Early presumptive diagnosis of DKA should be made at the primary care level, using reagent strips to test for glucose and ketones in both blood and urine.

A blood glucose level higher than 14 mmol/l on a Dextrostix®, in the presence of marked ketonuria, and in conjunction with a typical clinical state, may be used as a basis for immediate initiation of therapy before referral of the patient to a specialist centre.

Delay in diagnosis and inadequate management in the first few hours after presentation may markedly influence morbidity and mortality.

Emergency management
The characteristic biochemical abnormalities in DKA include hyperglycaemia, osmotic diuresis with water and electrolyte loss, intravascular volume depletion, hyperosmolality, decreased glomerular filtration rate, and excess production of ketones leading to metabolic acidosis and compensatory hyperventilation. Untreated patients die of ketoacidosis and circulatory collapse.

The availability of sophisticated laboratories and equipment is much less important than the institution of early basic emergency measures available in community health centres.

Very often even initial rehydration treatment is not started before referral, as the management is incorrectly perceived as too complex for that level of care.

The following measures should be taken:
◆ Careful examination is essential, noting presence of complicating infections and the degree of dehydration and shock.

◆ A blood specimen is taken for blood glucose, electrolytes, and acid-base status. Paper reagent strips are used immediately to screen the level of blood glucose and plasma ketones (spun serum necessary). The urine is examined for glucose and ketones, as well as for evidence of infection. The urine output is measured regularly and recorded.

◆ Usually dehydration and ongoing urine losses make intravenous therapy mandatory. An IV infusion of 0.9% saline is started at the rate of 15–25 ml/kg for the first hour to restore tissue perfusion. Potassium chloride (2 ml 15% KCl in each 200 ml IV fluid bottle or 10 ml/litre) is added once insulin has been given and the child has been seen to pass urine. The infusion rate is then slowed down to 10–15 ml/kg in the second hour, and to 5–10 ml/kg/hour for the next 3–4 hours. When the blood sugar has dropped to about 12–15 mmol/l, the IV fluid is changed to 0.45% saline in 5% dextrose, or to half-strength Darrow's in 5% dextrose.

◆ Short-acting regular insulin (a clear solution) is given: 0.1 u/kg IV stat into the infusion tubing and then 0.1 u/kg/hour either by repeated IM or IV injection, or by constant IV infusion. A peristaltic infusion pump should control the rate of the insulin IV infusion flow, to prevent iatrogenic disasters. Intermediate-acting insulin (a cloudy suspension) has no place in the treatment of DKA, and should never be given intravenously. The dose of insulin may be increased or decreased to achieve a steady return to normal of the blood glucose, acid-base status, and ketone levels. The premature discontinuation of insulin treatment because of declining glucose levels, however, often results in recurrence of the acidosis. Additional glucose should rather be infused to prevent hypoglycaemia, and the insulin continued, albeit at a lower dose. In the early hours of treatment, an insulin dose of less than 0.05–0.1 u/kg/hr will be insufficient to clear the ketosis.

◆ Intravenous bicarbonate has potential disadvantages including sodium overload, hypokalaemia, and decreased tissue perfusion. It should be limited to patients with severe acidosis (pH < 7.1) or those whose lives are threatened by respiratory or circulatory collapse. A dose of bicarbonate of 2–2.5 mmol/kg over 1–2 hours may be repeated till the acidosis is safely back to a pH of more than 7.1, but additional potassium requirements must be anticipated. If severe ketoacidosis does not improve, the intravenous lines, infusion pump, and connections should be checked. The 'freshness' of the insulin should be established, a new vial used, and the dose should be doubled every 2–3 hours until an adequate response is obtained. At the same time, the adequacy of the intravascular volume expansion should be assessed and the presence of severe underlying infection excluded.

◆ Complications such as hypoglycaemia, hypokalaemia, and hypernatraemia can usually be avoided by the judicious use of intravenous fluids and insulin. Close bedside observation has proved safer than frequent biochemical results from the laboratory. Often regular testing of blood and urine for glucose and ketones on paper strips is sufficient for a slow, steady titration of the insulin dose. Cerebral oedema with midbrain infarction may develop during treatment while clinical and biochemical improvement is taking place. Deepening coma, bradycardia, muscular hypertonicity, convulsions, and papilloedema may occur due to osmotic disequilibrium and brain hypoxia. It seems prudent therefore to avoid over-treatment with hypotonic fluids, too rapid an alkalinization, or too rapid a correction of hyperglycaemia. Cerebral oedema should be recognized immediately and reversed with IV mannitol 1–2 g/kg.

◆ As soon as the patient is fully conscious and has stopped vomiting, sugar-free drinks and milk may be offered. The IV infusion is discontinued when the patient is clinically stable and a substantial improvement in acidosis and ketonaemia has occurred. The daily estimated insulin requirements may be administered in a twice-daily 2:1 mixture of intermediate and regular insulins (total dose 0.5–0.7 u/kg/24 hours), given $^2/_3$ before breakfast and $^1/_3$ before supper. Any change should be made cautiously, and based on bedside blood glucose levels.

Long-term treatment

While stabilization is being attempted, the education of the child and his family should proceed as soon as the psychological impact of the diagnosis allows. It is essential to ensure proficiency of dose accuracy and injection technique. Also essential is an understanding of basic dietary principles, the proper use of urine and blood tests, and of the difference between ketoacidosis and hypoglycaemia and the steps to follow in each event. If possible, the family should be referred to a centre with special interest and expertise in childhood diabetes. To ensure long, healthy survival of these children and adolescents, particularly in the Third World environment, help from adequate professional and ancillary resources should be sought to offer the patients optimal care. Improved family education and co-ordinated care can decrease the need for hospitalization and prevent metabolic catastrophes which are often lethal or lead to permanent neurological damage.

Practical advice regarding food composition and timing should be given. Energy requirements should not be restricted, and should allow for the child's growth, e.g., 4 200 kj at one year of age, adding 420 kj for each additional year. Western-style 'junk foods', table sugar, and sweetened fizzy drinks should be avoided, and a return to traditional family foods rich in grains, vegetables, and fruit should be encouraged. Artificial sweeteners in moderate amounts are quite safe.

Ensuring the availability and proper storage of insulin — something so simple and at the same time so difficult — would have an enormous impact on reducing the morbidity and mortality associated with childhood diabetes in the Third World.

Local diabetes associations supported by the International Diabetes Federation can assist in pressurizing governmental health authorities to ensure a constant supply of insulin and of insulin syringes. The shelf-life of insulin at high environmental temperatures is unlikely to exceed 5–6 months, and exposure to direct sunlight will rapidly destroy it. Similarly, insulin must never be frozen. Insulin which has become yellowish or brown in colour, or which has flakes that do not dissolve, is unlikely to have retained its potency. As an international consensus has yet to be reached regarding a standardized insulin concentration — some countries use 100 u/ml, others have retained the old 40 u/ml — the use of syringes matched to the concentration has to be ensured to prevent tragic errors. It is safe for patients to use their own plastic insulin syringes repeatedly, and infection is rarely a problem. Test-strips tend to be scarce and expensive. They should be kept in a dark, air-tight bottle, and may be cut longitudinally in two without loss of accuracy. Every effort should also be made to equip each family with a vial of glucagon for subcutaneous use in case of hypoglycaemic coma.

Reasonable diabetes control is judged by normal growth and activity, lack of polyuria, and the absence of severe hypoglycaemic episodes. Glycosylated haemoglobin values close to the normal range are rarely achievable in a large proportion of children, and the test is invalid in the presence of a congenital haemolytic process. The successful management of these children — as judged only by the prevention of death or severe acute metabolic emergencies — still presents a formidable

challenge in the Third World, where the following problems are commonplace:

◆ insulin, syringes, and monitoring test strips are often scarce

◆ family resources make it impossible to adhere to a regulated life-style and predictable meals

◆ community health facilities are inadequate and people have no ready access to telephones or transport

◆ educational and cultural factors make it difficult for people to understand the complexities of the disorder and its management.

The primary health care worker must be prepared to provide a person-to-person supportive and educative service, if possible at or near the patient's home.

Acute acquired metabolic disturbances

These occur frequently in childhood, and often require correction in their own right, irrespective of the diseases causing them. Obviously there is considerable overlap with *inherited* metabolic diseases, as for example hypoglycaemia occurring in some glycogen-storage diseases, or acidosis in renal tubular disorders.

Disorders of acid base regulation

The pH of the body fluids is normally maintained within a fairly narrow range. Acidosis indicates a disturbance which can lead to a body pH below normal (7.4 ± 0.02). Conversely, alkalosis indicates a condition in which the pH may become higher than normal. A large number of hydrogen ions are produced daily from metabolic sources; these are mopped up by the body's buffer systems. While haemoglobin and the plasma proteins have the biggest buffering capacity, the bicarbonate/carbonic acid system is the most important buffer, because of the body's ability to excrete CO_2 through the lungs and thus rapidly adjust the hydrogen ion concentration:

$$H^+ + HCO_3 \leftrightarrows H_2CO_3 \leftrightarrows CO_2 + H_2O$$

If the primary disturbance lies in an altered pCO_2 through alveolar hypo- or hyperventilation, it is classified as respiratory acidosis or alkalosis. If the defect is primarily one of H^+ or HCO_3^-, it is classified as a metabolic disturbance.

Compensatory respiratory or metabolic mechanisms come into play in all disturbances to oppose the effect of the primary problem with the pH.

Assessment

The clinical circumstances indicate the possibility of a disturbance in acid-base regulation *(see Table 20.7)*.

Clinical examination is performed for evidence of dehydration or shock, for respiratory disease, and for cyanosis, ketosis, rickets, or other abnormality.

In metabolic acidosis, respiratory compensation results in deep, rapid respiration with pursed lips, but with no evidence of disease in the airways. In severe acidosis, peripheral vasoconstriction and poor capillary filling is often present even without other signs of shock. In neonates, significant acidosis may be unaccompanied by the usual physical signs. In severe metabolic alkalosis, the breathing pattern becomes shallow and infrequent.

The acid-base status is measured by means of a blood gas analysis (Astrup). The pH is the most important measurement, indicating the severity and need for treatment. The pCO_2 and HCO_3 levels indicate respiratory and metabolic components respectively.

Table 20.7   Acid-base disturbances

Disorder	Mechanism	Common associated conditions
Metabolic acidosis	Anaerobic Glycolysis Lactic acid	Tissue anoxia Shock
	Ketoacidosis	Starvation Diabetes mellitus Glycogen storage disease
	Organic acidaemia	Branch chain amino-aciduria, e.g., Maple syrup urine disease
	Administration of acidifying agents	NH_4Cl administration
	Reduced renal excretion of H^+	Renal tubular acidosis Renal failure Renal immaturity
	Gastrointestinal: Loss of HCO_3	Acute diarrhoea
	Renal loss of HCO_3	Chronic renal failure Renal tubular acidosis Acetazolamide treatment
Respiratory acidosis	Retention of CO_2 by the lung	Pulmonary disease Muscle paralysis or spasm
Metabolic alkalosis	Loss of H^+ from gut	Excess vomiting, e.g., plyoric stenosis, gastric drainage
	Loss of H^+ through kidneys	Diuretic: furosemide
	Excess renal HCO_3 retention	Hypochloraemia Hyperaldosteronism Hypokalaemia
	Administration of alkali	Bicarbonate administration Citrate administration Lactate administration
Respiratory alkalosis	Hyperventilation with exhalation of CO_2	Voluntary hyperventilation - emotional Central respiratory stimulation — drugs, e.g., salicylates — brain stem involvement

Often ancillary investigations help to elucidate the problem. The 'anion gap' refers to the difference between the sum of cation concentrations Na^+, K^+, Mg^{++}, Ca^{++} and the sum of the anion concentration Cl^-, HCO_3^-, $SO_4^=$, $PO_4^=$. This difference normally reflects the anionic contribution of plasma proteins and organic acid. An anion gap larger than 16 mmol/l indicates abnormal acid accumulation. A common cause for this is salicylate intoxication, but ketoacidosis secondary to starvation or diabetes, shock and hypoxia, and inherited disorders such as organic acidaemia are also associated with high anion gap metabolic acidosis.

The serum electrolytes may show hypokalaemia or hypochloraemia, while a high Cl^- out of keeping with the serum sodium is often a clue to a long-standing low plasma bicarbonate level.

Management

Appropriate treatment must be directed at the underlying disorder, e.g., fluid and/or glucose deficit, shock, vomiting, hypoxia, or respiratory failure. That is the only requirement in the majority of instances.

The pH must be corrected if outside the range 7.2–7.5, as this is important for cellular function. In **metabolic acidosis**, $NaHCO_3$ is given IV according to the formula: mmol HCO_3 = base deficit x 0.3 body mass (kg) (8.4% = 1 mmol/ml, 4.2% = 0.5 mmol/ml).

In severe **metabolic alkalosis**, NH_4Cl (5% solution = 1 mmol/ml) can be given according to the formula: mmol NH_4Cl = base excess x 0.3 body mass (kg).

In the absence of pH measurements, clinical signs of metabolic acidosis suggest a base deficit of 10 or more. $NaHCO_3$ may be given as a slow bolus intravenously (8.4%, 2 ml/kg).

Complications of treatment: Rapid administration of bicarbonate for correction of pH may result in fluid overload and a drop in serum ionized calcium level, causing tetany, as well as hypokalaemia and hypernatraemia, especially if over 8 mmol/kg is given (1 mmol bicarb = 1 mmol Na).

In neonates there is a well-documented association between the administration of bicarbonate and intraventricular haemorrhage.

Hypoglycaemia

The blood glucose level reflects the balance between glucose production and utilization. In the fasting state, glucose is produced by the process of glycogenolysis and gluconeogenesis. Intake of glucose from dietary sources or by intravenous administration contributes to the blood glucose level. Glucose utilization occurs obligatorily by red blood cells, brain, and kidney as their major source of energy, and by other tissues primarily under the influence of insulin.

The acute **symptoms** of hypoglycaemia result from deranged cerebral metabolism. In neonatal life they are non-specific and include lethargy, hypotonia, poor feeding, apnoea attacks, jitteriness or convulsions. In older children an acute fall of blood sugar results in sympathetic effects: there is a feeling of hunger and weakness, pallor, tachycardia and sweating; then headaches, visual disturbances, drowsiness, and coma or convulsions may occur. In those cases where the blood sugar level has been dropping gradually there may be very few warning signs before the patient becomes comatose or convulses.

Severe hypoglycaemia is a preventable cause of mental retardation in infancy, especially if recurrent.

In neonates, even asymptomatic hypoglycaemia may interfere with normal brain development. A whole blood glucose level less than 2.2 mmol/l constitutes hypoglycaemia *(see Chapter 5, Newborns)*.

Thus all seriously ill infants, especially while on restricted intake, need to have blood glucose levels monitored regularly, e.g., by Dextrostix®. This is especially true of malnourished patients who have decreased glycogen stores. In kwashiorkor, the development of hypoglycaemia is regarded as a serious sign, signalling severe substrate deficiency and inability to increase gluconeogenesis *(see Chapter 7, Nutritional Disorders)*.

Symptomatic hypoglycaemia calls for urgent treatment. Where an IV line is not available, oral glucose 10–25% solution should be given by nasogastric tube in a dose of 1 g/kg body mass. Otherwise 1 g/kg is given as a 50% solution IV. The symptoms should be rapidly relieved unless hypoglycaemia has been of long duration, or there are other complications such as liver failure. Thereafter it is important to confirm that the blood sugar has risen and is maintained within normal levels.

It is not sufficient to identify hypoglycaemia without explaining its pathogenesis, as only then can appropriate preventive therapy be instituted. The approach to investigation of a patient with hypoglycaemia depends on the history and examination. Particularly when hypoglycaemia is a recurrent unexplained finding, a blood sample should be obtained for glucose, urea, and electrolytes, liver function tests, insulin, lactate, ketones, and cortisol prior to giving intravenous glucose.

Blood sugar disturbances are summarized in *Table 20.8*.

Electrolyte disturbances

Electrolyte disturbances are summarized in *Table 20.9*.

Sodium is the principal extracellular cation. Thus major changes in serum sodium cause alterations in the osmolality of the extracellular fluid in relation to the intracellular compartment; hence water moves along the concentration gradient. The serum sodium level thus also reflects the state of the intracellular compartment.

Hyponatraemia

In hyponatraemia, water moves into the intracellular compartment with reduction of the extracellular volume and early development of circulatory insufficiency with any extra fluid losses.

Symptoms occur if there is an acute drop in the level of serum sodium. As the sodium level falls below 125 mmol/l, nausea, vomiting, muscle twitching, and lethargy may appear. If the level falls below 115 mmol/l, seizures and coma may occur. Where the sodium level has been falling

Table 20.8 Blood sugar disturbances

Disturbance	Mechanism	Common conditions
Hyperglycaemia	Insulin deficiency	Diabetes mellitus
	Defective glucose uptake	'Sick cell syndrome'
		Hypokalaemia
	Increased gluconeogenesis	Steroid therapy or excess
	Increased glycogenolysis	Stress-mediated catecholamine release
	Iatrogenic	High-concentration glucose administration
Hypoglycaemia		
Decreased availability or production of glucose	Subtrate deficiency	Small for gestational age
		Protein-energy malnutrition
		Chronic diarrhoea
		Starvation
		'Ketotic' hypoglycaemia
	Defects of glycogenolysis	Glycogen storage diseases
	Defects of gluconeogenesis	Endocrine deficiencies
		Enzyme deficiencies
	Mixed hepatotoxins	Liver disease and failure
		'Impila'
		Jamaican vomiting sickness
		Salicylates
Increased utilization of glucose	Hyperinsulinism	Infant of diabetic mother
		Beckwith's syndrome
		Erythoblastosis fetalis
		Leucine sensitivity
		Insulin treatment
		Oral hypoglycaemic agents
	Tumours of mesothelial orgin	Islet cell adenoma

slowly, many patients are relatively asymptomatic.

Severe hyponatraemia of less than 120 mmol/l requires correction. If the patient is dehydrated, the replacement fluid should have a sodium concentration equal to that of normal saline (e.g., Ringer's lactate, Normal Saline). In the absence of dehydration, the formula employed

Table 20.9   Electrolyte disturbances

Disturbance	Mechanism	Common conditions
Hyponatraemia < 130 mmol/l	Na⁺ deficiency in excess of fluid losses	Diarrhoea
		Water enema
		Burns
		Sweat losses
		Low solute feeding
		Malnutrition
		Hot climate
		Adrenal insufficiency
		Renal tubular dysfunction
	Water retention	Congestive cardiac failure
		Cirrhosis
		Nephrotic syndrome
		Syndrome of inappropriate ADH secretion
Hypernatraemia > 150 mmol/l	With dehydration water loss > Na loss	Diarrhoea
		Diabetes insipidus
		Osmotic diuresis
	Without dehydration	Defective thirst sensation
		Concentrated feeds
Hypokalaemia	Deficient intake	Protein-energy malnutrition
	Gut losses	Diarrhoea
		Enemas
		Congenital Cl-losing diarrhoea
	Renal wasting	Renal tubular disease
		Alkalosis
		Diuretic treatment
		Muscle wasting
		Endocrine disease
Hyperkalaemia	Alteration in cell metabolism	Acidosis
		Hypoxia
	Decreased renal excretion	Oliguria
		Acidosis
		Hypoaldosteronism
Hypocalcaemia	Lack of intake, lack of absorption, hyperphosphataemia	Neonatala hypocalcaemia,
		Hypoparathyroidism,
		pseudohypoparathyroidism,
		Rickets
		Renal disease
Hypomagnesaemia	Decreased intake	Protein-energy malnutrition
	Gut losses	Chronic diarrhoea
	Urine losses	Chronic diuretic therapy
Hyperphosphataemia	Decreased renal excretion	Renal failure
		Parathyroid hormone deficiency
Hypophosphataemia	Inadequate intake	Premature neonate
	Renal losses	Hyperparathyroidism
		Renal tubular disorder

for acute correction in small volumes is as follows: mmol Na^+ required = (125 minus serum Na level) x 0.6 x wt (kg). This may be administered as hypertonic saline. (*Note*: 1 ml 3% NaCl = 0.5 mmol Na^+; 1 ml 5%, NaCl = 0.87 mmol Na^+.)

Hypernatraemia

In **hypernatraemia with dehydration**, the osmotic gradient ensures water movement into the extracellular and intravascular compartments. This means that clinical signs of dehydration are masked.

Therefore the signs and symptoms of hypernatraemic dehydration are predominantly those of intracellular water loss from brain cells, with depressed sensorium, irritability, and even convulsions. The severity of neurological symptoms depends on the degree and the rate of rise of plasma osmolality. Therapy of hypernatraemic dehydration is directed at two goals: firstly, rapid restoration of intravascular volume by means of plasma expanders such as Ringer's lactate if circulatory insufficiency is present, and secondly, more gradual correction of the water deficit over 48 hours. Rapid correction of hypernatraemia at a rate faster than 1 mmol/l/hr carries the risk of water movement into brain cells down the osmotic gradient, with resultant cerebral oedema and convulsions. The rate of fall in the serum sodium depends on the speed of administration as well as on the sodium concentration of the infused fluid. For patients with a serum sodium above 160 mmol/l, the sodium concentration of the infused fluid is therefore initially raised to 90–105 mmol/l by adding sodium bicarbonate 8.4% to half-strength Darrow's/dextrose for about 6 hours. Thereafter half-strength Darrow's/dextrose can be used. The fluid is given at a steady rate of 10 ml/kg/hr, unless the patient has large continuing stool losses.

The treatment of the **hypernatraemic patient without dehydration** consists of an adequate water supply and salt restriction. If fluid overload is severe, peritoneal dialysis may remove a large amount of sodium.

Hypokalaemia

(*Also see Chapter 11, Gastrointestinal Disorders.*)

The symptoms of hypokalaemia depend to a certain extent on the rate of change of the serum potassium level. Heart, skeletal and smooth muscle, kidney, and brain are affected. Weakness, leading to hypotonia, and even paralysis and areflexia, occurs. This may be severe and resemble poliomyelitis with respiratory muscle depression. Cardiac arrhythmias and ECG changes may occur. Ileus may develop. Prolonged hypokalaemia leads to renal tubular changes, with reduced concentrating ability and subsequently interstitial nephritis. In treatment, oral potassium chloride 3–6 mEq/kg/24 hours is advised. In conditions of severe renal losses, e.g., Bartter's syndrome, up to 10 mEq/kg per 24 hours may be required. However, the concentration of potassium in intravenous fluids should not exceed 40 mmol/l. (1 mEq = 1 mmol; 1 g KCl = 13 mEq.)

Hyperkalaemia

Hyperkalaemia is a life-threatening condition and must be considered an emergency.

A substantial increase in total body potassium is incompatible with life. A moderate elevation of serum potassium is quite normal in the neonatal period, but thereafter a rise above 6.5 mmol/l is associated with a change in myocardial function, with a risk of ventricular fibrillation and death. The ECG will show peaked T waves, flattening of the P wave, prolongation of the PR interval, and progressive widening of the QRS complex.

As haemolysis of a blood specimen may cause an erroneously high potassium level, the decision to treat a patient for hyperkalaemia should be taken when a level of 6.5 mmol/l or above is associated with these specific ECG changes.

Treatment for hyperkalaemia:

♦ Eliminate all potassium intake.

♦ Administer sodium bicarbonate to correct metabolic acidosis.

♦ Inject 10% calcium gluconate, 0.5–1.0 ml/kg intravenously, slowly.

♦ Give intravenous glucose, 1–3 g/kg over 1 hour. Soluble insulin, 1 unit/3 g glucose, may be added to this infusion.

♦ Consider peritoneal dialysis if there is no improvement.

Hypomagnesaemia

Magnesium is an essential co-factor for many enzyme systems in oxidative phosphorylation, glucose utilization, and muscle contraction. It is required for the normal release of parathyroid hormone in response to hypocalcaemia. It is the second most important *intracellular* cation after potassium. Deficiency is common in conditions of protein-energy malnutrition and chronic diarrhoea, or with prolonged diuretic therapy. A dose of 250–500 mg of magnesium sulphate (0.5–1.0 ml 50% $MgSO_4$) given IM or IV daily for 3–5 days will usually correct the deficit.

Hypocalcaemia

Symptoms occur when there is a decrease in the ionized fraction of serum calcium. This accounts for about 50% of the total serum calcium if the serum albumin level is normal. The measured total serum calcium may be reduced by as much as 0.2 mmol/1 for every 10 g/l decrease in serum albumin, without any clinical features of hypocalcaemia.

In the presence of metabolic acidosis, the proportion of ionized calcium is increased, whilst in alkalosis, the reduction of the ionized fraction may result in symptoms despite near-normal calcium levels. Hypokalaemia can prevent the symptoms of hypocalcaemia from developing.

Sustained hypocalcaemia with onset in, or persistence beyond, the neonatal period is due to parathyroid hormone deficiency or resistance, vitamin D deficiency or resistance, chronic lack of calcium intake or absorption, and conditions leading to hyperphosphataemia, such as chronic renal disease.

The **clinical features** of hypocalcaemia are those of increased neuromuscular irritability, seizures and signs of raised intracranial pressure, eye and skin changes *(see below)*, and cardiac arrest. The latter may be preceded by ECG changes. The symptoms of neonatal hypocalcaemia include tremor or cyanotic attacks, and may resemble those of septicaemia, intracranial pathology, or metabolic disturbance.

Manifest tetany is when there are spontaneous spasms of motor muscles with sensory disturbances or central nervous excitability. This leads to jitteriness and convulsions. Typically, there is no depression of consciousness between convulsions. The characteristic carpopedal spasm consists of flexion and adduction at the wrist and metacarpophalangeal joints, with similar muscle spasms around the ankles. Laryngospasm *(laryngismus stridulus)* results in a stridulous, interrupted type of crowing inspiratory noise, or it may lead to apnoea. Sensory disturbances consist of tingling or numbness of the extremities.

Latent tetany may be detected by positive Chvostek's or Trousseau's signs. The former is elicited by tapping over the facial nerve anterior to the ear, and results in a twitching of the muscle of the ipsilateral side of the face. The latter consists of carpal spasm when a blood pressure cuff on the arm is kept inflated to just above the systolic blood pressure for 3 minutes.

Chronic hypocalcaemia leds to dystropic manifestations which include lenticular cataracts, dry and scaling skin, coarse hair, brittle nails, and enamel hypoplasia of teeth.

The **management** involves attention to rapid reversal of the underlying conditons. A slow intravenous injection of 2 ml/kg of calcium gluconate 10% is given, with monitoring of the heart rate during injection to detect and avoid bradycardia. Thereafter, oral calcium supplements may be prescribed, but this depends on the underlying or associated disorder.

Hyperphosphataemia

This occurs under the following main sets of circumstances:

♦ decreased glomerular filtration rate, as in acute or chronic renal failure

♦ increased load due to a large intake, e.g., cows' milk in young infants, or phosphate-containing enemas

♦ increased load from endogenous tissue destruction, e.g., cytotoxic therapy

♦ increased tubular reabsorption of phosphate due to deficiency of or resistance to parathyroid hormone.

Hyperphosphataemia depresses the serum calcium level and may lead to secondary hyperparathyroidism. A major clinical sequela of hyperphosphataemia is soft tissue calcification due to an increased Ca x P product.

Treatment involves identification of the predisposing cause. When renal phosphate excretion is reduced, intestinal phosphate-binding compounds such as magnesium trisilicate and aluminium hydroxide are used. The intake of dietary phosphate should also be reduced.

Hypophosphataemia

In view of the important role of phosphate in intracellular processes (ATP; CAMP; 2,3 DPG), as well as in mineralization of bone, phosphate deficiency can have a variety of effects. These include proximal muscle weakness with pain and hypotonia, neurological manifestations ranging from irritability and paraesthesiae to convulsions and coma, as well as diminished tissue oxygenation and decreased leucocyte function.

Hypophosphataemia is caused by excessive renal losses, e.g., familial hypophosphataemic rickets, renal tubular acidosis or hyperparathyroidism, inadequate intake (for example in premature infants), and rapid flux from extracellular to intracellular compartments (as for example during correction of diabetic ketoacidosis).

Treatment involves the correction of precipitating factors, as well as phosphate supplementation. This should be given several times a day to maintain aedquate phosphate levels.

Inherited metabolic disorders
Prevalence

The inherited metabolic diseases are rare. There are also wide regional variations in prevalence, due to factors such as genetic drift, founder effect, geographical and climatic influences, rate of consanguinous marriages, as well as heterozygote advantage. However, the rarity of inherited metabolic diseases in Third World countries may well be more apparent than real, due to lack of facilities and expertise for diagnosis. In addition, the true incidence may be masked by a high prevalence of nutritional and infective disorders and a high infant mortality rate.

(Also see Chapter 3, Genetics and Congenital Disorders.)

Pathogenesis

A genetically determined deficiency of enzymes, or of cofactors or other protein molecules leads to manifestations of disease in several ways *(see Fig. 20.3).*

Diagnosis

Traditional teaching has left many clinicians ignorant of the early manifestations of inherited metabolic disorders, and unprepared to take the necessary steps to diagnose them.

Neonates and young infants have a limited range of responses to severe illness, which are non-specific, viz., irritability, poor feeding, lethargy, vomiting, and failure to thrive.

Furthermore, these features tend to occur much more frequently in conditions which are not primarily metabolic. The picture is often that of an infant in deep coma or with vascular collapse, and the first impression is of septicaemia or cerebral haemorrhage.

Metabolic disease may mimic septicaemia, with coma and vascular collapse.

However, the *circumstances* under which the symptoms develop are usually more characteristic than the symptoms themselves:

♦ onset after several hours or days of good health
♦ occurrence in a full-term baby, following a non-traumatic delivery
♦ a relentless recurrence and progression of symptoms once they do appear
♦ a family history of consanguinity or unexplained early neonatal loss

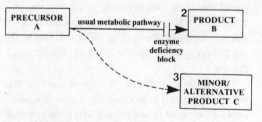

1 Substrate and precursor accumulation
Intracellular storage
Blood accumulation
Loss through gut or urine

2 Product Deficit

3 Utilization of minor or alternative pathways
Abnormal product accumulation.

Fig. 20.3 Genetically determined origins of disease

◆ a suspicious association of symptoms and biochemical abnormalities.

An inborn error ought to be seriously considered at an early stage in the presence of any suspicious clue, even when no obvious cause of the illness can be established. The laboratory tools available to investigate these conditions vary greatly in their complexity, but the screening methods for detecting them are few in number, comprising hypoglycaemia, electrolyte imbalance, metabolic acidosis with raised anion gap (serum chloride needs to be measured), ketonuria, ketonaemia, raised ammonia and lactate. Associating a persistent symptom with a persistent first-step biochemical abnormality is the first move in the right direction, both with regard to diagnosis and management.

Many late-onset presentations, usually occurring after 6 months of age, are preceded by insidious or intermittent warning symptoms which are commonly misdiagnosed or overlooked:

◆ gastrointestinal: failure to thrive, recurrent vomiting, hepatomegaly, jaundice
◆ neurological: developmental delay, progressive retardation, long-tract signs, lethargy, seizures
◆ musculoskeletal: floppiness, rickets
◆ general: abnormal odour
◆ specific entities: anaemia, cirrhosis, renal tubular disorder, cataracts, coarse facial appearance.

Screening and initial management

Table 20.10 lists some of the simple screening procedures which will facilitate the clinician's task when faced with a possible metabolic disorder. Instructions must be observed meticulously

Table 20.10   Screening procedures in the newborn nursery

Blood	Glucose
	Electrolytes
	Acid-base
	Ca, P, Mg
Urine	Colour
	Smell
	Reducing substances
	Ferric chloride and Phenistix®
	Acetest or Ketotest®
	2,4-DNP-hydrazine

Table 20.11   Classification of inborn errors into broad groups

1. Presentation with acute metabolic crisis (newborn or later onset)
   • neurological distress and signs of intoxication with ketosis and hyperammonaemia
   • neurological distress with emphasis on acidosis (lactic, organic)
   • signs of intoxication with severe hyperammonaemia
   • hypoglycaemic seizures with acidosis (lactic, ketosis)
2. Storage disorders excluding the central nervous system
3. Central nervous system storage disorders

and the reagents must be fresh. If recurrent hypoglycaemia is the main problem, it is important to take blood samples at specific times in relation to food intake. Thus, clinical and laboratory data can be assembled in a few hours, obviating long waiting periods for sophisticated results or inappropriate referrals. Classification of patients within a few broad groups *(see Table 20.11)* makes more sense than getting entangled in the complexity of metabolic pathways and their molecular defects.

As some of these metabolic disorders can cause irreversible brain damage, it is important to take interim measures once suspicion has been aroused and preliminary investigations are under way. While awaiting a more definitive diagnosis, a preliminary plan of management needs to be instituted *(see Table 20.12)*. What appears to be 'shot-gun' therapy will increase the infant's chances of survival and prevent major brain damage.

Whereas it may be impossible to implement the plan of action in its totality, every effort should be made to achieve as much as possible.

Access to special feeds, substrates, and megavitamins will undoubtedly be problematic in

Table 20.12   Plan for preliminary management of infant with suspected metabolic disorder

Total protein restriction
Ensure adequate calorie intake
Megavitamin cocktail
    folic acid, ascorbic acid, biotin, B_{12}
Sodium benzoate, lactulose, neomycin
Hormones or antagonists
Reintroduction of minimum protein intake

remote areas, but early contact with a referral centre may facilitate the treatment plan. Close dietary supervision and frequent biochemical monitoring may also not be feasible.

Precise diagnosis — resting on sophisticated biochemical investigations of blood, urine, or skin biopsy samples — is an essential prerequisite for genetic counselling; this may demand no greater effort than arranging transport of a few specimens to a distant laboratory.

Despite the rarity of these disorders and the perceived lack of relevance in the context of more pressing health needs of many communities, real benefit may be derived from a raised index of suspicion and the use of inexpensive preliminary screening tests with early access to experts.

F. Bonnici
D.F. Wittenberg

21

Metabolic bone disorders

Introduction

Metabolic bone disease in children may present clinically in one of several ways:

Osteomalacia and rickets, in which there is failure of, or delay in, mineralization of uncalcified osteoid or bone matrix. Thus the ratio of uncalcified osteoid to calcified bone is increased.

Osteoporosis, in which the total amount of bone per unit volume is decreased. The ratio of uncalcified osteoid to calcified bone is normal. The pathogenesis is related either to inadequate formation of bone matrix or to increased resorption of preformed bone.

Osteosclerosis, in which there is an increase in calcified bone per unit volume. It is generally due to a failure of normal bone resorption or an increase in bone formation.

It should be noted that osteomalacia and osteoporosis frequently may be found together in the same patient, and that in renal failure all forms of bone disease may occur together.

Rickets, osteomalacia, and the Fanconi syndromes

Rickets and osteomalacia refer to those bone diseases which present with a failure of mineralization of preformed bone matrix. Rickets manifests as a delay in mineralization at the growth plate, and thus only occurs in children whose epiphyses have not yet fused. Osteomalacia refers to a delay in mineralization at the endosteal bone surface, and thus occurs in both children and adults. In children, rickets and osteomalacia occur concomitantly.

Metabolism of vitamin D

In order to understand the pathogenesis of rickets, a knowledge of the role of vitamin D and its metabolites in the control of calcium homeostasis is necessary *(see Fig. 21.1).*

Humans acquire vitamin D either through the absorption of ingested vitamin D or by the conversion of 7-dehydrocholesterol to vitamin D in the skin under the influence of ultraviolet light. Most diets are deficient in vitamin D, so to prevent vitamin D deficiency, people rely heavily on that formed in the skin.

Once absorbed from the gastrointestinal tract or formed in the skin, vitamin D is either stored in muscle and fat, or transported to the liver where it is hydroxylated to 25-hydroxyvitamin D_3 (i.e., 25-OHD$_3$), the major circulating form of the vitamin. Both these compounds are inactive in people at physiological concentrations. 25-OHD$_3$ is transported to the kidney, where it undergoes further metabolism. Under the influence of parathyroid hormone (PTH) or hypophosphataemia, 25-OHD$_3$ is hydroxylated to 1,25-dihydroxyvitamin D_3 (i.e., 1,25-(OH)$_2$D$_3$), the active metabolite. Under the reverse set of circumstances an apparently inactive metabolite, 24,25-dihydroxyvitamin D_3 (i.e., 24,25-(OH)$_2$D$_3$) is formed. Both are excreted as 1,24,25(OH)$_3$D$_3$.

1,25-(OH)$_2$D$_3$ plays a central role in calcium homeostasis. Its principal sites of action are the gut, where it promotes calcium — and to a lesser extent phosphorus — absorption; and bone, where it acts synergistically with parathyroid hormone to increase bone resorption. Both of these actions increase the serum concentrations of calcium and phosphorus.

Causes of rickets
(See Table 21.1.)

The causes of rickets may be divided broadly into two groups:
- those primarily resulting in an inadequate supply of calcium
- those primarily producing hypophosphataemia.

Table 21.1 lists the common causes of rickets.

Calcium deficiency rickets
(See Fig. 21.2.)

455

Table 21.1 The causes of rickets/osteomalacia in children

Calcium deficiency rickets

a. ***Abnormalitites in vitamin D metabolism***

Nutritional rickets
- dietary defiency of Vitamin D; inadequate exposure to sunlight

Impaired absorption of vitamin D
- steatorrhoea, e.g., coeliac disease
- biliary obstruction, e.g., biliary atresia

Impaired hydroxylation of vitamin D to 25-hydroxy-vitamin D
- liver immaturity
- ?prematurity

Increased metabolism of vitamin D
- anticonvulsant drugs, e.g., phenobarbitone

Decreased renal synthesis of 1,25-dihydroxy-vitamin D
- renal failure
- vitamin D dependency rickets

End-organ resistance to 1,25-dihydroxyvitamin D

b. ***Dietary deficiency of calcium***
- e.g., prematurity

Phosphorus deficiency rickets

Decreased intake of phosphate
- prematurity

Decreased intestinal absorption of phosphate
- ingestion of large amounts of aluminium hydroxide

Increased renal losses of phosphate
- hypophosphataemic vitamin D resistant rickets:
  - X-linked
  - sporadic
- Fanconi syndrome
- mesenchymal tumours

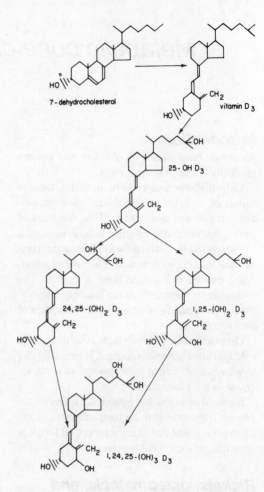

Fig. 21.1   The metabolism of vitamin D. Vitamin D is converted to 25-OHD in the liver, while both 1,25-(OH)₂D and 24,25-(OH)₂D are formed in the kidney

A. Abnormalities of vitamin D metabolism

Nutritional vitamin D deficiency

Aetiology: Rickets is generally thought of as a disease occurring particularly in countries in the northernmost latitudes, especially in large industrial cities, where cloudy skies and air pollution prevent an adequate exposure to ultraviolet light. However, rickets is well documented in India, the Middle East and Africa, and is seen frequently in infants in South Africa. The aetiology is an inadequate vitamin D intake, coupled with a lack of exposure to sunlight. Once

the infant is walking (1–2 years of age), vitamin deficiency is rarely seen in South Africa because of the abundant sunshine.

Breast milk contains only very small quantities of vitamin D or its metabolites. Their concentrations are normally insufficient to meet the daily requirements of the breast-fed infant, who is thus dependent on sun exposure or vitamin D supplementation to maintain an adequate vitamin D status. Cows' milk contains almost no vitamin D, so to prevent vitamin deficiency in infancy, all infant milk formulas in South Africa are supplemented with vitamin D (400 IU/litre). Except in rare cases where the mother is vitamin D deficient,

RICKETS

CALCIUM DEFICIENCY

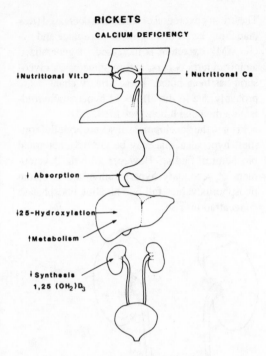

Fig. 21.2   Calcium deficiency rickets

rickets does not manifest in the first few months of life. The reason for this is that 25-0HD crosses the placenta, and at birth the neonate's levels correlate well with maternal concentrations.

Clinical features *(see Table 21.2)*: Rickets in the infant presents in its severest form with bone deformities, particularly involving the wrists, legs, chest-cage and skull. The extent and site of the deformities are determined largely by pressure effects such as those occurring during crawling. Leg deformities include knock-knees or bow-legs. In the young infant bowing of the distal tibia may occur. Chest deformities such as Harrison's sulcus involving the lower ribs, and the 'violin case deformity' of the upper ribs, are due to the effects of the diaphragm and intercostal muscles acting on abnormally pliable and soft ribs. Enlargement of the costochondral junctions produces the rickety rosary. The child who lies with his head frequently turned to one side may develop an asymmetric skull. The fontanelles are often large, and closure is delayed. Frontal and parietal bossing may give the typical 'hot-cross bun' appearance. Craniotabes, the sign elicited by being able to depress the skull bones above and behind the ears,

Table 21.2   The clinical features of vitamin D deficiency rickets

Signs of hypocalcaemia:
   Convulsions
   Apnoeic attacks
   Tetany
Signs of muscle weakness:
   Hypotonia
   Delayed motor milestones
   Prominent abdomen
Signs of delayed mineralization:
   Widened metaphyses (especially wrists and knees)
   Craniotabes in the young infant
   Delayed closure of fontanelles
   Enlarged costochondral junctions
   Harrison's sulcus
   Bowing of the long bones

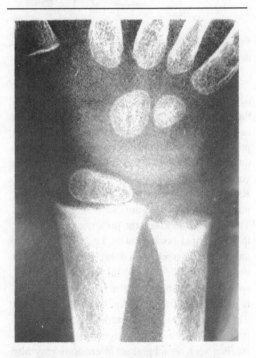

Fig. 21.3   Radiological features of rickets: widening of the epiphyseal plate, splaying and cupping of the metaphysis, irregularity of the metaphyseal plate and thinning of the cortices

is often present in young infants presenting with rickets, but is not pathognomonic of the disease. The metaphyses of the wrists, ankles, and knees may become palpably enlarged. Muscle weakness may be a prominent feature of vitamin D

457

deficiency, the weakness being more apparent in the proximal muscles. Knee and ankle reflexes may be increased in this condition. The severely affected infant has a protuberant abdomen and sweats excessively. Dentition may also be affected, with a delay in the eruption of primary dentition and, if rickets has been present for a prolonged period of time, enamel hypoplasia may occur. Signs of hypocalcaemia may also be present, and are usually associated with the classical features of rickets.

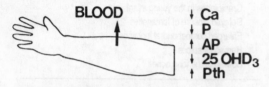

Fig. 21.4   Biochemical features of vitamin D deficiency rickets

In the early stages of vitamin D deficiency, bone deformities are not present. The infant may pass through this phase with no symptoms whatsoever, and present later with bone deformities; or may present early with apnoeic spells or convulsions due to hypocalcaemia. This is particularly so in the young infant.

Radiographic features: Radiologically, the features of severe rickets are diagnostic *(Fig. 21.3)*. The best sites to assess the presence of rickets are those of rapid bone growth, i.e., the wrists and knees. The features are a delay in epiphyseal development, widening of the epiphyseal plate, splaying and cupping of the metaphysis, and irregularity and fraying of the metaphyseal plate. The bones are osteopenic, with thin cortices and a coarse trabecular pattern. Signs of hyperparathyroidism such as subperiosteal erosions may also be found.

Early radiological features of rickets are difficult to detect, and may only manifest as decalcification of the skull bones or blurring of the metaphyseal plates at the wrists.

Biochemical features *(see Fig. 21.4)*: The typical biochemical features of vitamin D deficiency are hypocalcaemia, hypophosphataemia, elevated alkaline phosphatase concentrations, elevated parathyroid hormone levels, and low 25-0HD values.

The urinary excretion of calcium is decreased (less than 2 mg/kg/24 hours), while phosphate and cyclic AMP excretion is increased. A generalized aminoaciduria occurs, and in some cases glycosuria has been noted. These urinary changes are probably due to the effects of hyperparathyroidism on the renal tubule *(see Fig. 21.5)*.

Prior to the development of severe bone deformities, hypocalcaemia may be the only abnormal biochemical finding. However, with the development of secondary hyperparathyroidism, serum phosphorus values fall and alkaline phosphatase concentrations rise.

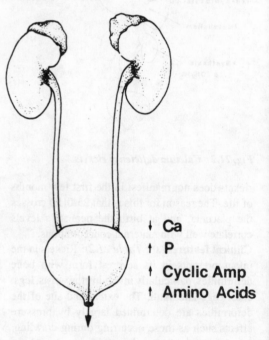

Fig. 21.5   Urinary abnormalities in vitamin D deficiency rickets

The normal values of certain parameters used to detect and classify the various types of rickets are age-dependent. Serum phosphorus concentrations are highest in the immediate neonatal period (1.8–2.6 mmol/l), falling rapidly over the next 6 months to a plateau (1.3–2.0 mmol/l) which persists until puberty, when values gradually fall to adult levels (< 1.3 mmol/l). The interpretation of alkaline phosphatase values is further complicated by the plethora of units used to measure this enzyme (IU/l, King Armstrong Units, Brodzansky Units, etc.).

In infancy concentrations may be slightly higher than throughout childhood (100–300 IU/l). During the adolescent growth spurt values rise (often up to 500 IU/l), and then fall rapidly to adult levels (< 100 IU/l). Serum calcium values (normal 2.25–2.75 mmol/l) change little throughout life, although there is a slight fall from childhood to old age. Total serum calcium values are dependent on albumin concentrations, so hypocalcaemia could be due to an actual decrease in ionized calcium levels or due to hypoalbuminaemia (of particular relevance in the malnourished child).

Treatment: Vitamin D deficiency is easily corrected by oral administration of vitamin D (1 000–5 000 IU/day) for a period of 6 weeks to 3 months. Within a month biochemical improvements will be observed and early evidence of radiological healing will be noted. If hypocalcaemia is a prominent feature, calcium supplements may be necessary in the early stages of treatment. If convulsions or apnoeic attacks occur, calcium gluconate (10%, 1–2 ml/kg) may be given slowly as an intravenous infusion, while the heart rate is closely monitored. In the young child, bone deformities may correct spontaneously over a period of months, thus orthopaedic correction of any deformities should be delayed as long as possible.

Prevention is as important as the curative treatment of vitamin D deficiency. Even in South Africa, with its abundant sunshine, an adequate vitamin D intake should be ensured, particularly during the first year of life. The average diet contains little vitamin D, and cows' milk almost none. It is thus recommended that all infants should be supplemented with vitamin D (400 IU/day) from birth, unless they are on a supplemented milk formula.

Impaired absorption of vitamin D

Vitamin D, being fat-soluble, is absorbed by a mechanism similar to that of dietary fats. Thus any condition causing steatorrhoea may impair vitamin D absorption. If adequate exposure to sunlight occurs, the reduction in vitamin D absorption may not produce any deleterious effects. However, in infants or sick children not exposed to ultraviolet light, vitamin D deficiency may develop. Large doses of vitamin D (10 000–50 000 IU/day) may be necessary to overcome the malabsorption. The problem is further compounded by a concomitant calcium malabsorption due to the formation of insoluble calcium soaps with the malabsorbed fatty acids. In infants, neonatal hepatitis and biliary atresia might lead to severe rickets through this mechanism.

Impaired hydroxylation of vitamin D to 25-hydroxyvitamin D

Impaired formation of 25-0HD in the liver may occur in severe liver disease, and it has been suggested as a cause of rickets in premature infants who have an immature hepatic enzyme system. This latter possibility has not yet been adequately documented.

Increased metabolism of vitamin D

Anticonvulsants, especially phenobarbitone, increase hepatic hydroxylation and excretion of vitamin D. Further, diphenylhydantoin directly blocks calcium absorption from the intestine and may also impair bone mineralization. Thus, anticonvulsants may predispose children to a higher prevalence of rickets in several ways. This is particularly so in institutionalized children, whose vitamin D intakes may be sub-optimal. The problem can be overcome by supplementing the diet with vitamin D (1 000 IU/day). The biochemical features of anticonvulsant rickets are similar to those described in vitamin D deficiency. However, the alkaline phosphatase concentration is a poor indicator of the presence of rickets, as alkaline phosphatase levels may be elevated due to an increase in the serum concentrations of the hepatic iso-enzyme. The latter rise is a manifestation of the hepatic effects of phenobarbitone rather than an indicator of bone disease.

Decreased renal synthesis of 1,25-dihydroxyvitamin D

Vitamin D dependency rickets is a rare, autosomal-recessive condition which presents in infancy with a picture similar to that seen in vitamin D deficiency. However, the bone disease only responds to large doses of vitamin D (25 000–50 000 IU/day). It has recently been demonstrated that despite normal serum levels of 25-0HD, 1,25-$(OH)_2$D concentrations are low. Further, the disease responds dramatically to physiological doses of 1,25-(OH)$_2$D (0.5 µg/day). It is postulated that there is an absence or abnormality of the 1 hydroxylase enzyme which converts 25-OHD to 1,25-(OH)$_2$D in the kidney. No cases of this form of rickets have been reported in South Africa.

Renal failure is associated with decreased levels of 1,25-(OH)$_2$D and may present with rickets and osteomalacia, but the bone disease of renal failure (renal osteodystrophy) has a complicated pathogenesis. Early on in the development of renal failure, decreased renal excretion of phosphorus leads to hyperphosphataemia, secondary hypocalcaemia and concomitant hyperparathyroidism. Long-standing hyperparathyroidism leads to osteoporosis, osteitis fibrosa cystica, and osteosclerosis. The secondary hyperparathyroidism can be partially controlled by the administration of an oral phosphate-binding agent such as aluminium hydroxide or calcium carbonate, which decreases serum phosphorus concentrations. Besides secondary hyperparathyroidism and 1,25-(OH)$_2$D deficiency, chronic acidosis may aggravate bone loss in chronic renal failure.

Radiologically, the features of renal osteodystrophy are variable, with signs of either secondary hyperparathyroidism or rickets and osteomalacia predominating. Epiphyseal slipping and epiphysiolysis may occur and lead to severe deformities of the limbs.

The **biochemical abnormalities** of renal osteodystrophy can be distinguished from other forms of rickets by the elevated serum creatinine and urea levels characteristic of renal failure. Further, although hypocalcaemia is a feature of other forms of vitamin D-related rickets, hyperphosphataemia is usually found only in renal osteodystrophy.

Treatment requires careful monitoring. Serum calcium and phosphorus concentrations should be maintained within the normal range by means of calcium supplementation and phosphate-binding agents. Vitamin D therapy may be required, particularly if osteomalacia is a prominent feature, but the dose needed varies widely from patient to patient, and therefore should be increased only slowly. More recently, 1,25-(OH)$_2$D has been used in place of vitamin D with good results. In some instances, partial parathyroidectomy may be required to control the hyperparathyroid bone disease.

End-organ resistance to 1,25-dihydroxyvitamin D

Recently a new rare syndrome of peripheral resistance to 1,25-(OH)$_2$D has been described (vitamin D dependency rickets type II). These children present with features of calcium deficiency rickets, do not respond to the usual therapeutic doses of vitamin D, and have markedly elevated serum concentrations of 1,25-(OH)$_2$D. This syndrome is not a single disease entity, as several different biochemical defects in the receptors for 1,25-(OH)$_2$D have been described. The net effect of these receptor defects is a failure of response of the target organs to normal circulating concentrations of 1,25-(OH)$_2$D. One apparently homogeneous disease entity within this syndrome is associated with total alopecia. Treatment of this condition is unsatisfactory, as the patients respond only partially to massive doses of 1,25-(OH)$_2$D or to large oral calcium supplements.

B. Dietary deficiency of calcium

Low dietary calcium intake is a recognized cause of osteoporosis in animals and has been implicated in the pathogenesis of involutional osteoporosis in humans. However, only recently has this deficiency been shown to lead to rickets and osteomalacia in vitamin D-replete individuals. Several cases of rickets in rapidly growing infants on very low calcium diets have been reported. In breastfed very-low-birth-weight (VLBW) neonates (< 1 500 g) the low phosphorus intakes are thought to be responsible for the elevated alkaline phosphatase values, osteopenia, and rickets which become manifest in these infants at about 12 weeks of age. It is now suggested that if VLBW infants are fed breast milk, their feed should be supplemented with calcium and phosphorus.

There is also evidence that rural black children in South Africa may suffer from a similar problem, due to the low calcium content of their diets (mainly maize-based), if milk is not consumed on a regular basis. Patients from the Transvaal and Natal have been reported with this condition. They generally present between 5 and 18 years of age, with leg deformities characteristic of rickets, hypocalcaemia, variable serum phosphorus concentrations, elevated alkaline phosphatase values, and normal serum 25-OHD levels. Radiographs reveal the presence of osteopenia and active rickets at the metaphyses of the long bones. The features of rickets on X-ray may be so mild as to be missed at a cursory glance, but all have histological evidence of osteomalacia on bone biopsy.

The biochemical and radiological abnormalities respond to a normal ward diet, and there is no evidence that vitamin D supplementation speeds the recovery. A number of these children had been previously diagnosed as having vitamin D-resistant rickets, as they were outside the age range in which vitamin D deficiency was common. Dietary calcium intakes are estimated to be between 100 and 300 mg/day in these children (recommended daily allowance: 800 mg/day). This condition is the most common cause of rickets in children between the ages of 4 and 18 years of age who are admitted to Baragwanath Hospital, Soweto, for investigation.

Phosphorus deficiency rickets
(See Fig. 21.6.)

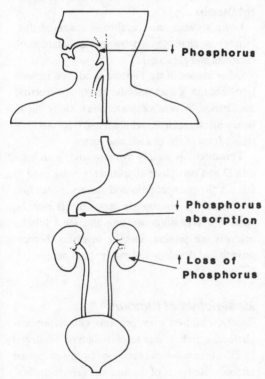

Fig. 21.6 Phosphorus deficiency rickets

Phosphorus depletion, despite an adequate vitamin D intake, may lead to the development of rickets. Unlike calcium or vitamin D deficiency, the disease is not accompanied by secondary hyperparathyroidism. Thus low urinary calcium excretion and a generalized aminoaciduria are generally not features of the disease. Furthermore, phosphorus depletion can be differentiated from vitamin D or calcium deficiency because phosphorus depletion is characteristically normocalcaemic.

Decreased intake of phosphorus
The average diet usually contains more than adequate phosphorus to meet requirements. However, premature infants fed on soya bean milk preparations have been reported to develop rickets, which has responded to phosphorus supplementation. Soya beans, like cereals, contain a portion of their phosphorus in the form of phytates, a complex phosphate molecule from which phosphorus is thought to be poorly absorbed. Very-low-birth-weight infants may also present with phosphorus deficiency rickets if they are exclusively breast-fed.

Decreased intestinal absorption of phosphorus
Unlike calcium, phosphorus absorption by the intestine is only partially controlled by body needs, and is generally very efficient. Although $1,25\text{-}(OH)_2D$ does increase phosphate absorption, it is little impaired in vitamin D deficiency states. Phosphorus absorption can be inhibited, however, by the ingestion of a phosphate-binding agent such as aluminium hydroxide, which is frequently used as an antacid in the treatment of peptic ulceration, or in the control of hyperphosphataemia in renal failure. If phosphate absorption is impaired sufficiently to induce hypophosphataemia, rickets and osteomalacia may occur.

Increased renal excretion of phosphate
Phosphate excretion by the kidney is controlled mainly in the proximal tubule. Although the mechanisms are not fully understood, two separate mechanisms have been described, one sensitive to parathyroid hormone and the other sensitive to calcium.

461

Hypophosphataemic vitamin D-resistant rickets

The classic example of this syndrome is X-linked hypophosphataemic vitamin D-resistant rickets. This disease is characterized by early growth failure, bone deformities, and excess renal phosphate loss. Biochemically, normocalcaemia and normal concentrations of parathyroid hormone distinguish it from the vitamin D-related causes of rickets. Further, unlike the Fanconi syndrome, there is no aminoaciduria and glycosuria is uncommon. In countries where vitamin D supplementation of all milks is routine, such as the USA, it has become the most common form of rickets seen in hospital. In South Africa it occurs in all racial groups, but the prevalence is unknown.

Although generally inherited as an X-linked condition, some 30% of cases appear to be the result of sporadic mutations. Affected males are always phenotypically abnormal, while females have a variable presentation, with some having only hypophosphataemia without bone deformities. The reason for the variable expression in females is explained by the Lyon hypothesis.

Radiologically, the picture is that of rickets, although signs of secondary hyperparathyroidism are absent. Osteopenia is also generally not seen. Muscle weakness, a feature of vitamin D-related causes of rickets, is absent in this condition.

The **diagnosis** is made by confirming a low tubular reabsorption of phosphorus in the absence of hyperparathyroidism.

Treatment is aimed at correcting the persistent hypophosphataemia. This is achieved by increasing the oral intake of phosphorus (1.5–3 g phosphorus/24 hours in 5 divided doses). As the increased phosphate load impairs calcium absorption and induces hypocalcaemia and secondary hyperparathyroidism, vitamin D (50 000 IU/day) is also given. Recently 1,25-$(OH)_2$D has been found to be more efficacious than vitamin D and is given in a dose of 0.5–1 μg/day. If treatment is adequate, growth rates usually increase and the bone disease heals. At present treatment is recommended until late adolescence, when growth has stopped and the epiphyses have fused. Treatment may be needed again in later life, when symptomatic osteomalacia may occur.

A rare, adult-onset form of hypophosphataemic osteomalacia has also been described. This is sporadic in nature, is associated with muscle weakness and, in some cases, with glycinuria. Treatment is similar to that used in the X-linked form of hypophosphataemic rickets.

Fanconi syndrome

The Fanconi syndromes do not constitute a single disease entity, but all are associated with proximal renal tubular dysfunction. In the severest form, the syndrome consists of phosphaturia, hypokalaemia, aminoaciduria, glycosuria, proximal renal tubular acidosis, and an absence of renal concentrating ability. Rickets and short stature are but two of the presenting signs, other features being more prominent depending on the aetiology.

Cystinosis, an autosomal-recessive disease characterized by the deposition of cystine crystals in many tissues, is associated with progressive renal failure, hepatomegaly, acidosis, and hypokalaemia.

Lowe's syndrome (cerebro-oculo-renal dystrophy) is characterized by mental retardation, cataracts and glaucoma.

Other causes of the Fanconi syndrome include tyrosinaemia, galactosaemia, hereditary fructose intolerance, Wilson's disease, and toxicity due to heavy metals such as cadmium and lead. An idiopathic form of the disease also exists.

Treatment is mainly symptomatic, with vitamin D and phosphate supplements being used to correct the phosphaturia and rickets. Potassium and citrate or bicarbonate supplements may be needed if potassium wasting and renal tubular acidosis are present. Despite vigorous therapy, growth and development may remain poor.

Mesenchymal tumours

Rarely, children may present with hypophosphataemic rickets due to phosphaturia produced by unknown substances secreted by mesenchymal tumours. Removal of the tumour corrects the biochemical abnormalities and heals the bone disease.

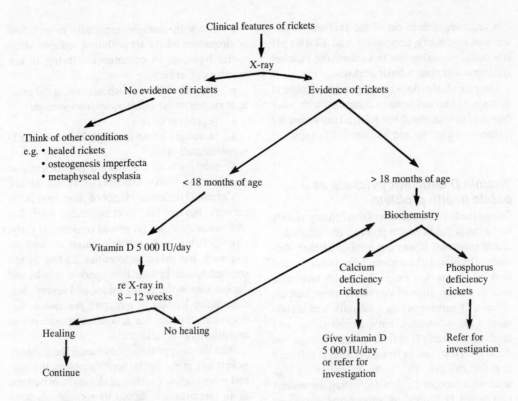

Fig. 21.7 Schematic approach to the diagnosis of rickets in a primary health care setting

The diagnosis of rickets in a primary health care situation

Fig. 21.7 provides a schematic approach to the management of a child with suspected rickets in a primary health care situation. Clinically, mild rickets is extremely difficult to diagnose accurately, as the signs are often difficult to assess, and are not pathognomonic of active rickets. In the child with gross bone deformities, other diseases such as osteogenesis imperfecta should also be considered. Craniotabes, although a sign which should alert the health care practitioner to the possibility of rickets, is frequently a normal finding in young infants, especially in those born prematurely. Rachitic rosary and widening of the wrists are difficult signs to interpret, especially in the thin child. It is therefore advisable not to treat a child for rickets without radiological confirmation of the disease. Further, if the child is walking, i.e., older than a year to 18 months, biochemical support should be obtained to help elucidate the aetiology of the rickets, as vitamin D deficiency is less likely in the child who can walk and therefore get out into the sun. In the infant, vitamin D deficiency is likely to be the cause, and a trial of therapy with vitamin D can be initiated without biochemical confirmation. It is important that the infant returns approximately 8 weeks after initiating therapy, for radiological confirmation of healing of the rickets. If healing is not evident on the radiographs, or if the child is outside the infant age group, then the following biochemical investigations are helpful in differentiating the various causes:

	Serum calcium	Serum phosphorus	Alkaline phosphatase
Calcium deficiency rickets	Low	Low/ normal	Elevated
Phosphorus deficiency rickets	Normal	Low	Elevated

A urine dipstick to detect the presence or absence of glycosuria, proteinuria, and alkaline pH is a useful screening test to exclude the Fanconi syndrome and renal tubular acidosis.

The patient who does not respond to vitamin D therapy, or who has features consistent with other causes of rickets, should be referred to a centre for further investigation and initiation of therapy.

Vitamin D deficiency rickets as a public health problem

During the first few decades of this century, rickets was a major public health problem in the industrialized countries. It was not until 1921 that Mellanby elucidated the anti-rachitic factor in cod liver oil. From then on public health measures, such as the provision of vitamin D drops, and the vitamin D supplementation of milk and certain other food substances, have almost completely eradicated vitamin D deficiency from Europe and America. However, in Britain rickets is still seen in Asian children. This is due in part to the high melanin content of the skin decreasing the amount of vitamin D formed by suboptimal ultraviolet light exposure, in part to the lack of skin exposed to sunlight due to clothing, and also to the lack of vitamin D in the diet.

In developing countries the problem of rickets has perhaps been largely neglected because attention is concentrated on more serious conditions such as malnutrition, gastroenteritis, and infectious diseases. It is possible that rickets was rare prior to the large movement of populations into the informal settlements and overcrowded dwellings of rapidly developing cities. Nevertheless, rickets and osteomalacia have been reported to be problems in China, Turkey, and more recently in Iran and India. In Africa, rickets has been described in a number of countries, and studies from Ethiopia exploded the fallacy that rickets does not occur in malnourished children. In southern Africa, accurate figures of the prevalence of rickets are not available, but data from Cape Town in the 1960s revealed that 17% of black and 8% of white infants had clinical rickets. It appears, however, that the prevalence of vitamin D deficiency has decreased dramatically over the last two decades.

Several factors predispose infants to rickets, perhaps the most important of which are:

♦ a lack of sunlight, especially in an urban environment where air pollution reduces ultraviolet light, or in communites living in the extremes of latitude

♦ cultural traditions such as keeping the pregnant mother or the infant away from sunlight

♦ vegetarian diets

♦ prolonged breast-feeding without vitamin D supplementation

♦ mothers who are vitamin D-deficient and therefore give birth to vitamin D-deficient infants.

Vitamin D deficiency is not of short-term interest only, but can lead to considerable morbidity and mortality if not prevented or detected early. Growth failure and limb deformities are well recognized, but pelvic deformities leading to obstructed labour in later life, apnoeic attacks and convulsions in the young infant, and severe chest deformities leading to recurrent pneumonia and respiratory failure, are less often considered as complications of rickets.

With the disappearance of vitamin D deficiency rickets as a major public health problem, the rarer and more complex causes of rickets have become more prominent. It should be recognized, however, that the prevalence of these other types of rickets is probably not becoming more *common*, but rather becoming more *apparent*.

Osteoporosis

Unlike rickets and osteomalacia, osteoporosis usually manifests clinically with fractures after minimal or no trauma. The diagnosis of osteoporosis is difficult, however, as in most hospitals the facilities for accurate assessment of bone mineral content are not available. Thus the diagnosis is dependent on the subjective impression of thin cortices and decreased bone density on routine X-rays. The picture is further complicated in older children, in whom growth has ceased, because osteomalacia may present with a similar radiological pattern to that of osteoporosis. However, the two syndromes can usually be differentiated biochemically, as osteoporosis is generally associated with normal serum calcium, phosphorus, and alkaline phosphatase concentrations.

Osteoporosis is an unusual problem in clinical paediatric practice, although a number of chromosomal abnormalities such as Down's syndrome have decreased bone density. *Table 21.3* lists the more frequent causes of osteoporosis in paediatrics.

Table 21.3 Causes of osteoporosis

Decreased bone matrix formation:
- osteogenesis imperfecta
- corticosteroid excess
- protein-energy malnutrition
- vitamin C deficiency
- copper deficiency

Increased bone resorption:
- immobilization
- marrow hyperplasia, e.g., thalassaemia
- juvenile osteoporosis
- hyperparathyroidism, e.g., renal failure

Decreased bone matrix formation

Osteogenesis imperfecta

Osteogenesis imperfecta is an inherited disorder characterized by decreased bone formation due to an abnormality in collagen synthesis. However, it is not a single disease entity, as it can be inherited as an autosomal-recessive or -dominant trait, and has several different clinical presentations. Studies utilizing the recent advances in molecular genetics have elucidated the genetic defects in a number of patients with osteogenesis imperfecta. Point mutations in the genes coding for the collagen molecules have been documented at a number of different sites. Because of the numerous different genetic defects possible, the diagnosis of osteogenesis imperfecta by means of gene probes is not a viable option at the present time.

Recently osteogenesis imperfecta has been divided into four clinical subgroups:

♦ OI I, which is usually a mild disease associated with blue sclera and deafness in adulthood. Fractures of the long bones may occur, but are relatively infrequent, and become less frequent once adolescence is reached. This form is inherited as an autosomal-dominant condition.

♦ OI II is the lethal form of osteogenesis imperfecta. It is inherited as an autosomal-recessive condition and usually presents with multiple intrauterine fractures, severe bone deformities at birth, and death in the neonatal period.

♦ OI III is also inherited as an autosomal-recessive trait, but is less severe than OI II. Fractures are frequent in this OI III group of children, and bone deformities may develop. The sclera are classically normal.

♦ OI IV is inherited as an autosomal-dominant trait, but tends to be more severe than OI I. The sclera in this form of the disease are normal.

Hydrocephalus may be a complication of osteogenesis imperfecta. The teeth may also be affected, being stained, translucent, and subject to early development of caries.

The radiographs in osteogenesis imperfecta may vary from a picture of mild to severe osteoporosis, with fractures, extremely thin cortices, and narrowing of the total width of the bone. The skull may show multiple wormian bones with platybasia.

No specific therapy is available for the child with osteogenesis imperfecta. Fractures heal well with adequate callus formation, but care must be taken to prevent deformities and limb shortening.

Corticosteroid excess

Cushing's disease, due to adrenal tumours or excess ACTH secretion, is relatively rare in children. However, corticosteroid therapy is used fairly frequently in a number of paediatric disorders. Osteoporosis is generally more severe in those children who receive corticosteroids daily than in those who receive alternate day therapy.

The **pathogenesis** is, firstly, a failure of adequate matrix formation due to a direct effect of the steroids on the osteoblast; and secondly, a block in calcium absorption from the gastrointestinal tract. Osteoporosis is further aggravated by the development of secondary hyperparathyroidism due to decreased calcium absorption, and by immobilization, which often results from the primary illness that is being treated with corticosteroids.

Treatment is difficult once bone loss is far advanced, but the block in calcium absorption can be overcome by the administration of large doses of vitamin D and calcium supplements. To be effective, this form of therapy should be started early in the course of the disease.

Protein-energy malnutrition

Although fractures are rarely a problem, most children admitted to hospital with protein-energy malnutrition have radiological evidence of osteoporosis. The aetiology of this is multifactorial, but protein deficiency probably plays a major role. Many of these infants are also on low calcium diets.

Treatment should be aimed at correcting the primary nutritional deficiency.

Vitamin C deficiency

Until recently, scurvy was not an uncommon diagnosis in the paediatric wards of hospitals in South Africa. Cows' milk is deficient in vitamin C, and levels are further decreased if the milk is heated. In paediatric practice, most cases of scurvy occur in the second half of the first year in those infants fed almost totally on cows' milk.

Clinically, scurvy presents in the infant with irritability, loss of appetite, and tenderness of the long bones. The latter may be associated with a refusal to sit or stand. Eventually the child refuses to move, lying with the arms and legs semi-flexed. Movement of the limbs elicits acute pain. Swelling and ecchymoses around the joints may also be noted.

The **radiographic changes** are usually characteristic: the bones are generally osteopenic, with a ground-glass appearance of the shaft. The cortices are thin but well-defined. The zone of provisional calcification at the growing ends of the bones is well demarcated, but beneath this line is an area of rarefaction. Subperiosteal haemorrhages, which produce the severe bone pain, are generally not visualized on admission; however, when healing occurs, the elevated periosteum calcifies, and the extent of the haemorrhages can be seen.

Treatment should be aimed at the prevention of vitamin C deficiency; so vitamin C supplementation of the diet should be recommended during the first year of life. Scurvy responds to vitamin C therapy (250 mg/day).

Copper deficiency

With the advent of prolonged intravenous alimentation for various gastrointestinal disorders, particularly chronic diarrhoea, cases of copper deficiency are now being reported. Copper deficiency leads to anaemia, neutropenia, and severe osteoporosis. Metaphyseal lesions may also be noted.

Increased bone resorption

Immobilization

Immobilization of any limb may produce marked osteopenia. In paediatrics this is most commonly seen in children with myelomeningoceles, with resulting paralysis of the legs. It is also seen in the affected limbs following poliomyelitis. Therapeutically there is little to offer.

Hyperplasia of the bone marrow

Chronic haemolytic anaemias, especially thalassaemia major, may be complicated by osteoporosis, with marked thinning of the cortices and extreme fragility of the long bones. Specific therapy is not available to correct the osteoporosis.

Hyperparathyroidism

Primary hyperparathyroidism is a rare disease in children. However, secondary hyperparathyroidism complicates a number of conditions, such as vitamin D deficiency and renal failure. Hyperparathyroidism may present with osteoporosis or osteitis fibrosa cystica (where resorbed bone is replaced by fibroblasts and connective tissue).

The characteristic **radiological features** of hyperparathyroidism are localized areas of subperiosteal resorption of bone, seen particularly along the metacarpals or phalanges. The lateral ends of the clavicles may also be severely demineralized. The lamina dura, a dense line of bone around the teeth, disappears due to resorption. Metaphyses may become ragged and frayed, so as to resemble the abnormalities seen in rickets.

The **treatment** depends on whether the aetiology is primary or secondary. Treatment of primary disease requires the removal of the parathyroid glands, while the treatment of secondary hyperparathyroidism is directed towards treatment of the primary cause, such as renal failure.

Juvenile osteoporosis

Juvenile osteoporosis is a disease of unknown aetiology, which presents in late childhood with symptomatic osteoporosis. The disease may be difficult to differentiate from mild cases of osteogenesis imperfecta, but the absence of any family history may be helpful. Symptoms usually subside once the patient reaches puberty, and at present there is no specific therapy.

Osteosclerosis

Osteosclerosis is characterized by increased density of bone, secondary to an abnormality in bone resorption and remodelling. Although dense, the bones may be abnormally brittle. Except for the patchy increase in bone density which may occur in renal osteodystrophy, osteosclerosis is uncommon, so only two of the causes will be discussed.

Osteopetrosis

Osteopetrosis may be inherited as either an autosomal-dominant or -recessive trait.

The **autosomal-recessive** condition is invariably fatal unless therapy is undertaken. It is associated with anaemia, neutropenia, thrombocytopenia, increased susceptibility to infections, extramedullary erythropoeisis, and complications due to nerve compression. Deafness and blindness occur due to the entrapment of the cranial nerves as they pass through the skull, and hydrocephalus may develop. Dental sepsis is frequent, with osteomyelitis of the jaw occurring as a complication.

Radiologically, all the bones are excessively dense, with tubular bones having no marrow cavity. Hand radiographs may reveal the classic 'bone within a bone' appearance.

Recently, bone marrow transplants have had some success in reversing this condition.

The **autosomal-dominant** variety of osteopetrosis is a milder disease, symptoms only becoming apparent in adolescence or adulthood. Skeletal X-rays show alternate zones of osteopetrosis and relatively normal bone, while in contrast to the recessive condition, the medullary cavity is maintained. Anaemia is unusual in the dominant form, but nerve compression, with associated deafness and blindness, still occurs.

Diaphyseal dysplasia

This disease usually presents in early childhood with tender swollen legs and muscle weakness. The diaphyseal portions of long bones are markedly thickened, and hyperostosis of the skull may occur. Anaemia and elevated erythrocyte sedimentation rates have been reported. No specific therapy is available, but corticosteroids may be helpful in relieving bone pain and improving muscle power.

J.M. Pettifor

Common allergic disorders

Definition

An allergic reaction is an altered or unusual reaction to the presence of an allergen. Allergy means altered reactivity. In essence this is a state of increased sensitivity or hypersensitivity to antigens or allergens, most of which are proteins in nature.

Epidemiology

Thousands of children in southern Africa — possibly as many as one in every five — have some sort of allergic disorder. This may be very mild, or may be a major problem for the affected child. There has been a three-fold increase in the prevalence of allergic disorders in this region over the last ten years, as well as in other countries overseas. The reason for this increase is unknown, but may be associated with socio-economic factors and rapid urbanization. Many environmental factors contribute to the sensitization of an allergy-prone individual in early life. The season of the year when the child is born, parental smoking, living in damp and overcrowded homes, or where there is high housedust, mite, and indoor fungal spore exposure are all factors associated with increased risk of developing allergies. An important factor may be increasing industrialization, with the associated rise in air pollution levels, and changes in the environment.

Recent genetic studies suggest that allergy is a strongly inherited tendency, and is carried on chromosome 11 as an autosomal dominant with variable penetrance. This is reflected in the fact that most allergic children have a strong family history of allergy.

Pathogenesis

Once an allergic individual has been sensitized to a specific allergen, e.g., grass pollen or housedust mites, specific antibodies of the IgE subclass develop. The combination of allergen and IgE anti-body located on specialized cells, called mast cells — situated in the respiratory and gastrointestinal tracts and in the skin — results in the release of potent chemical mediators from granules contained in these cells (see Fig. 22.1). Among these mediators released are histamine, serotonin, eosinophil chemotactic factor (ECF), and neutrophil chemotactic factor (NCF). This part of the reaction occurs rapidly, and is known as the early phase of the allergic reaction. Some hours later, metabolic products of arachidonic acid metabolism occurring in the mast cell membrane release potent smooth muscle constrictors and inflammatory agents. Depending on the metabolic pathway of arachidonic acid metabolism, i.e., cyclo-oxygenase or lipoxygenase, leukotrienes or prostaglandins are released into the surrounding tissues.

The recruitment of inflammatory cells such as eosinophils and neutrophils to the site of the reaction results in local tissue damage and inflammation through the release of substances such as major basic protein. This phase of the reaction is the late phase allergic reaction, and occurs 6 – 8 hours after initiation of the allergic process. Prolonged inflammation of the affected tissues occurs, which accounts for the characteristic pathological changes associated with the common allergic disorders. These include asthma, allergic rhinitis or nasal allergy, atopic or allergic eczema, urticaria and angioedema, and food allergies.

Factors influencing allergy

The influence of genetic factors has already been mentioned. Other important factors include age, climate, and the intensity and frequency of exposure to allergens.

Age

Allergic manifestations tend to vary with the age of the child. Atopic eczema is usually the first of the disorders to present in infancy, and often manifests in the first few weeks of life. Food allergies

Mast cell or basophil

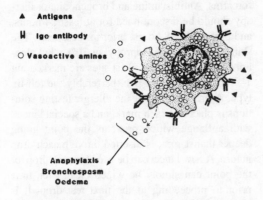

▲ Antigens

Ⴙ Igᴇ antibody

○ Vasoactive amines

Anaphylaxis
Bronchospasm
Oedema

Fig. 22.1 Hypersensitivity Type 1 reaction

are also more common in infants. Both of these conditions tend to become less severe by the second or third year of life. At this stage, asthma and allergic rhinitis usually present for the first time. Fully 80% of asthmatic children have had their first attack by the age of 5 years. There is a strong tendency for many children who have atopic dermatitis in infancy to develop allergic rhinitis and asthma later.

Climate, weather, location

Climatic conditions have a great effect on allergic diseases. The climate will determine which pollens and fungal spore exposures occur, and the weather conditions themselves, e.g., cold air, may strongly affect susceptible children. A damp climate favours the growth of highly allergenic fungal spores. Many children sensitive to fungal spores will be at their worst during humid spells. Sudden weather changes also cause worsening of symptoms in many allergic children.

Intensity and frequency of exposure to allergens

The intensity and frequency of exposure to allergens plays a large part in the development of allergic disorders. It is not enough to have an allergic individual and potentially-sensitizing allergens. The two must be in close contact for a long enough period for sensitization to occur. The most significant allergens are those encountered most often — either at home, out of doors, or at school.

These allergens are found in abundance in the air or in foods, and some have their effect through bodily contact, such as clothing, leather articles, dyes, or metals.

Detection of allergens

A careful allergic history *(see Fig. 22.2)*, which should almost always be obtained from the child's mother, will help to identify the child's allergic disorder as well as to identify possible allergens in his or her environment. Skin tests or radioallergosorbent tests (RAST), provocation tests, and elimination diets will help to identify those allergens most likely to be causing clinical symptoms. Four areas need to be carefully considered:

♦ the home, especially the child's bedroom
♦ the classroom
♦ the diet
♦ the circumstances, place, and timing of the onset of symptoms.

Table 22.1 lists the most common allergens affecting allergic children, and their usual place of occurrence.

Table 22.1   Allergens of importance in allergic children and their source

Home	School	Diet	Outdoor or seasonal
Housedust	Dust	Milk	Trees
Mites	Small pets	Wheat	Grasses
Cats	e.g., guinea pigs,	Eggs	Weeds
Dogs	mice, hamsters	Soya	e.g., plantain
Birds	Fungal spores	Peanuts	Fungal spores
Fungal spores		Fish	Flowers
		Nuts	Shrubs
		Pork	

Allergy testing

The common allergy tests are:

♦ skin tests
♦ radioallergosorbent tests (RAST)
♦ provocation tests
♦ elimination diets.

Of these, skin tests are the simplest, cheapest, and most accurate.

Allergy history form

Name:

Address:

Date: Age: Sex: Birth date:

Chief Complaint: Asthma Cough Hayfever Eczema
Urticaria Blocked nose Nasal discharge Croup
Headache Cold G.I. upsets Sinus infections
Onset and course:

Season:
Family history:

Aggravating factors: Weather change Dampness Heat
Cold Humidity Pollution Housedust Exposure to animals
Parents' occupations:
When and where free of symptoms:

Foods suspect:
Exercise:
Known sensitivities:
Drug sensitivities: Penicillin Sulphas Aspirin Others
Which medicines help:
Home environment: Age of house and type
Area   Pets: Cats Dogs Birds Other
Pillow   Mattress
Bedcover   Heaters
Carpets   Houseplants
Trees near house   Cooking arrangements
Previous allergy test and hyposensitization:

Past medical and surgical history:

Emotional status:
Physical examination

Laboratory: Blood count
                     Nasal
                     IgE level   Other immunoglobulins
                     RAST
                     X-rays
                     Stool
Skin test results
Inhalents   Ingestants
Diagnosis: 1.
                          2.
Management: 1.
                          2.
                          3.

Fig. 22.2 Allergy history form

Skin tests

Skin tests are usually performed on the child's forearms. Antihistamine and bronchodilator therapy should be discontinued for at least 24 hours, and preferably 48 hours, prior to these tests. The skin is cleaned with isopropyl or 70% ethyl alcohol and allowed to dry. Test sites are marked out 1–2 cm apart using a pen, preferably the felt-tip type. A drop of each of the allergic testing solutions is placed at each mark, and a special lancet, with a flange which prevents the point going deeper than 1 mm, is inserted through each drop in turn. A new lancet can be used for each drop, or the point can simply be wiped clean each time prior to proceeding to the next test drop. It is important not to prick too deeply, and not to draw blood. Many false positive reactions may occur because of poor technique. After 15 minutes, observe the test sites for erythema and weal formation. The average (taken between greatest and smallest) or largest diameter of the weal should be noted in millimetres, and compared with controls.

If a large weal (15 mm) appears in less than 10 minutes, wipe the allergen from that test site.

A negative control using the saline diluent solution alone should always be included, to assess excessive local skin reaction to mechanical trauma. This occurs especially in children with the tendency to develop dermatographism. A 0.1% histamine solution serves as a positive control. This histamine positive control aids in interpreting skin tests (a standard 3+ reaction) and demonstrates diminished or absent skin reactivity to histamine found in many infants, some African children, and especially in children who have inadvertently taken antihistamines.

Skin tests for foods are less accurate than for the inhalant allergens, and a careful history, limited RAST tests, or elimination diets may be required for diagnosis. Provocation tests require specialized facilities, and are not advised where adequate facilities and expertise are not available.

Physical examination of the allergic child

The physical examination of allergic children should always include particular attention to growth and development. Height and weight need to be carefully recorded on growth charts.

Children with severe nasal obstruction due to allergic rhinitis, and those with chronic asthma, are often small for their age. Those with atopic eczema are likely to be underweight. Many allergic children are unhappy or irritable, and many have the characteristic allergic facies. They are often extremely pale and have dark blue rings under their eyes — the so-called 'allergic shiners'. A nasal crease is often noted where the bony and cartilagenous portions of the nose meet. This is due to the child continuously rubbing the tip of the nose in an upward direction to relieve nasal itching and obstruction. This manoeuvre is one of the common allergic mannerisms, and is known as the 'allergic salute'. Face-pulling and twitching of the nose are also common. Allergic children are often mouth-breathers, and their mouths are usually open in order to breathe. Their lips are often dry and cracked.

The ENT and respiratory systems require careful examination. Assessment of the appearance of the nasal mucous membrane will only become accurate with experience. Nasal mucosal swelling, changes in colour of the mucosa, and the nature of the mucus discharge should be noted. Post-nasal mucus drip is common, as is a rather uneven appearance of the posterior pharyngeal wall due to lymphoid hyperplasia. Serous otitis media (also known as 'glue ear') is commonly associated with nasal allergy. Air bubbles may be noted behind the ear drum in the early stages of this condition. A geographic tongue is said to be more common in allergic children, and may be a helpful pointer to diagnosis.

Chest deformities are fairly common. Barrel chest, pigeon chest, and pectus excavatum are the most common in asthmatic children. Hyperinflation of the chest is often present even between attacks of asthma. Unless the chest is carefully auscultated with the child breathing out forcibly, an expiratory wheeze may be missed.

Table 22.2   Special investigations in the diagnosis of allergic disorders

Diagnostic tests	Positive result	Interpretation
Phadiotop	Positive or negative	A new screening test to detect the allergic child. Eliminates problems of interpretation found with total IgE estimation. Rather expensive
Blood eosinophils	> 6% on peripheral count or 400 cells/mm^3 on total count	Suggests allergy. Not specific. Parasitic infestation will also cause elevated counts. Examine stools
Nasal mucus stained with Hansel's stain	Clumps of eosinophils seen on slide	Allergic rhinitis, but normal in young infants
Sweat test	Raised sweat chloride, above 70 mEq/l	Suggests cystic fibrosis - important in differential diagnosis
Immunoglobulins		
IgA	Range for age	If low, may account for recurrent respiratory infections
IgG	Range for age	
IgE	Range for age	If raised, indicates allergy or worm infestation. Examine stools
Radiographs		
Chest	Hyperinflation in quiescent periods	Chronic asthma (always hyperinflated in acute attacks)
Postnasal space	Enlarged adenoids	Common cause of nasal obstruction
Paranasal sinuses	Mucosal thickening or opacification	Infection, or associated with allergic rhinitis
RAST	++ to ++++	Detects specific IgE directed against common allergens. May be useful in young children, those with extensive eczema, or where antihistamines have not been discontinued. Expensive. Use appropriately.

The skin and exposed mucosal surfaces are often affected in allergic children. The conjunctivae should be checked for 'pavement slabbing', which is typical of allergic conjunctivitis. Special note should be taken of the flexures of the arms and legs, the neck, feet, and nappy area for possible atopic eczema.

Children with chronic asthma may develop a poor posture. They are often round-shouldered and pull their shoulders up because they are using the accessory muscles of respiration.

Other helpful investigations in allergy diagnosis

There are many conditions which may mimic allergic disorders in children. This is especially the case with asthma, allergic rhinitis, and suspected food allergies. Further special investigations are directed towards establishing that the child is definitely an allergic individual, and also towards excluding some of the more common conditions encountered in southern Africa which should always be included in the differential diagnosis of allergic disorders (see Table 22.2).

Common allergic diseases

Asthma, allergic rhinitis, and food allergy will be discussed. (Also see Chapter 14, Ear, Nose, and Throat Disorders; Chapter 24, Dermatological Disorders and Chapter 25, Disorders of the Eye.)

Asthma

Definition

Asthma is a chronic condition in which there are episodes of *reversible* narrowing of the airways in response to various stimuli. It is characterized by cough, wheezing, and dyspnoea. Recently a new definition has been proposed: any child, regardless of age, with recurrent (three or more) episodes of wheezing and/or dyspnoea should be considered as having asthma until proved otherwise.

An essential feature of asthma is extreme sensitivity of the airways to environmental and other factors. This increased sensitivity is known as bronchial hyperreactivity.

The onset of asthma may be as early as the first few weeks of life, but is most common between the ages of 2 and 5 years. It is often confused with bronchiolitis in infants.

A health professional in the field faced with a wheezing child should establish whether there is a family history of asthma and other allergic disorders. Most helpful in diagnosis is the recurrent nature of asthma.

The old saying that 'all that wheezes is not asthma' is certainly true in developing countries, but to this should still be added 'but usually is in children over 3 years (having excluded the possibility of a foreign body)'. Children must be referred for maintenance treatment of asthma as attacks become more frequent and severe, and where there is interference with schooling, sport, exercise, and sleep.

Prevalence

Asthma is not a notifiable disease, and accurate statistics for its prevalence in the childhood population are difficult to determine. Limited field studies indicate a prevalence of between 3.5 and 6% in South African children. Asthma is probably less common in rural children than in urban areas. Admissions to hospital of children with acute asthma attacks appear to be on the increase, a trend which has been reported in many developed countries as well.

Pathology

Asthma is considered to be an inflammatory disease of the airways. Airway narrowing and obstruction is caused by a combination of the following abnormalities:

◆ airway smooth muscle spasm
◆ oedema of the airway mucosa
◆ mucus plugging of smaller airways
◆ inflammation, which may involve:
  — eosinophil and lymphocyte infiltration
  — mast cell activation
  — subepithelial collagen deposition
  — damage to the airway epithelium.

Following exposure to allergens and other irritants, pulmonary mast cells appear to initiate both an immediate bronchospastic response and a late inflammatory response, which result in a two-phase alteration in the airway hyperactivity. Mast cell-derived mediators such as histamines and leukotrienes produce immediate

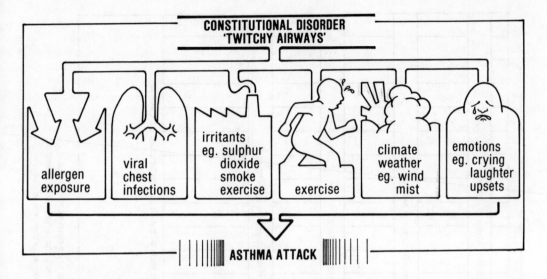

Fig. 22.3   Factors precipitating asthma attacks

bronchoconstriction. This appears to be the major feature of the immediate response *(see Pathogenesis, above)*. Chemotactic factors such as NCF, ECF, and leukotrienes attract eosinophils and neutrophils to the airway mucosa. Eosinophils release major basic protein, which damages airway epithelium and induces mast cell mediator release. Platelet activating factor (PAF) activates platelets which release thromboxanes, and these aggravate inflammation.

Precipitating factors

There are many factors which may precipitate asthma attacks *(see Fig. 22.3)*.

Diagnosis

The first approach to diagnosis should always be to take an adequate history, followed by the physical examination. The history includes the family history and the patient's symptoms. This helps to exclude conditions which mimic asthma *(see Table 22.3)*.

Investigations should include simple pulmonary function tests using a peak flow meter. The Mini-Wright Peak Flow Meter® is reasonably priced and gives accurate readings. If airflow obstruction is present, the diagnosis can be confirmed by showing significant improvement (> 15%) in peak flow following an inhaled beta 2 agonist bron-

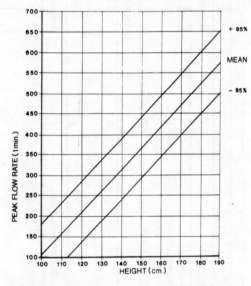

Fig. 22.4   Peak expiratory flow rates in normal children. From Godfrey et al., *British Journal of Diseases of the Chest,* vol. 64, no. 15, (1970).

chodilator. From the age of about 5–6 most children are able to perform these tests well, but younger children are often unable to blow adequately on the peak flow meter *(see Fig. 22.4)*.

Another diagnostic technique is a therapeutic trial with a bronchodilator. A record of changes in peak flow rates measured at home and entered in

Name _____ Age _____ Height _____ cm

MONTH _____ Day

WHAT SORT OF NIGHT DID YOU HAVE?

Write down the appropriate number for each night

Good night. No coughing or wheezing 0
Slept well but coughed or wheezed once or twice 1
Woke up two or three times due to cough or wheeze 2
Awake most of the time due to cough or wheeze 3

ACTIVITY DURING THE DAY

Write down the appropriate number for each day

Quite normal 0
Only able to run short distances 1
Limited to walking 2
Too breathless to walk. 3

PEAK FLOW METER READING (best of three readings)

Record the reading for each category

(Normal range for size _____ to _____)
On waking, before medicine ....
Midday, before lunch or sport .....
Before evening medicine ....

MEDICATION

Record the number of doses used in the last 24 hours

Name of medicine   Dose

COMMENTS

Write down your comments on anything that may be related to the asthma

i.e. To what do you attribute the attack?
What causes the wheeze (weather? diet? cold? dog? exercise? etc.)
Lots of phlegm? Is phlegm coloured?
Nebulization? Hospital admission?

Use this diary to keep a record during the month.
You can photocopy this page and show it to your doctor at your next appointment.
Write the score in the box provided.

Try and be as regular as you can in recording the score,
but don't worry if you cannot complete all the information.
The diary will help your doctor to see how you are
progressing.

Fig. 22.5 Asthma diary

a carefully-kept asthma diary *(see Fig. 22.5)* will show response to medication. This approach yields as much definitive information as an exercise or histamine challenge.

Skin tests

Most asthmatic children are allergic subjects. Limited skin testing to determine possible sensitization to environmental allergens is useful. Once the offending allergen is identified, parents can be advised on ways to limit exposure. Recommended skin tests for this region include housedust mites *(D. pteronyssinus),* cats, dogs, and South African grasses. RAST tests are a useful alternative where skin tests cannot be performed, but their expense needs to be kept in mind.

Treatment of asthma: the acute attack

Do not underestimate the severity of an asthma attack *(see below).*

Beta agonist bronchodilators in inhaled form are the most useful drugs for treating the child with an acute attack. Using metered dose inhaler (MDI) bronchodilators such as salbutamol (Ventolin®) or fenoterol (Berotec®), two puffs (200 mcg) may be administered every 2 – 3 hours. The powder forms of these inhalers require active inhalation, which may be beyond the ability of a child with a bad attack of asthma, and they are expensive.

In young children a hole may be cut in a paper cup large enough to take the mouthpiece of a MDI. The cup is held over the child's mouth and three to four puffs of the MDI fired into it. The cup usually fits snugly over the face, and little medication is lost. Excellent bronchodilation results when this method is used.

If there is no response to the inhaler either initially or after several doses over a period of one hour, the child should be treated as for acute severe asthma *(see below).*

Nebulization

Several home nebulizers are available. They are simple air compressors which can nebulize salbutamol or fenoterol respirator solution via a face mask nebulizer. This form of treatment has revolutionized the management of acute asthma. It should be noted that air, and not oxygen, is being

---

Table 22.3 Differential diagnosis of asthma in infants and children

Foreign bodies in the airway — unilateral wheezing may be noted, but not in all cases
Supraglottic causes
    Retropharyngeal abscess
    Tonsillar abscess
    Epiglottitis
Laryngeal causes
    Croup
    Stenosis
    Tetany
    Vocal cord paralysis
    Angioedema of larynx
Tracheal causes
    Tracheomalacia
    Tracheitis
    Vascular rings
    Lymph node compression
Bronchial causes
    Bronchiolitis
    Bronchitis
    Bronchiectasis
    Lymph node compression, e.g., tuberculosis
Pulmonary causes
    Pneumonia
    Cystic fibrosis
    Tuberculosis
    Pertussis
    Atelectasis
    Congenital lobar emphysema
    Hypersensitivity pneumonitis
    Loeffler's syndrome
Other causes
    Congestive cardiac failure
    Vascular ring
    Gastro-oesophageal reflux
    Hyperventilation

---

used to nebulize the bronchodilator, and this may be a disadvantage.

In infants and children under 2 years: Add 0.5 ml ipratropium bromide solution (Atrovent®) to 1 ml of normal saline and nebulize 3- to 4-hourly. Salbutamol or fenoterol solution 0.5 ml may be combined with the ipratropium bromide.

Over 2 years of age: Add 1 ml salbutamol or fenoterol respirator solution to 1 ml normal saline and administer 3- to 4-hourly. Ipratropium bromide solution 1 ml may be added to this mixture.

If there is no response to two nebulizations

given 1 hour apart, the child must be managed as for acute severe asthma.

Acute severe asthma (status asthmaticus)

This is diagnosed when:
◆ there is no response to two puffs of beta 2 agonist bronchodilator given 30 minutes apart, or
◆ there is no response to two nebulizations with a beta 2 agonist bronchodilator.

Acute severe asthma may occur in any asthmatic child, usually quite suddenly. There is no response to the usual methods of treatment, probably because of severe inflammation of the airway mucosa and plugging by thick tenacious mucus. Precipitating factors include allergen exposure, viral infections, weather changes, or emotional upsets. Not uncommonly, no cause is found.

Acute severe asthma must be regarded as a medical emergency.

Physical findings include:
◆ an anxious patient with laboured breathing, audible wheeze, and tachypnoea, which interfere with speech
◆ marked hyperinflation of the chest with use of the accessory muscles of respiration
◆ markedly diminished breath sounds with intense wheezing noted on auscultation
◆ pulsus paradoxus > 10 mm Hg during inspiration.

Treatment of acute severe asthma

The child must be admitted to hospital, preferably to an intensive care unit. A simple way to remember which treatment is required is to use the '4hs':
◆ **h**ospitalize
◆ treat for **h**ypoxaemia
◆ administer **h**ydrocortisone, and
◆ **h**ydrate the child adequately.

Therapeutic policy: Give oxygen by face mask or nasal prongs. Set up IV drip with 5% dextrose water at 60–80 ml/kg/24 hours.

Medications

◆ Nebulize beta 2 agonist preparations. Give 1 ml of salbutamol or fenoterol respirator solution diluted with 1 ml of normal saline in the nebulizer. Repeat 2- to 3-hourly.

◆ Hydrocortisone 2 mg/kg IV (irrespective of whether or not the child has previously had steroid therapy). The dose is repeated every 6 hours. The majority of children improve by this time. Change to an oral prednisolone course for 5–10 days after an episode of acute severe asthma. Improvement should be monitored using a peak flow meter.
◆ Aminophylline must be used with caution, as severe side-effects may occur in children. It should only be used where facilities for measuring the serum levels are available.

Doses used are as follows:
Loading dose: Aminophylline 6 mg/kg IV over 10 minutes (if the child has not had any theophylline therapy in the previous 24 hours). If the child has had theophylline previously, following measurement of the serum level, a constant infusion of 0.5 mg/kg/hour is used. This infusion rate can be achieved by using the following guide:
◆ weight of patient
◆ add 2 ml of aminophylline (250 mg/10 ml) to 100 ml 5% dextrose water
◆ select a 60 drops/ml drip administration set
◆ set the drip rate to equal the patient's weight in kg.

Notes:

1 If the patient responds poorly to therapy, arterial blood gases should be monitored as necessary.
2 ECG monitoring is essential if IV aminophylline is being given.
3 Continuous low-flow oxygen via nasal prongs must be administered to keep the PaO_2 above 60 mmHg.
4 Do not overhydrate the patient.
5 Monitor peak flow levels at least every 6 hours.

Danger signs in acute severe asthma
◆ Rising $PaCO_2$ (> 45 mmHg)
◆ PaO_2 of 50 mmHg or less
◆ Restlessness
◆ Rising pulse rate
◆ Peak flow < 60% predicted
◆ 'Silent chest' on auscultation
◆ Chest pain (intrathoracic air leak)
◆ Disturbance in level of consciousness

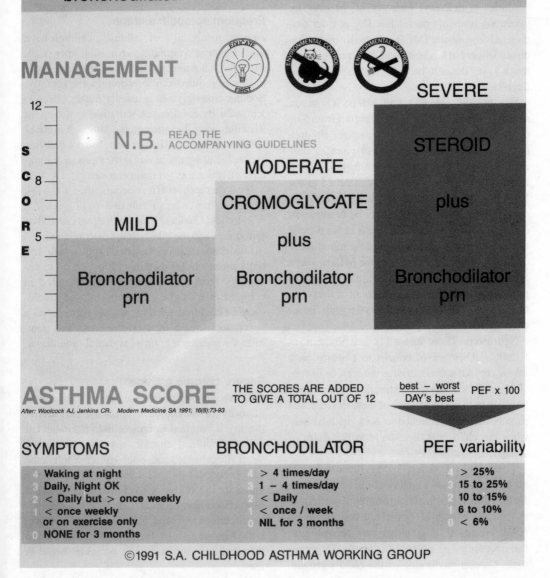

Childhood and Adolescent Asthma
CONSENSUS 1991

DIAGNOSIS

Asthma must be diagnosed whenever a patient has recurrent wheezing or cough which responds to a bronchodilator

MANAGEMENT

EDUCATE FIRST

ENVIRONMENTAL CONTROL

ENVIRONMENTAL CONTROL

SEVERE

N.B. READ THE ACCOMPANYING GUIDELINES

STEROID

plus

MODERATE

CROMOGLYCATE

plus

MILD

Bronchodilator prn

Bronchodilator prn

Bronchodilator prn

SCORE 12 8 5

ASTHMA SCORE

After: Woolcock AJ, Jenkins CR.   Modern Medicine SA 1991; 16(8):73-93

THE SCORES ARE ADDED TO GIVE A TOTAL OUT OF 12

$$\frac{best - worst}{DAY's\ best}\ PEF \times 100$$

SYMPTOMS	BRONCHODILATOR	PEF variability
4 Waking at night	4 > 4 times/day	4 > 25%
3 Daily, Night OK	3 1 – 4 times/day	3 15 to 25%
2 < Daily but > once weekly	2 < Daily	2 10 to 15%
1 < once weekly or on exercise only	1 < once / week	1 6 to 10%
0 NONE for 3 months	0 NIL for 3 months	0 < 6%

©1991 S.A. CHILDHOOD ASTHMA WORKING GROUP

Fig. 22.6   Childhood and adolescent asthma treatment

Asthma maintenance treatment programme

(See Fig. 22.6.)

Maintenance treatment of asthma falls into two main categories:

◆ bronchodilators, which include beta 2 agonists, methylxanthines, and anticholinergics, and

◆ anti-inflammatory or prophylactic agents such as sodium cromoglycate, ketotifen, and corticosteroids (inhaled or oral).

Modes of delivery: Delivery of the drug by inhalation is always preferable. Dry powder or a metered dose inhaler (MDI) are usually used. This direct delivery of medication to the airways allows much lower doses to be used, which reduces the likelihood of side-effects.

Dry powder inhalers and MDIs: These are simple devices ideal for use in children from 5 or 6 years of age onwards. Many younger children can also use them effectively. For younger children, and older ones with poor inhalation technique, a spacer device should be attached to the MDI, e.g., Aerochamber® with soft face mask. A very effective spacer device may be constructed out of a plastic cola bottle. A hole is cut in the end of the bottle large enough to take the mouthpiece of a MDI. Three to six puffs of the MDI are then introduced into the bottle. The child simply has to pant or breathe in and out in the spout of the bottle to inhale an adequate dose of beta 2 agonist bronchodilator.

Nebulizers: These are used both at home and in hospitals. They are of benefit to children with severe chronic asthma, in acute attacks, or in very young children. Careful instruction must always be given as to the limitations of these devices, and parents must be cautioned to seek medical help when the child fails to respond to this form of therapy.

Treatment schedules: Asthma therapy aims at achieving as normal a quality of life as is possible for the child: she or he should be able to participate in sport, attend school regularly, and sleep well at night. Treatment programmes vary according to the frequency and severity of the child's symptoms. Careful monitoring of the child's growth, and attention to possible side-effects of treatment are essential.

Mild infrequent asthma

Most children with asthma experience only mild and infrequent episodes of wheezing and coughing in the course of a year. Their quality of life is unaffected, and their symptoms are easily controlled using intermittent beta 2 agonist therapy. Prophylactic agents such as sodium cromoglycate are indicated only in anticipation of possible precipitating events such as exercise, cold air, and exposure to animals or pollen.

Frequent episodic asthma

Approximately 20% of asthmatic children have more frequent symptoms (> 6 episodes per year), such that schooling and sleep are affected. These children require daily prophylactic therapy. Sodium cromoglycate is usually highly effective and safe in children. Alternatively, a trial of ketotifen may be attempted. Although inhaled steroids are highly effective, they are not first-line prophylactic agents in this context, as their long-term effects are as yet undetermined.

If no therapeutic effect occurs after a 6-week trial of sodium cromoglycate or 8- to 12-week trial of ketotifen, (Zaditen®) inhaled steroids should be introduced and the other agents discontinued.

Low doses of inhaled steroids appear safe. Initially doses of 400 mcg/day (200 mcg bd to encourage compliance) may be administered in conjunction with a beta 2 agonist. Inhaled steroids should be administered in powder form or via a spacer to increase their effectiveness and minimize the incidence of oropharyngeal candidiasis.

Severe chronic asthma

Children with severe chronic asthma form a small minority of childhood asthmatics. Aggressive therapy is required in these children to alleviate daily symptoms, chronic airways obstruction, sleep disturbance, and poor exercise tolerance. Larger doses of inhaled steroids (> 800 mcg/day, upper limit 1 600 mcg/day) are often indicated. Side-effects may occur at these levels, and should be carefully monitored. If bronchodilation is poor with beta 2 agonist therapy, sustained-release theophyllines or ipratropium bromide should be used.

If oral steroids are needed, alternate day prednisone is best, using the lowest dose possible.

Common problems in asthma management

Infants and small children: Treatment may be difficult for various reasons. A face mask nebulizer is probably the most effective way of delivering drugs effectively. In mild cases, oral beta 2 agonists may be quite effective.

In more severe cases, nebulized beta 2 agonists constitute the first line of therapy. If there is no clinical improvement, ipratropium bromide may be added. Should symptoms persist, nebulized sodium cromoglycate or oral ketotifen is used. If there is still poor control, sustained-release theophylline products may be tried. Oral steroids (using particularly the alternate day regime) may be required in severe cases. Nebulized or inhaled steroid preparations should also be useful in this difficult group.

Exercise-induced asthma (EIA)

EIA is best controlled with an inhaled beta 2 agonist used 3–5 minutes before exercise. Sodium cromoglycate administered 20 minutes prior to exercise is also very effective. Lack of response to these measures implies poor asthma control.

Nocturnal asthma

Regular episodes of coughing and wheezing at night (usually in the early hours of the morning) indicate poor asthma control and the need for more effective therapy. Once appropriate daytime therapy has been prescribed, attention should then be paid to any possible nocturnal symptoms. Long-acting beta 2 agonists or theophyllines taken at bed-time are often effective. Attention to environmental control should be recommended in those children with sensitivity to household allergens.

Allergic rhinitis

There are two forms of allergic rhinitis; the seasonal form known as hay fever, and the perennial form with persistent symptoms. Intense sneezing, watery rhinitis, nasal congestion, and conjunctivitis are the main symptoms. Itching is found particularly in the seasonal form. Symptoms may often mimic a cold, but the persistence of symptoms or their seasonal nature helps in making a diagnosis.

Seasonal allergic rhinitis or hay fever

Symptoms are usually precipitated by exposure to seasonal wind-borne pollens, e.g., grass and tree pollens or fungal spores. These usually occur in spring, early summer, and at the change of seasons. There is intense sneezing, watery nasal discharge, and itching. Not only the nose itches, but also the palate and the ear canals. The diagnosis is usually easily made.

The allergen is identified by means of a history, skin testing, or RAST. Clumping of eosinophils will be seen on smears of nasal mucus stained with Hansel's stain.

Treatment

It is usually impossible to avoid the allergens causing seasonal allergic rhinitis.

Antihistamines: The older preparations with their sedative side-effects are no longer recommended. Successful results may be obtained using the new short-acting, non-sedating antihistamines such as cetirizine (Zyrtec®) and loratidine (Clarityne®).

Sodium cromoglycate (Rynacrom®) nasal spray or drops may be effective in the seasonal form of allergic rhinitis.

Beclomethasone (Beconase®) or **budesonide** (Rhinocort®) **nasal spray** is also effective. Children prefer the aqueous form of these preparations.

Desensitization: This is very effective, especially for grass pollen allergy, where virtually all children desensitized will benefit.

Depot steroid injections are not necessary to control symptoms.

Perennial allergic rhinitis

(See Chapter 14, Ear, Nose, and Throat Disorders.)

Perennial allergic rhinitis is usually due to sensitivity to allergens present in the environment throughout the year, e.g., housedust mites, pet allergens, or fungal spores.

Treatment

Environmental control is an essential component of treatment. Simple schemes to reduce indoor mite, mould, and pet allergen exposure are often very effective.

Antihistamines: The newer, non-sedating antihistamines such as cetirizine, loratidine, or the longer-acting astemizole may be effective in controlling symptoms.

Sodium cromoglycate nasal spray or drops are not very effective in perennial allergic rhinitis, but younger children may respond well.

Beclomethasone or budesonide nasal spray is highly effective in this form of rhinitis.

Desensitization is often very successful, especially if the child is sensitive to a single, unavoidable allergen. The procedure is ineffective when more than two allergens are combined in the vaccine. It is not intended as a substitute for removal of avoidable allergens, e.g., allergy to dogs and cats.

Oral steroids are not recommended unless symptoms are very severe and response to therapy is poor; this is unlikely with the range of treatments now available.

Note: Nasal decongestant drops of any type should not be used for prolonged periods. Even though the danger of rebound chemical rhinitis is unlikely, with some preparations prolonged use is not recommended.

Food allergy

Food allergy is thought to affect between 1 and 4% of the paediatric population, and is especially common in infants and young children. It becomes less common beyond the age of 2–3 years. True food allergy always involves an immune mechanism, and should not be confused with the many cases of intolerance to foods such as tyramine in cheeses or toxins contained in contaminated foods.

There is often a family history of food allergy or other atopic disorders which helps in the diagnosis.

Gastrointestinal symptoms such as vomiting and diarrhoea are the most common manifestation of food allergy, but skin reactions such as urticaria and atopic dermatitis, and angioedema and respiratory symptoms including nasal obstruction or wheezing may occur.

Few foods have been implicated in true food allergy in infants. These include egg white, cows' milk, soya and other legumes, wheat, and fish.

Later, sensitivity to shellfish and nuts may occur, and persist throughout life.

A careful history, skin test, or RAST may be of some help in establishing the diagnosis and the offending food. Where there is any difficulty, elimination diets, oligoallergenic diets, or occasionally double-blind, placebo-controlled food challenge tests may be indicated. The latter is used in special units only.

Treatment is usually effective if the offending food is eliminated from the diet, e.g., a milk- or egg-free diet. Where the food cannot be identified, good results have been obtained using sodium cromoglycate powder (Nalcrom®) administered in a small amount of warm water 10–20 minutes prior to feeds. Alternatively, ketotifen given twice daily has been of some use.

Advice for the parents of the allergic child: Housedust and mite control

Housedust is a special kind of dust, and is an important factor in many allergies. It is especially the presence of housedust mites in this dust which makes it such a problem for the allergic child. Dust mites are so tiny that you cannot see them without a microscope. They are quite harmless, except to those who are allergic to them. Mites are found on the surfaces of mattresses, bedclothes, armchairs, and carpets. They feed on human skin scales, and on mould in damp places. They constantly re-infest bedding and houses, however new. Mites multiply during late spring, and in summer and autumn. Sunlight kills them.

If you follow these instructions carefully you can eliminate much of the troublesome dust in your home, and at the same time control the housedust mites. Remember that the dust mites hide in the dust you will find in even the cleanest bedroom — deep in carpets and curtains and the seams of mattresses — where even the most house-proud person will not spot them.

Helpful habits

The mattress

Bedding is the dust mites' favourite haunt. They are especially fond of a nice cosy mattress. But you can beat them by wrapping your mattress in a fitted plastic cover.

The bedding

Dust mites are choosy. They have a decided preference for wool and cotton. So you can deter them by using only synthetic bedding materials, and by washing all sheets every week. A duvet reduces laundry, but with this and with pillows you must avoid feathers, down, or kapok.

Mites hate the sun!

Get your blankets and mattresses out in the sun whenever you can — there is nothing better to kill mites. Make the most of sunshine to dry sheets and pillow cases. Place the bed in a sunny position in the room.

The vacuum cleaner is your best weapon

A daily attack with the vacuum cleaner will help to get rid of dust mites. Vacuum all carpets, especially in bedrooms and under beds. If you can, choose vinyl rather than carpets. Vacuum upholstery, curtains, and even blankets.

Curtains are dust collectors

It is best to use lightweight materials for curtains. Remember to vacuum them often. Wash them regularly — at least once every 6 weeks.

You can't be too tidy

Put clothes away in wardrobes; do not hang clothes behind doors. When you dust, never use a completely dry duster. A damp duster is like a wet blanket to dust and the dust mite, and it could save your child a wheezy or sneezy night.

Keep bedroom furniture simple

Avoid bookcases, shelves, ornaments, and other dust-collecting surfaces if possible.

General hints for allergic children

1 Do not keep plants, dried flowers, books, or stuffed toys in the child's bedroom.
2 Your child must not make the bed or help with dusting.
3 Avoid candlewick bedspreads and heavy curtains.
4 If there is a double bunk, let the allergic child sleep on the top bed.
5 Do not allow animals or birds in the bedroom, and preferably not in the house.
6 When visiting or on trips, take the child's pillow.
7 Do not use enzyme-containing washing powders.
8 Avoid using insecticide or deodorant sprays in the child's presence.
9 Avoid ice-cold drinks and drinks preserved with sulphur dioxide.
10 Do not let your child eat in bed.

Natural history of allergic conditions

The vast majority of children with atopic eczema and asthma will outgrow their illness before they reach their teens. This applies particularly to boys and to those children in whom the illness first manifests in early childhood. The more severe asthmatics, especially those who have required steroid therapy, are less likely to outgrow their asthma. For reasons which are not clear, female asthmatics have a poorer chance of outgrowing their asthma.

Children with hay fever and perennial allergic rhinitis are often troubled by these illnesses in adult life unless they are adequately treated in their early years.

Pulmonary eosinophilia

See Chapter 13, Respiratory Disorders.

Allergic emergencies

Anaphylaxis

Anaphylaxis is an acute hypersensitivity reaction caused by the administration of an allergen or antigen to which the patient is sensitive. These include many drugs, antibiotics (especially penicillin), vaccines, sera, and insect bites and stings.

The onset is usually unexpected, and may occur within seconds or minutes of exposure to the allergen. The child will collapse, and rapidly enter a state of shock and possible respiratory arrest. In general, allergic reactions which occur abruptly are the most severe, and may well be fatal.

Treatment

A successful outcome depends on immediate therapy.

In the following order give immediately:

1 Adrenaline 1:1 000 0.3–0.5 ml IM. This must be injected immediately. May be repeated at 20-minute intervals if necessary.
2 Antihistamine, e.g., promethazine (Phenergan®) 0.25–0.5 mg/kg IM.
3 IV fluids: Shock is due to hypovolaemia secondary to massive exudation of intravascular fluid. Maintenance of normal intravascular volume by IV fluids is essential, e.g., Ringer's lactate, normal saline, or 5% dextrose in saline.
4 Oxygen is given by face mask or nasal catheter to prevent hypoxaemia.
5 Aminophylline is administered if bronchospasm develops in spite of adrenaline therapy. It must be given slowly IV in a dose of 4 mg/kg.

6 Intubation or tracheostomy if there is airway obstruction due to angioedema.

Later:

1 Steroids are only administered following the immediate and urgent steps outlined above. Steroids have a slow onset of action. Administer hydrocortisone 100–200 mg IV 4- to 6-hourly for 24 hours, or longer if required.
2 Isoprenaline HCL (Isuprel®) is infused at a rate of 1–4 mcg/minute if cardiovascular collapse occurs.

E.G. Weinberg

23

Juvenile chronic arthritis and vasculitides

Introduction

The rheumatic diseases are characterized by chronic or recurrent non-suppurative inflammation of connective tissues. The exceptions are the vasculitic syndromes of Kawasaki disease and Schönlein-Henoch purpura, which are mostly self-limiting acute disorders. The common target organs are the musculo-skeletal system and the vascular endothelium, because of their preponderance of connective tissue. The aetiology of the rheumatic diseases is unknown, but genetic susceptibility, an association with infective trigger factors, and an exaggerated or aberrant immune response — including autoantibody production — all play a role in the pathogenesis to varying degrees.

Diagnostic criteria are based on clinical signs and symptoms because of the lack of defined aetiological agents. Laboratory studies provide supportive evidence of the inflammatory process, and in some cases may demonstrate autoantibody production or genetic markers.

Two broad groups of autoantibodies may be present — rheumatoid factors which are serologically detected by their binding to IgG, and antinuclear antibodies which are detected in tissue sections by their binding to various constituents of cellular nuclei.

The differential diagnosis of the rheumatic diseases is vast, and includes infections, malignancies, allergic disorders, bleeding, and traumatic conditions. Critical to the diagnosis of rheumatic disorders, which occur infrequently among blacks in Africa, is the positive exclusion of such conditions, as they often require early and specific treatment.

Juvenile chronic arthritis

Juvenile chronic arthritis (JCA) is defined as objective arthritis which has been present for longer than 3 months (chronic) and occurs before 16 years of age (juvenile). The diagnosis of all forms of JCA is based almost entirely on clinical grounds, and it is therefore most important to exclude other known causes of arthritis, of which the most important include:

◆ infections, e.g., viral, bacterial, and tuberculous
◆ post-infective arthritis, e.g., viral, rheumatic fever, bowel infections
◆ other rheumatic diseases, e.g., SLE, dermatomyositis, Schönlein-Henoch purpura
◆ haematological, e.g., haemophilia
◆ neoplastic diseases, e.g., leukaemia
◆ trauma and non-rheumatic conditions of bones and joints.

There are three major groups of juvenile chronic arthritis. Features of this disease seen in African and Indian children in Durban are shown in *Fig. 23.1*.

Systemic onset disease (Still's disease)

This condition presents at any age with high intermittent fevers, chills, and an erythematous rash which comes and goes but is most prominent in intertrigenous areas and when the fever is high. The rash may be produced by rubbing the skin (Koebner phenomenon) during spikes of fever. Diffuse lymphadenopathy, hepatomegaly, splenomegaly, and serosal inflammation including arthritis, pericarditis, pleuritis, and peritonitis are present to a varying degree. The children look, and are, systemically ill and have a leucocytosis, raised ESR, and anaemia. The joints most commonly affected are the wrists and ankles, although multiple joints may be involved. Following this initial phase, the clinical presentation is very variable. Resolution may occur after about 6 months with or without treatment, but recurrences are not uncommon, and chronic arthritis may ensue.

Polyarticular arthritis

About 30–40% of cases of JCA present with multiple, progressive joint involvement including the finger joints, the spine, and the temporomandibular

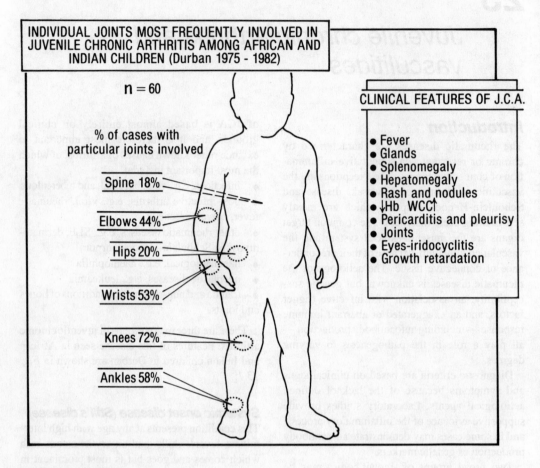

INDIVIDUAL JOINTS MOST FREQUENTLY INVOLVED IN JUVENILE CHRONIC ARTHRITIS AMONG AFRICAN AND INDIAN CHILDREN (Durban 1975 - 1982)

n = 60

% of cases with particular joints involved

Spine 18%
Elbows 44%
Hips 20%
Wrists 53%
Knees 72%
Ankles 58%

CLINICAL FEATURES OF J.C.A.

- Fever
- Glands
- Splenomegaly
- Hepatomegaly
- Rash and nodules
- ↓Hb WCC↑
- Pericarditis and pleurisy
- Joints
- Eyes-iridocyclitis
- Growth retardation

Fig. 23.1 Juvenile chronic arthritis

joints. Severe joint deformities may result. Girls are more commonly affected, and autoantibodies — including rheumatoid factor — are negative. In a minority of older children rheumatoid factor may be positive and the clinical picture resembles adult rheumatoid arthritis in that there are more systemic symptoms, rheumatoid nodules may be present, and there is often progression to severe chronic rheumatoid arthritis.

Pauciarticular arthritis

By definition less than five joints are involved, and these are usually large joints, especially the knees. Although chronic inflammation of the eye can occur in any form of JCA, iridocyclitis is present in about 30% of children with pauciarticular arthritis at some time in the course of the disease. This

is a serious complication which will lead to cataracts, visual impairment, and blindness if not specifically treated. Six-monthly diagnostic slit lamp examination is essential.

Iridocyclitis affects 30% of children with pauciarticular JCA. This may cause blindness.

Geographical variations

The pattern of JCA is not uniform throughout Africa. In Nigeria it resembles the forms of JCA described above, while in Uganda and Zambia certain unusual features have been detected. In southern Africa the most common presentation of JCA is polyarticular. Pauciarticular disease, the rash of systemic onset JCA, subcutaneous nodules, and iridocyclitis are not frequent. There is a relatively high incidence of rheumatoid factors in African children with JCA.

Prognosis

The prognosis for JCA is extremely variable, but is improved by early diagnosis and comprehensive management, and is generally better than adult rheumatoid arthritis. Complete recovery can take place.

Treatment

Treatment of JCA includes anti-inflammatory drug therapy, prevention of complications (iridocyclitis, contractures, etc.), and an integrated approach to the management of disability. Many children have a good clinical response to high doses of aspirin — 80 mg/kg/day in divided doses. If this is ineffective in controlling symptoms of swelling, pain, and stiffness, indomethacin 1.5 mg/kg given at night may be helpful. Care should be taken to monitor children for the toxic and adverse effects of these drugs. Iridocyclitis requires long-term, topical corticosteroids. Severe systemic disease and intractable joint pathology calls for corticosteroids as the next step in treatment. Those cases in which other drugs such as penicillamine and gold may be indicated should preferably be assessed at a paediatric centre.

The prevention of contractures and the maintenance of maximal mobility are very important, and physiotherapy or occupational therapy should be initiated at an early stage. In the latter stages, orthopaedic surgery is often helpful to correct deformity and enhance mobility. As in all chronic diseases of children, long-term support and education of the family and child are essential.

Systemic lupus erythematosus

Systemic lupus erythematosus (SLE) is rare in childhood. It most commonly affects adolescent girls, and the clinical picture closely resembles SLE in adults. In children under 10 years it is exceedingly rare, but affects both sexes, and has a very poor prognosis. The prevalence of SLE is higher among black adults and children than among whites in the USA, the UK, and the Caribbean. In Africa however, the disorder has been infrequently reported among black adults and is rare in black children; the exception is the Western Cape, where the disease occurs more often in coloured and black women than in white women.

Presentation

SLE usually presents as chronic arthritis or arthralgia, fever, and a characteristic rash. The rash is typically chronic, maculo-papular, erythematous, and distributed over the malar area of the face and bridge of the nose in a butterfly distribution.

SLE is a multisystem disease in which the underlying pathology is a widespread vasculitis affecting small blood vessels associated with circulating soluble immune complexes.

Areas of infarction and thrombosis due to the underlying vasculitis may be evident in the fingers, palms, soles, and mucous membranes.

The renal system is commonly affected by the vasculitis and this can progress to chronic nephritis and renal failure. Hepatomegaly, lymphadenopathy, pericarditis, polyserositis, and neurological and haematological dysfunction are also frequent complications.

Diagnosis

The diagnosis is usually suspected when chronic arthritis is associated with the typical rash, or in adolescent girls with multisystem disease including purpura, nephritis, and migraine. Laboratory tests may provide confirmatory evidence, antinuclear and anti-DNA antibodies are often present, and the Coombs' test may be positive. In the acute phase, complement levels may be low, the ESR is raised, and there is often anaemia, leucopenia, and thrombocytopenia.

Treatment

SLE is difficult to treat and the prognosis is not good. Arthritic symptoms can be controlled by non-steroidal anti-inflammatory drugs, but high dose corticosteroids are usually required for renal, haematological, and neurological involvement. The disease usually progresses, and renal failure frequently develops. Immunosuppressive drugs may be used, but as with steroids, side-effects are serious, and children with SLE should be referred to a specialist centre for assessment and advice.

Neonatal SLE is seen in infants whose mothers have SLE, which may be unrecognized. It is due to the placental transfer of maternal autoantibodies.

The infant may develop a fever and skin rashes in the first few weeks, but the most important consequence is congenital heart block, which can be permanent. Congenital heart block can be detected *in utero* and the mothers of all newborns with congenital heart block should be investigated for SLE.

Juvenile dermatomyositis

Dermatomyositis should be suspected in children with progressive symmetrical muscle weakness who have characteristic skin lesions. The typical skin changes are a violaceous or purplish discoloration of the upper eyelids associated with periorbital oedema, and chronic, atrophic, scaly, mauve lesions over the dorsal surfaces of the metacarpo-phalangeal and inter-phalangeal joints, elbows, and knees.

The myositis may be painful, and affects mainly proximal muscles. The onset may be acute, subacute or chronic, but it is insidiously progressive and may affect swallowing and breathing. There is often a low-grade fever and these children are irritable and miserable. The underlying pathology is a vasculitis of small blood vessels.

Diagnosis

The diagnosis is largely clinical, and all laboratory tests may be negative. However, a raised creatine phosphokinase (CPK), an increased urinary creatine/creatinine ratio, an abnormal EMG, and muscle biopsy may help to confirm the diagnosis. Subcutaneous and muscular dystrophic calcinosis may develop later in the disease.

Treatment

The prognosis without treatment is bad, and it is most important to make the diagnosis early and to start high dose corticosteroids (2 mg/kg/day). This usually prevents progression, controls symptoms, and leads to long-lasting remission. Failure of steroid treatment, or steroid dependency forces the use of other immunosuppressive drugs. Careful monitoring of muscle weakness, respiratory failure and swallowing problems is essential, and early physiotherapy and occupational therapy prevent contractures. All patients should be referred to a unit specializing in management.

The differential diagnosis includes other forms of myositis (viral infections, trichinosis, toxoplasmosis) and infectious polyneuritis.

Scleroderma

Scleroderma may be localized, with areas of fibrosis, atrophy, and synovitis. The rarer systemic form, or systemic sclerosis, has signs of generalized fibrosis of the subcutaneous tissues, skin, oesophagus and internal organs, and Raynaud's phenomenon is common.

Mixed connective tissue disease

This is an overlap syndrome which combines some of the features of SLE, dermatomyositis, scleroderma, and JCA. Antibodies to ribonucleoprotein (RNP) give a speckled antinuclear pattern in tissue sections and are frequently but not invariably present.

Therapy of both scleroderma and mixed connect-ive tissue diseases is difficult, but corticosteroids may control symptoms.

Table 23.1 Classification of vasculitides

Size of blood vessel	Site of lesion	Diseases
1. Small vessels		
Venules	Skin, subcutaneous tissue	Erythema nodosum, viral illness (e.g., rubella,
Arterioles	Intra-organ vessels	infective endocarditis, Schönlein-Henoch purpura, dermatomyositis, systemic lupus erythematosus
2. Medium-sized muscular arteries	Subcutaneous tissue, organ arteries, e.g., coronary, hepatic, mesenteric arteries	Polyarteritis nodosa, Kawasaki disease
3. Large arteries	Large vessels, e.g., aorta, renal, vertebral arteries	Takayusu's disease, cranial arteritis

Vasculitides

The common underlying pathology is a vasculitis of unknown cause in which immune mechanisms and immune complexes have been implicated. A classification based on the size of the affected blood vessel is shown in *Table 23.1* and *Fig. 23.2*.

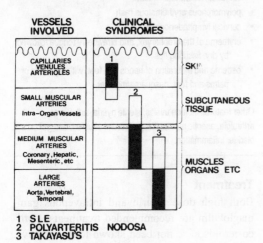

Fig. 23.2 Site of the lesion and clinical syndromes of vasculitides

Polyarteritis nodosa

This is a rare multisystem disease characterized by fever, Raynaud's phenomenon, arthralgia, myalgia, and erythematous skin rashes. The underlying pathology is a generalized inflammatory vasculitis of medium sized vessels which may affect any organ, but renal and neurologic involvement are the most serious. The aetiology is believed to be immune-complex mediated, and evidence of preceding streptococcal and hepatitis B infection may be obtained in some cases. The prognosis is not good, but steroid treatment helps to control symptoms, and cytotoxic drugs such as cyclophosphamide are sometimes indicated.

Takayusu's arteritis

This form of arteritis is confined to the aorta and large vessels, and occurs mainly in older girls. The condition is found world-wide, but the highest prevalence is in Japan and the Far East, and it is not uncommon in southern Africa. Many affected children are undernourished and are from impoverished communities. Immune deposits have been

detected in affected vessels, but the relative roles of infection, immunity, nutrition, and genetics are not known. An association has been noted with a strongly reactive tuberculin test, but no other signs of tuberculosis are usually present.

In the acute phase the condition is often missed because the symptoms are non-specific — fever, arthralgia, myalgia, and fatigue. Laboratory studies show a raised ESR and IgG. Most children present late in the disease when the underlying vasculitis has led to stenosis, thrombosis or aneurysmal dilation of the aorta and its branch vessels, and symptoms secondary to arterial occlusion develop. When the abdominal aorta and renal arteries are affected, severe hypertension and its complications develop, as well as symptoms of visceral ischaemia. Involvement of the carotid arteries leads to cerebral anoxic symptoms and focal neurological signs. Absent or reduced pulses are frequently detected (pulseless disease) in one or more of the limbs, and bruits may be heard.

A classification based on site and extent of the disease is given below *(see Fig. 23.3)*.

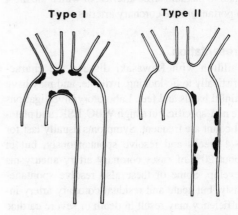

Fig. 23.3 Takayusu's arteritis. Classification based on site and extent

Type I: disease of aortic arch and its branches
Type II: disease of thoracic and abdominal aorta and their branches
Type III: extensive disease (this is a combination and extension of Types I and II).

The only useful investigation is angiography to assess the extent of the arterial disease. Treatment is aimed at controlling symptoms, e.g., hypertension and seizures, although corticosteroids have been used if there are signs of active inflammation. Antituberculous therapy has been advocated, but there is no evidence that it alters the course of the disease, which is slowly progressive but may arrest at any stage. Surgical correction of vascular stenosis or the removal of an ischaemic kidney may be indicated, particularly when reno-vascular hypertension is present.

Kawasaki disease (mucocutaneous lymph node syndrome)

(See Table 23.2.)

Kawasaki disease is an acute multisystem disease predominantly affecting children under 5 years of age. It has a world-wide distribution. Cases have been seen in South Africa, especially in the Western Cape. The aetiology is unknown, although the occurrence of epidemics and clustering of cases suggests that an infectious agent may be implicated.

The pathology is due to a vasculitis affecting small to medium sized arteries, of which the most important are the coronary arteries.

Presentation

Children with Kawasaki disease are characteristically toxic-looking, irritable, and may have painful hands and feet. Laboratory investigations are non-specific, but a high WBC, ESR, and platelet count are frequent. Symptoms usually last for 2–4 weeks and resolve spontaneously, but in about 20% of cases coronary artery aneurysms develop. Some of these also resolve spontaneously, but acute and residual coronary artery insufficiency may result in death or severe cardiac disability.

Diagnosis

The diagnosis is based on clinical criteria *(see Table 23.2)*. The differential diagnosis includes group A streptococcal infections, staphylococcal toxin syndromes, measles, drug reactions, rickettsial infections, infectious mononucleosis, and other rheumatic diseases.

Table 23.2   Criteria for the diagnosis of Kawasaki disease

A spiking fever of more than 5 days' duration plus four of the five following signs:

- conjunctivitis without exudate
- polymorphous erythematous rash
- cervical lymphadenopathy
- erythema of the oropharynx, and strawberry tongue followed by dry, fissuring lips
- oedema and induration of hands and feet, with erythema of palms and feet, desquamating later

Other features include uveitis, sterile pyuria, arthritis or arthralgia, aseptic meningitis, pericardial effusion, and gall bladder inflammation.

Treatment

Both high dose aspirin and intravenous gammaglobulin are recommended treatments. Corticosteroids have not been shown to be effective. High dose aspirin (80–100 mg/kg/day) is given for 2 weeks, followed by low dose aspirin (3–5 mg/kg/day) for a further 6–8 weeks to inhibit platelet aggregation. Aspirin reduces the duration and severity of symptoms, but has no effect on the development of coronary artery vasculitis.

Intravenous immunoglobulin (IVIG) has been shown to significantly reduce the incidence of coronary artery aneurysms when given in the first 10 days of the illness. IVIG can be given as a single dose of 2 g/kg over 10 hours as soon as the clinical diagnosis has been established, or as 4 consecutive daily doses of 400 mg/kg. The single dose regime appears to be slightly more effective, but care must be taken to prevent fluid overload.

Coronary artery involvement is detected by echocardiography, and follow-up studies should be performed at 6–8 weeks. Most children recover completely when treated promptly, but the long-term effects of the coronary artery vasculitis have not been established.

D.W. Beatty

24
Dermatological disorders

Introduction

Bacterial infections and eczema, either alone or in combination, are the most common causes of rashes in children and should always be considered first in the differential diagnosis of any skin disorder.

Table 24.1   Skin disorders in children

	Approximate percentages
Eczema	20
Staph. & Strep. infections	20
Scabies	15
Insect bites + papular urticaria	5
Warts	5
Fungal infections	5
Other	30

Attention to the following points in the history and examination should help to diagnose a puzzling skin disease:
- The **duration** of the present attack and the number and duration of previous rashes, if any.
- A **family history** of skin disease, or contacts at home, school, or elsewhere.
- The **whole skin surface** should be inspected in a good light. This examination should include the skin folds (neck, behind the ears, armpits, groin, and perineum) and the hair, nails, and teeth.
- The site of the **first lesion** and the **distribution** of the rash on the body. Are the lesions diffuse, localized, grouped, or symmetrical?
- The **morphology** of the primary lesion and its localization in the skin. Is it a macule, papule, nodule, vesicle, pustule, or burrow? Is it situated just under the horny layer, in the epidermis, or under it? Does it extend into the dermis or subcutaneous tissue? Palpatation of the skin is just as

important as inspection for establishing the level of the lesion.
- **Secondary effects** such as scratch marks, thickening of the skin due to rubbing, infection, and pigmentary changes must be distinguished from primary lesions due to the skin disease itself.
- **Examination of the mouth, throat, ears and perineum.** Underlying infections such as tonsillitis or gastrointestinal candidiasis may be the cause of seemingly unrelated skin rashes.

Eczema

Eczema is the most common skin disease and occurs with equal frequency in all races. The term dermatitis is synonymous, but is usually reserved for eczema due to contact.

Definition: Eczema is an inflammatory skin disease which affects mainly the epidermis, resulting in the formation of an intra-epidermal vesicle in the acute stage.

Common causes of eczema in babies:
- dryness of skin
- atopic eczema
- seborrhoeic eczema
- napkin dermatitis
- bacterial infection.

Clinical features
(See Table 24.2.)

Eczema has many different causes, but the lesions are similar in all types. Itch is a common symptom. The clinical features of eczema can be divided into three stages, any of which may be present at the same time or at different times in the same patient.

Acute: The skin is red and swollen. Vesicles are visible on the surface and may open to discharge a clear, serous fluid — so-called 'weeping eczema'. The fluid dries up to form pale crusts. This vesicular stage may be followed by scaling or the formation of pustules.

Subacute: Primary lesions consists of papules, with or without scaling.

Chronic: The epidermis is thickened and the normal skin furrows are prominent, referred to as lichenification. Papules, nodules, and scaling may also be found.

Secondary changes: Because of the itch, excoriations are common and may lead to secondary infection. Constant rubbing of the skin causes it to thicken and increases the itch. Pigmentary changes are prominent, particularly in dark-skinned races, and may consist of hyper- or hypopigmentation. Once the eczema has healed the skin colour and texture gradually return to normal.

Table 24.2 Clinical signs in eczema

Acute
Swelling (oedema)
Vesicles
Erythema
'Weeping'

Subacute
Papules
Scaling

Chronic
Papules
'Lichenification'
Scaling

Secondary changes
Excoriations
Secondary infection
Hyper- or hypopigmentation

Types of eczema in children
Dryness of the skin
This is perhaps the most common cause of eczema in infants, in whom dryness is often aggravated by too much bathing, soaps, and powders. It is worse in the winter months. *Pityriasis alba* is a form of dry eczema which occurs commonly on the faces of children of all races. It results in depigmented, scaling patches which are cosmetically disturbing. It is often mistakenly ascribed to vitamin deficiency.

Infection
Skin infections causing damage to the epidermis may result in a secondary eczematous rash. A fairly common cause is purulent otitis externa.

Eczema following trauma of various kinds, including burns, is usually also due to secondary infection. Secondary eczematization may occur around the lesions of scabies and *molluscum contagiosum*.

Atopic eczema
This is a constitutional form of eczema in which there may be a history of hay fever, asthma, and urticaria in the family. These atopic manifestations may also occur in the patient with eczema. In the infant with atopic eczema, a papular and scaling eruption usually starts on the cheeks and extensor parts of the limbs, but may become generalized *(see Fig. 24.1)*. Itch is usually severe, and excoriations and secondary infection are common. At times the eczema may become more acute and oozing. Atopic eczema commonly starts at the age of about 3 months and recurs in a fluctuating

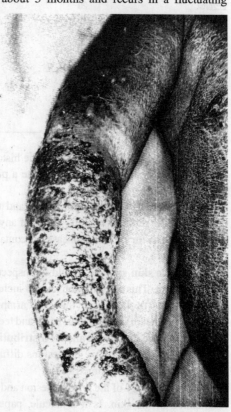

Fig. 24.1 Atopic infantile eczema: Lichenification and scaling (trunk), secondary infection with oozing and crusting (arm)

manner. In older children the eczema tends to become localized in the flexures of the elbows and knees or around these and other joints.

Atopic eczema in babies is often wrongly ascribed to an allergy to cows' milk. In the small number of cases where milk allergy does play a role, gastrointestinal signs such as vomiting and diarrhoea are also present.

It is important that infants with eczema should continue to be breast-fed.

Older children may be allergic to other foods such as eggs or fish. The fluctuating nature of the disease must be explained to parents, who should be warned that the eczema is likely to recur until the child outgrows it, usually by the time he goes to school. Until then it should be kept under control, as untreated it tends to disseminate. Any foods which appear to aggravate the eczema should be temporarily avoided and re-introduced later.

Nummular eczema is the name given to round or coin-shaped patches of eczema which may occur in patients with atopic eczema.

Hand and foot eczema: In older children with atopic eczema, the lesions are often confined to the hands and feet, particularly the palms and soles. In some children the skin is very dry and cracked and this is called keratotic eczema. In others the eczema consists of vesicles and pustules which may recur at intervals for years.

Follicular eczema: Toddlers sometimes develop a fine papular eczematous rash on the limbs, which does not respond well to treatment, but disappears after several months.

Seborrhoeic eczema

This condition is often familial and is considered to be one of the inborn or constitutional types of eczema. The characteristic lesions consist of yellowish scales on the scalp, so-called 'cradle cap'. The flexural areas such as the axillae, groins, perineum, folds in the neck and behind the ears are commonly affected, and the distribution is thus similar to that of the seborrhoeic dermatitis of adults. The lesions often become moist and secondarily infected, and in severe cases the rash may become generalized. It usually starts during the first few weeks of life and may recur for several months, but seldom persists beyond the first year

(see Fig. 24.2). Seborrhoeic eczema is easier to treat and not as persistent as atopic eczema. However, it is not always possible to differentiate between atopic and seborrhoeic eczema in a young infant.

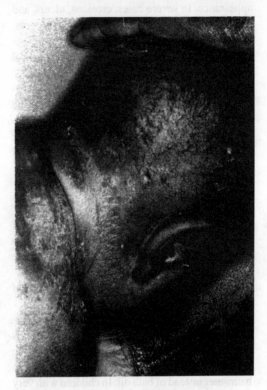

Fig. 24.2 Seborrhoeic infantile eczema: Erythema, scaling, and depigmentation in flexures, and involvement of scalp

Contact dermatitis

Objects such as school benches, car seats, and shoes are sometimes suspected of causing contact dermatitis in children. It may be difficult to decide whether the rash is due to an allergy or to mechanical irritation in a patient with atopic dermatitis. Patch tests may be helpful in the diagnosis. Contact dermatitis due to plants is seen in children of the older age group. The lesions of plant dermatitis are characteristically linear in shape and may be intensely irritating.

Napkin dermatitis

Irritant or eczematous rashes due to soap powders, rinses, or infrequent changing of soiled napkins are easily recognized if it is remembered that the affected skin corresponds to the area in contact with the napkin and the folds in the groins and perineum are spared. The affected skin may be red, glazed, and shiny or have an eczematous appearance. In severe cases, erosions, ulcers, and nodular lesions may occur. Seborrhoeic eczema, candidiasis, and bacterial infection must be excluded. Maximal involvement is seen in the inguinal and intergluteal folds in seborrhoeic dermatitis, and around the anus in candidiasis. Perineal cellulitis is characterized by redness and pain. The term 'napkin psoriasis' is used to describe well-circumscribed, erythematous, smooth or scaling patches which may be an early manifestation of psoriasis in some cases *(see below)*.

Treatment

Any patch of eczema should receive attention; if left in a state of activity, the eczema is likely to spread to other parts of the body and even become generalized.

Treatment of the child with eczema consists of the following:

◆ Relieve dryness of the skin by using an ointment such as ung. emulsificans BP which contains white vaseline, liquid paraffin, and emulsifying waxes. It may be rubbed into the skin or used in bathwater instead of bath oil. In children with very dry skins, it may even be used instead of soap. Vaseline is also useful to relieve dryness.

◆ Any secondary infection always retards healing of the eczema and should be treated. For small areas of infected eczema, a combined antibiotic-steroid cream should be used. If there are hard crusts which need to be removed, a greasy ointment will do this more effectively than a cream. If the infection is widespread or severe, a systemic antibiotic such as erythromycin or cloxacillin should be given in addition.

◆ Moist weeping areas of eczema should be treated with lotions, or wet dressings where bandaging is easy. Saline can easily be made at home by adding 2 teaspoons of salt to a litre of water. It is seldom necessary to use a wet dressing for more than a few days. If an area of weeping eczema looks infected, weak potassium permanganate solution or diluted eusol may be used instead of saline.

◆ Choose the most suitable topical corticosteroid preparation. If the skin is dry, a greasy ointment should be used; if the skin is not dry, and particularly under hot, humid conditions, a cream may be better tolerated. If necessary a trial of each separately may be helpful.

◆ Decide what strength the topical corticosteroid preparation should be. In infants with large areas of eczema, the steroid should be diluted in order to minimize side effects through absorption, and also to make the ointment or cream go further. A corticosteroid preparation such as betamethasone valerate may be diluted up to ten times in ung. emulsificans if a greasy preparation is required; or in ung. emulsificans *aquosum* if a cream base is preferred.

◆ Use undiluted corticosteroid preparations where the eczema is chronic and the skin thickened. If some patches of eczema are still resistant to treatment, occlusive dressings may be tried. The cream or ointment is covered with plastic overnight and left open during the day. This method is particularly useful for keratotic eczema on the palms and soles. Occlusive dressings should not be used if there is any sign of infection, as they will cause it to spread.

◆ In napkin dermatitis the first measure should be to stop the use of nappy creams and disposable diapers, as they may occasionally be the cause of the rash. Napkins should be changed frequently, rinsed well, and left off for as long as possible. Mild corticosteroid creams may be used for a short period in the acute stage.

Bacterial diseases

Staphylococcal and streptococcal infections

Staphylococci and streptococci commonly cause primary and secondary skin infections in children, particularly if they are malnourished and live in overcrowded, unhygienic conditions.

Staphylococcal infections result in the formation of pus and tend to be localized. Neonates are, however, particularly susceptible to *Staph. aureus*, and easily develop generalized infections. Streptococcal infections tend to spread diffusely with very little, if any, suppuration. In the newborn, infection by group B β-haemolytic streptococci from the birth canal may cause a bacteraemia,

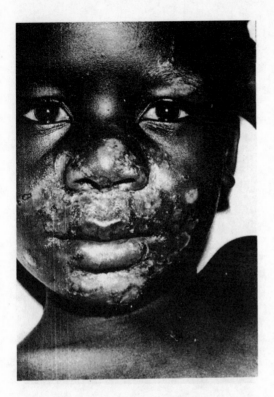

Fig. 24.3 Impetigo: Round, confluent, oozing, and crusted lesions extending into nostrils

which may present in the skin as cellulitis or a purpuric rash. In older children, skin infections are caused by group A β-haemolytic streptococci and may be followed by glomerulonephritis. Infections with strains of streptococci and staphylococci which produce an erythrogenic toxin may result in widespread or localized erythema followed by desquamation.

Treatment: Antibiotic ointments are usually sufficient for localized superficial infections. In widespread staphylococcal infections and for most streptococcal infections, a systemic antibiotic should be given in addition. Erythromycin and cloxacillin are usually safe and effective where sensitivity tests are not available.

Impetigo

This is a very common, superficial, contagious skin infection which may be caused by either staphylococci or streptococci, but usually both. Infection often starts in the nostrils, and the face is most commonly affected, but any part of the skin may be involved. The lesions, which may be single or multiple and confluent, start as small blisters and spread to form round, moist, eroded or crusted areas, at the periphery of which the remains of the blister are usually visible *(see Fig. 24.3)*. Treatment consists of antibiotic ointments such as Polysporin® or Terramycin®, which should include the nostrils if necessary. Where lesions are widespread, an antibiotic should be given by mouth in addition.

Impetigo (pemphigus) neonatorum

In the newborn, staphylococcal impetigo may spread rapidly to form large, superficial bullae, often containing pus. Swabs for culture should be taken from an unbroken blister. Epidermolysis bullosa and bullous congenital syphilis should be excluded by biopsy and serology.

Staphylococcal scalded skin syndrome

The clinical picture resembles that of very superficial burns and is due to a toxin which causes erythema and desquamation. The site of the staphylococcal infection may be the nose, eyes, or skin. Staphylococci may be isolated from the primary infection, but are not found in the distant skin lesions due to the toxin *(see Fig. 24.4)*.

Ecthyma

This is a deep form of impetigo in which the infection extends into the dermis, resulting in the formation of crusted ulcers, followed by depressed scars. It usually occurs on the legs following trauma or insect bites. Antibiotic or antiseptic ointments or wet antiseptic dressings such as eusol will remove the crusts and disinfect the ulcer. An antibiotic should always be given by mouth in addition, as the infection is too deep to respond to topical treatment only.

Boils (furunculosis)

Boils are due to a staphylococcal infection in and around hair follicles. They present as painful, raised, red nodules in which the centre is hard at first, but later softens and discharges pus. Isolated boils heal spontaneously and do not require treatment. In some children they are recurrent, however, and often associated with styes. These

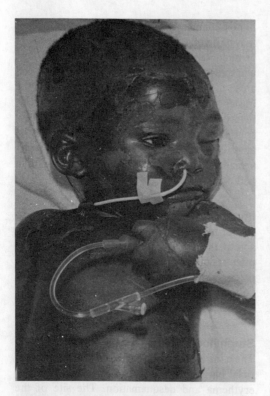

Fig. 24.4   Staphylococcal scalded skin syndrome.
Note abscess in left orbital region, the focus of
infection

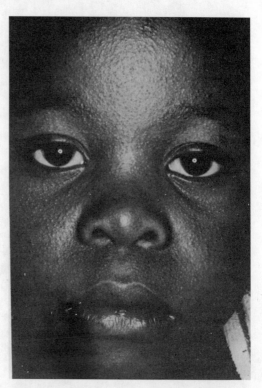

Fig. 24.5   Streptococcal eruption: Fine follicular
rash associated with streptococcal tonsillitis

children and other members of the family are
usually nasal carriers of staphylococci. Treatment
of numerous and recurrent boils consists of systemic and topical antibiotics, which should be
given for at least 2 weeks. If sensitivity tests are
not available, cloxacillin is preferred. Nasal carriers should be treated with an antibiotic ointment,
applied in both nostrils for at least 2 weeks.

Cellulitis

This is an infection of the dermis and subcutaneous tissues. The affected skin is red, tender, swollen, and warm, and regional lymph glands are
enlarged and tender.

Erysipelas is a superficial form of cellulitis
caused by streptococci. A raised, red, advancing
margin is seen on the skin and sometimes blisters
form on the surface.

Perianal cellulitis due to group A β-haemolytic
streptococci is a cause of erythema and pain in the
perineal area in young children.

Skin eruptions secondary to streptococcal tonsillitis

Desquamation of the skin, particularly the palms
and soles, may be the only complaint in a patient
who is otherwise well and has not had scarlet
fever. It is thought to be due to a previous asymptomatic infection with streptococci which produce
an erythrogenic toxin. A fine rash, consisting of
very small, diffuse, suerpficial papules, occurring
in children with a fever, may be due to streptococcal tonsillitis *(see Fig. 24.5)*. The rash and fever
respond rapidly to an oral antibiotic. Streptococcal
tonsillitis may precipitate an attack of guttate psoriasis or seborrhoeic dermatitis, and streptococcal
infection is probably the most common cause of
urticaria in children.

Disseminated intravascular coagulation (DIC)

Gram-negative septicaemia following gastroenteritis is the most common cause of DIC in infants,

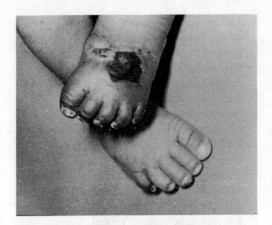

Fig. 24.6 Disseminated intravascular coagulation: Angulated skin infarct and gangrene of toes

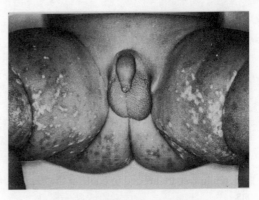

Fig. 24.7 Congenital syphilis: Scaling, pigmented maculo-papules

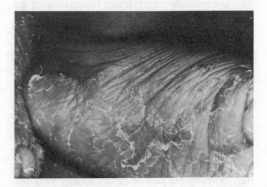

Fig. 24.8 Congenital syphilis: Confluent scaling macules on soles of feet

but it may also follow septicaemia due to strepto-coccal and staphylococcal infections. Skin lesions in DIC are characteristic and consist of angulated purpuric macules which may be followed by the formation of large blisters and skin infarcts *(see Fig. 24.6)*. Biopsy of these lesions shows necrosis of the epidermis and multiple fibrin thrombi in the dermal vessels. Occlusion of deeper vessels may cause gangrene of larger areas such as the ears or digits. Skin biopsy is very useful for the diganosis, as blood tests are often normal. Intensive treatment with broad spectrum antibiotics should start immediately, before results of tests are available.

Syphilis
(Also see Chapter 8, Infectious Disorders.)

Congenital syphilis
Early congenital syphilis occurs within the first 2 years of life. The time of onset of lesions in the baby and their severity depends on the activity of the maternal infection during pregnancy. Bullous lesions with an infiltrated base may be present at birth or appear soon after, and commonly involve the palms and soles. Widespread, scaling, maculo-papular eruptions, mucous patches in the mouth, and moist condylomas in the perineum resemble those of early adult secondary syphilis *(see Figs 24.7 and 24.8)*.

Late congenital syphilis is rarely, if ever, seen, but the possibility of a gumma should be borne in mind in any patient with a chronic ulcer of un-known cause.

Endemic syphilis
This uncommon, non-venereal, *Treponema palli-dum* infection spreads in children by direct skin contact. A primary chancre is rarely seen. Skin and mucous membrane lesions correspond to those of early and late secondary syphilis, and gummas may occur at a later stage. Sexually transmitted disease must always be considered.

Venereal syphilis
Primary chancres may occur as a result of sexual abuse of infants and young children. The charac-teristic firmness of the ulcer and enlarged, rub-bery, regional lymph nodes suggest the diagnosis. Serological tests may be negative in the early stage

and should be repeated after 3 months. Secondary syphilis, although rare in children, should be considered in any infiltrated, papular rash of unknown cause.

Tuberculosis

(Also see Chapter 9, Tuberculosis.)

Skin lesions may be due to direct infection with *Mycobacterium tuberculosis* or to hypersensitivity reactions called tuberculides. Biopsy and a tuberculin test are needed to confirm the diagnosis.

Tuberculous chancre

This is extremely rare. Primary inoculation of the skin results in a nodule which soon ulcerates. The important feature is enlargement of the regional lymph glands.

Lupus vulgaris

This is the most common type of tuberculous skin infection, occurring in a partially-immune patient who has previously had tuberculosis elsewhere. Lesions may be single or multiple, and occur on any part of the body. They may present as soft, flat, or warty plaques or raised spongy nodules. The most common type occures around the nose and has a raised, slowly advancing edge and ulcerating centre. Destruction of the nasal cartilage may result in severe deformity. Patients should be investigated for other foci of tuberculosis.

Tuberculides

These are multiple disseminated lesions resulting from an underlying tuberculous focus which is not always demonstrable. They are due to hypersensitivity reactions, to *M. tuberculosis*, and the tuberculin test is usually strongly positive. There are three clinical types, which may occur singly or together in the same patient:

1 **Papulonecrotic tuberculide:** Lesions consist of papules and pustules which ulcerate, and heal to form oval-to-round depressed scars. They are symmetrically distributed and occur mainly over the extensor aspects of the limbs, particularly the elbows and knees and on the buttocks. Biospy shows a vasculitis due to a type III (Arthus) hypersensitivity reaction.

2 **Lichen scrofulosorum:** Lesions consist of small, firm papules which are commonly grouped together in round patches, but may be diffuse and widespread. Biopsy shows tuberculoid granulomas which are due to cell-mediated immune response.

3 **Nodular tuberculides:** Lesions occur mainly on the lower legs. In the acute form, known as erythema nodosum, nodules appear when the tuberculin test becomes positive in a primary infection. Chronic forms are known as nodular vasculitis, or erythema induratum if they ulcerate. They tend to recur until the underlying tuberculous infection is treated.

Leprosy

See Chapter 8, Infectious Disorders.

Viral infections

Herpes simplex

(Also see Chapter 8, Infectious Disorders.)

Primary infection in infants usually results in gingivostomatitis, consisting of either a few or numerous painful, round or oval ulcers, which heal within 2–3 weeks. In older children, herpes simplex takes the form of 'fever blisters', with clusters of vesicles grouped together on a red base. The blisters become crusted and heal within 2 weeks. The lesions usually occur on the face, mostly on or near the lips, and are preceded by a tingling sensation. In some individuals, lesions recur at intervals for many years; the virus is thought to remain dormant in cutaneous nerves between attacks.

Herpes simplex infection is sometimes followed after 1–2 weeks by erythema multiforme. Disseminated cutaneous herpes simplex consists of a few or many scattered vesicles without any herpetiform grouping. Direct spread of the virus in skin lesions is a rare but serious complication of atopic eczema, known as eczema herpeticum or Kaposi's varicelliform eruption. Herpes simplex infection should be considered in any vesicular rash of unknown cause.

Treatment

Treatment of skin lesions consists of drying, antiseptic applications such as spirits, ether, or eusol.

Antibiotics are indicated only if secondary infection is present.

Severe and generalized infections call for oral or intravenous acyclovir.

Herpes zoster

This is caused by the varicella-zoster virus. Primary infection results in chickenpox. Reactivation of a latent infection in the dorsal ganglion of the spinal cord results in herpes zoster. Children exposed to herpes zoster may develop chickenpox. The lesions of herpes zoster consist of grouped vesicles arranged along the cutaneous distribution of a spinal nerve; they heal within 2–3 weeks. Zoster is relatively rare in children, and neuritis seldom a problem as it is in adults. A severe attack of herpes zoster, whether localized or disseminated, is suggestive of underlying immunosuppression. Treatment consists of acyclovir.

Hand, foot and mouth disease

This infection, due to a coxsackie virus type A, usually occurs in toddlers who have few systemic symptoms. The lesions consist of round or oval vesicles which heal within 2 weeks. The lesions are found commonly, but not exclusively, in the mouth and on the palms and soles. Symptomatic treatment suffices for this self-limiting condition.

Molluscum contagiosum

Caused by a pox virus, the lesions are usually numerous and consist of umbilicated dome-shaped papules containing a cheesy material. The older co-operative child can be treated by inserting the tip of a sharpened match stick, which has been dipped into liquified phenol, into the central pore. In young children, tretenoin (Airol®, Retin A®) or benzyl benzoate emulsion (Ascabiol®) can be rubbed into the affected area 3 times a day until the skin is red and scaling. The lesions become inflamed and then disappear.

Warts

Warts are caused by the human papilloma virus and are extremely common in children of school-going age. The ordinary wart (verruca vulgaris) may be single or multiple and is recognizable by its papillomatous surface. **Plane warts** are small, flat warts which occur in large numbers on the face

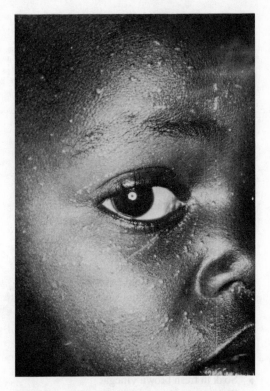

Fig. 24.9   Plane warts: Multiple small papules, some in lines along scratch marks

and limbs *(see Fig. 24.9)*. **Condylomata accuminata**, or genital warts, occur on the genitalia or around the anus and have a moist, vegetating papillomatous surface. The possibility of sexual abuse must be considered.

Treatment

Until children develop immunity against the virus, warts are likely to spread and recur after any form of treatment. Most warts will, however, eventually undergo spontaneous healing, which may be preceded by the appearance of haemorrhagic dots in the centre of the warty projections.

Scarring and unnecessary pain must be avoided: the aim of conservative treatment is to cause irritation of the wart. The resultant inflammatory reaction is usually followed by disappearance of the wart.

Many topical treatments are available, but perhaps the most useful is a common home remedy. Pieces of lemon peel, cut to the size of the warts,

497

are left to soak in brown vinegar for the duration of the treatment, which may take several weeks. Every night a fresh piece of soaked peel, white side next to the skin, is affixed to the wart by means of a plaster. Applications are repeated until the wart becomes inflamed.

For plane warts, the easiest form of treatment is to rub them with 25% benzyl benzoate emulsion (Ascabiol®), 2–3 times a day until the skin becomes red and scaly. It may be necessary to repeat the treatment several times.

Condylomata accuminata are painted with 20% podophyllin in tincture of benzoin, which is dusted with talc powder to protect surrounding skin, and washed off after 6 hours, or earlier if painful. Treatment may be repeated at weekly intervals if necessary.

In general, warts should never be excised, but currettage, with or without preceding light electrodesiccation, is at times justified.

Home remedy for warts
- Pieces of lemon peel cut to size of wart
- Soak in fresh brown vinegar
- Fix to wart with plaster, white side to skin
- Repeat daily until wart is inflamed

Fungal infections

The yeast *Candida albicans* and many of the dermatophytic fungi, which grow in the horny layer of the epidermis, are common causes of infection in children. In all of these the diagnosis may be confirmed by microscopical examination. Skin, hair, and nail scrapings are covered with 30% potassium hydroxide, to which a droplet each of blue Parker Super Quink® fountain pen ink and glycerine are added. The specimen should be re-examined after a day if nothing is seen initially.

Candidiasis

Eruptions due to *Candida albicans* are common in babies, often appearing soon after they have been treated with antibiotics for an infection. The rash usually starts around the anus and spreads to the perineum, groins, and intergluteal fold. Other moist, flexural areas such as the axillae and neck folds may also be involved. The rash is well-circumscribed with a moist, eroded surface and bright red colour. Small discrete, outlying papules

and pustules are a characteristic finding *(see Fig. 24.10)*. The pustules contain a whitish exudate, and being very superficial, soon break to form erosions surrounded by a small peripheral scale. Occasionally a widespread secondary rash consisting of scaling papules occurs on the trunk and limbs. The mouth should always be examined for the presence of 'thrush' (white flecks which cannot be rubbed off without causing bleeding), as this and the extension of the rash into the anus are indicative of a gastrointestinal infection.

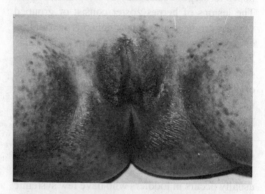

Fig. 24.10   Candidiasis: Perineal involvement in gastrointestinal candidiasis. Note outlying pustules and scaly macules

Treatment

Topical applications of nystatin (Mycostatin®) amphotericin B (Fungizone®), or one of the imidazole preparations (Daktarin®, Canesten®, Pevaryl®) soon clear any skin lesions, but these will recur if any underlying gastrointestinal infection is not treated simultaneously. Oral suspensions of nystatin and amphotericin B are available for this; the latter being more effective.

Ringworm (tinea)

Ringworm infections in children are caused by members of the microsporum and trichophyton species. As a general rule, scalp ringworm occurs only before puberty, and 'athlete's foot' only after.

Scalp ringworm (tinea capitis)

T. violaceum, the most common cause of ringworm in black children, is widespread in disadvantaged communities, spreading easily among household contacts. The lesions consist of patchy or diffuse areas of scaling and hair loss, which may, however, be mild and hardly visible. Mild infections may heal spontaneously without leaving a trace, but in some children secondary bacterial infection results in scarring and patchy permanent hair loss. *M. canis* infections, which are more common in white children, usually cause well-circumscribed, round, scaly areas of hair loss *(see Fig. 24.11)*. Occasionally a lesion may undergo an inflammatory reaction with the formation of a boggy swelling studded with pustules, known as a kerion.

Kerion is due to a hypersensitivity reaction, not to secondary bacterial infection, and should not be incised.

Close inspection of a scalp affected with ringworm reveals thickened, white, opaque hair stumps in which the fungus is easily seen in scrapings taken for microscopical examination.

Body ringworm (tinea corporis)

The lesions are characteristically ring-shaped, with active, raised, scaly margins which spread outwards. Sometimes more than one advancing edge is present and concentric rings are formed.

Nail ringworm is rare in children, and thickened, irregular, or crumbly nails are more likely to be due to diseases such as eczema or psoriasis.

Treatment

Many topical anti-fungal preparations are available. Whitfield's ointment is much cheaper than, and probably as effective as, most of them. The imidazoles (Canesten®, Daktarin®, Pevaryl®) have a broad spectrum antifungal and antibacterial action. Nystatin and amphotericin B, useful for candida infections, are not effective against dermatophytes. Griseofulvin (Grisovin®, Fulcin®), used only by mouth, is specific for dermatophyte infections and is used to treat tinea of the scalp and nails. Topical treatment alone is usually sufficient to clear body ringworm, but widespread infections are easier to control if griseofulvin is given in addition. Use of Whitfield's or other antifungal ointments helps to prevent spread of infection.

Sporotrichosis

The causative organism, *Sporothrix schenckii*, is found in the soil and on plant material, and enters

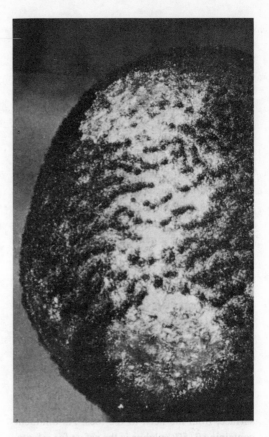

Fig. 24.11 Scalp ringworm: Broken-off white hair stumps in scaling patches of hair loss

the skin through minor injuries. This deep fungal infection should be suspected in any chronic purulent, ulcerative or granulomatous skin lesions which do not respond to antibiotic therapy. Lymphatic spread often results in a centrally-extending row of nodules which may ulcerate. The diagnosis may be confirmed by culture and biopsy. Response to potassium iodide, given by mouth, is specific and may be used as a therapeutic test. Marked improvement is evident within 1–2 weeks, but treatment must be continued for 2–3 months, until the lesions are quite inactive. If the patient is allergic to potassium iodide, ketoconazole (Nizoral®) may be used instead.

Infestations

Scabies

The mite *Sarcoptes scabiei* causes periodic epidemics of an intensely itchy rash, which is common in all races. The characteristic lesions consist of small vesicles and short, superficial burrows, often seen between the fingers. Skin scrapings to demonstrate mites are best taken from these sites. The most common lesions, however, are small, superficial papules which may be widespread on the trunk and limbs but tend to cluster around the axillae and on the buttocks. The papules may be few or numerous, and invariably show evidence of scratching. They heal to leave small white spots with a dark rim, which take several months to fade. Larger nodular lesions, so-called persistent scabies papules, are sometimes found in the axillae and groin and on the genitalia. Young babies often have a widespread rash which may include the face and scalp; vesicles and pustules on the palms and soles are a characteristic finding in babies. Often the diagnosis is suggested when one or more household contacts have a similar itching rash.

Treatment

Three preparations are available, and each is curative provided that it is applied over the entire skin surface, from the neck to the toes. An ointment containing 2–5% sulphur is the safest for infants. It should be applied for 3 consecutive nights and include the head if this is involved. Ascabiol® (25% benzyl benzoate emulsion), also applied for 3 nights, is not tolerated by young children, as it causes a burning sensation on raw areas. Gamma benzene hexachloride (Quellada®, Gambex®) requires only one application, but is toxic and not recommended for babies, or for young children with many excoriated lesions. To avoid reinfection, close household contacts should be treated at the same time. Scabicidal soaps alone are not effective in an established infection, but are probably useful for prevention. At the end of the treatment period, clothes and bed-linen are laundered in the usual way and do not require any special disinfestation.

Skin lesions and itch decrease immediately, but take 3–4 weeks to clear completely. Persistence of itch after proper treatment is likely to be due to dryness and even eczema resulting from the topical applications, all of which may irritate the skin.

Insect bites

Insect bites cause itchy papules, in the centre of which a small punctum (the bite) can usually be seen. Vesicles or large blisters may form on some of them. Insect bites are invariably scratched and often secondarily infected. Flea bites tend to be small, are often grouped in short lines, and although they occur mainly on exposed parts of the limbs, are often found around the waist. Mosquito and bedbug bites are larger, and the latter usually have a prominent, haemorrhagic punctum. Jassids — small, hard, green flying insects found on grass — are an infrequently recognized source of insect bites. Jassid bites are small, intensely itchy, and largely confined to the lower extremities.

Papular urticaria (lichen urticatus)

In some children who are hypersensitive to insect bites, numerous, intensely itchy papules occur on the limbs, particularly during the months when insects abound. Unlike true urticaria, which is fleeting, the lesions are fixed, scratched, and often secondarily infected. Children between the ages of 2 and 6 years are affected, and attacks may recur during several successive summers.

Treatment

Prevention of insect bites is difficult. Insect repellents and mosquito nets should be used and pets should be treated for fleas and kept out of doors. In mild cases, calamine lotion may suffice. Severely itching lesions are best treated with a corticosteroid cream covered with a waterproof plaster to enhance penetration. An antibiotic ointment should be prescribed if there is any sign of infection.

Sandworm (larva migrans, creeping eruption)

Larvae of the cat and dog hookworm (Ankylostoma braziliense) penetrate any part of the skin which comes into contact with soil contaminated with the eggs. The characteristic lesions are severely itchy, superficial, relatively large winding burrows. Secondary infection is common. Thiabendazole (Mintezol®) rubbed into the skin 2–3 times a day is curative. It is most readily available as an oral veterinary suspension (Thibenzole®), but crushed tablets may be incorporated into a cream base.

Myiasis

The fly *Cordylobia anthropophaga* lays her eggs on clothing hung out to dry. Larvae burrow into the skin from infected clothing, causing red painful nodules. These are mistaken for boils until the larvae are seen moving in the central opening. Application of vaseline cuts off their air supply and causes them to wriggle outwards. Once the larvae have been removed, the lesions heal quickly. Infestation can by prevented by ironing clothes before they are worn.

Lice

Head lice cause periodic epidemics among white and Indian school children. The easiest form of treament is to shampoo with gamma benzene hexachloride (Quellada®, Gambex®).

Immunologically mediated skin disorders

Urticaria

Skin lesions appear within seconds, are intensely itchy, and disappear within hours without leaving a trace. They may be few or numerous, and may consist of flat, red papules or large, confluent plaques or rings. Crops of new lesions may continue to appear for days or years.

The lesions are due to oedema, resulting from increased permeability of blood-vessels following the release of histamine and other substances in the skin *(see Table 24.3)*. When deeper vessels are involved, diffuse, ill-defined swellings result. These are known as angio-oedema, and often affect the eyelids or lips. Larynx involvement may be a life-threatening complication.

The term dermographism is used to describe the production of raised weals by firm stroking of the skin. It is often found in patients with urticaria, but may occur as an isolated finding in perfectly normal individuals.

Urticaria may be due to a variety of causes such as parasites, infections, foods or drugs; but the aetiology is often unknown. Routine investigations in chronic urticaria should include blood count, bilharzia serology, examination of urine and stools for infections and parasites, and X-rays

Table 24.3   Some causes of urticaria in children

Infections	Tonsillitis
	Urinary tract infection
	Sinusitis
	Dental sepsis
Parasites	Worms
	Schistosomiasis
Drugs	Aspirin
	Penicillin
Foods	Eggs, fish
	Preservatives

of the chest. Occasionally X-rays of teeth and sinuses are necessary.

Acute urticaria in children is usually due to infections such as streptococcal tonsillitis. Penicillin and aspirin, commonly used in infections, are the most common drugs which cause urticaria. It is often impossible to decide whether a drug, or the infection for which it is given, is the offender.

Treatment

An antihistamine by mouth is all that is needed in a mild attack of unknown cause. A systemic antibiotic should be given in addition if an underlying infection is suspected. Severe attacks of urticaria may require systemic corticosteroids as well. If laryngeal oedema threatens, adrenalin should be given subcutaneously and the antihistamines by IM or IV injection. Corticosteroids have a more delayed action.

Allergic vasculitis

(See Chapter 23, Juvenile Chronic Arthritis and Vasculitides.)

Erythema multiforme

Lesions consist of small papules or vesicles, which spread outward to form one or more concentric rings with dark centres — so-called target or iris lesions. They vary in appearance from small, flat papules with raised edges and a dark central crust, to large, haemorrhagic bullae. The rash is symmetrical and occurs mainly on the face and extensor surfaces of the limbs, particularly over the elbows and knees. Drugs, and bacterial and viral infections (notably *Herpes simplex*) are known causes of erythema multiforme, but often the aetiology is obscure.

Stevens-Johnson syndrome is a severe form of erythema multiforme in which the lesions are large, bullous, and crusted, and the mucous membranes of the mouth, genitalia, and eyes are involved *(see Fig. 24.12)*. Some cases of Stevens-Johnson syndrome are due to infections such as *Mycoplasma pneumoniae*, others to drugs such as sulphonamides or phenolphthalein, but the cause is often unknown.

Toxic epidermal necrolysis is a severe form of erythema multiforme in which blistering of the skin resembles burns. It may be found in association with other forms of erythema multiforme. The epidermal blister is deeper than in staphylococcal scalded skin syndrome, from which it should be distinguished, if necessary by biopsy.

Treatment

Erythema multiforme takes 3 weeks to clear and no specific treatment is required for mild cases with no underlying cause. Severe cases are given systemic antibiotics and corticosteroids, although the steroids probably do not alter the course of the disease. The lips and genitalia should be treated with greasy, antibiotic ointments to soften crusts and prevent infection.

Erythema nodosum

Lesions consist of painful, deep nodules on the lower legs, mainly over the shins. They are usually bilateral and tend to recur for 2–3 months. The overlying skin may be red and oedematous and the condition is often misdiagnosed as cellulitis. In children, streptococcal infections are the most common cause, and they should be examined for possible tonsillitis, sinusitis and dental infection. Tuberculosis and sarcoidosis should be excluded. Often no cause is found, and a viral infection suspected.

Genetic disorders

Ichthyosis

The term ichthyosis is used for a group of inherited disorders of the epidermis which are characterized by dryness and scaliness. The degree of scaling

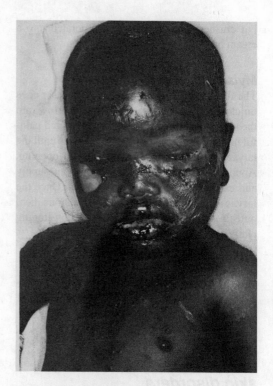

Fig. 24.12 Stevens-Johnson syndrome: Erosion of mucous membranes (mouth and eyes), erythema multiforme with target lesions (chest) and toxic epidermal necrolysis (cheeks)

varies from a mild superficial desquamation to an appearance resembling the scales of a fish.

The term **collodion baby** is used to describe a neonate covered with a shiny, glazed membrane, which cracks and peels off within a few days. This may be an early manifestation of one of the persistent forms of ichthyosis.

Harlequin fetus is the most severe form of ichthyosis, in which marked hyperkeratosis and rigidity of the skin over the whole body results in the formation of deep fissures. It is rare, recessively inherited, and usually results in death before or shortly after birth.

Treatment

Treatment of ichthyosis consists of the regular use of greasy ointments such as ung. emulsificans BP. The retinoic acid derivative, etretinate (Tigason®) results in temporary improvement, but long-term treatment is limited by serious side-effects.

Epidermolysis bullosa

This is a group of inherited disorders with varying age of onset and severity, in which blisters form under the epidermis. The only type commonly encountered in South Africa is the recessively inherited **epidermolysis bullosa letalis**, seen in black neonates. At or soon after birth, blisters appear on any part of the skin and in the mouth. Some blisters heal, but new ones appear, and the child dies within a few months. Impetigo neonatorum and congenital syphilis must be excluded.

Miscellaneous skin disorders

Erythema toxicum

Lesions appear within the first few days of life and clear spontaneously within 3 days. They consist of small pustules on an erythematous base and occur on any part of the body, but mainly on the trunk and proximal parts of the limbs. The cause is unknown and no treatment is required.

Pityriasis rosea

This condition is thought to be due to a viral infection. It occurs sporadically or in small epidemics, affecting mainly children and young adults. The rash is usually confined to the trunk and proximal parts of the limbs, but in younger children may be more widespread, involving even the face and scalp. The lesions start as small papules, which soon enlarge to form oval macules covered with fine, superficial scales. On the back and chest they are arranged in lines which follow the direction of the ribs *(see Fig. 24.13)*. The generalized rash may be preceded by a large, round, scaling macule, the so-called herald patch, which is usually misdiagnosed as ringworm. The rash clears spontaneously within 2 months. Treatment consists of a bland cream such as ung. emulsificans aquosum, with or without a corticosteroid diluted to 10%. Atypical forms may need to be differentiated from seborrhoeic dermatitis and secondary syphilis.

Psoriasis

This chronic, usually recurrent, skin disease is common in all races. The cause is unknown, but genetic factors play a role. Skin lesions consist of raised, well-circumscribed plaques with rather shiny scales which become white and opaque on being scratched. The whole scale can often be scraped off in one piece, revealing a brownish, glistening membranous under-surface and small bleeding points on the exposed underlying dermis. The lesions are usually large and round, occurring mainly over the knees and elbows and on the scalp;

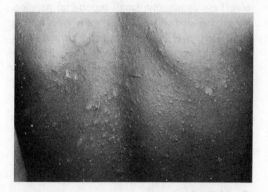

Fig. 24.13   Pityriasis rosea: Herald patch, papular and scaling lesions on back

but they may vary in size and shape and occur on any part of the body. Involvement of the nail bed results in pitting, thickening, and friability of the nail plate.

Guttate psoriasis consists of a widespread eruption of small lesions which may appear rather suddenly on the trunk, usually after an acute infection, particularly streptococcal tonsillitis.

Treatment

Treatment of psoriasis remains a problem. Guttate psoriasis usually clears after a precipitating infection is treated, but the disease may recur later in a chronic form. Psoriasis may respond to full strength or diluted corticosteroid ointments, particularly under occlusive dressings, but the lesions tend to recur. Ointments containing coal tar (e.g., 5% coal tar and 10% salicylic acid in ung. emulsificans) usually give better results and longer remissions. Some patients improve if they are given an antibiotic for a long period, even if there is no evidence of a focus of infection. Fortunately psoriasis may also undergo spontaneous remission.

Lichen planus

This disease of unknown cause occurs twice as commonly in blacks as in whites. Children are sometimes affected. Characteristic lesions consist of purplish, well-demarcated, polygonal, flat-topped papules with a shining, scaly surface. The lesions are very itchy and somtimes spread along scratch marks — the so-called Koebner phenomenon. Less commonly, small superficial papules, larger ring-shaped lesions, or warty nodules are seen. They may be few in number or numerous and widespread, and can involve any part of the skin. Lichen planus in the mouth appears as milky-white lines or spots. Involvement of the nail bed may cause permanent loss of the nail plate. New crops of lesions usually appear for many months, and further attacks are common. When healing, lesions develop a slate-coloured hyperpigmentation and itching subsides.

Treatment

Treatment consists of corticosteroid creams, full strength or diluted, depending on the size of the area involved. Occlusive dressings greatly enhance their effect and should always be used on the limbs. Systemic corticosteroids are reserved for widespread lesions which are unresponsive to topical treatment.

Chronic bullous dermatosis of childhood

The cause of this chronic disease and of the related but less common condition, **dermatitis herpetiformis** is unknown. Skin lesions consist of itchy subepidermal bullae, which heal to leave round confluent patches of hyperpigmentation. They are symmetrically distributed on the trunk and extensor surfaces of the limbs. Crops of new blisters may continue to erupt for many years. Dapsone is used to treat both disorders. Some patients with dermatitis herpetiformis improve on a gluten-free diet.

Vitiligo

Lesions consist of well-circumscribed symmetrical white patches which tend to spread progressively. The skin is otherwise normal. The loss of pigment is due to destruction of melanocytes, probably an autoimmune phenomenon. An association with other autoimmune diseases such as thyroiditis and diabetes has been described in adults, but children with vitiligo are invariably healthy. There is a family history of vitiligo in about one-third of patients. Vitiligo-like depigmentation may follow trauma and inflammatory skin diseases.

Treatment

Corticosteroid creams may be tried for 3 months and sunscreens should be used for large areas of depigmentation. Results of treatment are unsatisfactory and difficult to assess, as lesions may repigment spontaneously.

Alopecia areata

Like vitiligo, with which it is sometimes associated, alopecia areata may be autoimmune in origin. It is characterized by round, well-circumscribed areas of hair loss, which occur most commonly on the scalp, and in which the skin is smooth and lax. Sometimes the eyebrows or eyelashes are affected, with or without scalp involvement. In most patients the hair regrows within a few months, but in some, the patches of alopecia may recur and spread. Usually no cause is found, but in some children stress plays a definite role, and the possibility of problems at home or at school should be investigated.

Treatment

Corticosteroid creams or preparations causing inflammation of the skin such as tretinoin (Airol®, Retin A®) are worth trying. Systemic corticosteroids should not be given, as they cause only a temporary regrowth of hair.

Acne

Although this common condition is seldom a problem before puberty, some children with large sebaceous glands and an inherited tendency to acne may develop blackheads as early as the age of 10 years. The first and most important measure is to wash the face twice daily with a mild toilet soap and a face cloth, and to avoid the application of creams and ointments of any kind. Drying agents such as 2% sulphur in calamine lotion may be applied to greasy areas and actual lesions.

E.J. Schulz

25

Disorders of the eye

Introduction

Striking advances in ophthalmology over the last decade or two have made this speciality popular with would-be specialists. Unfortunately these advances often require an expensive support system not available in underserved areas. This causes reluctance on the part of young ophthalmologists to move into areas where they are sorely needed. However, primary health care workers can do much to alleviate the problem.

Paediatric ophthalmic examination

History

The mother should be questioned about the visual milestones such as fixing and following. Smiling at mother usually occurs by the time a baby is 8 weeks old. Motor milestones should also be checked, as these are often dependent on vision. Children often do not complain of visual loss, but a squint or other signs may have been noted.

Clinical examination

(Also see Chapters 1 and 2).

Every effort should be made to put the child at ease. Small children are best examined on the mother's lap. Visual alertness should be noted, with any obvious abnormalities such as proptosis, ptosis, abnormal head posture, squint, or nystagmus. The use of a penlight torch, finger puppet, or toy is useful in determining central fixation and following. Each eye should be assessed using the examiner's thumb as an occluder.

Visual acuity in pre-school children may be assessed with the Illiterate E Chart *(see Fig. 25.1)*. The Snellen chart is used for older children but may also be used for pre-school children, surprisingly effectively, in the following way. A white card showing regular letters such as HOT, etc. is given to the child. The examiner then points to these letters on the Snellen chart and the child is

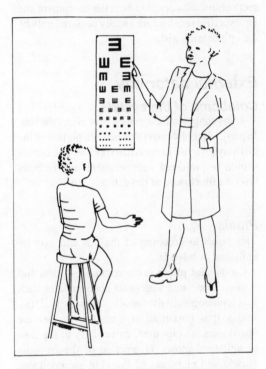

Fig.25.1 Testing acuity of a non-literate child: The child is taught to point his finger in the same direction as the horizontals of the E

asked to 'find the letter on the card'. Even small children often enjoy this 'reading game'.

The external eye should be examined as carefully as possible using the penlight torch and, when necessary, a loupe. Fluorescein strips should be used for staining the cornea, in preference to liquid fluorescein which may become contaminated with pseudomonas. The slit lamp should be used where available. A lid speculum may be necessary. Dilatation of the pupil for examination of the fundus may be performed in neonates with phenylephrine 1% and cyclopentolate hydrochloride 0.5% (Cyclogyl®). In older children phenylephrine 2.5% cyclopentolate hydrochloride 0.5% (Cyclogyl®), and tropicamide hydrochloride 1%

Mydriacyl®), may be used. Fundoscopy with the direct ophthalmoscope is often difficult. An assistant should attempt to obtain the child's attention at a distance in order to allow visualization of areas other than the macula. Speed is essential. Fundoscopy in children is best performed with the indirect ophthalmoscope, but both the instrument and the expertise required are usually acquired only by the ophthalmologist.

External deformity

Coloboma of the eyelids

Various congenital anomalies may affect the lids. In particular coloboma (absence of a portion of the lid) may give rise to corneal exposure. The cornea should be protected with ointment and the baby referred for closure of the defect.

Ptosis

This refers to drooping of the lids and may be unilateral or bilateral.

Congenital ptosis is the commonest form and is often associated with other abnormalities such as blepharophimosis (small interpalpebral fissures). It is important to ascertain whether the visual axes are obscured, particularly in the case of unilateral ptosis. Overaction of the frontalis muscle and elevation of the chin are common. Where the ptosis is unilateral and the visual axis is obscured, surgery is urgent to prevent amblyopia.

Usually, however, surgery is best deferred until the child is older.

Third nerve palsy causes ptosis, but there are almost always other signs such as extraocular muscle weakness. The pupil may be involved.

Horner's syndrome (a lesion of the sympathetic pathway) gives rise to a mild ptosis with a small pupil on the same side. In congenital cases the affected iris may be paler.

Myasthenia gravis should always be included in the differential diagnosis.

Haemangioma of the lid may grow with alarming rapidity in infancy and may give rise to a mechanical ptosis with occlusion of the visual axis and resultant amblyopia. Corticosteroid injection may be helpful in inducing regression. Most haemangiomata do resolve before 5 years of age.

Inflammatory conditions of the lids

Stye (hordeolum): This is caused by inflammation of the lash follicle. It is commonly associated with chronic lid margin inflammation due to staphylococcus. Pus points at the lash, which should be removed. Hot compresses and antibiotic ointment should be applied.

Meibomian cyst (chalazion): This is a chronic lipogranulomatous inflammation of the meibomian gland. A firm, round lump is felt on the lid, and on everting the eyelid a dark or yellow lesion is seen on the palpebral conjunctiva. An incision along the meibomian duct at right angles to the lid margin on the palpebral surface, followed by curettage, is curative. Unfortunately this usually requires a general anaesthetic in children. Small lesions may occasionally disappear spontaneously. Where a meibomian abscess has developed there may be marked lid swelling and surgical incision over the pointing area is necessary.

The danger of cavernous sinus thrombosis should always be borne in mind with severe infections of the lid area.

Proptosis

Proptosis implies forward displacement of the globe, and is not common. It may be congenital and bilateral, occurring with shallow orbits or in association with craniofacial abnormalities. Sinus pathology, orbital abscess, and tumours such as rhabdomyosarcoma should all be included in the differential diagnosis. Signs of inflammation, presence or absence of ocular movement, and presence of masses palpated through the lids are helpful in making the diagnosis. Any sudden onset of proptosis, particularly if unilateral and associated with pain and loss of vision, should be referred for urgent assessment. Computerized tomography is almost always necessary. All patients with proptosis require referral to the ophthalmologist.

The red eye (with discharge or watering)

Conjunctivitis

This is an acute inflammation of the conjunctiva which is usually bacterial or viral.

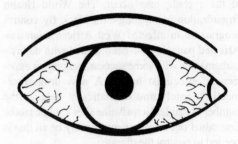

Fig. 25.2a Conjunctival injection: The blood vessels are large, superficial, and emanate from the periphery

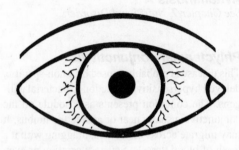

Fig. 25.2b Ciliary injection as seen in keratitis, uveitis, etc.

Conjunctival injection must be differentiated from ciliary injection, which indicates more serious, deeper pathology *(see Fig. 25.2a and b)*.

Bacterial

Common causative organisms are *Staphylococcus epidermidis*, *Staphylococcus aureus*, haemophilus and streptococcus. The eyes are diffusely red with dilatation of the superficial vessels. There is often a discharge and the eyes may be stuck together in the morning. The cornea is clear and the vision good. Frequent treatment with chloramphenicol drops, hourly at first and decreasing to 4 times a day, usually results in cure. Neomycin may cause sensitivity and gentamicin should not be used as a first line drug, to prevent development of resistant strains. Patients who show no improvement within 2–3 days, or in whom the cornea becomes hazy or the vision deteriorates, should be referred for specialist treatment.

Viral

Adenovirus infection is the commonest cause of viral conjunctivitis. Pharyngo-conjunctival fever (PCF) is due to adenoviruses 3 and 7. Children are often affected and have a simultaneous upper respiratory tract infection. Epidemic kerato-conjunctivitis (EKC) is due to adenoviruses 8 and 19. There is commonly an associated keratitis as well as enlarged pre-auricular nodes. Both viral conditions are highly contagious and it is very important to avoid hand–eye contact. Hand-washing by health care professionals is essential between cases.

Treatment is supportive, and topical chloramphenicol may be used to prevent secondary infection. Antiviral agents and corticosteroids should *not* be used. Patients should be strongly discouraged from the practice of washing their eyes with their own urine, which may lead to secondary gonococcal conjunctivitis with eventual loss of the eye.

Ophthalmia neonatorum

Gonococcal infection causes hyperacute purulent conjunctivitis between days 2 and 4 after birth. Treatment with one intramuscular dose of ceftriaxone 62.5 mg usually effects a cure.

Chlamydia trachomatis is also a cause of ophthalmia neonatorum, presenting between 5 and 14 days after birth with an acute mucopurulent conjunctivitis. Treatment is with topical tetracycline and oral erythromycin for 14 days (50 mg/kg/day) in four divided doses.

Gonococcal or chlamydia conjunctivitis in a child should give rise to suspicion of sexual abuse *(see Chapter 4, Community Paediatrics)*.

Vernal conjunctivitis (spring catarrh)

This is an allergic, extremely itchy, kerato-conjunctivitis common in atopic patients. There is associated watering and photophobia. On examination there are raised limbal nodules often associated with increased pigmentation at the limbus. Eversion of the upper lid reveals the typical cobblestone mucosa. The two manifestations may occur separately or together. The lids may be hyperpigmented due to itching and rubbing. Treatment is prophylactic, with the use of cromoglycate drops. Topical cortisone may be required, but this treatment should be reserved for the specialist centre. The disease is usually mild, but can be severe and blinding.

Uveitis

This inflammation may affect any portion of the uveal tract, viz., iritis, cyclitis, or choroiditis. Generally, though, one speaks of an anterior, posterior or pan-uveitis (i.e., involvement of the whole uveal tract). Symptoms include pain, redness, photophobia, and blurred vision. Infection is usually more prominent in the area of the limbus, giving rise to the so-called 'ciliary flush' as opposed to the diffuse redness of conjunctivitis *(see Figs 25a and b)*. Careful examination with a bright penlight and the loupe may reveal keratic precipitates (KPs) on the endothelial surface of the cornea. Iris nodules may also be present.

Investigation

Investigation may require sophisticated testing.
♦ **Tuberculosis** should always be ruled out.
♦ **Blunt trauma** may give rise to a chronic traumatic uveitis.
♦ **Juvenile chronic arthritis,** particularly the pauciarticular type, is commonly associated with bilateral chronic anterior uveitis *(see Chapter 23)*.
♦ **Toxocara larvae** infestation is one of the commonest causes of unilateral uveitis in children of poor socio-economic background *(see Chapter 8, Infectious Disorders)*. Ocular *larva migrans,* may give rise to endophthalmitis and macular or peripheral retinochoroidal granulomas. Treatment with oral thiabendazole may exacerbate the condition when the worm dies, and should not be used without concurrent systemic steroid therapy. Sophisticated vitreous surgery at specialized institutions may sometimes save the sight of the eye. The condition may be difficult to differentiate from retinoblastoma *(see below)*.
♦ **Cysticercus,** the encysted form of *taenia solium*, and other parasites may cause posterior uveitis *(see Chapter 8, Infectious Disorders)*.
♦ **Onchocerciasis (river blindness)** is a chronic parasitic infection due to the microfilariae of *Onchocerca volvulus*, with the black fly as the vector. The disease may give rise to chronic uveitis associated with corneal and retinal scarring. Secondary cataract, glaucoma, and phthisis bulbi (shrinkage

of the eyeball) may occur. The World Health Organization has a long-term black fly control programme in affected West African countries. Affected patients have been treated with diethylcarbamazine with some success, but only in experienced specialist hands. A new drug, Ivermectin®, safely and dramatically reduces the number of viable microfilariae after a single tablet. One tablet once a year may possibly be all that is needed to control the disease.

The red eye (with corneal involvement)

Avitaminosis A
See Chapter 7, Nutritional Disorders.

Phlyctenular conjunctivitis
This disease is probably caused by a non-specific, delayed hypersensitivity reaction to bacterial antigens. The condition presents as a nodule on the conjunctiva, usually near or astride the limbus. It may migrate across the cornea, dragging with it a leash of blood vessels. Severe ulceration or even perforation can occur. Treatment is with topical corticosteroids. Tuberculosis must always be excluded.

Herpes simplex keratitis
Herpes simplex is a common cause of corneal ulceration which is often not recognized in Third World situations. A classic dendritic ulcer which stains well with fluorescein may occur, as may a geographic atypical stromal ulcer which is less easy to diagnose.

Recurrent episodes lead to corneal scarring and sometimes blindness. Precipitating factors include ultraviolet light and fever — hence the common occurrence in children with malaria or measles. Symptoms include pain, photophobia, and tearing. The diagnosis should be suspected where the ulcer has lasted for longer than a week and where there is a history of repeated corneal ulcers.

Disciform keratitis may also occur due to an immune response to the viral antigen within the stroma. It is usually unilateral, but in young, poorly-nourished children bilateral disease is common.

Treatment

Antiviral topical treatment should be used, such as idoxuridine (IDU) 1% drops hourly until the ulcers heal, but not for more than 2 weeks. Trifluor-thymidine (TFT) 1% may be instilled 4- hourly. Acyclovir is effective but expensive. It is available as a 3% ointment which can be used 3-hourly. Topical steroids encourage proliferation of the virus.

Disciform keratitis requires the use of steroids. Treatment of this condition requires specialist care, as active viral disease may recur with the steroid treatment.

Trachoma

The disease is caused by chlamydia and is spread mainly by flies and by direct contact. In the early stages of the disease there is an acute inflammation of the lid conjunctiva, which progresses to mature follicles on the lids and subsequently results in scarring. Scarring of the cornea is caused by constant scratching of the eyelashes from inturned lids (entropion). The main thrust of treatment should be prevention. Improved sanitation and decreasing the fly population are very important. Daily washing of the face leads to marked decrease in the incidence of the disease — 'Every child should have a clean face every day'. Sharing of face-cloths and towels should be discouraged in endemic areas.

In active stages tetracycline ointment may be applied 4 times a day for 6 weeks, together with oral tetracycline or erythromycin. Severe entropion should be corrected with lid surgery.

White pupil (leukocoria)

Cataract

Cataract occurs when the lens of the eye becomes cloudy and presents as a grey or white appearance in the pupil. It may be unilateral or bilateral, and present in varying degrees from birth and during childhood. The cause is often not found (*see Table 25.1 for causes*).

Management

Management may be difficult in unsophisticated populations. Patients with dense bilateral cataracts should be referred for surgery as soon as possible, before the development of nystagmus (before 6 weeks of age). Where cataracts are bilateral and immature, surgery may be postponed until vision

Table 25.1 Causes of cataract in childhood

Hereditary

Congenital rubella (may be associated with microphthalmia and /or retinopathy)

General conditions, e.g., atopic dermatitis, diabetes, galactosaemia, and Down's syndrome

Trauma (sudden, usually unilateral development of cataract)

deteriorates. Unilateral cataracts are probably best left alone except where parents are strongly motivated and where there is a possibility of wearing contact lenses.

It is most important to differentiate cataracts from the leukocoria of retinoblastoma.

Retinoblastoma

Retinoblastoma is a primary malignant neoplasm of the retina and is the commonest intraocular malignancy of children. About a third of cases are bilateral. A small percentage have a positive family history. The commonest presenting sign is a white pupil (leukocoria). Frequently small blood vessels will be noted on the white surface, which is never the case with uncomplicated cataracts. Other presenting signs are painful red eye, squint, buphthalmos and proptosis. Urgent referral to hospital is mandatory. Advanced pathology is seen when there has been a delay in identification of the problem in the home or at primary level. The mainstay of therapy for these patients is enucleation or exenteration, with or without radiotherapy and/or chemotherapy. Treatment at a specialized centre is necessary. Further delays occur when parents do not agree to enucleation and take their children to traditional healers first. Delay in diagnosis or treatment greatly increases the risk of spread, initially via the optic nerve and locally, but later to other sites such as the skull and long bones. Genetic counselling in patients with a family history is essential.

Retinopathy of prematurity (formerly retrolental fibroplasia)

This disease occurs in premature infants, especially those under 1.5 kg birth weight who have had oxygen therapy. Its incidence is increasing again owing to the improved survival of premature babies. In advanced cases fibrous tissue causes a white appearance in the pupil. The peripheral retina is incompletely vascularized and fibrovascular proliferation may occur in response to oxygen damage. Progression gives rise to retinal detachment and fibrosis. Fortunately, spontaneous regression occurs in about 80% of infants.

Management

Preventative measures require that infants at risk should be screened between the 7th and 9th weeks of life, as retinal detachment seldom occurs before 7 weeks and retinopathy of prematurity usually does not occur for the first time after 9 weeks. The pupil should be dilated with phenylephrine 1% and cyclopentolate hydrochloride 0.5% (Cyclogyl®). The lids are retracted with an infant speculum. The periphery should be carefully examined for evidence of a white line or new vessel tufts. Dragging of the macula towards the temporal periphery may be seen.

    Treatment in the early stages is with prophylactic cryotherapy and in the late stages with complicated and sophisticated vitreoretinal techniques. The outlook for vision in advanced cases is very poor.

Lacrimation (tearing)
Nasolacrimal duct obstruction

A membranous obstruction at the terminal end of the duct is common, and may result in a clear or pussy discharge. Spontaneous canalization occurs in the majority of cases. Massage four times a day over the lacrimal sac is helpful, particularly if the common canalicus is blocked with the index finger. Sulphacetamide drops four times a day may be prescribed. Probing is recommended in cases which fail to canalize by the age of one year. However, difficult cases may require silicone tube itubation or dacryocystorhinostomy.

Glaucoma

Glaucoma occurs when the intraocular pressure is raised above the normal 21 mmHg.

    Primary glaucoma due to congenital abnormalities in the drainage angle is the commonest cause. (Causes are listed in *Table 25.2*.) An enlarged

Table 25.2　Causes of glaucoma in childhood

Primary glaucoma
Anterior chamber abnormalities
Neurofibromatosis
Sturge-Weber syndrome
Trauma
Secondary glaucoma (after blunt trauma or other serious eye
   pathology)

cornea (buphthalmos — ox-eye) during the first 3 years of life should always raise the suspicion of glaucoma. The normal corneal diameter before one year of age is 10 mm. A steamy cornea, tearing, and photophobia may precede or accompany these signs. In an older child, sudden onset of glaucoma may cause pain and vomiting together with loss of vision.

    Retinoblastoma may masquerade as buphthalmos.

    Any child suspected of having glaucoma should be immediately referred to an ophthalmic centre. Surgery is usually required to control the intraocular pressure. However, the visual outcome is often poor.

Squint (strabismus)

This occurs when the visual axes of the eyes are not aligned. The commonest form of squint in children is congenital esotropia (eyes turning inwards). *(See Table 25.3 for causes of squint.)* It is important to establish the age of onset, family history, and whether the squint is intermittent or constant. The diagnosis is made by shining a light onto the eyes from a distance. Any deviation of the corneal light reflex from the centre of the pupil is noted *(see Fig. 25.3)*. This allows assessment of the angle of deviation and will help to rule out the false diagnosis of strabismus in a baby with large epicanthic folds *(see Fig. 25.4)*. When the fixating

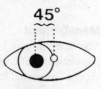

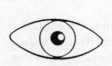

Fig. 25.3　Left esotropia of 45 ° with the light reflex at limbus

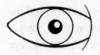 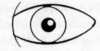

Fig. 25.4 Large epicanthic folds cause pseudostrabismus. Light reflexes central in both eyes

eye is occluded, the deviated eye should quickly take up fixation. Failure to do so implies amblyopia ('lazy eye'). A head turn or tilt may imply a paralytic squint or other syndrome where there is deviation of the eyes in one position of gaze only.

Table 25.3 Causes of Squint in childhood

Congenital deviations, e.g., esotropia

Hypermetropia (far-sightedness)

Paralytic squints (exclude intracranial pathology)

Special syndromes, e.g., Duane syndrome

Retinoblastoma or other serious ocular pathology

Management

All children with a squint must first be assessed by the ophthalmologist.

◆ Underlying pathology must be excluded. Retinoblastoma commonly presents first as a squint.

◆ Amblyopia due to squint in children up to 7 years of age must be reversed by patching. Occlusion of the good eye is done for approximately 1 week per year of age until each eye is used alternately, i.e., the child is *alternating*.

◆ If alternation is present or has been achieved, surgery may be delayed if necessary until the child is older. When appropriate the eyes may be straightened by recession or resection of the extraocular muscles.

◆ Hypermetropic (far-sighted) children may develop esotropia at about 2 years of age, and glasses may correct these squints.

Early referral, exclusion of serious pathology, and reversal of amblyopia with conscientious

patching are very important in squint management.

Trauma

Eye trauma is extremely alarming to both child and parent. Reassurance and calm handling is important. In severe injuries the general condition should be assessed to exclude intracranial injury.

The possibility of a non-accidental cause must always be borne in mind.

Chemical burns

This is a dire emergency, especially if alkali burn is suspected. These burns progress to penetrate the cornea and involve the anterior chamber, iris, and lens. Copious washing with water or saline, if available, should be commenced immediately, and in the case of alkaline burns should be continued for several hours while the patient is being transported to hospital for specialized treatment.

Blunt injuries

Subconjunctival haemorrhage may present a frightening appearance but it is generally not of a serious nature and clears within 7–10 days. However, it is imperative that more serious injury is ruled out. Pertussis is a common cause of subconjunctival haemorrhage.

The external eye should be carefully inspected. Hyphaema in the anterior chamber will present as a level of blood behind the cornea. Severe hyphaema may appear absolutely black, so that no anterior chamber details are visible. The eye should be padded and the patient kept at bed rest for several days. If the intraocular pressure rises, a washout of the hyphaema is indicated. Sequelae of blunt trauma include secondary glaucoma, dislocated lens, and macula holes.

Penetrating injuries

Laceration of the cornea is usually obvious, sometimes with a presenting knuckle of iris. Obscure penetrating injury may be suspected when the eye is very soft to digital palpation. This can be done by very gentle alternating pressure on the upper lid, using both index fingers and with the eye in a downward gaze. X-ray of the orbit is mandatory where an intraocular foreign body is suspected.

Referral of all patients with penetrating injuries is imperative.

Corneal foreign body

These can be very irritating and should be carefully looked for. They are difficult to remove in a child without a general anaesthesia. When deeply embedded they should be removed with a disposable needle, taking care not to cause a perforation.

If not deeply embedded, topical benoxinate anaesthetic drops (Novesin®) may be instilled, and the cornea gently wiped with a cotton bud. Topical antibiotic drops should be instilled, and the eye padded for 24 hours. Epithelial defects usually heal rapidly.

A.L. Peters

26

Orthopaedic problems

Disturbance of gait

This may be due to ataxia or to a limp. Ataxia is of neurological origin and the patient has an incoordinated, awkward, unbalanced gait with the feet set wide apart (wide-based).

Limp

This may be due to:

◆ shortening of a limb
◆ pain in some part of the limb
◆ weakness of the muscles
◆ stiffness of a joint.

By carefully observing the patient while he is walking, it is often possible to localize the cause of the limp before proceeding further with the examination of the limb.

Shortening may be due to a true discrepancy in length (as measured from the anterior superior iliac spine to the medial malleolus), or it may be apparent because of an adduction deformity of the hip, causing a pelvic tilt. The latter would cause a reduced measurement from the umbilicus to the medial malleolus, but would not affect the true length from the anterior superior iliac spine to the malleolus.

With a **painful joint**, the patient will naturally be reluctant to bear weight on it, and in walking will get his weight off that limb as quickly as possible, giving a characteristic limp.

Muscle weakness will result in poor joint control. For example a weak quadriceps muscle will allow the knee to hyperextend, or a weak tibialis anterior will cause a foot-drop deformity, with consequent high-stepping gait, so that the drop-foot will clear the ground as the patient swings the limb forward.

Joint stiffness (ankylosis) may be partial or complete.

It may be:

◆ intra-articular due to joint disease, in which case movement in all directions is reduced, or

◆ extra-articular due to contractures arising from muscle imbalance, such as is commonly seen in poliomyelitis (*see Chapter 8, Infectious Disorders*). This will affect some, but not all, of the different movements in a joint.

The sudden onset of a limp due to pain in a joint can be the first sign of bone or joint infection, and therefore calls for immediate investigation and treatment.

Painful joints

The common causes are:

◆ trauma
◆ pyogenic (septic) arthritis
◆ non-pyogenic arthritis
◆ tuberculous arthritis
◆ juvenile chronic arthritis (juvenile rheumatoid arthritis)
◆ haemophilia (the least common).

Pyogenic arthritis

The joint may be invaded via a penetrating wound, by blood spread, or from an adjacent osteitis (e.g., the upper metaphysis of the femur is actually intracapsular, and osteitis here would therefore occur within the hip joint).

Pathology

The disease goes through three successsive stages

1. *Pyoarthrosis:* The joint becomes filled with pus.
2. *Suppurative synovitis:* The synovium and capsule become thickened and inflamed.
3. *Suppurative arthritis:* The vascular granulations spread across the articular cartilage, destroying it.

As healing occurs, fibrous tissue may be formed across the joint, limiting movement (fibrous ankylosis); or bone may grow between the joint surfaces, resulting in total rigidity of the joint (bony ankylosis). *(See Fig. 26.1.)*

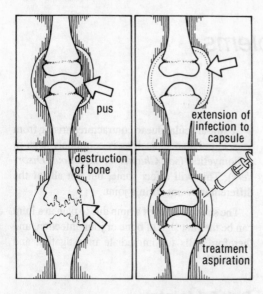

Fig. 26.1   Pathology and treatment of pyogenic arthritis

Clinical features

The patient may be very ill, with a high temperature and rapid pulse. In a superficial joint such as the knee, the swelling will be obvious and the skin will be red and hot. There will be marked tenderness with fluctuation, and all movements will be restricted.

Pyogenic arthritis in neonates may be painless.

Investigations

The white cell count and ESR will be raised, and the patient may be anaemic. In the haematogenous variety, a blood culture may indicate the causative organism, which is often *Staphylococcus pyogenes*. Radiology in the early stages will show no abnormality, although there may be some increase in the joint space. After approximately 10 days there will be osteoporosis, areas of erosion of bone, and diminution of the joint space.

Treatment

This must commence early, and one should not wait for radiographic confirmation, which will be too late to begin effective treatment.

♦ The effusion should be aspirated and the pus sent immediately for microscopy, culture, and sensitivity.

♦ Antibiotic therapy is commenced, preferably using sodium fusidate or a combination of penicillin and cloxacillin administered intravenously for the first 72 hours and then given orally. Subsequent laboratory investigation may suggest more effective antibiotics. This treatment must be given for at least 6 weeks.

♦ Blood transfusion and/or other intravenous fluid may be needed.

♦ Splint the affected limb (e.g., a Thomas splint to immobilize the knee, or skin traction for the hip joint). The aim is to keep the joint in its optimal position, so that if it does become permanently stiffened, it will be in the best position for function; a markedly flexed knee cannot be used for walking.

♦ Even with upper limb infections, patients should be kept in bed until the temperature has settled and the general condition is satisfactory, which usually takes about a week.

Non-pyogenic arthritis

In children this can occur with a number of infectious diseases, including rubella, measles, pneumonia, typhoid, and brucellosis. There is pain and effusion of one or more joints. It is often no more than a mild synovitis, which responds to aspiration and analgesics. In rheumatic fever the pain flits from joint to joint.

Tuberculous arthritis
Pathology

The condition is usually spread through the blood to the synovium, but less often is transmitted directly from bone. The synovium becomes thick, grey, and oedematous, spreading as a pannus across the articular surface, destroying it and invading the sub-chondral bone. If treatment is commenced early, while the disease is still in the synovial stage, it can be cured medically. Once there has been bony erosion or destruction, the granulation tissue converts to fibrous tissue and traps the bacilli within it. The bacteria may remain quiescent for many years, but an injury could cause a flare-up. This fibrous tissue also restricts joint movement.

The joints most commonly affected by tuberculosis are the hip, knee, elbow, and wrist, although any joint can become infected.

Occasionally the synovium of a tendon sheath can become involved in a tuberculous process. This can also happen in a bursa, particularly the one overlying the greater trochanter of the femur.

Clinical features

Pain is usually slight, and the major features are swelling, stiffness, and deformity. The swelling is due to synovial thickening rather than effusion, and therefore it is not fluctuant. With intra-articular disease, the movements in *all directions* are reduced. Later the necrotic material forms a cold abscess which may break through the skin, leaving a chronic, discharging sinus.

Investigations

The full blood count is not usually of value, but the ESR will be raised and the tuberculin test is significantly positive in a certain percentage of patients. Initially the X-rays will show generalized rarefaction and later there will be joint space narrowing as the articular cartilage becomes eroded.

Bony erosions will be seen once the subchondral bone becomes invaded: this will lead to progressive destruction of the joint surfaces, and sometimes even dislocation of the joint.

Whilst the X-ray signs help, they are not diagnostically definitive, because similar changes are seen with other chronic arthritides, e.g., pyogenic, rheumatoid, and brucellosis. It is therefore also necessary to examine the synovial fluid or perform a synovial biopsy. In a certain percentage of patients even the histology is equivocal, and a therapeutic trial is advisable.

Treatment

General: Bed-rest is required, with a nutritious, high-protein diet, as well as the administration of the appropriate antituberculous drugs *(see Chapter 9, Tuberculosis)*. The latter are administered until the ESR is normal and there is radiological evidence of healing, which may take up to a year.

Local: The diseased joint must also be rested, by splinting it in the position of function. Surgical treatment may be needed to drain a very tense cold abscess, or to arthrodese a severely damaged joint.

Juvenile chronic arthritis

See Chapter 23, *Juvenile Chronic Arthritis and Vasculitides.*

Haemophilia

(Also see Chapter 18, Blood Disorders.)

In this disease, bleeding into the joints is a common manifestation and may cause:

Acute haemarthrosis: Even a minor injury can cause a very painful and swollen joint, with raised skin temperature similar to a pyogenic arthritis. The usual joints involved are the hinge joints, namely the knees, elbows, and ankles.

Haemophilia must be considered where there is acute arthritis of the elbow, knee, and ankle.

Treatment is to stop the bleeding by Factor replacement, compression bandages, and a back-splint.

It is important to be aware of this condition, although it is uncommon, because it can be dangerous to aspirate the knee joint without suitable Factor replacement.

Chronic haemarthrosis: Recurrent intra-articular bleeding leads to synovitis and later to joint surface destruction. This results in swollen, stiff, and deformed joints, such as are seen clinically with chronic joint infections. However, there are radiological differences between the two. In the knee joint, for instance, the femoral intercondylar space is widened.

Acute osteitis (osteomyelitis)

Pyogenic infection of the bone demands early and intensive therapy if it is not to leave serious and debilitating sequelae.

Adequate primary health care of the child with osteitis, with good referral channels, will make the difference between complete recovery and crippling complications.

It may be caused by:

◆ blood-borne organisms, of which the most common is *Staphylococcus pyogenes*. Skin sepsis causes a predisposition to this source of infection;

◆ direct spread, which occurs from a wound such as a compound fracture, and the diagnosis is usually obvious. The infection may be less severe, and can be caused by a large variety of organisms, such as staphylococci, streptococci, *E. coli* or proteus.

Pathology

In the haematogenous type, the infection begins in the metaphysis, where pus forms, spreads into the marrow cavity, and forces its way under pressure to the surface of the bone. Here it elevates the periosteum and then spreads along this sub-periosteal plane. If the pressure is not relieved, the bone dies because its blood supply is cut off, and this dead bone forms a sequestrum. The elevated periosteum forms a new layer of bone called the involucrum.

Clinical features

In small infants, systemic reaction to the infection may be mild, so that pseudoparalysis may be the only feature. In the older child, the onset may be insidious, with a limp being the only feature.

The child may be extremely ill, with a rapid pulse and high temperature, and become toxic, with confusion and restlessness. The affected limb will be held immobile and be extremely tender. Sometimes if one merely touches the bed, it will cause the child to scream. At first there will be no tell-tale swelling, redness, or local warmth to in-dicate the site of the infection. More than one bone can be involved, especially in immunodeficiency and sickle-cell anaemia. The pelvic bones are occasionally affected, with severe pain and sys-temic reaction, and late onset of local signs making diagnosis difficult initially.

Investigations

The ESR and white cell count will be elevated. As the X-ray will probably be normal for the first 10 days, one must make the diagnosis and commence treatment long before radiological changes are seen. Later, there is patchy rarefaction at the meta-physis and new periosteal bone formation occurs, followed by the development of areas of sclerosis.

Treatment

◆ Intravenous replacement of fluids and electro-lytes must commence immediately, and anaemia must be corrected by blood transfusion.

◆ Antibiotics such as sodium fusidate (the most effective) or a combination of penicillin and clox-acillin are prescribed intravenously for 72 hours and then given orally.

◆ The affected limb is splinted.

◆ If there has not been a dramatic improvement in the clinical condition after 24 hours, with a reduction of temperature and pulse rate, then inci-sion and drainage are imperative. The affected metaphyseal region is exposed, and holes are drilled through the cortex to release the pus and decompress it. This surgical approach is often necessary *ab initio* where there is obvious local swelling.

◆ Laboratory examination of the pus may indi-cate a change of antibiotics.

◆ Antibiotic therapy must be continued for at least 6 weeks, while the limb remains in splints.

Chronic osteitis

Chronic osteitis is the result of inadequate treat-ment of acute osteitis.

The bone may have been partially destroyed and may contain sclerotic areas, as well as abscess cavities. There may also be chronic discharging sinuses, but little or no pain is felt. These changes are permanent and *incurable*.

It is pointless to give antibiotics during this quiescent phase of chronic osteitis, because the bone is sclerotic (avascular) and blood-borne antibiotics will not reach the diseased region.

The disease is liable to acute exacerbations, when there will be recurrence of pain, swelling, and pyrexia. These may occur many years later. In such an attack, antibiotics and bed-rest may sub-due the infection, but an abscess must be drained and any sequestra removed.

There are also three types of osteitis which are chronic from the start:

◆ **Brodie's abscess:** The patient presents with chronic pain at the end of a long bone, but there is little clinical abnormality. An X-ray, how-ever, shows an abscess cavity in the metaphy-seal region.

◆ **Syphilitic:** *See Chapter 8, Infectious Disor-ders.*

◆ **Tuberculous:** This most commonly occurs in the spine, but it is occasionally seen in the hands and feet (dactylitis). *(See Chapter 9, Tuberculosis).*

Spinal tuberculosis

This was originally described by Percival Pott, and is sometimes called Pott's disease.

Pathology

The infection begins in a vertebral body, which becomes softened and collapses. This causes an angulation in the spine, (kyphos or gibbus), which will be more obvious in the thoracic spine, where there is a normal kyphosis, than in the cervical or lumbar spine where the natural curve is in the opposite direction, i.e., lordotic. *(See Figs 26.2–26.4.)*

As the infection progresses, necrotic caseous material forms a cold abscess around the spine (paravertebral swelling on X-ray). This pus may either compress the spinal cord, causing paraplegia, or it may track through the soft tissue planes and appear subcutaneously at some site remote from the original lesion. Thus a lumbar spinal lesion could present as a psoas abscess in the groin.

Clinical features

There is a gradual onset of vague ill-health, with slight aching in the back. Often in younger children the first thing noticed by the mother is a gibbus. Spinal movement is restricted by the pro-

tective muscle spasm; so when picking up an object the hips are flexed rather than the back being bent. Later, spinal cord compression may occur and will cause weakness or complete paralysis of the lower limbs, with upper motor neurone features. Occasionally, due to nerve compression and 'girdle' pain, the presenting feature is abdominal pain mimicking an acute abdomen.

Radiological features

The region is osteoporotic, and an area of erosion is seen in the vertebral body, with narrowing of the disc space. Progressive destruction is associated with spread into adjacent vertebral bodies, causing further collapse and gibbus formation. A paravertebral abscess is seen in the antero-posterior view as an increased density of the soft tissues around the affected vertebrae.

Treatment

Active stage: The patient's resistance to the disease must be increased by bed-rest and a nutritious, high-protein diet, whilst antituberculous drugs are given to subdue the infection.

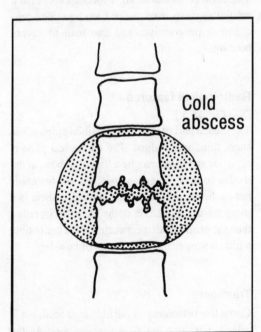

Fig. 26.2 Tuberculosis of the spine: Cold abscess formation

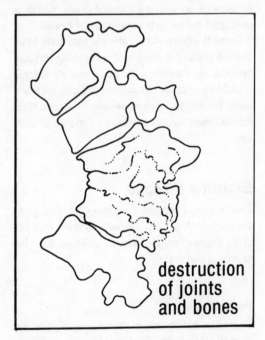

Fig. 26.3 Tuberculosis of the spine: Destruction of the vertebrae and joints

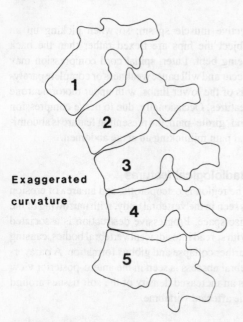

Fig. 26.4 Bone changes in rickets in contrast to tuberculosis

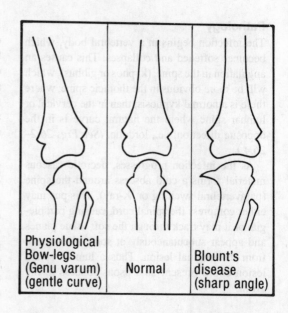

Physiological Bow-legs (Genu varum) (gentle curve) | **Normal** | **Blount's disease (sharp angle)**

Fig. 26.5 Physiological bow-legs and Blount's disease. Note the sharp medial angle and lip

Healing stage: Once the general health has improved and the lesion is healing, the child can be allowed up wearing a spinal brace, which is used until the lesion is radiologically healed.

Complications: A cold abscess may have to be drained if there is danger of it breaking through the skin and forming a chronic sinus. Paraplegia in children usually responds to conservative treatment, but surgical decompression is needed if no improvement has occurred after a month of therapy.

Blount's disease

This is one of the less common causes of genu varum (bow-legs), but warrants mention here because it is seen mainly in black children. It is also known as tibia vara.

Pathology

There is a disturbance in the development of the medial part of the tibial metaphysis, and with growth, the bone angulates medially at this site. It is usually bilateral, but may be unilateral.

Clinical features

The child is normal in all respects, except for a medial angulation of one or both legs. The condition is progressive, and can lead to severe bowing.

Radiological features

(See Fig. 26.5.)

The medial part of the proximal tibial epiphysis is short, thin; and wedged. The epiphyseal plate is irregular and there may be a 'beak' of bone at the medial edge of the metaphysis, but this feature is not exclusive to tibia vara. Classically, there is a sharp medial angulation of the metaphysis, rather than the gentle medial curvature of the entire tibia which is seen in the other forms of bow-leg.

Treatment

Corrective osteotomy of the tibia is needed, but is usually not done before 4 years of age. As the condition is progressive, the osteotomy may have to be repeated in later years, and the parents should be warned of this before treatment is commenced.

Congenital talipes equinovarus (club foot)

Causes
◆ Idiopathic: This is thought to be due to mixed genetic and environmental causes. It is the most common type.
◆ Occurs with myelomeningocele and congenital muscle abnormalities, e.g., arthrogryposis multiplex congenita.
◆ May be associated with major skeletal defects, e.g., an absent or shortened tibia.

Pathology
There is an equinus adduction and inversion of the hind foot, with adduction and inversion of the forefoot. Initially bone and joint changes are minimal, but they become more evident if the deformity is not corrected. In the early stages there may be histological changes in the muscles, whilst later there is obvious calf muscle atrophy.

Types
Extrinsic: This variety corrects easily with passive manipulation and is probably due to the intrauterine position of the fetus.

Intrinsic: These patients have a small inverted heel and the deformity is more difficult to correct by passive stretching. This type has a worse prognosis, will require more treatment, and may relapse.

Treatment
This must be commenced as soon as possible, preferably on the first day of life. Various methods are advocated, but basically they all involve passive stretching to correct the deformity, followed by splintage with strapping, plaster of Paris or a J-splint.

In the first week of life only frequent manipulations are carried out, but thereafter manipulation is combined with immobilization.

Manipulation must be done with care, and if possible the mother should be taught to do this so that it can be done frequently. The heel is held between the thumb and index finger, whilst the other hand is used firstly to correct the adduction deformity of the forefoot, and then to correct the inversion. Finally, efforts are made to overcome

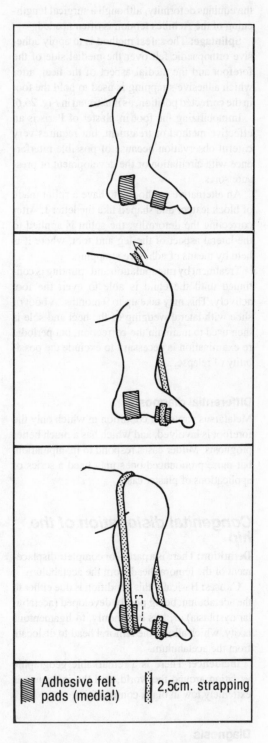

| ▨ Adhesive felt pads (medial) | ▥ 2,5cm. strapping |

Fig. 26.6 Strapping of foot in congenital talipes equinovarus

the equinus deformity, although a surgical lengthening of the Achilles tendon is often needed.

Splintage: The safest method is to apply adhesive orthopaedic felt over the medial side of the forefoot and the medial aspect of the heel, after which adhesive strapping is used to hold the foot in the corrected position, as illustrated in *Fig. 26.6.*

Immobilizing the foot in plaster of Paris is an effective method of treatment, but requires very careful observation because of possible interference with circulation or the development of pressure sores.

An alternative method is to have a splint made of block leather and shaped like the letter J. After correcting the deformity, the splint is applied to the lateral aspect of the leg and foot, where it is held by means of adhesive strapping.

Treatment by manipulation and splinting is continued until the child is able to evert the foot actively. This may take up to 9 months. A boot or shoe with lateral wedging of the heel and sole is then used to maintain the correction, but periodic re-examination is necessary to exclude the possibility of relapse.

Differential diagnosis

Metatarsus varus is a condition in which only the forefoot is involved, and which has a much better prognosis. Milder cases respond to manipulation, but more pronounced ones may need a series of applications of plaster casts.

Congenital dislocation of the hip

Definition: There is a partial or complete displacement of the femoral head from the acetabulum.

Causes: Basically this condition is due either to the acetabulum being poorly developed (acetabular dysplasia) or, less commonly, to ligamentous laxity, which allows the femoral head to dislocate from the acetabulum.

Incidence: There is a remarkable geographic variation around the world, and the incidence is extremely low in black communities.

Diagnosis

If the condition is diagnosed early, the treatment is simple and effective; but if diagnosed late, the

treatment is complicated and the results are not good.

It is therefore important to examine the hips of all newborn infants, using Barlow's modification of the Ortolani test.

This is done with the baby supine and both the hips and the knees flexed to 90 °. The examiner holds the limbs, with the thumb in front of the hip and the middle finger behind the greater trochanter. The hips are then abducted slowly with gentle backward pressure on the femur. The test is positive if a click is felt during this manoeuvre, as the dislocated femoral head slips into the acetabulum.

In severe cases it is impossible to abduct the hips.

Treatment

The sooner the treatment is commenced, the better the prognosis. The hip is reduced, held flexed and abducted in a splint.

If conservative measures fail (as may happen with late diagnosis), open reduction, and sometimes acetabular reconstruction, will be needed.

Orthopaedic pitfalls

'Pseudo-trauma'

In children presenting with a painful limb, there is nearly always a history of trauma, but one may be misled by this. Thus, if no bony injury is seen on X-ray of the painful limb, one should suspect a pyogenic osteitis or arthritis, and the patient's temperature, white cell count, and ESR should be checked. If there is still any doubt, the child should be given a simple analgesic and re-examined the next day, to be quite certain that more serious pathology is not being overlooked.

Cellulitis

This is a serious diagnosis in children. It is best to suspect the inflammation as being due to an underlying osteomyelitis, and to treat it as such. Even if the diagnosis does prove to be cellulitis, less harm will have been done than if one had misdiagnosed an acute bone infection. If one does not treat acute osteomyelitis early and correctly, the patient will be left with a grave, permanent disability due to an incurable chronic osteitis.

▶ ## *Perthes' disease*

This condition is due to an avascular necrosis of the femoral head, which is uncommon in black patients. Radiological changes similar to those caused by Perthes' disease are sometimes seen in black children, but usually prove to be the result of chronic infection such as tuberculosis. The diagnosis of Perthes' disease should therefore not be made unless biopsy of the joint has ruled out other causes.

Plaster casts

Enclosing a swollen limb, or a limb liable to become swollen, in a plaster cast is dangerous

because of the possibility of circulatory embarrassment. The cast should therefore always be split before the patient is allowed to go home. The entire length of the cast, as well as the deeper layers such as bandage or wool, must be split so that the skin is exposed. Furthermore, an injury around the elbow should *never* be enclosed in a plaster cast, and can be very adequately controlled with a collar and cuff combined, with a posterior plaster slab if necessary.

J.N. Bear

27

Poisoning

Introduction

After road accidents, burns, drowning, and abuse of children, poisoning is the fifth most common cause of non-natural deaths in childhood in South Africa. Approximately 3% of all non-natural deaths in childhood are caused by poisoning. Larger hospitals treat over a thousand children per year who have accidentally ingested a potentially poisonous substance. Hence accidental ingestion of harmful substances is common and appears to be increasingly frequent in childhood, but fortunately is seldom fatal. More boys than girls are treated, and children between the ages of 1 and 5 years are the most vulnerable.

The majority of poisons are swallowed. Contamination of eyes and skin are other sites through which children can be harmed by toxic substances. Most cases are accidental. Should an older child, especially a teenager, be treated for poisoning, one should consider the possibility of attempted suicide. Parents have been known to administer poisons to their children intentionally, either to murder them, or as part of the 'Munchausen-syndrome-by-proxy', where adults inflict illness on a child or falsify symptoms so that the child requires medical evaluation. Poisoning may also take place through contamination of skin, clothing, or food by agricultural and industrial products such as insecticides. Inadvertent administration of an overdose of a prescribed drug by doctors, nurses, and parents can also occur. Carbon monoxide is of course inhaled.

Poisoning depends primarily on the availability of toxic substances in the child's surroundings. In regions where households do not have electricity, paraffin is the most common serious poison. In agricultural areas, insecticides and plants are more common. The incidence of salicylate poisoning has declined in many parts of the world. The reasons are that aspirin is less frequently prescribed, and

is often dispensed in bottles which are difficult for children to open.

In general about 60% of the substances ingested are drugs, of which psychotropic preparations, tranquilizers, sleeping tablets, anticonvulsants and analgesics are most common. In South Africa the commonest plants involved are syringa, mushroom, oleander, and *Datura stramonium*. Some herbal remedies administered to children can be extremely poisonous. One of these is a tuber, *Callilepsis laureola*, otherwise known as 'impila'. A form of poisoning which is likely to become more common is drug abuse, including solvent sniffing. *(Also see Chapter 4, Community Paediatrics.)*

Acute poisoning

In practice, children are usually brought with a history of having ingested a substance which may be poisonous. The following information should be obtained:
- symptoms present
- name of substance, amount ingested, time of ingestion
- the exact name and the container of the putative poison
- first aid treatment given
- assessment of whether the event was an accident, an overdose of a prescribed drug, or a suicide attempt.

Immediate treatment, where necessary, should be given for shock, respiratory distress, airway obstruction, aspiration, depression of the central nervous system, paralysis, convulsions, arrhythmia, or dehydration.

Equally important is to remove the poison. If the eyes have been exposed to the poison, they should be irrigated with copious amounts of water or saline solution. If skin is affected, the clothes should be removed and the skin, hair, and nails thoroughly washed with soap and water. Young children absorb substances through the skin more rapidly than adults, as they have a thinner epidermis and stratum corneum. The skin should not be scrubbed. If the substance ingested is innocuous, no treatment is necessary. Advice can often be obtained from a poison information centre. When in doubt, vomiting should be induced or gastric lavage performed.

Emesis should be induced even 6 hours after ingestion, as tablets can take several hours to pass from the stomach into the duodenum. Aspirin and tricyclic antidepressants can remain in the stomach for up to 24 hours.

Contraindications to inducing vomiting are:
◆ loss of consciousness,
◆ absence of protective airway reflexes
◆ presence of convulsions
◆ poisoning with paraffin
◆ poisoning with caustics, acids or corrosives
◆ haematemesis.

Emesis is more efficient than lavage in removing gastric contents. The lumen of the tube used for lavage is often too narrow to allow the passage of whole or partially-dissolved tablets, leaves or seeds. Contraindications to lavage are identical to those for emesis. In children who have depressed consciousness, endotracheal intubation before lavage can prevent aspiration.

The best way to make the child vomit is to administer syrup of ipecac by mouth or via a small nasogastric tube.

The dosages for syrup of ipecacuanha (USP) are:
6 – 9 months: 5 ml
9 – 12 months: 10 ml
1 – 10 years: 15 ml
over 10 years: 30 ml.

It is probably useful to give tepid water orally (5 ml/kg body weight) thereafter. The child should then be encouraged to walk around. Some authorities advise against giving syrup of ipecac to infants and suggest that gastric lavage should be used instead. Most children vomit within 20 minutes. The syrup of ipecac may be repeated once if vomiting does not occur within 20 minutes. When the child vomits the head should be held lower than the body to prevent aspiration. If the second dose does not induce vomiting, gastric lavage should be performed.

When performing gastric lavage, the patient's arms and legs should be restrained and the child should be positioned on the left side with the head slightly lower than the body. The largest bore tube that can safely be inserted orally is used. Half strength tepid normal saline (0.45% Na Cl) in amounts of up to 50 ml at a time is alternatively instilled and drained until about 500 ml has been used. After the stomach has been emptied, activated charcoal can be given orally or via the stomach tube. A mixture of 30 ml activated charcoal and 240 ml of water is made, and about 5 ml/kg body weight given. It should be given for all poisonings except paracetamol, alcohol, caustics, hydrocarbons, and iron.

Some substances are excreted from the blood into the bile or into the intestinal tract and thereafter reabsorbed. In such cases repeated doses of charcoal are necessary. This is especially so with ingestion of phenobarbital, salicylates, theophylline, digoxin, and carbamazepine.

Administration of a cathartic can shorten transit time in the intestines and thus reduce absorption of the poison. If the child has taken a poison with anticholinergic or narcotic properties, sodium sulphate or magnesium sulphate (250 mg/kg body weight) or sorbitol (1 g/kg body weight) can be given. Magnesium sulphate is contraindicated in the presence of renal failure.

Milk or water may be given to dilute swallowed caustic or corrosive agents, provided the child is capable of swallowing, is not shocked, and does not have a perforated oesophagus. No more than 15 ml/kg should be used, to a maximum of 250 ml, to prevent vomiting.

Vinegar (for caustic soda) or alkalis (for acids) should *not* be given, as the chemical reaction can cause thermal burns.

If there is a delay, give nothing orally, administer fluids intravenously, and refer all cases for specialist care.

Whether children who have been poisoned should be admitted for observation and treatment depends on the symptoms and signs and on the nature of the poison, as some poisons have a delayed or prolonged effect. Methods to enhance elimination of toxic substances include forced diuresis, alkalinization of the urine, peritoneal dialysis and haemodialysis.

Common signs and symptoms of poisoning

It is often necessary to consider the possibility of poisoning in a child who presents with features of other illnesses. *Table 27.1* is an incomplete list of possible symptoms and signs and the common poisons that cause them:

Table 27.1 Signs and symptoms of common poisonings

Signs or symptoms	Poison
Ataxia	Organophosphate insecticides, antihistamines, alcohol, phenytoin
Arrhythmia	Digitalis, tricyclic antidepressants, theophylline
Bradycardia	Digitalis, mushrooms, barbiturates, organophosphates
Coma	Narcotics, barbiturates, phenothiazines, alcohol, benzodiazepines, mushrooms, carbon monoxide, salicylates
Constricted pupils	Barbiturates, organophosphates, phenothiazines
Convulsions	Camphor, atropine, organophosphates, mushrooms, theophylline, tricyclic antidepressants
Delirium	Atropine, *Datura stramonium*
Dilated pupils	Atropine, belladonna alkaloids
Dry mouth	Atropine, belladonna alkaloids, antihistamines
Fever	Atropine, salicylates
Haematemesis	Iron, caustics
Haemorrhage	Warfarin
Hot, dry skin	Atropine, belladonna alkaloids
Hypoglycaemia	Alcohol, impila
Methaemoglobinaemia	Nitrates, nitrites
Jaundice	Mushrooms, paracetamol
Pneumonia	Paraffin
Respiratory depression	Alcohol, barbiturates, organophosphates, carbon monoxide benzodiazepines
Salivation	Caustics, mushrooms, organophosphates
Tachycardia	Atropine

Poisons and drugs can be identified in specimens of blood, urine, or vomitus. Expert assistance is required for this.

Specific antidotes to certain poisons are available. They are described in the following section.

Specific poisons

Paracetamol

Pathological effect: Centrilobular necrosis of the liver.

Clinical features: Nausea, vomiting, and malaise occur for a brief period and are followed after 2–3 days by hepatic dysfunction. Plasma levels can be determined.

Treatment: Induce vomiting. Do not give charcoal. Administer acetylcysteine when indicated. Obtain advice.

Tricyclic antidepressants

Pathological effect: Anticholinergic.

Clinical features: Dry mouth, blurred vision, tachycardia, arrhythmia, irritability, constipation, excessive sweating, tremors, coma, and convulsions.

Treatment: Induce vomiting. Give activated charcoal and a cathartic. Monitor heart and respiration. Refer to intensive care unit. Physostigmine is an effective antidote.

Benzodiazepines

Pathological effect: CNS depression.

Clinical features: Impaired consciousness, ataxia, depressed respiration.

Treatment: Induce vomiting. Give activated charcoal. Monitor and support respiration.

Salicylates

Pathological effect: Stimulation of respiratory centre with respiratory acidosis, followed by uncoupling of oxidative phosphorylation, increased oxygen demand, metabolic acidosis, and ketonuria.

Clinical features: Fever, tachypnoea, tachycardia, and sweating initially; followed by dehydration, vomiting, hypoglycaemia, renal failure, convulsions, and coma.

Treatment: Induce emesis. Give activated charcoal. Treat for dehydration, acidosis, and hypoglycaemia. Forced alkaline diuresis. Dialysis for severe poisoning.

Carbon monoxide

Pathological effect: Carbon monoxide has a high affinity for haemaglobin and causes decreased tissue oxygen delivery.

Clinical features: Confusion, headache, nausea, vomiting, syncope, and coma. Skin and mucous membranes may be pink.

Treatment: Pure oxygen inhalation at higher than atmospheric pressure if possible. Respiratory and cardiac monitoring, and ventilation if necessary.

Iron

Pathological effect: Vasodilatation, increased capillary permeability, hypotension, acidosis. Hepatocellular necrosis. Haemorrhagic necrosis of stomach and small bowel.

Clinical features: Vomiting, diarrhoea, haematemesis, malaena, and shock; followed after about 2 days by metabolic acidosis, hypoglycaemia and liver damage. Gastrointestinal strictures may develop after several weeks. Diagnostic tests include serum iron and total iron binding capacity. Iron tablets are radio-opaque.

Treatment: Induce vomiting if no contraindications exist. Activated charcoal should not be given. After emesis, perform gastric lavage with 2 g desferrioxamine in 1 litre of water to which sodium bicarbonate has been added. After lavage, desferrioxamine can be left in the stomach. Admit to hospital and obtain advice.

Hydrocarbons

Pathological effect: Chemical damage to alveoli and pulmonary capillaries and toxic action on CNS. Paraffin has a far greater effect on the lungs than on the central nervous system.

Clinical features: Burning sensation in mouth, and perhaps choking. If aspirated, signs of respiratory distress develop. Agitation, coma, and convulsions may occur.

Treatment: Induction of vomiting of paraffin is contraindicated, as this can lead to aspiration; moreover, the neurological effects of paraffin are relatively uncommon and seldom serious. If the substance is likely to have serious systemic effects, gastric lavage is undertaken only after the insertion of an endotracheal tube.

Hydrocarbons are occasionally used as carriers for pesticides and herbicides.

Turpentine, benzine, toluene, and mineral spirit have greater systemic effects than paraffin. Cases of hydrocarbon poisoning must be treated with caution, and carefully observed rather than discharged promptly.

Mushrooms

Pathological effect: Mushrooms contain a variety of toxins.

Clinical features: They can cause cholinergic symptoms, atropine-like symptoms, and hepatorenal failure.

Treatment: Vomiting should be induced and activated charcoal administered. All cases should be admitted to hospital, as the serious toxic effects are often delayed.

Phenothiazines

Pathological effect: Phenothiazine overdosage usually produces extrapyramidal signs.

Clinical features: Rigidity, tremor, and dyskinesis, but may also cause arrhythmia and convulsions.

Treatment: Vomiting should be induced. Gastric lavage may be necessary, as phenothiazines have an anti-emetic action. Activated charcoal should be given. Cardiac monitoring may be necessary. Biperiden can counteract the dystonic effects of phenothiazines.

Organophosphate insecticides

Pathological effect: Organophosphates inhibit acetylcholine.

Clinical features: Sweating, salivation, increased bronchial secretions, constricted pupils, bradycardia, vomiting, diarrhoea, muscular weakness, fasciculations, convulsions, and coma.

Treatment: It is imperative that the patient be rid of the poison by the quickest route and the most thorough means. If gastric lavage is likely to work more quickly than emesis, it should be used. Activated charcoal should be administered. Treatment with atropine and if necessary oxygen and ventilation must be started. The dose of atropine is 0.05 μg/kg by slow intravenous infusion. This may be repeated under careful monitoring at a dose of 0.02–0.05 μg/kg every 5–10 minutes until the patient shows distinct signs of atropine effects and bronchial secretions are diminished. Intensive care is indicated. Repeat the atropine periodically to maintain atropinization for at least 24 hours, and then taper the dose before discontinuing. Aminophylline, theophylline, and tranquilizers should be avoided. Convulsions can be treated with diazepam and ventilatory support. Rebound effects of the poison can occur, because organophosphates are taken up by lipids and slowly released. Monitoring may therefore be necessary for a few days.

Alcohol

Pathological effect: Alcohol damages, *inter alia,* the nervous system and liver. All alcohols can be absorbed from the intestinal tract, from the skin, and through the lungs.

   Clinical features: Alcohols can cause ataxia, slurred speech, vomiting, hypoglycaemia, acidosis, coma, and respiratory arrest. Some solvents, cleaning fluids, and antifreeze contain isopropyl alcohol, methanol, and ethylene glycol, which are especially poisonous.

   Treatment: Vomiting should be induced if it is not contraindicated. Activated charcoal and a cathartic can be given. Monitoring of cardiorespiratory status, hydration, acid-base status, and blood glucose is necessary. The toxic effects of methanol and ethylene glycol can be diminished by the careful administration of ethanol.

Herbal toxins

The number and variety of plants which can be poisonous when swallowed, or irritate the skin and eyes, is very large. *Datura stramonium* contains belladonna alkaloids. The treatment is very similar to that for the tricyclic antidepressants.

   The tuber *Callilepsis laureola*, which is also known as 'impila', is contained in some herbal medicines. It causes hypoglycaemia, renal damage, and centrilobular necrosis of the liver. Patients presenting with impila poisoning are predominantly young African children of variable nutritional status, with a short history of diminishing level of consciousness, convulsions, and gastrointestinal symptoms. They are usually tachypnoeic and have acidotic-type

breathing, and are often profoundly hypotonic and hyporeflexic, but there is no evidence of jaundice, hepatic foetor, or focal neurological signs of meningeal irritation. Hypoglycaemia is invariable, and is very frequently accompanied by signs of renal impairment, with hyperkalaemia, uraemia, and acidosis. There are always biochemical indices of hepatic failure, with liver function tests showing disturbances which include elevated serum enzyme levels, prolonged prothrombin time, and a raised CSF glutamine level. Evidence of renal failure may accompany and sometimes precede the development of hepatic failure. Management is for the hypoglycaemia, hepatic failure, and renal failure.

   Health workers are encouraged to become familiar with the varieties of plants which are poisonous in the area where they work, and to learn the effects and treatment of these poisons.

Prevention

As in all things, prevention of poisoning is better than cure. Regulations should be drawn up by the authorities with regard to the safe use and storage of noxious substances. Health workers can contribute by educating the community, particularly parents. Cases of child abuse or attempted suicide will need appropriate management.

   All containers of medicines should be labelled with the name and correct dosage of the contents. Medical practitioners and other health workers should tell patients to keep all drugs safely away from children. This applies not only to parents, but to all patients, especially the elderly. Many children are poisoned while visiting grandparents. Paraffin should never be stored in bottles normally used for food or beverages, and should always be kept out of reach of children.

   Every health worker should have a ready supply of syrup of ipecacuanha, labelled with the correct doses and easily available for use in an emergency.

   Every year new medicines, chemicals, herbicides, and insecticides become available and old ones are discarded. No health worker can therefore keep abreast of current diagnoses and treatment of poisoning. Accordingly it is imperative that an accessible source of rapid information be available, such as an up-to-date reference book *(see bibliography)* or contact with a poison information centre.

R.E. Cronje

28

Surgical problems

Introduction

Paediatric surgery in the Third World is sufficiently different to 'standard practice' to justify
separate consideration. Not only do diseases
unique to tropical and subtropical environments
present, but they do so in a host frequently ravaged
by nutritional and other diseases. Late presentation and advanced disease are common. Amongst
neonates, maternal disease or placental insufficiency may complicate surgical presentation.

Health professionals at primary and secondary
level will continue to be responsible for the bulk
of the care of surgically-ill children in the Third
World.

This chapter discusses separately neonatal problems and those affecting the older child. Disorders
which are seen at both ages are discussed under
the age of most common presentation, but the
division is clearly arbitrary and indistinct.

Transportation

One important consequence of the centralization
of paediatric surgical services is the need to transport surgically-ill neonates and children. The
principles of preparation of a patient for transportation are independent of the length of journey or
mode of transport. Such preparation is the responsibility of the referring staff, and diligence ensures
the maximum chance of the patient arriving in a
condition fit for further investigation or early surgery. Pre-transfer communication between sending and receiving units is essential.

Two sides

The simple mnemonic 'TWO SIDES' serves as a
reminder of the essential aspects of transportation:
◆ *Tube (nasogastric):* Prevents vomiting if
properly supervised, and maximizes respiratory
excursion.
◆ *Warmth:* Maintenance of body temperature is
vital. Babies can be kept warm without sophisticated technology by wrapping them, including the

head, in aluminium foil. For exposed viscera *see
below*.
◆ *Oxygen* can safely be provided by headbox.
◆ *Stabilization:* As transportation does not improve a patient's condition, it is mandatory to start
out with a fully resuscitated child. A stable patient
has unobstructed ventilation, is normovolaemic as
measured by a urine output of 1 ml/kg/hr, has
warm peripheries, and is normoglycaemic.
◆ *Intravenous fluids:* Fluid replacement is essential, and intravenous cannulae rather than needles are preferred, with the drip site available to
inspection. Professional supervision is required.
◆ *Documentation:* Details of presentation, investigation, and primary management should be
provided to prevent duplication.
◆ *Escort:* The surgically-ill child needs professional monitoring and management by the most
senior personnel available during transport.
◆ *Specimens:* Where the mother is not accompanying her newborn, ideally a clotted specimen of
her blood should be sent to allow a safe blood
cross-match.

Care should be taken in selecting a mode of
transport. Flight in an unpressurized aircraft,
either fixed-wing or helicopter, allows gas within
body cavities to expand. This may be critical
where such expansion compresses vital structures
(e.g., in diaphragmatic hernia) or is enclosed (e.g.,
closed loop obstruction).

Neonatal surgery

There is infrequently justification for any surgery
in the neonatal period, other than that required to
alleviate life-threatening congenital anomalies.
Surgical pathology often occurs with premature
birth, when adaptive processes to extrauterine life
may be incomplete and reflexes immature.

Of vital surgical concern are:
◆ energy stores and temperature homeostasis
◆ defence mechanisms against infection
◆ hepatic maturity and clotting factor deficit

- pulmonary maturity and control of breathing
- circulatory stability.

These factors are important determinants of surgical management in as much as they increase anaesthetic and surgical risk. Postoperative management is an essential component of success. It must be appreciated that neonates experience pain which makes a significant contribution to the stress of an operative procedure, therefore pain relief is an important component of postoperative care.

Surgical lesions cannot be treated in isolation. Success is based upon an accurate history and examination, and upon the orchestrated input of a team which includes the surgeon, paediatrician, anaesthetist, and nursing staff. As parents are an important component of the team, their input should be encouraged.

Congenital abnormalities

Surgically-correctable abnormalities are either overt or covert. Whilst the former are revealed by inspection of the patient, covert anomalies are manifested by abnormal function in the affected system in an apparently normal neonate. Both varieties will only be revealed with certainty if routine examination and observation is applied to *all* newborns.

The causes of some anomalies are well known (e.g., thalidomide — phocomelia), but in most patients the cause remains a mystery. However, it is well established that interference with fetal blood supply may result in major defects in the affected part, and this is well demonstrated in small bowel atresia. Many other fetal insults — maternal alcohol, smoking, drugs, physical trauma, or infections — may result in anatomical defects if applied during the critical first trimester when organ development is proceeding rapidly. Any insult at such an embryologically busy time is likely to affect more than a single anatomical structure and result in non-random associations of defects (e.g., duodenal atresia in trisomy 21, or the VATER association, an acronym for **V**ertebral abnormality, **A**norectal malformation, **T**racheo-oesophageal fistula associated with **E**sophageal *(sic)* atresia and **R**adial dysplasia. Secondary associations include cardio**V**ascular defects and **R**enal anomalies). Such mnemonics serve to

remind the clinician to seek further defects when one is discovered.

Combinations of defects, particularly when a chromosomal abnormality is included, present cumulative management and ethical difficulties.

Overt anomalies

Overt anomalies are revealed by diligent clinical examination. Those requiring urgent attention are shown in *Table 28.1.*

Table 28.1   Overt anomalies requiring urgent intervention

Body wall defects
Absent or misplaced orifices
Neural axis defects
Neonatal tumours
Facial clefts
Ambiguous genitalia

Body wall defects

Babies are occasionally born with anterior thoraco-abdominal defects allowing herniation of viscera, either covered by a membrane of amnio-peritoneum (exomphalos, syn., omphalocele) or unprotected, with a thick fibrinous exudate over the herniated bowel (gastroschisis). Such defects represent failure of the embryonic cephalic or caudal parieto-visceral folds. Subjacent visceral developmental anomalies are common (e.g., cardiac lesions), and may be exposed on the surface of the body, e.g., ectopia vesicae, cloacal extrophy. Due to the antenatal evisceration the abdominal cavity fails to develop its full capacity. It may be impossible to safely return the evisceration to the patient. The sequelae of such defects are hypothermia, hypovolaemia, and peritonitis due to exposure. There may be associated intestinal malrotation and obstruction, or hypoglycaemia (Wiedemann-Beckwith syndrome).

Primary management is directed towards excluding associated defects and maintaining body temperature. This can be achieved most readily by enclosing the herniated viscera or sac in a non-adhesive plastic (e.g., Klingfilm®) or Gladwrap® inside a covering of Gamgee® and aluminium foil. Gastric decompression by nasogastric tube to prevent vomiting and postnatal herniation of previously enclosed bowel is essential. The blood sugar level must be maintained within normal limits. Antibodies should be commenced at the time of diagnosis.

Definitive management: Emergency surgery is necessary in all babies at risk of peritonitis. Where the abdomen cannot be stretched to accommodate the viscera, a temporary Silastic® tent must be manufactured to enclose it. Where an intact sac presents, surgery may still be desirable, particularly if the sac volume is small. Nonoperative treatment by tanning the sac with daily applications of 0.5% mercurochrome will allow epithelialization over a period of weeks. The resultant ventral hernia can be electively repaired later.

Anorectal malformations

These anomalies are common, both singly or as part of a syndrome, particularly in association with oesophageal atresia and defects of the lower abdominal wall. The absence of an anus at the usual site is diagnostic. The diagnosis is rarely delayed in babies born at home, as most mothers are careful to examine their newborn child thoroughly. Diagnostic delay is almost exclusively a phenomenon of institutional care.

Anorectal malformations are classified as high or low, describing the relationship of the bowel end to the muscles of continence.

Low lesions: The bowel ends distal to the muscle of continence. Frequently in females an ectopic orifice exists which allows intestinal decompression. In males a fistula may run from an occluded anus along the median raphe of the scrotum to the penis. It is recognizable as beads of white desquamated cells, or meconium, along the line of the raphe. Such a fistula rarely allows adequate intestinal decompression. In some males there is no evidence of fistula or anal orifice, which calls for radiography to distinguish it from a high lesion. Where effective decompression exists there may be no signs of intestinal obstruction.

High lesions: In high lesions the bowel either ends blindly above the pelvic floor, or more commonly ends as a fistula into the bladder or posterior urethra in males, and in females into the uterus or upper vagina. Diagnostic delay allows the signs of low intestinal obstruction to develop, with abdominal distension leading

eventually to vomiting, respiratory embarrassment, caecal perforation and death. Meconium may be evacuated in small quantities via the vagina or in the urine, and its presence in the napkin may mislead attendants. Diagnosis rests upon noting the absence of a patent anus.

Primary management: For both high and low lesions the child is in danger of intestinal obstruction. Following diagnosis, nasogastric decompression will minimize bowel distension and thus maximize diaphragmatic excursion. Intravenous replacement of loss through gastric aspirates or vomitus will be required. Careful examination must be carried out to exclude other defects or disorders.

Definitive management: In low lesions a perineal exploration and anoplasty is performed, with a good prognosis for subsequent continence. In high lesions an initial colostomy is followed by definitive surgery at 6–9 months. The prognosis for continence must be guarded, as several elements required for normality (e.g., internal sphincter, and anal canal lined with skin) will be absent, and the function of existing elements may be compromised by surgery or secondary defects, e.g., sacral abnormalities.

Neural axis defects

Whilst these lesions are discussed in detail elsewhere, it is appropriate to discuss here indications for surgery. There is clearly no place for surgery in anencephaly or severe microcephaly which may be accompanied by a large meningoencephalocele.

In the more usual dilemma of the baby with a spinal meningomyelocele, it would be cruel to subject to surgery a baby for whom such surgery carries no prospect of any benefit. Congenital hydrocephalus, a large lesion on the back, a thoraco-lumbar situation, patulous anus, urinary dribbling, spastic diplegia, club feet, and kyphosis are all individually and collectively poor prognostic signs. Surgery may be indicated in any baby without hydrocephalus who can control the hips, but many babies fall into a grey area between two obvious extremes. In referring such babies for specialist opinion it is important not to encourage unrealistic expectations in family members.

Surgery never improves the existing neurological deficit.

Neonatal tumours

Tumours may appear virtually anywhere, and should always be investigated. The commonest lesion is the sacrococcygeal teratoma. The features include a large cystic swelling attached to the coccyx, with anterior displacement of the anus, and frequently intrapelvic extension, which is palpable rectally. The condition is rarely seen in males, and is commonly associated with prematurity. These tumours are often larger than the host, and bleeding into the tumour may cause anaemia or fetal death. Early complete removal along with the coccyx is essential to prevent recurrence and malignant transformation, and surgery in the neonatal period is appropriate.

Cleft lip and palate

These defects are quite obvious, excepting incomplete palatal clefts, which must be actively sought. Whilst some units are achieving excellent results with neonatal surgery for cleft lip, conventional wisdom suggests that lips be repaired at 10–12 weeks and the palate at 10–12 months. Secondary surgery in later life may be needed as growth distorts the anatomy. Feeding problems can be overcome either by spoon-feeding, by using special teats where clefts are partial, or, as a last resort, tube feeding. A facial cleft does not always prevent sucking, and a trial of breast-feeding is worthwhile.

Ambiguous genitalia

(Also see Chapter 20, Endocrine and Metabolic Disorders.)
Failure of sexual differentiation may not be an emergency in the usual meaning of the word. It is, however, important to recognize and investigate urgently in order to exclude adrenogenital syndrome with electrolyte abnormalities and allow gender assignation for normal psychosocial development. It is important to realize that gender assignation depends not only on chromosomal sex but, perhaps more importantly, on phenotypic sex, and this latter depends upon normal gonadal development and end organ sensitivity to sex hormones. One can rarely tell the appropriate gender by looking at ambiguous genitalia. It is preferable to avoid assigning a gender until a definitive plan of management has been designed. Altering an inappropriately-assigned gender can be difficult, traumatic, and in some instances impossible. Referral to a tertiary centre for investigation is thus imperative.

Covert anomalies

By their very nature, covert abnormalities are not obvious to inspection, and their diagnosis depends upon the recognition of disordered function, which may be present at the time of birth, or may be delayed for hours, days, or in some cases months or years.

Functions commonly disturbed by covert anomalies include:
- ventilation (respiratory distress)
- feeding (vomiting)
- micturition (oliguria, anuria)
- defecation (constipation)
- movement (paralysis).

Ventilation

The causes of disordered breathing in the neonate are legion *(see Fig. 28.1)*.

Abdominal distension: The commonest 'surgical' disorder presenting with breathing difficulty is abdominal distension. As the neonate is an obligate diaphragmatic breather, fatigue and respiratory distress will ensue if increased intra-abdominal pressure has to be overcome. Intestinal distension will reduce with nasogastric decompression. Occasionally in ascites or pneumoperitoneum paracentesis is justified to improve respiratory excursion.

Space-occupying lesion: Any space-occupying lesion within the chest will compromise ventilation. The commonest such lesion is the congenital diaphragmatic hernia *(see below)*. Pneumothorax behaves as a space-occupying lesion, and even without 'tension' may present as respiratory embarrassment.

Pneumonia: Consolidation of lung tissue secondary to aspiration pneumonitis or pneumonia will prevent adequate gas exchange. Inhalation of vomitus, sometimes associated with intestinal obstruction, is the commonest surgically-related cause. Nursing patients prone or in the lateral

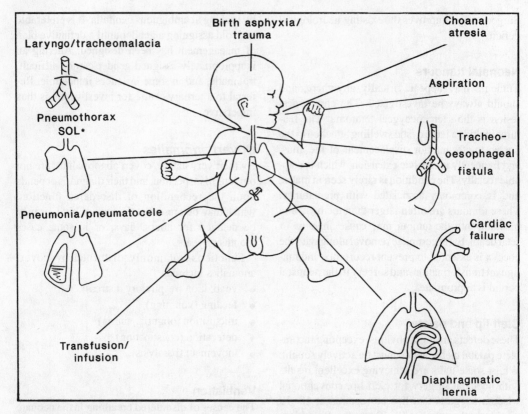

Fig 28.1 *Common surgically-related causes of neonatal respiratory distress*
* SOL = space occupying lesion

position rather than supine will minimize the risk of aspiration in otherwise-healthy individuals. Aspiration of saliva or gastric juice is a common presenting feature in oesophageal atresia, a lesion excluded by the ability to pass a nasogastric tube *(see below). Also see Chapter 5, Newborns.*

Airway obstruction: *See Chapter 5, Newborns.*

Diaphragmatic hernia: Because intrathoracic pressure is lower than intra-abdominal pressure, any defect in the diaphragm will allow abdominal viscera to herniate into the chest. The possible sites are:

◆ posterolateral diaphragm (Bochdalek hernia)

◆ retrosternal (Morgagni hernia)

◆ oesophageal hiatus (hiatal hernia)

◆ muscular diaphragm ('eventration').

Bochdalek hernia: The posterolateral defect in the diaphragm represents persistence of the pleuro-peritoneal canal. Because abdominal

viscera — principally bowel and liver or spleen — have been present in the chest throughout intrauterine development, the abdominal cavity will be small, never having been stimulated to maximal development. Furthermore, the ipsilateral lung will be small (hypoplastic) having been physically restrained, and the contralateral lung will be less severely abnormal.

Pathology: Although the obvious defect is in the diaphragm, a secondary problem lies in the wall of the pulmonary arteries and arterioles where, in conjunction with pulmonary hypoplasia, there is hypertrophy of the muscle. This hypertrophied muscle responds to a variety of stimuli, e.g., cold, acidosis, hypoxia, and pain, by constriction, thereby causing pulmonary hypertension. Although the ipsilateral lung is predominantly affected, in fact both lungs are abnormal. With acidosis and hypoxia pulmonary hypertension ensues. This in turn results in persistent fetal circulation *(see Chapter 5, Newborns)*. Although closure of the diaphragmatic defect will contribute little to correction of the basic pathology, it will give the hypoplastic lung the opportunity to expand and grow.

Presentation: Patients present with dyspnoea and cyanosis at a variable time after birth. Early onset of symptoms of respiratory distress implies gross pulmonary inadequacy and hence a bad prognosis. Those babies in whom presentation is delayed for 24 hours or more have demonstrated the adequacy of their lungs and have a good prognosis. Presentation may be expedited by allowing bowel within the chest cavity to become filled with air, as may happen during ventilation by mask, crying, or swallowing. This causes the herniated bowel to dilate, further compressing any ipsilateral lung tissue, displacing the mediastinum, and impeding the contralateral lung.

Diagnosis: In these babies respiratory distress is accompanied by a scaphoid abdomen and the mediastinum may be clinically deviated. Bowel sounds in the chest are an unreliable sign, but a chest radiograph shows multiple loops of bowel, usually on the left side. Very rarely, staphylococcal pneumonia or congenital lobar emphysema may produce somewhat similar appearances.

Primary management: Surgery is not a 'fire-engine' emergency, but transfer to a paediatric surgeon is required.

Early postnatal presentation: Many patients with virtual pulmonary aplasia are unable to sustain postnatal life, and may die before diagnosis. When the diagnosis is made, a nasogastric tube is passed and allowed to drain freely. The factors known to exacerbate pulmonary hypertension are avoided, particularly cold and hypoxia. Ventilation may mandate endotracheal intubation. No attempt should be made to 'expand' the compressed lung by increasing ventilation pressure, as this will simply cause contralateral pneumothorax. Transfer may be indicated if the patient's condition is stabilized.

Unpressurized air transport is not advised, as this may cause air in bowel within the chest to expand, with potentially disastrous results.

Delayed presentation: Where symptoms begin after 24 hours, pulmonary function is clearly adequate to sustain life, and the prognosis is good.

Similar primary care is instituted, but endotracheal intubation is rarely necessary.

Definitive management: On arrival at a paediatric unit patients are reassessed and adverse factors (e.g., cold) which are frequently associated with transportation are corrected. Surgery is delayed until the patient is stable. Intra- and postoperative epidural anaesthesia may be used in addition to general anaesthesia, to obviate the effects of pain on pulmonary artery pressure. Transabdominal repair is performed, and closure of the diaphragm is rarely problematic. Closure of the abdomen may be more difficult, and stretching is sometimes needed. Postoperative care is directed to preventing pulmonary hypertension. The return of a fetal circulatory pattern, often after a 'honeymoon period' of satisfactory progress, represents treatment failure.

Morgagni hernia: Retrosternal or Morgagni hernias are rare, and usually not large enough to seriously compromise ventilation. Bowel may occasionally incarcerate in such a defect. Diagnosis is made by lateral chest X-ray when the anterior disposition of mediastinal bowel shadows becomes clear.

Oesophageal hiatal hernia: This is further discussed under gastro-oesophageal reflux. Not all hiatal herniae result in reflux however, and they may present with mass effect or incarceration.

Eventration: Massive eventration is pathologically identical to a Bochdalek hernia, and is more properly described as a diaphragmatic hernia with a sac. Lesser degrees of eventration may result in recurrent or chronic chest infection, or may remain asymptomatic to be revealed as an irregular diaphragm on a routine chest X-ray. Most eventrations of any significance should be repaired.

Oesophageal atresia

Congenital obstruction of the oesophagus occurs in approximately 1 in 2 500 live births. Although several patterns are seen *(see Fig. 28.2)*, in 90% of cases the oesophagus ends blindly in the upper mediastinum, whilst the lower oesophagus ends in the trachea. This tracheo-oesophageal fistula is usually at the level of the carina.

Pathophysiology: The effects of this anatomical derangement can be deduced from a study of *Fig. 28.2(3)*. Firstly, at each breath a proportion

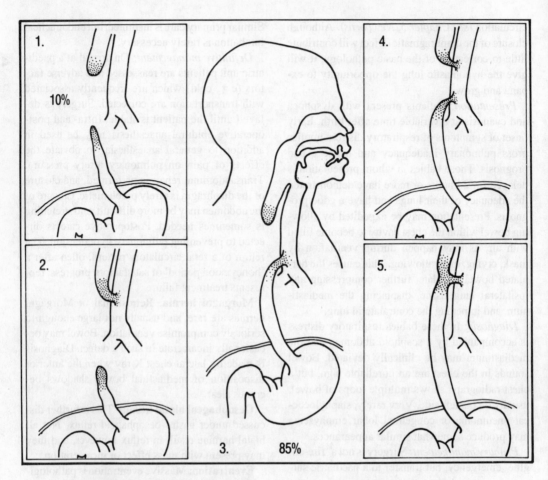

Fig. 28.2 Oesophagal atresia: Five varieties, with approximate distribution in percentages

of the tidal volume will be diverted into the oesophagus and thence the stomach. Gaseous distension results, with effective splinting of the diaphragm. Gastro-oesophageal reflux is promoted, and gastric juice will reflux into the trachea and lungs. Pneumonitis and pneumonia rapidly result. Saliva and any feeds will accumulate in the upper blind pouch and then spill over into the trachea, enhancing the pneumonitis. As the baby is breathing through an oesophago-pharyngeal pool of saliva, bubbles and froth appear at the lips. Finally, any attempts at feeding will promote massive aspiration, often with cyanosis and bradycardia.

Clinical presentation: Oesophageal atresia may be seen as an isolated anomaly or as part of a syndrome, e.g., VATER association *(see above).*

Given the dramatic nature of the abnormality, it is surprisingly often missed. Maternal polyhydramnios is often reported, and prematurity affects 50% of patients. The babies usually look perfectly normal and have normal Apgar scores, but a high index of suspicion should be stimulated by the presence of any other anomaly, particularly anorectal malformations.

The babies are typically 'bubbly' and choke on feeding. It is impossible to pass a stiff nasogastric tube beyond 11–12 cm. (It is possible to cause a soft tube to curl up in the upper pouch, giving a false impression of oesophageal continuity.)

An erect chest and abdominal radiograph is taken with the tube in place, confirming its arrest in the upper thorax. No other investigations are necessary, but an air contrast oesophagogram can be performed, if desired, outlining the upper pouch. Contrast media other than air are dangerous. Invariably a tracheobronchogram results, with deterioration of the respiratory status.

Progressive pneumonia occurs if the diagnosis and primary management is delayed. Starvation and depletion of energy stores further worsen the prognosis.

Primary management: A baby with oesophageal atresia can be made 'safe', allowing time for improvement of general condition, transportation, or surgery. All feeding attempts are stopped immediately the diagnosis is suspected. A wide tube (preferably double lumen) is passed into the upper pouch, which is kept dry by frequent aspiration or continuous suction. Gastro-oesophageal reflux may be reduced by nursing the patient 'head up', and its effects minimized by intravenous cimetidine or an equivalent. Pneumonitis or pneumonia is treated with antibiotics and oxygen supplementation, physiotherapy, or occasionally intubation and mechanical ventilation. Intravenous fluids are required, as no oral intake is possible.

Definitive management: At a paediatric surgical unit any associated abnormalities are evaluated. Ideally surgery is performed as soon as possible, but time can be spent preoperatively improving the condition of babies in whom pneumonia or other problems have arisen.

In developing countries where parenteral nutrition is impracticable and staffing levels are less than ideal, and where babies present late with existing malnutrition, a preliminary gastrostomy may be performed for subsequent access for feeding. At thoracotomy the fistula is divided and the trachea repaired. Oesophageal continuity is restored where possible. A cervical oesophagostomy or salivary fistula may be necessary if the oesophageal ends cannot be brought together without unacceptable tension. In patients with oesophageal atresia without a fistula there is rarely sufficient distal oesophagus to allow an anastomosis.

Postoperative care consists of a continuation of preoperative management. Gastrostomy feeds are generally begun at 48 hours, and are introduced at low pressure lest feeds reflux into the oesophagus. A contrast swallow is usually performed on the

fifth to seventh day, and if satisfactory, graded oral fluids are commenced.

Prognosis: Low birth weight, other major anomalies, and pneumonia have an important bearing on survival. Large, healthy babies with no other anomalies have a 95% chance of survival. If diagnosis is delayed and pneumonia allowed to develop, the survival drops to 75%. In the presence of other anomalies the overall survival is 65%, but major cardiac, neural axis, or pulmonary anomalies carry a much worse prognosis.

Patients with recognizable chromosomal lesions which are in themselves life-limiting are offered no active treatment.

Vomiting

Whilst some regurgitation of feed may be sufficiently common as to be regarded as normal, true vomiting is always pathological. Bile-stained vomitus is indicative of intestinal obstruction, and always warrants the attention of a surgeon. Non-bilious vomiting is less commonly due to a 'surgical' cause, but if persistent requires investigation.

Intestinal obstruction: Obstruction of the bowel, whether mechanical or paralytic, is characterized at any age by cessation of progression of intestinal content and nutrient absorption, resulting in starvation. There is distension of bowel above the obstruction by secretions and swallowed air, resulting in abdominal distension to a degree dependent upon the level of obstruction *(see Table 28.2)*. Fluid within static bowel loops is effectively lost from the total body fluid, and dehydration results. Once the bowel distal to the obstruction has emptied, no further passage of faeces or flatus occurs, i.e., absolute constipation. Bacterial proliferation in the stagnant fluid above the obstruction may result in 'faeculent fluid' in the small bowel. Distension may be sufficient to compromise intestinal mucosal blood flow, thereby breaching the mucosal barrier to luminal organisms and toxins. Periodic decompression of the proximal bowel is provided by vomiting, which will be bilious or faeculent if the obstruction is distal to the ampulla of Vater. There will be additional features of toxaemia or peritonitis where a strangulating obstruction is present.

Table 28.2 Clinical features of intestinal obstruction

Level of obstruction	Vomiting	Distension	Constipation
High	Early	Minimal	Late
Mid	Variable	Moderate	Variable
Low	Late	Marked	Early

▶ Features of respiratory distress may dominate the picture, due to aspirated vomitus, often aggravated by abdominal distension.

Primary management: Whatever the cause of intestinal obstruction, the patient can best be served by:

◆ Passage of a nasogastric tube: If properly supervised this prevents vomiting, reduces abdominal distension (and thus improves respiratory function) and maximizes intestinal blood flow. Nasogastric tubes should never be closed, but allowed to drain freely, with frequent intermittent aspiration.

◆ Intravenous fluids: Except in unusual circumstances, isotonic fluid losses can be replaced by an isotonic fluid such as Ringer's lactate with added dextrose. The volume replaced is guided by signs of fluid deficit, particularly pulse rate, blood pressure, and urine output.

◆ General care: This includes maintenance of body temperature, relief of pain, and antibiotic therapy where indicated.

Diagnosis of intestinal obstruction is clinical. Radiology may help to localize the site and occasionally the nature of the obstruction. Both supine and erect films are required, and the hallmark of 'obstruction' is the presence of air-fluid levels within the bowel, and an absence of air shadows in the pelvis. Unfortunately the presence of air-fluid levels is not pathognomonic of intestinal obstruction, and they may be seen in inflammatory bowel disorders, particularly gastroenteritis and dysenteries. Clearly the clinical picture in such conditions precludes a diagnosis of obstruction, but the distinction can at times be taxing. Despite these reservations, the cardinal investigation of all neonates with bilious vomiting remains the erect chest and abdominal radiograph. Abnormal air-fluid levels or evidence of a large fluid-filled stomach should prompt surgical referral.

Specific causes of intestinal obstruction in the neonate are discussed here. Pathology more characteristic of infants and children is discussed under *General Paediatric Surgery, see below.*

Intestinal atresia: Congenital occlusion of the bowel lumen can affect any part of the gut, but most commonly affects the duodenum or proximal jejunum.

Duodenal atresia: Occurs at the level of the ampulla of Vater, and is thought to represent a failure of recanalization of the embryonic duodenum. There is a non-random association with Down's syndrome, which of itself increases the risk of congenital heart lesions and other associated anomalies. Clinically patients present with early onset of bilious vomiting with little, if any, epigastric distension. The stigmata of Down's syndrome may be present. An erect chest and abdominal radiograph reveals the 'double-bubble' caused by a large gastric air-fluid level on the left and a large air-fluid level in the duodenum on the right. There is no gas distally. These babies are often small, and maintenance of body temperature is vital. A nasogastric tube is passed, and the proximal bowel decompressed. This fluid is replaced, in addition to the baby's maintenance requirements. Where multiple abnormalities do not preclude an acceptable prognosis, surgical bypass of the atretic area is performed at laparotomy. Postoperatively, gastroduodenal inertia may delay feeding such that parenteral nutrition is required.

Jejuno-ileal atresia: In a classic series of experiments in Cape Town, Louw and Barnard showed that atresia results from interference with the fetal blood supply to the bowel. Atresias may be multiple, associated with a mesenteric defect, or result in the apparent disappearance of a considerable length of bowel. Small bowel atresia is most common in the proximal jejunum. Bilious vomiting is the principal symptom. Abdominal distension will depend upon the site of obstruction. Babies with atresia may pass inspissated meconium on one or two occasions, with consequent diagnostic delay. Radiographs will show air-fluid levels in proportion to the length of bowel above the most proximal obstruction. Management is as in duodenal atresia. Resection of atretic areas with intestinal anastomosis is usually required. The prognosis depends upon the nature of the defect and general state of the patient at presentation.

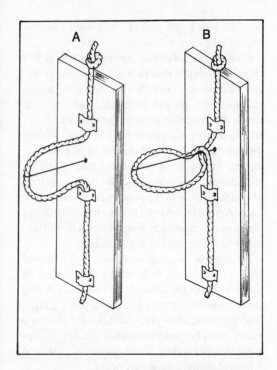

Fig. 28.3   Normal intestinal rotation occurring counter-clockwise around the axis of the superior mesentric artery
a. Prior to rotation
b. The proximal limb representing duodenum comes to lie posterior to the distal limb representing transverse colon

However, as a rule the more distal the obstruction, the more favourable the prognosis.

Meconium ileus: One way in which patients with cystic fibrosis present is with neonatal intestinal obstruction. In this condition intraluminal obstruction of the distal ileum is caused by tacky meconium with the consistency and tenacity of chewing gum. The clinical features of ileal obstruction are present, but radiologically the viscid intestinal content prevents the formation of air-fluid levels and gives a 'ground glass' appearance to the lower abdomen. Volvulus of the ileum may supervene. The cystic fibrosis gene is prevalent amongst whites. Black patients may present with 'meconium ileus equivalent', but subsequent testing fails to confirm true cystic fibrosis. Gastrografin, which is hygroscopic, instilled *per rectum* may enter the terminal ileum and relieve the obstruction. Sometimes operative clearance is re-

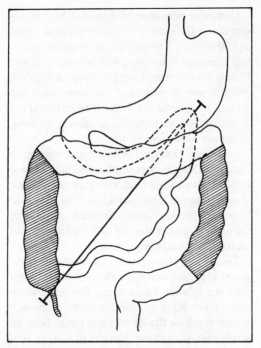

Fig. 28.4   Normal rotation, demonstrating the long posterior attachment of the midgut loop

quired, which may involve intestinal resection. The ultimate prognosis depends upon the expression of other features of cystic fibrosis, particularly respiratory.

Intestinal malrotation: As the intestine outgrows the fetal abdominal cavity it herniates into the base of the umbilical cord. During its return, at approximately the tenth week of pregnancy, the midgut undergoes rotation about the axis of the superior mesenteric artery *(see Fig. 28.3)*. The effect of this 270° counter-clockwise rotation is to provide the midgut loop with a long attachment to the posterior abdominal wall extending from the left upper quadrant to the right lower quadrant, minimizing the risk of volvulus *(see Fig. 28.4)*. Any abnormality of rotation will result in a shorter posterior attachment of the midgut loop and a higher incidence of volvulus. Any such volvulus presents as a duodenal obstruction. It is doubtful whether peritoneal bands extending from a displaced caecum to the lateral abdominal wall (Ladd's bands) cause extrinsic duodenal obstruction.

Clinical presentation: Midgut volvulus can present at any age, with 80% occurring below a year and 30% below 1 month. The presentation is of a high intestinal obstruction with bilious vomiting. Bloody stools strongly suggest bowel infarction, which is usually associated with prostration and toxaemia. Volvulus can occur without bowel necrosis, and may be intermittent, causing recurring symptoms over a long period.

Diagnosis: Duodenal obstruction, complete or incomplete, may be seen on plain abdominal films. Confirmation comes from a contrast meal which shows abnormal configuration of the duodenal loop and a duodeno-jejunal flexure to the right of the midline, even when the radiological signs of obstruction are absent.

Treatment: Malrotation is a surgical emergency. Presentation with duodenal obstruction implies that volvulus has occurred. Should volvulus proceed to midgut necrosis, the bowel from duodenum to splenic flexure becomes gangrenous, an unsalvageable situation. The aim of surgery is to devise a stable arrangement and to recreate a long posterior midgut attachment to prevent future volvulus, obviously before necrosis occurs. This is achieved by derotating the bowel to the fetal position of nonrotation, wherein the small bowel lies to the right of the abdomen, and the colon to the left.

Constipation

Most newborns pass meconium during the first 24 hours of life, and failure to do so requires investigation, particularly if there is accompanying abdominal distension. Causes include:

◆ *Mechanical:*
   Proximal atresia or other obstruction
   Ectopic or stenotic anus
◆ *Functional:*
   Meconium plug
   Aganglionosis/neuronal dysplasia
   Small left colon syndrome.

Meconium plug: Where delay in passage of meconium is recognized, rectal examination or gentle saline enema may reveal an inspissated plug of pale meconium followed by the passage of apparently normal meconium associated with clinical decompression. However, a diagnosis of meconium plug obstruction can only be made with any confidence once colonic aganglionosis has been excluded. All patients with such histories require long-term follow-up.

Congenital intestinal aganglionosis (CIA) (Hirschsprung's disease): CIA is underdiagnosed in neonates in a Third World environment, and may still present in infants and children. Rarely the condition presents for the first time in adulthood, in patients who have been unaware of their bowel habit being abnormal. In all patients a diligent interrogation will reveal that symptoms started in the neonatal period, the most consistent of which is delay in the passage of having meconium. Approximately one in three patients initially diagnosed as meconium plug obstruction will turn out to have intestinal aganglionosis.

An absence of ganglion cells in the neuronal plexi of the bowel wall results in a failure of transmission of the wave of relaxation which precedes peristaltic contraction. Embryonic ganglionic migration takes place caudally and may stop at any level, but most commonly reaches the sigmoid or upper rectum. Total colonic or even total intestinal aganglionosis may occur.

Clinical presentation: In neonates delay in stooling is cardinal. Older patients may present with failure to thrive, abdominal distension secondary to megacolon, or simply with chronic constipation. Rectal examination in such patients may be followed by explosive decompression as the unrelaxing aganglionic internal sphincter is forced to dilate by the examining finger. Aganglionosis may result in perforation of the caecum due to increasing pressure within the colon secondary to distal obstruction, or to fulminating enterocolitis. In view of this, neonatal management is of some urgency. In sophisticated environs the distal bowel may be kept empty by daily enemas, suppositories, or lavages. In the Third World a more satisfactory solution is a colostomy placed in a ganglionic portion of colon. Definitive surgery can be performed around the age of six months, and normal bowel function can be anticipated thereafter.

Diagnosis: Following clinical suspicion the diagnosis can be confirmed by plain X-ray films or contrast enema which will reveal a rectum and sigmoid of apparently normal calibre with dilated proximal bowel above. Pressure studies will show an absence of physiological internal sphincter relaxation in response to rectal distension. This investigation may be difficult to interpret in neonates, but is a useful screening test in older children. Rectal biopsy will show hypertrophied nerves and absence of ganglion cells in both Auerbach's and Meissner's plexi.

Small left colon syndrome: Infants of diabetic mothers, or of those taking certain psychotropic drugs, may present with a meconium plug-like syndrome. Contrast enema reveals an apparently unused colon from splenic flexure distally. A gastrografin enema is therapeutic, and colonic function thereafter appears normal, but there may be some difficulty distinguishing this condition from long segment aganglionosis. There is clearly a spectrum of neonatal colonic dysfunctional states with similar clinical and radiological appearances, and correct diagnosis may well involve manometry and biopsy.

Micturition

In the absence of hypovolaemia normal babies pass urine within 4– 6 hours of delivery. Failure to do so may be indicative of a urinary tract abnormality. Such abnormalities may reflect abnormalities of urine production or excretion. It is important that in all neonates the time of first micturition, and where possible the nature of the urinary stream are noted. There is a clear association between abnormalities of fetal urine production and excretion and pulmonary development. Urine production starts at around the eighth to tenth intrauterine week, and is an important contribution to amniotic fluid volume. Hence urinary dysfunction will have been present for 6 months or more before presentation with consequent renal damage at birth which governs the overall prognosis.

Urinary obstruction: Unilateral obstruction such as pyeloureteric junction obstruction causes no interference with micturition, and overall renal function is protected by a contralateral normal kidney. In females bilateral obstruction may rarely be due to bilateral ureteroceles obstructing the ureterovesical junction. In males, in whom lower urinary obstruction is many times more common, the most singular cause is valvular urethral obstruction.

Posterior urethral valves: In the normal urethra small mucosal folds spread from the veru montanum to the side walls of the prostatic urethra. Exaggeration of these folds results in 'valves' which obstruct, partially or totally, the passage of urine. There is dilatation of the prostatic urethra proximal to the obstruction, hypertrophy and trabeculation of the bladder with diverticula, dilatation of both ureters, and bilateral hydronephrosis. At the time of birth this urinary obstruction is of long standing, and the prognosis depends entirely upon the number of residual nephrons, which in turn depends upon the degree of valvular obstruction. Patients who present early have the most complete obstruction, most renal damage, and poorest prognosis. Patients who survive into childhood have a correspondingly good prognosis.

Clinical presentation: A neonate may have been noted to have failed to pass urine or to have passed with a poor stream. Bilateral hydronephrosis may be palpable, as may an hypertrophied, thick-walled bladder. Abnormal renal function will be evidenced by raised urea and creatinine. A small proportion of patients will present with urinary ascites, and oedema of the abdominal wall and lower limbs.

Primary management: Valvular obstruction is truly valvular. There is no obstruction to passage of a catheter or feeding tube. This should be passed under sterile conditions, as nephrons can be as surely destroyed by infection as by persisting obstruction. Upper tract obstruction, manifest by failure of improvement in renal function and persistently poor output, may be due to secondary vesico-ureteric obstruction caused by the tremendously thickened bladder wall. In such patients, upper tract diversion may be needed. Most patients will improve on catheter drainage alone.

Radiology: Sonography is often diagnostic, but a voiding cysto-urethrogram is more readily interpretable.

Definitive management: Disruption of the valves can be performed in the neonate if small calibre optics are available. In their absence, urinary diversion, either cystostomy or ureterostomy, must be performed as a temporary measure. When the urethra is large enough to admit a cystoscope the valves can be destroyed by diathermy or disrupted by a balloon catheter.

Movement

Nerve damage and paralysis as a result of birth injury, abnormal tone, jitteriness, and convulsions are discussed in *Chapter 5, Newborns.*

Neonatal GIT bleeding

Blood may be present in vomitus (haematemesis) or in the stool (haematochezia).

Haematemesis: *See Chapter 5, Newborns.*

Haematochezia: Bleeding *per rectum* is most frequently a manifestation of haemorrhagic disease of the newborn *(see above),* particularly in an otherwise healthy baby. Bloody stools are, however, an important feature of intestinal mucosal necrosis secondary to necrotizing enterocolitis, volvulus neonatorum, and neonatal dysenteries.

Necrotizing enterocolitis (NEC): The intestine bears the brunt of any hypoxic or hypovolaemic insult, as blood is diverted from the splanchnic circulation to vital organs, especially the heart and brain. Within the bowel blood is shunted away from the mucosa to preferentially perfuse the muscle layers. This compromises the mucosal barrier and allows luminal toxin and organisms access to the deeper layers of the bowel wall, giving rise to the clinical features of NEC, including bloody stools in many patients. Thus NEC represents the final common pathway of many primary pathologies. The clinical and radiological features are described elsewhere *(see Chapter 5, Newborns),* and treatment in the majority of patients is non-operative.

Surgery is required where there is evidence of full-thickness bowel necrosis, viz., pneumoperitoneum, intra-abdominal mass (omentum and small bowel loops), peritonitis (manifested often by abdominal wall oedema and erythema), and failure to respond to medical treatment. This is the most difficult indication to define, but falling platelet and white cell counts are helpful indicators. Late surgery may be required to deal with strictures which result from the healing of circumferential ulceration.

Volvulus neonatorum: *See Malrotation, above.* It must be remembered as a cause of bloody stools in the neonate, but such a presentation suggests that intestinal necrosis has already occurred, and the prognosis is poor.

Neonatal dysenteries: *See Chapter 5, Newborns.*

Other neonatal surgical problems

Labial fusion

Baby girls are often seen with a normal anus but covered vagina, giving rise to a misdiagnosis of vaginal atresia. These girls pass urine normally and are otherwise healthy. This appearance is due to midline fusion of the labia minora, and the defect can be painlessly corrected by gentle separation using an ear swab or blunt probe. Once separated, a non-adherent dressing keeps the labia apart to prevent refusion.

Amniotic bands

Congenital constriction rings affecting fingers and toes, or more commonly ankles and wrists, are not uncommon. The aetiology remains unclear, but fibrous bands within the amniotic fluid are held responsible. Often there is spontaneous amputation of the digit or limb distal to the constriction.

Surgery in the form of multiple Z-plasties is required. This can safely be performed in the neonatal period, with good results.

Circumcision

There are few, if any, indications for neonatal circumcision. There are some absolute contraindications, however *(see below).*

The controversy surrounding circumcision stems from the incorrect use of terms such as 'phimosis' and 'pinhole meatus' as well as a lack of awareness of preputial physiology. It is unnecessary to retract the prepuce to wash the glans. It is also untrue that removal of the prepuce prevents masturbation and that circumcision is necessary to prevent penile cancer. The profession should adopt a stance of reassurance and re-education, both of the laity and of professionals who perpetuate such myths.

The prepuce forms a protective cover for the glans penis and prevents excoriation of the glandular epithelium by nappies and urine.

The prepuce is retractable in less than 5% of newborns, and it should never be forcibly retracted *(see Phimosis, below).*

The prepuce and glans are joined by a viable cell layer which breaks down with time, leaving epithelial debris in the coronal sulcus. This debris is *not* pus, and is not associated with inflammation. Ballooning of the prepuce during micturition will occur in all boys until the urinary meatus can be exposed, and may in fact be the natural force causing separation.

Attempts to retract the prepuce will reveal the line of cell union which may appear 'pinhole'. However, if it allows the passage of urine at this age it is adequate.

At 4–6 years the prepuce is retractable in 90% of boys.

Contraindications:

◆ *Hypospadias:* The prepuce provides useful and sometimes essential tissue for reconstruction and should never be discarded prematurely.

◆ *Buried penis/microphallus:* In this condition assessment of an appropriate resection is impossible, and inadequate skin may be available for future surgery.

◆ *Napkins (diaper):* No matter how careful a mother may be, her infant will spend some time each day in a wet nappy. Glandular mucosa thus treated becomes ulcerated and scarred. Occasionally the meatal orifice is affected in this way, leading to stenosis requiring further surgery.

Maternal advice: Mothers should be told to keep the genital area socially clean and not to retract the prepuce for hygiene or any other purpose. They should be reassured about 'ballooning', and that the 'pinhole meatus' will mature into a wide channel of communication. Social or traditional circumcision can be performed at or around the age of puberty with the understanding and consent of the individual.

Phimosis

Phimosis represents the end result of the healing of skin trauma caused by forced retraction. This manoeuvre produces longitudinal splits in the inner preputial layer which result in severe burning dysuria or 'crying on micturition', and ultimately in fibrosis and stricturing of the preputial orifice. Circumcision may be indicated. The condition is largely preventable by parental and professional education.

Inguinal hernia

In children, with rare exceptions, inguinal herniae are of the indirect variety, representing persistence of the processus vaginalis. This outpouching of peritoneum extends as a sleeve to the upper pole of the testis and is thought to play an important role in testicular descent. Patency of this tube either wholly or in part will allow abdominal contents to descend into the scrotum.

The condition is more common in males. However, when present in girls herniae are more often bilateral. Most commonly bowel or omentum is found as sac content, but ovaries, Fallopian tubes, and even free ascaris worms have been encountered.

Clinical presentation: Usually the mother notices an intermittent inguinal swelling, often initially during crying. When examined, the inguino-scrotal region may appear quite normal. It may, however, be possible to appreciate a slight thickening of the cord on the affected side. Even when examination is unhelpful, the maternal history is relied upon and elective surgery booked. In females an irreducible 'node' — in fact the ovary — may remain, although the child is otherwise asymptomatic.

Complications: The presence of a hernia is of itself a benign condition, but is the necessary precursor of potentially lethal complications — incarceration (irreducibility) and strangulation (gangrene of the hernial content). Herniae should be repaired to prevent these complications. The younger the patient, the higher the risk of complications, and therefore the earlier surgery should be prescribed.

Incarceration presents with a fixed inguino-scrotal swelling, usually in a patient with prior experience of a similar but reducible swelling. Intestinal obstruction follows any prolonged incarceration, and is associated with abdominal distension and vomiting. The increased intra-abdominal pressure tends to perpetuate and exacerbate the incarceration, which proceeds inexorably to intestinal gangrene if not treated. This may affect a whole bowel loop or just an arc of the bowel circumference. The final result of either event is intestinal perforation, toxaemia, and death.

Strangulation is heralded clinically by local signs of inflammation, often to the point where an abscess is seriously considered. Intestinal obstruction, toxaemia, and dehydration are present to a variable degree.

Management: When incarceration is diagnosed the treatment aim is early reduction of the hernia followed by later elective repair. This is done because acute repair implies a greater anaesthetic risk and the oedematous friable tissues add to the surgical hazard. Thus a nasogastric tube is passed, intravenous fluid therapy initiated, and the child is given a sedative (e.g., Vallergan®) or a caudal anaesthetic. The foot of the cot is elevated and the child is watched for 60 minutes *after* falling asleep, whereafter gentle pressure is applied to reduce the hernia. Repair is arranged when convenient after a 48-hour period. The child should be kept under observation during this time lest incarceration recur. Should reduction fail, or if the initial impression is of strangulation, there is no alternative but to resuscitate the patient for emergency surgery. Bowel infarction requires intestinal resection, but timeous surgery may allow ischaemic bowel to survive, hence surgery is urgent.

Hydrocele

In children hydroceles usually communicate with the peritoneal cavity. In other words they are in fact herniae, but the communication is too narrow to allow bowel to descend to the scrotum. Peritoneal fluid tends to accumulate in the scrotum by day and flow back to the abdominal cavity at night. The child presents with a painless scrotal swelling which is often worse in the evening. One can get above the swelling and perhaps appreciate thickening of the spermatic cord. Transillumination cannot be relied upon in small children, as even herniae containing bowel will allow the passage of light. The testis is often impalpable.

Hydrocele which persists after 12 months of age may be treated by herniotomy. Before 12 months, only exceptional hydroceles require any attention, as most resolve spontaneously.

Pyloric stenosis

Hypertrophic pyloric stenosis is a condition of unknown aetiology in which the thickened pyloric ring causes an incomplete gastric outlet obstruction. It is rare in the Third World, and the diagnosis

is often delayed due to the similarity of some of the clinical features to gastroenteritis.

Clinical presentation: Symptoms start at around 3 weeks of age. The cardinal symptom is bile-free vomiting which increases in frequency and forcefulness until it occurs after every meal and is truly projectile. Occasional flecks of blood in the vomitus are a reflection of underlying gastritis. In the Third World 30% of patients will have diarrhoea at presentation, making differentiation from gastroenteritis particularly difficult. Associated features are weight loss due to failure of adequate intake, dehydration secondary to fluid loss in vomitus, and obvious hunger unless the patient is moribund. On examination, which ideally is performed while the baby is feeding, visible peristalsis crossing the epigastrium from left to right may be seen. A palpable pyloric mass may be felt, at the right edge of rectus abdominis, midway between the umbilicus and costal margin, when it is forced into prominence by an antral peristaltic contraction.

Biochemistry: Due to late presentation and diagnosis, severe nutritional and biochemical deficits are frequently seen. Pure loss of gastric juice results in a metabolic alkalosis with hyponatraemia, hypochloraemia and hypokalaemia. There is usually a paradoxical aciduria. Recognition of the biochemical lesion and the importance of correcting it preoperatively have reduced the mortality of pyloric stenosis to less than 1% in most units.

Diagnosis: A clinical diagnosis may require no confirmation in experienced hands. However, the rarity of the disorder in the Third World, and the difficult differential diagnosis, mean that confirmation will be required in many cases. Barium meal is the most accurate diagnostic tool, allowing visualization of a large stomach with vigorous peristalsis and a long, very narrow pyloric channel (string sign). Ultrasound scanning has a false negative rate of 10–20%.

Treatment: The management of pyloric stenosis is surgical, but it is not an emergency. Alkalosis is corrected by infusion of normal saline made up to a 10% dextrose solution. When sufficient volume has been infused to stimulate a urinary output, potassium is added to the infusion. In shocked patients an initial infusion of colloid may be necessary to restore circulating volume. Serial checks of the electrolyte profile allow an optimal time to be selected for surgery, usually within 48 hours of admission. Gastric lavage to remove sour curds from the stomach may ameliorate gastritis. Ramstedt's pyloromyotomy, first performed in 1912, remains the ideal operation. The hypertrophied pyloric muscle is split, allowing the mucosa to pout out. If care is taken to avoid perforating the mucosa, no further procedure is necessary.

Postoperative care: Patients may start taking small volume feeds as soon as fully awake following surgery, and well-nourished babies may be home by the third postoperative day. In patients with marked gastritis, postoperative vomiting may delay resumption of full feeds. The sequelae of malnutrition — particularly wound infection and dehiscence — and chest infections complicate recovery in up to 10% of patients. Deaths, however, should be rare, even in the Third World.

Umbilical problems

Umbilical granuloma: A dull, reddish, polypoid lesion appearing at the umbilicus at the time of cord separation is likely to be an umbilical granuloma — exuberant granulation tissue representing healing of the umbilical cicatrix. Frequently there is a modest mucopurulent exudate. Very much less frequently vitello-intestinal or urachal remnants may present, distinguishable by faeculent or urinary discharge.

Umbilical granulomata are satisfactorily treated by one or two applications of silver nitrate. It is important to protect surrounding normal skin with petroleum jelly or equivalent, and to cover the umbilicus with a dressing to prevent indelible staining of the baby's clothes.

Omphalitis: Umbilical infection, manifested locally by tenderness and erythema with or without a discharge, is a serious condition. Because infection may spread via the umbilical vein to the portal vein, with resultant thrombosis, the lesion is of surgical interest. Aggressive antibiotic therapy is vital, and the risk of tetanus must be remembered. Drainage and debridement with umbilical vein division may be required in occasional instances.

Umbilical hernia: Contraction of the umbilical ring occurs as a normal postnatal event. Delay in closure of the ring results in a defect, allowing herniation of abdominal viscera. Defects just above the umbilical ring — supra-umbilical hernia — have a different natural history. Umbilical hernia is common, affecting up to 50% of black South African children and a considerable but lesser percentage of other ethnic groups. As the pathology is one of 'delay', spontaneous 'closure' of the hernia can be predicted. Whilst these herniae, like any other, are subject to incarceration and strangulation, such events are rare and do not justify routine surgical repair. Umbilical herniae which persist after 6 years should be closed electively. Supra-umbilical herniae do not disappear spontaneously and always require surgery, which is best deferred until 2–3 years of age.

The umbilical hernia is unique in providing a window into the abdomen and, where the size of the defect permits, palpation of the viscera through the hernia may be particularly rewarding. Similarly, as the hernia represents skin lined with peritoneum, the signs of peritonitis are readily elicited by gently 'tapping' the hernia.

General paediatric surgery
General trauma
By virtue of their natural curiosity, inexperience, and incomplete physical development, children of all ages are particularly prone to trauma. Whilst it may be trite to repeat that children are not merely small adults, nowhere is this better demonstrated than in consideration of trauma.

As childrens' bones bend rather than break, a normal X-ray at presentation may misrepresent the considerable bony and soft tissue deformity which occurred at the moment of impact. Conversely, bones which do break suggest major distortion at injury, particularly with regard to ribs.

Childrens' heads are proportionately larger than adults, and are supported by less developed neck muscles. In infants with open sutures the skull can expand to accommodate increasing intracranial pressure, and the neurological signs of a space-occupying lesion may develop late.

The relatively small blood volume of the child exposes him to risks of hypovolaemia after apparently trivial bleeding.

The relatively large and unprotected upper abdominal viscera are prone to both blunt and penetrating injury. Injured children tend to swallow air, causing significant gastric dilatation and necessitating nasogastric decompression.

Due to their large surface area, children rapidly become hypothermic.

Indirect concerns deserve attention; such as the adequacy of tetanus immunization, the pyschological well-being of the injured child who must be separated from his family during treatment, and occasionally guilt experienced by the family after childhood injury.

A further responsibility of the professional caring for paediatric trauma victims is the spectre of non-accidental injury, which introduces further ethical dilemmas onto an already crowded stage.

Mechanisms of injury

Children are exposed to blunt injuries from falls, blows, or motor vehicle accidents. Penetrating injuries result from civil violence, dangerous playacting or fighting, and falls onto sharp objects. Patterns of injury characteristic of non-accidental injury are described in *Chapter 4, Community Paediatrics.* However, recurrent injury and/or delay in seeking professional help should increase suspicion.

Significant trauma in childhood frequently results in multiple injuries with more than one organ system affected. In major trauma head injury is an invariable associate.

Burns, drowning, electrical shock, and ingestion of foreign bodies or corrosives are more common amongst children, and are important causes of morbidity and mortality.

Burn injury

Mechanisms

Burns commonly occur in the home, where hot liquids may be poured over a child (e.g., by pulling over a kettle or cup of beverage) or spilt onto a floor where a child is sitting. Occasional burns result from such accidents as failure to test the temperature of bath water. Houses may be set alight, resulting in flame burns in addition to the inhalation of smoke particles and noxious gases. Open-fire cooking carries similar risks. In fair-skinned babies overlong exposure to the sun can result in significant injury. Chemical burns may result from contact with acids, alkalis, or petroleum products.

Pathology: Dermal injury in a burn is characterized by a central zone of maximum damage and concentric zones of lesser damage until uninjured skin is reached. Burns are classified according to the surface area affected and the depth of burn in the zone of maximum necrosis.

Superficial burns: There is no dermal involvement. Such burns are characterized by erythema and blistering. Sensation is intact and spontaneous healing can be expected.

Partial thickness burns: Superficial layers of dermis are involved. Deeper structures such as sweat glands and hair follicles are unaffected, and represent a source of new epithelial cells. Spontaneous healing is possible if infection is prevented.

Full thickness burns: Full depth of skin and appendages are burned. Clinically flesh may be charred or dead white. Sensation is absent. These burns are characterized by the development of slough, which separates after 2–3 weeks leaving granulation tissue. Skin grafting is inevitable.

Body surface area (BSA): Children's body proportions vary with age *(see Fig. 28.5).* As a rule the area of the palmar surface of the hand represents 1% of total surface area.

Primary management

At the scene: The immediate need is to minimize the extent of the injury. Obviously it is important to remove the patient from the fire or hot liquid, but burn injury continues for some time after removal of the exogenous source, and generous soaking or immersion in cold water is beneficial up to as long as an hour after injury. The burned area should then be dressed in any clean cloth, and the patient taken to a health facility.

Health professional: Burn injury assessment must allow a search for other injuries and exclude inhalation injury. The burn depth and surface area are estimated.

Indications for mandatory admission of a child with burns
- burn in any child younger than 3 months
- > 8% BSA burned
- involvement of hand, face, or perineum
- circumferential limb burn.

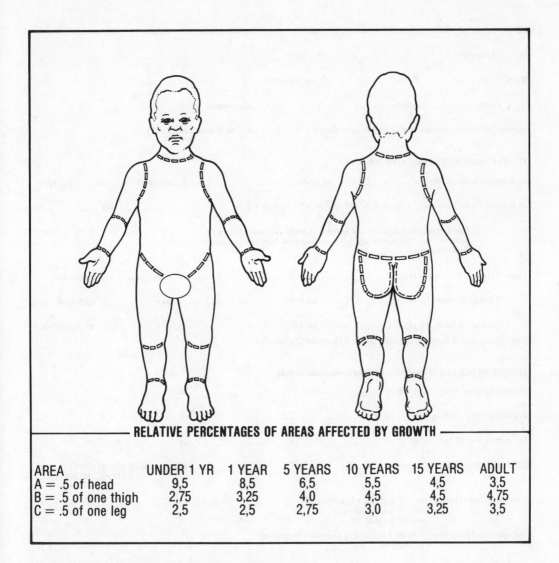

RELATIVE PERCENTAGES OF AREAS AFFECTED BY GROWTH

AREA	UNDER 1 YR	1 YEAR	5 YEARS	10 YEARS	15 YEARS	ADULT
A = .5 of head	9,5	8,5	6,5	5,5	4,5	3,5
B = .5 of one thigh	2,75	3,25	4,0	4,5	4,5	4,75
C = .5 of one leg	2,5	2,5	2,75	3,0	3,25	3,5

Fig. 28.5 Body surface proportion and relative change with growth

Systemic care: Intravenous fluid replacement is urgent, taking consideration of the fact that fluid loss started at the time of injury and may precede arrival at hospital by several hours. The volume required can be estimated from the formula provided *(see Burn management chart, Fig. 28.6)*. Regular clinical assessment of the patient, including urine output and haematocrit, is essential.

Analgesia and tetanus prophylaxis must not be forgotten. Antibiotics as prophylaxis are probably unhelpful, but they may be indicated for associated problems. Ileus accompanies any major burn, and nasogastric decompression is important. Antacids minimize stress ulceration.

A common gastrointestinal complication of burn injury is asphyxiation by ascaris worms, particularly in infants wearing occlusive dressings around the chest and upper arm which prevent them from turning over or getting their hands to their mouths. Prophylactic vermifuge should be considered when ileus resolves.

Name: .... Age: .... · Weight: ....

Date of Admission: .... IP number: ....

Burn: Date: .... Time: .... Time first seen: ....

     Cause: .... Area: .... %   Clean/Septic

Measles prophylaxis: Measles vaccine/immunoglobulin/nil   (delete those not applicable)

FLUID REPLACEMENT during first 36 hours

a) Basic requirement: Weight: .... kg x Area: .... % (max 30 %) = ... ml (a)

b) Supplement for raised PCV: (Actual PCV – Normal PCV*) x5 x (age + 1) = ... (b) .... ml

               This supplement is adjusted and added to 0, 8 and 18 hours, and may be necessary more frequently depending on severity of burn and response to fluid replacement.

From   0 hours – 8 hours give (a) .... ml + (b) .... ml = ... ml plasma

       8 hours – 18 hours give (a) .... ml + (b) .... ml = ... ml plasma

    18 hours – 36 hours give (a) .... ml + (b) .... ml = ... ml plasma/blood

Use blood instead of plasma during third period if Hb below 12 g/100 ml.

MAINTENANCE FLUID required in addition to replacement fluid

For each kg up to 10 kg   give 100 ml = ... ml
+
For each kg from 11-20 kg give 50 ml = ... ml
+
For each kg over 20 kg   give 20 ml = ... ml

Total maintenance fluid requirement = ... ml / 24 hours IN ADDITION TO
                                                      REPLACEMENT FLUID

Give IV for large burns: ie. over 8 % if under 1 year of age
                               over 10 % for children
                               over 15 % for adults

Recommended fluid: Electrolyte No 2 (depending on serum electrolytes).

INVESTIGATIONS

	Admission	8 hours	12 hours	18 hours	24 hours	36 hours
Hb	....	....	....	....	....	....
PCV	....	....	....	....	....	....
Urea	....	....	....	....	....	....

*GUIDE TO ADEQUACY OF FLUID ADMINISTRATION

i) Urine output. Minimum = 1 ml/kg/hour.

ii) PCV (haematocrit). Normal PCV: Neonate 60 %, Child 38 %, Adult 42 %.

Fig. 28.6 Burn management chart

Local care: The ideal is to provide a clean, atraumatic environment for burn healing. *Infection effectively deepens the extent of a burn.* Many efficacious creams, impregnated tulle gras and ointments are available. Where facilities exist, early tangential excision of deep burns, effectively cutting out the burn, is desirable. Few centres in developing countries enjoy such luxury. Skin grafting usually follows the separation of slough at about 21 days.

Psychological care: All burns cause scars. Some scar the body as well as the mind, others just the mind. The sequelae of pain, separation from family, altered body image, and effects of visible scarring can be minimized by starting support early. The family may deserve equal consideration, as guilt feelings may arise.

Ingestion of foreign bodies and corrosives

Foreign bodies

An infant will put any interesting object into her mouth as part of her exploration of the environment. Older children contrive to ingest a variety of objects, the most common being coins, but also razor blades, needles, safety pins, broken glass, and fish bones.

◆ If a foreign body sticks in the oesophagus it should be urgently removed.

◆ If a foreign body reaches the stomach it is likely to pass uneventfully.

Oesophageal foreign bodies

Three physiologically 'narrow' areas in the oesophagus are the common sites of foreign body impaction, viz., cricopharyngeus, level of aortic arch, and oesophageal hiatus.

If a foreign body is allowed to remain impacted, ulceration and perforation will result, hence removal should be arranged urgently. Smooth objects (e.g., coins) which have been impacted less than 24–48 hours are conveniently removed using a Foley catheter. Under X-ray control the persistence of the coin is confirmed. A suitably-sized, lubricated Foley catheter (usually size 8–10) is passed like a nasogastric tube. Once it has passed the impacted object the balloon is inflated, and under an X-ray screen the catheter is pulled back to engage the coin. The patient is turned prone and

the coin and catheter withdrawn together. Ideally oesophageal integrity is confirmed at the same sitting by performing a limited barium swallow.

Sharp objects, pins, or chronically impacted coins should be removed under general anaesthesia using a rigid oesophagoscope.

Gastric or more distal foreign bodies

Once an object reaches the stomach, and invariably once it has negotiated the pylorus, it will pass atraumatically. The author has observed double-edged razor blades and broken glass pass without comment, and the patient has been totally unaware of their eventual elimination. There is no need to hospitalize such patients. An X-ray check in 2–3 days to confirm progress or evacuation is all that is required. Rarely abdominal symptoms develop or progress is halted, and referral for surgery may be appropriate.

Fish bones may stick into or through the oesophageal wall and are usually not visible on plain X-rays. Diagnosis can be achieved by contrast swallow or oesophagoscopy. The history is usually diagnostic.

Strictures: It should be remembered that in patients with pre-existing oesophageal strictures an unchewed food bolus may constitute a foreign body which impacts. Such patients clearly need further evaluation when the obstruction has been relieved.

Corrosives

Proprietary drain cleaners, pool acids, bleach, etc. are freely available and represent a continual hazard to a child. The storing of acids or alkalis in containers attractive to children, within reach of children, and which can be opened by children contributes significantly to this hazard.

Pathology: Strong alkalis cause more damage than acids as they tend to stick to mucosa, prolonging contact. For this reason solid particles or granules tend to cause more significant, though more focal, damage than liquids.

Presentation: Rarely, if ever, is ingestion witnessed by an adult. Any suggestion of corrosive ingestion must therefore be taken seriously. In florid cases there may be burns of the lips and chin, salivation, and obvious mouth ulceration. Alternatively the oral mucosa may escape unscathed while the oesophagus or stomach is severely injured.

Management: All patients are admitted to hospital. Oesophagoscopy is the only way of diagnosing oesophageal injury, and this should be done as early as possible. Pending oesophagoscopy, antibiotics and fasting are advised. In those patients where oesophagoscopy reveals no injury, these measures are discontinued and the patient discharged. Where injury is present they are continued, and although the role of steroids remains debatable, their use may be of value. Feeding may continue via a fine bore tube. Some patients will develop oesophageal scarring and stenosis requiring dilatation, and rarely late oesophagectomy may be necessary. Immediate surgery may be required in patients with oesophageal perforation manifested by mediastinitis, toxaemia, and frequently pleural effusion.

Prevention is much easier than cure, and simple education campaigns have worked wonders in the United States and United Kingdom.

Blunt abdominal injury

The realization that there are no disposable abdominal organs, and particularly that splenectomy creates a state of life-threatening immuno-compromise, has revolutionized attitudes to trauma management in children. Viscera may be divided into:
◆ *solid viscera:* liver, spleen, pancreas, kidneys
◆ *hollow viscera:* alimentary tract, urinary tract, biliary tree
◆ *diaphragm.*

The principal morbidity of trauma to solid viscera stems from blood loss, and in the case of hollow viscera it is peritonitis.

Solid viscera

The aim of surgery in solid visceral injury is to stop bleeding, which usually occurs spontaneously. Management depends entirely upon the patient's clinical status. Instability which fails to respond to resuscitation is the only indication for intervention. When surgery is indicated, every effort is made to prevent organ resection, particularly of the spleen, and many techniques have evolved to assist the surgeon.

Hollow viscera

Injury to hollow viscera is manifest by the development of peritonitis, and the early detection of progressive clinical signs forms the rationale for the frequent re-evaluation of the trauma victim by a single observer.

A confident diagnosis or strong clinical suspicion justifies laparotomy, as the morbidity of delay is significant.

Diaphragm

Injuries of the diaphragm are frequently missed, both clinically and radiologically, but blunt injury often causes massive disruption with gross clinical features of herniation of abdominal viscera into the thorax. Diaphragmatic injuries require immediate repair through a transabdominal approach.

Multiple trauma

The child with multiple injuries creates major diagnostic and therapeutic challenges. Invariably a head injury co-exists, and response to painful stimuli and examination may be obtunded. Abdominal examination may be difficult in the presence of pelvic or rib fractures. Multiple sites of bleeding may conceal the need for surgery to arrest bleeding at one particular site.

Management

A detailed account of trauma management is beyond the scope of this chapter. However, the **principles** are based on:
◆ resuscitation
◆ evaluation
◆ observation
◆ operation.

Because of clinical difficulties, evaluation may involve the adjunctive use of radiology, sonography, or radioisotopes. Where staff shortages and lack of facilities make observation hazardous, consideration must be given to early surgery to both diagnose and manage intra-abdominal injuries. Successful management may depend upon the input of specific surgical disciplines (e.g., faciomaxillary surgeons), but the child with multiple injuries should remain under the care of the general surgeon or paediatric surgeon whether in a district hospital or trauma centre.

Snake bite

There are few corners of the planet not exploited by snakes. They are found from high mountains to deserts, from temperate zones to the tropics, and range from the strictly arboreal species of forest areas to those which spend their entire life underground. Several varieties have adapted well to urbanization, and can be found in and around houses in suburban and village areas. Given this enormous contact with people, it is perhaps surprising that snake bite is not a more frequent injury, and that death from venomous snake bite remains rare. Several factors account for this apparent paradox. Firstly, few species of snake are aggressive towards prey as large as human adults or children, and unless provoked or cornered are inclined to withdraw strategically, minimizing confrontation. Furthermore, of all the world's snakes, less than 20% are even mildly venomous, and of those, few are life-threatening to humans. Even bites by venomous species do not always lead to envenomation of the victim, or to the injection of lethal doses.

Small children, by virtue of their insatiable curiosity and small size, are doubly at risk. In areas where young boys are employed as herdsmen, especially barefoot, the risks are increased. They should be warned of the dangers of probing crevasses in rocks or tree-stumps, termitaries, etc. with bare hands. Many bites occur at night, when barefoot individuals tread on or near an unseen snake. This is particularly common with regard to the puffadder, *Bitis arietans,* whose reluctance to move until trodden on is characteristic. Regular paths around dwellings or villages should be as well illuminated as possible. Most importantly, people must be educated not to chase and kill snakes on sight. Children are again at increased risk, as their often playful aggression is likely to be misunderstood by the reptile. A correct approach and slow withdrawal will allow the snake to move off. One should be aware of the ability of many snakes to feign death convincingly, and approach apparently-dead snakes with caution.

Mechanisms

Snakes 'bite' by ejecting a viscous salivary secretion, which is stored in venom sacs, through hollow fangs into the victim. This secretion is species-specific, but contains a variety of enzymes and toxins. Certain species, notably the cobras, may also 'spit' venom onto an epithelial surface where it may be locally irritating, or rarely, absorbed through abrasions or mucous membranes, e.g., conjunctiva.

The effect of a standard injected venom dose is related to the mass of the victim. Small snakes, injecting a lower volume, are generally less dangerous than large snakes. Small victims, however, exhibit toxic effects earlier and these are more serious than in larger individuals.

Snake identification

The clinical expression of envenomation by any given species is predictable. In order to design appropriate therapeutic interventions, therefore, it is desirable to know the species responsible for the injury. Accurate identification of non-venomous species is equally important in order to allay anxiety and obviate the need for expensive and hazardous therapy. Due to similarities in size and colouring between quite unrelated species, accuracy can only be assured if the snake, complete with head, is brought with the victim.

Venomous snakes have fangs, situated either at the front of the mouth or towards the back of the jaw, below the eye *(see Fig. 28.7).* Fangs may be 'fixed' or 'hinged'. The latter variety are not obvious to inspection but can be 'unhinged' by drawing a thin stick from the angle of the mouth forwards. Do not look for fangs with the fingers; even when the snake is dead, envenomation can occur. 'Back-fanged' snakes tend to cling on after striking, and a history of difficulty in removing the assailant is typical of this variety. Non-venomous snakes have numerous small teeth, but lack fangs.

Clinical features of snake bite

Whilst nearly all victims give a history of snake attack, it is as well to recognize objective signs of injury to assist in the assessment of preverbal children, the comatose, and inaccurate historians.

Non-venomous snakes, lacking fangs, truly 'bite'. They leave a ragged wound in which their teeth may be shed. The effects of such a bite are entirely non-specific. Local tenderness and cellulitis may be present by the time of presentation, but there are no symptoms suggestive of

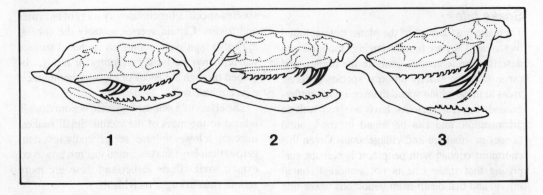

Fig. 28.7   Snake fangs: 1. Posterior   2. Anterior-fixed   3. Anterior-hinged

envenomation. Non-specific signs such as nausea and vomiting may however be present, but rarely predominate.

Paired fang marks are the hallmark of assault by a venomous species. In swollen tissue a magnifying glass may be needed to demonstrate the lesion. Single or paired 'scratch' marks may result from a 'side-swipe' strike.

The majority of bites occur on the foot or ankle, with the hand and arm next in frequency. Since back-fanged species need to draw the affected part into their mouths in order to strike, they rarely, if ever, bite more proximally than the wrist or ankle. Bites over the head, neck, and trunk are sufficiently uncommon to raise clinical suspicion. In these circumstances bites by a spider or scorpion should be considered.

Anxiety is an almost universal response to snake attack in adults, but small children may be deceptively calm about their experience.

Venomous snakes

In order to cause any significant effects, venomous snakes have to inject an adequate dose of venom into the victim. Protective clothing, an abrading strike, immature snake, broken fangs, or recently-emptied venom sacs all compromise the snake's ability to inject adequate volumes of venom. Thus a snake attack does not necessarily imply envenomation.

As aggressive treatment for envenomation is hazardous and occasionally lethal, there must be objective evidence of envenomation before its use.

Whilst snake venoms are all highly complex chemically, a broad division is possible depending on the principal system affected — viz., cytotoxic, neurotoxic, and haemotoxic.

All snakes have each element represented in their venom, but the gross effect depends upon the proportion of each component.

Cytotoxic venom fixes locally at the site of injury, causing swelling and local tissue necrosis, and often intense pain.

Neurotoxic venom is disseminated along venous and lymphatic channels, causing a non-depolarizing neuromuscular blockade. These effects may be relatively mild, e.g., transient ophthalmoplegia, or potentially lethal, e.g., respiratory paralysis.

Haemotoxic venom may cause red cell destruction by phosphatases, resulting in haemolysis, jaundice, and thrombosis; or may interfere with clotting mechanisms, resulting in clot instability or frank bleeding from mucous membranes or urinary or gastrointestinal tracts, due to capillary endothelial damage.

In all cases, secondary effects due to the liberation of chemical fractions such as histamine, kinins, and prostaglandins add to the clinical picture.

The three important groups of venomous snakes are:

- *Viperidae* — vipers, adders
- *Elapidae* — cobras, mambas
- *Colubridae* — boomslang, bird (vine) snakes.

This classification is along anatomical lines, and there is overlap of toxin secretion patterns between the groups.

Primary management

The aims of 'first-aid' are to preserve the patient's life, minimize morbidity, and to avoid the use of potentially lethal treatment methods.

The absorption of toxins via lymphatics and veins is enhanced by exercising the affected limb. Immobilization delays the onset of symptoms. Tourniquets should *never* be used.

They increase the effects of cytotoxic venom by concentrating it at the site of injury, and there are safer ways of diminishing venous and lymphatic drainage in situations such as elapid bites, where such effects may be desirable. Ideally the limb should be immobilized on a splint and firmly bandaged with crepe or similar material. There is no place for incising, sucking, cauterizing, or bleeding the site of injury. The risk of local and systemic sepsis, injury to major nerve, vessel, or tendon, or, rarely, the absorption of venom by the intervener, is increased.

Antivenom should only be administered in the field if:

- accurate identification shows the snake to be venomous
- the afflicted person is showing signs of envenomation
- the offending snake's venom is known to be included in the antivenom
- the antivenom has been correctly stored and transported (which usually implies refrigeration), *and*
- the patient is known not to be sensitive to horse serum.

Antivenom should then be injected intravenously, preceded by a test dose. Local injections have little effect on already-fixed cytotoxic venom, and absorption of systemically-active venom occurs rapidly, requiring systemic antivenom for its effective eradication. Thereafter transportation to a medical facility should be expedited.

Hospital management

All patients referred with snake bites should be detained for no less than 48 hours, as late manifestation of injury, particularly by colubrid snakes is common. Confirmation of injury is obtained by history and examination. Depending on the delay in referral and on snake identification, antivenom administration may be appropriate. Facilities for managing anaphylaxis should be to hand, and antivenom injected only after the response to a test dose has been assessed. Antivenom is rarely necessary in cases of adder bites where the local cytotoxic damage is already established, but may be indicated in elapid and colubrid bites. Supportive measures such as ventilation, transfusion, and nutrition are provided as necessary. Fasciotomy may occasionally be necessary where venom has been injected into deep fascia. Within tight, fibrous compartments swelling initially affects the nerves, before progressing to vascular obstruction. By the nature of injury such compartment syndromes usually affect only one compartment, and radical measures (fibulectomy, etc.) are inappropriate, but decompression of the affected area is urgent. The surgical management of necrosis and ulceration will proceed when the risk to life by the original envenomation has passed. However, joint mobility should be maintained initially by passive, and then later active, physiotherapy.

Cardiac depressant effects are seen in some of the more dangerous elapid bites, and monitoring is essential. It is important to recognize apparent 'relapses' after clinical improvement, and to maintain vigilance for 24–48 hours after the restoration of normal function. Regular monitoring of crude clotting time will rapidly unveil the effects of haemotoxic envenomation. Clinical monitoring of ocular and respiratory muscle function is essential.

Simple measures such as tetanus prophylaxis, wound management, and antibiotics where appropriate, should not be forgotten.

Infections
General

Much of Third World surgical practice involves the management of patients with infection. The surgeon's contribution to such management lies in the drainage of pus and excision of necrotic tissue. Factors within the community which predispose to infection, such as poverty, poor hygiene, malnutrition, and deficiency diseases also complicate management.

Soft tissue abscesses

An abscess is a localized collection of pus within the tissues, and may occur at any site and be due to any organism or combination of organisms. Soft tissue abscesses are the commonest cause of surgical admission in paediatric practice, and the majority are due to *Staphylococcus aureus*. The formation of an abscess implies some degree of host defence against the invading organism, allowing localization of the innoculum and a polymorph response.

Common sites for abscess formation:

- skin and dermal appendages — furunculosis
- regional nodes — suppurating lymphadenitis
- muscles — pyomyositis.

Visceral abscesses are discussed under the appropriate organ system elsewhere.

Clinical signs: The classical signs of inflammation may be readily appreciated in superficial abscesses. However, deep-seated abscesses may be associated only with pain and loss of function. Pain is typically throbbing, and disturbs or prevents sleep. The sign of fluctuation is difficult to elicit in these exquisitely tender lesions, and superfluous to the diagnosis. Similarly, diagnostic 'aspiration' is rarely indicated and can be misleading, as a negative aspiration cannot be held to mean an absence of pus. Aspiration of tender inflammatory lesions, with the necessarily wide-bore needle, in awake children is not conducive to good doctor–patient relationships.

Patients may be well, apart from the local lesion, suggesting adequate localization. However, many patients will be constitutionally unwell, with fever, malaise, and often cellulitis surrounding an obvious abscess. Such signs suggest poor localization and continuing bacteraemia.

Management principles: The treatment of an abscess is surgical drainage, and this should be performed as soon as possible. Antibiotics play an adjunctive role and are indicated in patients in whom signs of poor localization are present and in immunosuppressed patients, including neonates and diabetics. Their use is also justified in abscesses affecting the face, to minimize the risk of cavernous sinus thrombosis. Where an antibiotic is to be used, one which is effective against community strains of staphylococcus should be selected. Analgesia is important, and must be remembered.

Suppurating lymphadenitis: Abscesses within lymph nodes are commonly seen in the inguinal, axillary, occipital, and submental groups. Invariably a portal of entry is evident. The causative lesion should be addressed. It must be remembered that the inguinal nodes drain the lower anal canal and perineum, and a primary lesion should be sought at these sites in addition to the lower limbs.

Pyomyositis: It is believed that most intramuscular abscesses result from minor trauma which leaves a haematoma within the muscle. This then becomes infected during a transient bacteraemia thereafter. Muscles commonly affected include quadratus femoris, anterior abdominal wall muscles and iliopsoas. Diagnostic difficulty occurs frequently in abdominal wall abscesses, where intra-abdominal pathology may be suspected at first, and in iliopsoas abscesses, where hip pathology is often the admission diagnosis. Spasm of psoas causes the adoption of the classical position of flexion, adduction, and internal rotation. All movement, active or passive, is resisted, as any stretching of psoas causes severe pain. Sonography is usually diagnostic. Drainage is performed via the most direct route. Psoas is reached via an extraperitoneal approach which allows additional access to iliacus.

Post-operative treatment: With adequate drainage, an abscess cavity will heal by granulation. Dressings and drains are used to prevent the skin wound from healing before the cavity is obliterated, and to contain any exudate. Packing the cavity is counterproductive, and is used only to control bleeding from the abscess wall. A host of proprietary and nonproprietary dressings are available.

Unusual abscesses

From time to time abscesses may be encountered that do not follow the rules. Non-tender abscesses should provoke suspicion of tuberculosis. Non-healing abscesses may be due to TB or perhaps a foreign body. Recurrent abscesses may be a manifestation of a specific immunological deficit. An unusual odour or character of pus may suggest an exotic organism. Whenever an unusual abscess is encountered the pus must be sent for culture and the abscess wall must be biopsied.

Cellulitis

Cellulitis represents a spreading infection of the skin and subcutaneous tissue and is clinically associated with local erythema, pain and tenderness, and frequently with fever, malaise, and non-specific nausea and vomiting. Any area may be affected, and the condition is classically associated with penicillin-sensitive streptococci, but may be due to *Staphylococcus aureus.*

As the clinical features of cellulitis and osteitis are identical, it is wiser to treat all such patients as if the pathology were osteomyelitis *(also see Chapter 26, Orthopaedic Problems).* Radiographs are of no help in this dilemma, as they are completely normal for the first 10–12 days of osteomyelitis. Thus all patients with inflammatory changes over any bone, but particularly the leg, are admitted. Blood cultures and white cell count are drawn, and a high dose penicillin active against community staphylococci is given, preferably intravenously. Temperature recordings are made 2-hourly, and analgesics provided. Within 6–12 hours improvement in local signs and in the temperature chart should be evident. If there is no change, or deterioration, it is safer to explore the affected area to make certain the bone is infection-free. To miss or partially treat acute osteomyelitis sets in motion a series of events that often results in prolonged morbidity and even limb amputation or death.

Peritonitis

Inflammation of the peritoneum may be due to a primary infection, but more commonly follows a primary pathology of the bowel or female genital tract. Non-bacterial peritonitis is much less common, but may be due to insults such as the presence of urine in the peritoneal cavity following rupture of the bladder, the presence of CSF secondary to ventriculo-peritoneal shunting, or occasionally intraperitoneal bleeding.

Clinical presentation: Bacterial peritonitis, whether primary or secondary, presents with signs and symptoms colloquially known as 'acute abdomen'. Patients are usually moderately or severely ill, with prostration. Enquiry may reveal an underlying predisposing or preceding pathology. Examination will reveal marked tenderness which is either generalized or maximal over the affected quadrant. Involuntary spasm of the abdominal wall muscles (guarding) will be present, and percussion tenderness or rebound tenderness may be elicited. Tenderness on rectal examination is present when the pelvic peritoneum is inflamed. There is rarely sufficient free fluid to be clinically appreciated, but there is commonly abdominal fullness secondary to bowel stasis and dilatation. Umbilical herniae are helpful, as at the umbilicus skin and peritoneum are closely associated. In patients with a patent processus vaginalis, pus or inflammatory exudate may present in the scrotum as an acute hydrocele.

In the neonate, signs of peritonitis may be misleading, and diagnosis is often delayed until features such as abdominal wall oedema or erythema present. The diagnosis may also be delayed in paraplegics, children with spina bifida, and following trauma, particularly if a head injury coexists. In these groups special vigilance is required.

Differential diagnosis: The differential diagnosis of the acute abdomen is broad and includes extra- as well as intra-abdominal pathology. However, the presence of peritonitis, with very rare exceptions, is an indication for laparotomy. Preoperative preparation must cater for commonly occurring pathologies, particularly appendicitis, typhoid, and other causes of small bowel perforation, amoebiasis and its sequelae in both the colon and liver, as well as the commonly encountered late manifestations of ascariasis, intussusception, and trauma.

Pathophysiology: With peritoneal inflammation, there is massive fluid exudate into the peritoneal cavity, with proliferation of organisms usually of bowel or female genital tract origin — including both Gram-positive and Gram-negative aerobic and anaerobic bacteria. The faeculent aroma of the peritonitic abdomen signifies the presence of anaerobes, amongst which will be penicillin-resistant bacteroides species. The omentum, appendices epiploicae and loops of small bowel become oedematous and attempt to localize the pathology, creating intraperitoneal abscesses. Intraperitoneal fluid loss is quite sufficient to cause shock and requires urgent replacement. As the volume lost cannot be directly measured, replacement is effected using clinical signs as a guide.

Serosal inflammation of the bowel provokes an ileus, with further concealed fluid losses within the lumen. This ileus contributes to the abdominal distension and is responsible for associated vomiting. The massive absorptive area of the peritoneum ensures absorption of toxins and organisms leading to septicaemia and all its sequelae.

Primary management: Without exception patients in whom peritonitis is diagnosed should be prepared for theatre. Such preparation should include:

◆ *Intravenous fluid replacement:* In shocked patients an initial plasma bolus should be followed by a balanced electrolyte solution to restore pulse, blood pressure, and a urine output of at least 1 ml/kg/hr.

◆ *Intravenous antibiotics:* Peritonitis is a mixed infection and antibiotics effective against aerobes and anaerobes are necessary. Where metronidazole is available this is an ideal antianaerobic agent. Elsewhere chloramphenicol is useful. Gram-negative cover can be provided by an aminoglycoside, and ampicillin covers a wide range of Gram-positive organisms and is effective against *Salmonella typhi*.

◆ *Analgesia:* Once peritonitis is diagnosed, no useful purpose is served by leaving a child in pain. Indeed relief of pain may have important therapeutic benefit. As the pain is severe, opiates are frequently employed.

◆ *Nasogastric decompression:* Ileus secondary to peritonitis will lead to vomiting, which is distressing and particularly painful in children with peritonitis. Nasogastric drainage further relieves abdominal distension.

Primary peritonitis

In developed communities primary peritonitis has been virtually eliminated by the widespread use of antibiotics for respiratory and other infections. In the Third World primary peritonitis remains a significant problem and is seen in otherwise healthy children (especially females) and immunosuppressed children, typically with nephrotic syndrome.

Primary peritonitis is usually due to a single organism, particularly pneumococcus or *Haemophilus influenzae*, and may be associated with a previous respiratory tract infection. In girls,

organisms may ascend via the Fallopian tubes, and *E. coli* or other Gram-negatives may be encountered. The pus of primary peritonitis never smells faeculent.

Management: Many patients are diagnosed at operation by the findings of thin, non-odorous pus with no other intraperitoneal pathology. Where clinical suspicion is aroused preoperatively (for example in renal units), a short trial of high dose penicillin is justifiable. Should no clinical response be evident in 6–12 hours, surgery is advisable.

Typhoid

Typhoid fever is discussed fully in *Chapter 8, Infectious Disorders*. Surgical interest in typhoid relates to the complications of ileal perforation and bleeding.

Typhoid perforation

Aggressive resuscitation and surgery for typhoid perforation has seen mortality fall from over 60% to less than 10% over the last 20 years. Clinical deterioration in a patient being treated for typhoid, with onset of abdominal pain and peritonitis is sufficient to justify surgery. Nonoperative management carries a prohibitive mortality. Peritonitis may be the presenting feature of typhoid, which must always be considered in the differential diagnosis in endemic areas.

Investigations: Half of the patients with perforation show evidence of pneumoperitoneum on X-ray. It is important to note that absence of pneumoperitoneum does not exclude intestinal perforation. Similarly, whilst a relative leucopenia may be suggestive of typhoid, any white cell count is compatible with perforation. Anaemia is found in half of the patients.

Pre-operative treatment: Resuscitation is the key to operative success. Antibiotic cover must be extended to encompass not only *Salmonella typhi*, but also enteric organisms which are now released into the peritoneal cavity. Fluid, electrolyte, and acid base balance should be corrected.

Surgery: Excision of the affected lymphoid patch, or patches, is required, with repair of the bowel. Thorough peritoneal lavage is performed to remove pus and debris. 'Near' perforations are oversewn.

Post-operative care: Complications are frequent, including chest and wound infections. The most serious complications are intestinal fistulae and intraperitoneal abscesses. Recurrence or relapse of typhoid may be seen in 5% of patients.

Typhoid bleeding

Bleeding from typhoid ulcers in the ileum or caecum may be torrential. It must be acknowledged that in many patients with typhoid a clotting disorder exists relating to typhoid hepatitis and thrombocytopenia. Before any surgery is planned, correction of clotting defects using vitamin K, plasma, or platelet infusion is mandatory. Blood transfusion is required to correct anaemia and hypovolaemia. At operation, localization of a bleeding site may be difficult, and it may be necessary to perform a right hemicolectomy to be sure of resecting the causative lesion.

Appendicitis

Appendicitis can no longer be regarded as a rare disease in the Third World, but recognition is often delayed. Whilst any age may be affected, the disease is typically seen in the older child, from 6 years to adolescence. Inflammation of the appendix follows luminal obstruction, which may be due to lymphoid hypertrophy secondary to viral infection, or to a faecolith. In the Third World, additional obstructive factors include pin worms, round worms, bilharziasis, and amoebiasis. Luminal obstruction of whatever cause is followed most frequently by progressive necrosis of the appendix wall, perforation, and peritonitis. Initially a perforation may be locally contained by loops of bowel and omentum, so that an appendix mass or abscess develops. However, general peritonitis frequently arises, with a marked deterioration in the prognosis.

Presentation: The great variation in signs and symptoms is partly responsible for the high diagnostic error rate. This variation may be due to some extent to the highly variable position of the appendix and contiguous inflammation of a number of possible organs. Late presentation, when the symptoms of appendicitis are superseded by the signs of generalized peritonitis, is common, and under such circumstances accurate preoperative diagnosis may be impossible and is largely academic. During the early phase of luminal obstruction the visceral pain of appendiceal distension is appreciated at the umbilicus. As transmural inflammation reaches the serosal surface, which is somatically innervated, allowing accurate localization, the pain is felt at the site of inflammation, usually the right lower abdomen. Thus the pain appears to move from the umbilicus to the iliac fossa.

With the onset of pain, nausea and vomiting are common. Loss of appetite is an almost constant symptom, and mucoid diarrhoea may occur, particularly if the rectum is secondarily inflamed. Other features are those of cystitis, and apparent hip irritability. Fever is frequent, but rarely above 38.5 °C.

Examination may reveal a furred tongue and foetor, but more specific signs include localized iliac fossa tenderness and involuntary guarding. Percussion tenderness over McBurney's point is a convincing finding, but the site of maximal tenderness will vary with the position of the appendix. Rectal examination will be tender on the right when the appendix is adjacent or the pelvic peritoneum inflamed. Without treatment the pain worsens until the appendix ruptures, when temporary relief may occur before the pain of peritonitis supervenes.

No objective investigations are available to confirm a diagnosis of appendicitis, which remains a clinical responsibility.

Treatment: All patients in whom appendicitis is seriously suspected should be admitted and watched for progression or regression of symptoms and signs. In many patients iliac fossa pain disappears rapidly and a formal diagnosis is never achieved. For those with convincing signs at admission, or who deteriorate during observation, emergency appendicectomy is appropriate treatment. The patient is prepared for surgery as for peritonitis. Surgery through an iliac fossa incision is acceptable where a confident diagnosis has been made and signs are localized.

Postoperative care: Potential complications are numerous, but uncommon except for wound infection and intraperitoneal abscesses. Deaths are related not to appendicitis *per se,* but to the sequelae of peritonitis and septicaemia.

Amoebiasis

Amoebic disease and its complications are fully discussed in *Chapter 8, Infectious Disorders*. Only transmural amoebic colitis is considered here.

Pathology: These patients are frequently chronically depleted with pre-existing malnutrition, hypoproteinaemia, and anaemia. Contamination of the peritoneal cavity by colonic organisms which have leaked through areas of full-thickness amoebic necrosis is a devastating additional burden. The omentum initially attempts to seal areas of necrosis and prevents the clinical signs of peritonitis from developing, and the enormity of the colonic mischief may be concealed for a long time.

Clinical presentation: Amoebic colitis must be suspected in any malnourished, toxic child with a current or recent history of profuse diarrhoea. Proctosigmoidoscopy will show typical ulcers with slough. Fresh scrapings will show haematophagous amoebae in patients without prior exposure to metronidazole. Abdominal distension with tenderness on deep palpation suggest transmural colitis temporarily sealed by omentum. Frank peritonitis will inexorably follow.

Management: Before peritonitis develops, surgery may be avoided in some patients by aggressive non-operative management. Thus all patients are given amoebicidal drugs and antibiotics against coliform aerobes and anaerobes. Full supportive care is instituted, including transfusion of blood, plasma, or albumin. Only if symptoms abate is surgery deferred.

Surgery: Resection of the entire colon in these children carries a prohibitive mortality, and recent experiences suggest that pancolonic disease is as well managed by ileostomy diversion and prograde colonic lavage.

Localized disease that can be encompassed by a limited resection should be excised. The bowel ends are exteriorized rather than risk an anastomosis in such depleted patients.

Postoperatively: These patients need intensive nursing and medical care postoperatively, particularly to prevent intractable pulmonary oedema. Late colonic strictures may occur where affected areas have been left unresected.

Motility disorders

Intussusception

Intussusception occurs when proximal bowel (the intussusceptum) invaginates into the bowel immediately distal to it (the intussuscepiens). In the First World this is almost exclusively a disorder of infants under one year of age, and may be associated with viral respiratory tract disease or a weaning diet. In the Third World the condition is seen at any age, with at least 50% of patients being over the age of 2 years, and is frequently associated with non-specific diarrhoeal illness. Late presentation is a feature of tropical intussusception, which further alters management.

Pathophysiology: As the proximal bowel passes within the distal bowel the mesentery becomes compressed. Initially lymphatic, and then venous obstruction occurs, causing oedema and congestion of the mucosa, with bleeding into the distal lumen. This blood and mucus is passed as a typical 'red currant jelly' stool. Ultimately arterial occlusion leads to gangrene of the intussusceptum. Very rarely is there a pathological mural lesion which acts as a lead point, and most cases are 'idiopathic'. The intussusceptum may start at any point in the bowel — most usually the ileo-caecal region (but in children over 2 the transverse colon is commonly implicated, *see Table 28.3*) — and may pass a variable distance along the bowel, even prolapsing through the anus. The distinction between prolapsing intussusception and rectal prolapse is vital, and is discussed below (*see under Rectal Prolapse*).

Table 28.3   Site of intussusception in 77 children

	Under 2 yrs	Over 2 yrs	Total
Ileocolic	37 (80%)	11 (35%)	48 (62%)
Colocolic	5 (11%)	17 (55%)	22 (29%)
Enteroenteric	4 (09%)	3 (10%)	7 (9%)

Clinical presentation: In approximately 30% of patients symptoms begin during, or soon after, an acute diarrhoeal illness. Initially intestinal colic and reflex vomiting are seen in association with a somewhat tender, sausage-shaped mass. As the pathology progresses, bloody mucoid stools are passed, and pain becomes continuous. Ultimately bowel perforation with peritonitis occurs. In 25% of patients the apex of the intussusceptum is palpable on rectal examination.

Differential diagnosis: In the Third World intussusception must be differentiated from intestinal ascariasis, amoebiasis, and dysenteric illness, particularly in view of the clinical association with diarrhoea.

Investigation: Clinical suspicion may be confirmed by:
◆ *ultrasound,* which shows a characteristic bull's-eye appearance of the bowel on transverse section;
◆ *barium enema,* demonstrating a mass effect within the colon and the 'coil spring' of barium between mucosal folds;
◆ *laparotomy* in those patients presenting with peritonitis.

Management: In the First World many patients may be treated nonoperatively by reducing the intussusception with a barium or air column at the diagnostic enema. Patients suitable for such treatment in the Third World are uncommon, as the length of history, presence of intestinal obstruction, or peritonitis are contraindications. Most patients are treated operatively with open reduction of the intussusception. Resection of gangrenous bowel will be required in up to 30%.

Post-operative care may be complicated by endotoxaemia which results from flooding the portal circulation with bacteria and toxins which had previously been confined within the intussuscepted loop by the venous and lymphatic obstruction. Pre-operative use of anti-endotoxins or plasma may reduce the associated morbidity.

Special intussusceptions

Post-operative intussusception may follow any operative procedure, and diagnosis is often delayed as usually only the small bowel is involved.

Chronic intussusception: Intussusception may rarely be present for several days without signs of intestinal obstruction or progression to intestinal necrosis, and in such cases there is a higher than usual incidence of lead points.

Recurrent intussusception: Following nonoperative or operative treatment, intussusception may recur in 1–2% of patients, either because a lead point has been overlooked or because the original reduction was incomplete. Treatment of the recurrence is the same as for primary intussusception.

Rectal prolapse

'Something coming down' during defecation or other straining, or persisting independent of bowel function, is a distressing symptom. Rectal prolapse must be differentiated from prolapsing intussusception and prolapsing polyp. In prolapsing intussusception it is possible to pass the examining finger alongside the protruding mass into the rectum. Prolapsing polyps may be palpable and hooked down by the examining finger. Histologically they are benign juvenile polyps in the overwhelming majority.

True rectal prolapse is a symptom of an underlying disorder, not a disease in its own right. The causes are shown in *Table 28.4.*

Table 28.4 Causes of rectal prolapse

Functional	Diarrhoea
	Parasites
Anatomical	Malnutrition with loss of supporting ischiorectal fat pad
	Pelvic floor paralysis, e.g., myelomeningocele
	Congenital anomalies
Others	Cystic fibrosis. 5–10% of children with cystic fibrosis will develop rectal prolapse at some stage
	Idiopathic

Management: The management of the prolapse is the recognition and management of the underlying disease. In a Third World environment, nonspecific diarrhoeal diseases and parasites predominate. Surgery is reserved for the correction of anatomical abnormalities. Conservative measures, pending primary disease control, may include raising the foot of the cot, sedation, and manual reduction. Gallow's traction, buttock strapping, and encircling perianal sutures are unlikely to be sufficiently secure to resist the *vis a tergo* of intra-abdominal pressure, and may complicate any subsequent prolapse. Recurrent or resistant idiopathic prolapse may justify some intervention, be it submucosal injection or other manoeuvre, but such instances are extremely uncommon.

Gastro-oesophageal reflux

Reflux of gastric acid into the oesophagus may occur when the mechanisms which control gastric continence fail. The effects of such reflux will depend upon the pH and duration of each episode, the frequency with which reflux occurs, and the height within the oesophagus at which low pH is recordable. Prolonged gavage feeding is a potent contributor to oesophageal inflammation and strictures. Sliding hiatal hernia may be associated with reflux.

Clinical presentation: Gastro-oesophageal reflux may present at any age, and is certainly underdiagnosed in a Third World environment. This is due firstly to a nonspecific symptomatology which is shared with many common disorders, and secondly to the difficulty in confirming a clinical suspicion.

Presentation may be principally due to:

◆ *vomiting* which is non-bilious and may be confused with pyloric stenosis and cause failure to thrive;

◆ *aspiration* giving rise to recurrent sporadic bronchospasm indistinguishable from asthma. Genuine aspiration pneumonia, which tends to recur or fails to clear, is frequently seen;

◆ *anaemia* secondary to blood loss from oesophagitis, which is common as the presenting feature;

◆ *dysphagia* due either to the pain of oesophagitis or to oesophageal stricture. This is the presenting feature in some late cases;

◆ bizarre *athetoid movements* (Sandifer's syndrome), which are presumably caused by the gastro-oesophageal reflux. These are occasionally encountered amongst children with cerebral palsy.

Diagnosis: Oesophagoscopy may reveal oesophagitis which can be histologically confirmed and graded. Barium meal may reveal an associated hiatal hernia, but unfortunately reflux can be provoked in many normal children, and the demonstration of reflux under the artificial conditions of the X-ray suite is unreliable. Radioisotopes instilled directly into the stomach via a nasogastric tube may be picked up later in the lung fields, confirming aspiration. The gold standard, however, is 24-hour pH monitoring using an intra-oesophageal electrode, although this is rarely available.

Management: Medical management can be instituted on clinical suspicion, and includes thickening feeds, posture, and the judicious use of prokinetic agents. Antacids will minimize damage to the oesophagus and give symptomatic relief in Sandifer's syndrome. Surgery is necessary to deal with oesophageal strictures and patients with life-threatening complications, e.g., aspiration. Medical management failures and neurologically impaired children should also be offered surgery in the form of a transabdominal fundoplication.

Paralytic (adynamic) ileus

Many insults provoke the intestine into a state of hypotonic inertia, particularly inflammation, hypokalaemia, prolonged obstruction, and surgery.

Pathophysiology: Generally the whole bowel is affected. Fluid loss into the bowel lumen may be considerable. Abdominal distension, vomiting, and hypovolaemia result. Bowel sounds are usually absent.

Clinical presentation: The presentation is usually that of the underlying pathology, with the onset of the signs and symptoms of intestinal obstruction. A particular dilemma arises in the small child with severe gastroenteritis who after some days of profuse diarrhoea ceases to pass stool and develops abdominal distension. The distinction between mechanical and paralytic ileus in such patients may be clinically impossible. Following correction of any electrolyte deficit, further investigation is justified.

Diagnosis: As in mechanical obstruction (*see below*), air-fluid levels within distended bowel loops are seen on X-ray. Such air-fluid levels tend to occur at one level within the abdomen rather than in a stepladder pattern, and are all much the same length, with no disproportionately dilated loops. In some individuals contrast enema may be required to exclude intussusception.

Management: The underlying pathology must be aggressively treated. Postoperative ileus can be expected to resolve in 24–48 hours. Persistent ileus should prompt consideration of a 'relook' laparotomy. Intravenous fluids and nasogastric drainage are indicated in all patients.

Genitourinary tract
Testicular maldescent
It is believed that spermatogenesis is greatest at temperatures lower than core temperature. The testis, having developed in the retroperitoneum, is forced into the scrotum through the inguinal canal by abdominal pressure transmitted to the upper pole of the testis via the processus vaginalis. Should the testis fail to descend, the processus persists, and then constitutes a patent processus vaginalis or potential inguinal hernia.

The empty scrotum, unilaterally or bilaterally, may be due to anorchia, abdominal wall paralysis, or commonly to obstruction to the neck of the scrotum causing the testis to divert to an ectopic (usually inguinal) site. If clinical examination reveals testes, even if they cannot be induced to enter the scrotum, the prognosis is good. If no testes are palpable even in ectopic sites, the prognosis must be guarded pending the results of exploration.

Testicular malignancy and maldescent
There is a higher than normal risk of testicular malignancy in the undescended testis, as well as in the normally-situated contralateral testis. Placing the testis surgically in the scrotum does not diminish the risk of malignancy, but may make surveillance easier. These risks justify removal of an intra-abdominal gonad which cannot be brought into the scrotum.

Management: Surgery is generally deferred until 2 years of age. The operation performed is an orchidopexy, part of which is a herniotomy of the inevitable accompanying hernia.

The prognosis for fertility in bilateral undescended testes is poor. In unilateral cases fertility may be slightly reduced or normal.

The retractile testis
An apparently undescended testis that can be coaxed into the scrotum is termed 'retractile'. Clinically, the empty scrotum looks well developed, unlike the flat, hypoplastic scrotum of genuine maldescent. The retractile testis is normal in all respects and has simply been drawn up by a strong cremaster muscle. No treatment is indicated.

Testicular torsion
Torsion of the testis is usually in fact torsion of the spermatic cord in patients in whom the tunica vaginalis invests the lower part of the cord, leaving the testis hanging freely, and aptly described as a 'bell clapper'. Occasionally torsion of the testis proper on a long mesorchium occurs. The diagnosis must be firmly established, as any anatomical abnormality allowing torsion will be bilateral and both testes are at risk. Thus whilst early operation is desirable to salvage the affected testis, even when this opportunity has passed, late operation is justifiable to protect the remaining testis.

Clinical presentation: Torsion may occur at any age — even antenatally — but is usually associated with adolescence. Acute onset of lower abdominal or inguinal pain is frequently associated with vomiting. A mild pyrexia may suggest an inflammatory lesion, and tenderness, swelling, and erythema of the affected hemiscrotum may mimic orchitis.

No sexually inactive male should be diagnosed as having epididymo-orchitis without operative exclusion of torsion.

Management: The scrotum must be explored. If the history is short, detorsion may salvage at least some testicular function. A gangrenous testis should be removed. In any event the contralateral side must be explored and the testis anchored to prevent torsion of the remaining gonad.

Paraphimosis
In this condition a retracted prepuce is prevented from returning to its normal position by an often mild stenosis of the preputial orifice. Oedema of the distal prepuce results in an alarming ring of swollen tissue at the base of the glans. Proximal to this on the penile shaft the constricting ring can be identified. The glans itself is quite unaffected.

Management: Using a penile block the swollen prepuce can be so compressed that the oedema is forced under the constricting band and dispersed. This takes time and patience, but once achieved, allows the constricting ring to slip distally over the glans into its normal position. Should this manoeuvre prove unsuccessful, incision of the constricting band in the midline dorsally may be necessary. Following reduction the prepuce is inevitably swollen and oedematous for some time, and any decision with regard to future management should be deferred until all swelling has disappeared and a full assessment of any causative or provocative lesion can be made. Circumcision is not always necessary.

Balanitis

Inflammation of the preputial sac results in oedema of the prepuce and dysuria with a purulent discharge. Retraction of the prepuce is impossible. Antibiotics and local toilet are prescribed. Recurrent attacks may lead to preputial scarring and the need for circumcision.

Hypospadias

In hypospadias the urethral meatus may be situated at any site from the perineum to the penile tip. There is usually an abnormal hooded prepuce with chordee (ventral flexion) of the penile shaft. In perineal or penoscrotal hypospadias the bifid scrotum may be associated with genital ambiguity. In patients with hypospadias other genitourinary abnormalities are more common than in the normal population, and full urinary evaluation is indicated. The hypospadic orifice may be narrow, and its adequacy must be reviewed. Surgical correction begins at age 3–4 years and may involve a number of procedures. As the prepuce is essential to the reconstruction of the distal urethra, these patients should *not* be circumcised.

Prune belly (abdominal muscle deficiency) syndrome

This peculiar disorder is aptly named, as the wrinkled skin of the abdomen is draped over the subjacent viscera with no muscle intervening. The classical case is unmistakable, but occasionally only a single abdominal quadrant is affected, altering the clinical appearance. The condition is almost exclusively seen in males, and the deficient abdominal wall results in undescended testes, broad substernal angle, and poor cough predisposing to chest infections. The sinister effects of the syndrome are found in the urinary tract, where megacystis, ectatic ureters, and hydronephrosis are seen, often with urethral atresia and patent

urachus. Prognosis depends upon residual respiratory and renal function.

Parasites

Ascaris lumbricoides
(Also see Chapter 8, Infectious Disorders.)

Large numbers of adult worms may be present, and stool ova counts of more than 50 000 ova/gram of stool are not unusual. Ascariasis may present in the following ways.

Asymptomatic carriers

Patients with quite unrelated pathology may be found to harbour ascaris worms. Their presence does not always mean that they are the cause of disease, and the vomiting of worms or rectal passage of worms should be viewed with circumspection.

Subacute intestinal obstruction (worm colic)

A large, entangled bolus of worms may impact, commonly in the distal ileum, causing an incomplete obstruction. Clinically, abdominal colic with vomiting (often containing worms) and a palpable mass are present. The condition can be distinguished from intussusception if:

♦ more than one mass is present

♦ the palpable mass coincides with a radiologically evident mass of worms

♦ the mass is seen on ultrasound to be composed of worms.

It may occasionally be necessary to perform barium enema to confidently exclude intussusception.

Management: Left alone, the worms will disentangle themselves and distribute themselves evenly along the bowel. Management consists of observation, with nasogastric drainage if vomiting is significant. Intravenous fluid replacement and antispasmodics must be given. Usually symptoms abate overnight and oral intake can be resumed. Stool examination will reveal any cohabitors, so complete eradication of parasites can be achieved when all symptoms have settled.

Small bowel volvulus

A bolus of worms in the small bowel may act as the apex of a volvulus. Early recognition of this complication and surgical detorsion before intestinal necrosis occurs is an important aim of the observation of patients with worm colic. All patients with worm colic in whom obstructive symptoms persist after 12–24 hours should be re-evaluated radiologically to exclude volvulus.

Hepato-biliary ascariasis

A worm may enter the ampulla of Vater during ascent towards the stomach. A single worm will dilate the ampulla so that the likelihood of further worms finding access to the biliary tree is increased. Within the biliary tree, worms ascend into hepatic radicles, where they form 'nests' or abscesses. Surprisingly, biliary worms may be entirely asymptomatic, and discovered only on sonography. More often, hepatic tenderness and fever present in a patient with known intestinal ascariasis, suggesting a degree of hepatocholangitis. Operative intervention is indicated for

♦ intractable pain
♦ cholangitis persisting despite antibiotics
♦ obstructive jaundice
♦ pancreatitis
♦ persistence of intrabiliary worms on sequential sonographic examination over an empiric 4–6 week period.

Pancreatitis

A worm passing through the ampulla into the biliary tree may cause a transient hyperamylasaemia, probably due to oedema of the ampulla. There is rarely clinically significant evidence of pancreatitis. Occasionally a worm will impact in the pancreatic duct, resulting in acute pancreatitis with compelling symptoms justifying laparotomy. Pancreatic resection may be required.

All patients admitted for complications of ascariasis must be advised to take regular vermifuge whilst asymptomatic, in order to minimize the worm load. Appropriate measures to improve sanitation must be advocated.

Abdominal pain

Pain is a common indicator of surgical pathology, but may also occur in syndromes for which operative treatment is inappropriate. As such disorders form part of the differential diagnosis of intra-abdominal surgical pathology, syndromes of abdominal pain without physical signs other than mild tenderness are briefly discussed here.

Nearly all children suffer from abdominal pain at some time. Rarely is pain sufficiently severe or persistent to warrant medical attention. Pain that is of sufficient intensity or of such a character to prompt hospital admission may similarly remain undiagnosed in 10–20% of patients. Adding a speculative label to such patients is unhelpful, and may inhibit the investigation of recurrent attacks.

Investigations

It may be difficult to decide how much investigation is justified in a given setting, particularly as the yield is extremely low. A complete physical examination is the minimum. Depending upon clinical findings, a full blood count, stool parasitology, urinalysis, and occasionally abdominal ultrasound may be worthwhile.

Acute nonspecific pain: This diagnostic category can include all pain that settles without specific treatment, and is typical of patients who are admitted for observation lest more typical signs of appendicitis develop. Pain may be severe, is usually central, and may be associated with vomiting. Most importantly, it disappears rapidly. The cause or causes are unknown.

Cyclical abdominal pain: Recurrent pain is not unusual, and if it results in disruption of school or social activities, may present to the clinician. Although any age may be affected, it is common amongst girls aged 8–12 years. Specific features include:
 – identical pattern to each recurrence
 – normal between attacks
 – periodicity usually weeks or months
 – may be accompanied by nausea, vomiting, sweating, and pallor
 – bouts of pain usually less than 48 hours
 – tendency to reduced frequency with age.
The aetiology is unknown, but may be indirectly related to migraine, or may have an hormonal basis. Attacks settle spontaneously and treatment is purely symptomatic. Investigations are negative, although there may be considerable parental

pressure to continue with them. Children 'grow out' of the condition.

Psychosocial pain: Undoubtedly in many children pain is a response to stress, either at home or at school. Such pain may be recurrent, but lacks the periodicity of cyclical pain. Although presumably nonorganic in origin, pain is nonetheless real, and may justify symptomatic treatment. If the social environment of the child is known, a correct diagnosis may be possible. It must be remembered, however, that children in stressful environments can also develop appendicitis, and clinicians should be reticent to ascribe symptoms to nonorganic causes unless the evidence is incontrovertible. Thus the diagnosis is frequently made in retrospect.

Referred pain: Pain originating in organs of foregut origin will be referred to the epigastrium, and thus oesophageal, pulmonary, and occasionally cardiac pain may present as abdominal pain. Frequently lower lobe pneumonia causing pleuritis is referred to the upper abdomen. The paucity of objective signs will stimulate enquiry beyond the abdomen.

Miscellaneous

A wide variety of diseases may occasionally present with abdominal pain:

- juvenile diabetes
- meningitis
- tetanus
- ovulation
- viral respiratory infection (mesenteric adenitis).

In many instances the diagnosis is only made clear by the natural evolution of the disease.

Diabetes occurs with sufficient frequency to justify urine testing for glucose on all patients admitted with abdominal pain.

Gastrointestinal bleeding

Gastrointestinal (GI) bleeding in older children may be acute or chronic, and may present as upper gastrointestinal haemorrhage with haematemesis and melaena, or as lower tract haemorrhage with haematochezia.

Chronic GI bleeding

By its very nature chronic bleeding is never massive, and secondary symptoms such as anaemia predominate. Anaemia is usually of an iron deficiency type. Important causes include intestinal parasites, e.g., ancylostomes, gastro-oesophageal reflux *(see above)* and gastrointestinal polyps. Whilst symptoms suggestive of gastrointestinal disease are often present, screening of anaemic patients for the presence of occult faecal blood has an acceptable yield. Investigation may include endoscopy once the secondary symptoms are controlled.

Acute GI bleeding

Bleeding above the duodeno-jejunal flexure may present as haematemesis often resembling coffee grounds. Melaena represents blood which has been partially digested during its passage through the bowel, and has a characteristic tarry appearance and consistency as well as a distinctive odour. In any bleeding situation the priorities are patient resuscitation and making a precise diagnosis after excluding a bleeding diathesis. Thereafter definitive treatment must be planned.

Endoscopy: Making a precise diagnosis is to a large extent dependent upon upper GI endoscopy. When the patient has been stabilized, and circulating volume restored, endoscopy should be performed. Children over the age of 7 or 8 years tolerate endoscopy under sedation and mucosal anaesthesia. Younger children are best examined under general anaesthetic.

Radiology: Plain radiographs and barium studies are unhelpful other than in portal hypertension.

Peptic ulcers

Acute ulcers are associated with head injuries, burns, or any severe stress. Chronic ulcers are uncommon.

Antacids given regularly to patients at risk minimize the incidence, and treatment must include relief of the stress whether it is caused by sepsis, hypovolaemia, or other factors. Surgery is occasionally necessary if bleeding continues.

Mallory–Weiss tear

A gastro-oesophageal mucosal tear can be produced during vomiting. The diagnosis can only be confirmed endoscopically, and this must be performed early. Conservative measures are usually successful.

Portal hypertension

Surgical treatment may be indicated for the sequelae of portal hypertension, viz., oesophagogastric varices (often), hypersplenism (occasionally), ascites (rarely).

Clinical presentation: Haematemesis may be the presenting complaint. Stigmata of portal hypertension, notably splenomegaly, ascites, or abdominal wall collaterals, may be present. Endoscopy will confirm variceal bleeding. Barium swallow will demonstrate the varices but cannot confirm them as the site of bleeding.

Management: The patient is resuscitated and early endoscopy performed. A bleeding varix may be sclerosed by injecting an irritant such as ethanolamine oleate into the lumen. Definitive management may include further sclerotherapy or some form of porta-systemic shunt surgery.

Gastritis/oesophagitis

Mucosal damage may result from drugs (particularly aspirin), inflammation trauma (particularly from poorly-managed gastric tubes), or acid injury in the oesophagus. Whilst haematemesis is not common, such mucosal injury must always be considered in the differential diagnosis, and a history of recent aspirin ingestion sought. Endoscopy is essential to the diagnosis. Rarely is surgery necessary to control bleeding.

Lower GI bleeding

Blood *in* the stool is indicative of colonic or lower small bowel pathology. Blood *on* the stool suggests rectal or anal blood loss. Enterocolonic disorders presenting with bleeding include: inflammatory conditions, mechanical disorders such as intussusception, and neoplastic disease, particularly colonic polyps.

Anal bleeding may be painless, suggesting polyps, or painful, suggesting fissures or haemorrhoids.

Rectal examination and sigmoidoscopy are pivotal investigations. All polypi must be histologically evaluated.

Jaundice
Prolonged neonatal jaundice

A comprehensive account of neonatal jaundice is given in *Chapter 5, Newborns.* It is important to recognize timeously small proportion of jaundiced neonates who require operation, lest the chances of surgical success be negated by progressive biliary cirrhosis. The need for surgical intervention should be diagnosed before 8 weeks of age. Delay proportionately reduces the chances of success.

Biliary atresia

The term biliary atresia is a misnomer, as it is now believed that the biliary system scleroses perinatally in response to an agent presumed to be viral. Thus sclerosing cholangio-hepatitis would more accurately describe the pathology. Both the intra- and extra-hepatic biliary tree may be affected, and usually the entire ductal system and gall bladder are sclerotic. In addition there is an associated hepatitis with progression to cirrhosis and liver failure.

Jaundice is late in onset and prolonged beyond the physiological period. Untreated, the condition rapidly results in cirrhosis, with portal hypertension, ascites, and progressive liver dysfunction, although death may be delayed for 2–3 years.

Diagnosis: Investigations cannot reliably distinguish between neonatal hepatitis alone or with an associated sclerosing cholangitis, as they are expressions of the same disease process. A patient with prolonged jaundice requires ultrasound examination to exclude choledochal cyst, and other special investigations at a tertiary centre. Operative cholangiography must be planned with a view to a Kasai hepato-portoenterostomy if biliary atresia is confirmed, before the tenth week of life.

Progressive liver disease is not halted by biliary drainage, and even where a Kasai procedure has been successful, there may still be an indication for later liver transplantation, which currently offers the best chance of longevity to these children.

Choledochal cyst

Cystic dilatation of the extra-hepatic bile ducts, with loss of the normal epithelium, must be suspected in any jaundiced infant. In the Third World most patients present under 6 months of age. Recognition is important, as the lesion is eminently correctable provided that surgery is performed before biliary cirrhosis develops. Cardinal symptoms are obstructive jaundice with a sub-hepatic mass lesion.

Other surgical disorders
Tongue tie
The lingual frenulum is a normal structure which secures the mobile tongue to the floor of the mouth. It is not necessary to protrude the tongue in order to speak normally or to suck, and mothers

should be so advised. If it is considered that lingual mobility is seriously impaired, the frenulum may be divided. As the frenulum is avascular save a clearly visible vessel at its base, it is safely divided in the clinic using sharp scissors.

Parents must not be allowed to expect that such 'surgery' will improve diction or compensate for delayed vocal milestones.

L. Hadley

29

Oral health

Introduction

In spite of their high frequency, oral and dental diseases are often overlooked in the training and practice of health professionals. Yet the pain, discomfort, anxiety, and restriction of activity that accompany dental disease are very real. The health of the oral and dental tissues is related to the health of the whole individual; the health of each person relates to the health of the whole community. This concept of 'whole community–whole patient–whole mouth' care is significant for prevention, treatment, and cure.

There has been an unfortunate separation of oral health from general health care. The two major dental diseases — caries and periodontal disease — are diseases arising from problems of nutrition and hygiene, and are therefore preventable.

This chapter cannot be an in-depth review of paediatric dentistry; it can only be an overview of the major problems likely to be encountered, with an emphasis on prevention and primary intervention. Non-dentally-trained personnel can undertake a variety of interventions and preventive measures which can be of great benefit to under-served communities.

Normality

See Figs. 29.1 and 29.2.
There are some common misconceptions about the teeth, two of which are worth mentioning. The first is colour: perfectly healthy teeth vary in colour both between individuals and in the same individual. The reason is that the tooth is made up of different hard tissues. The bulk of the tooth consists of dentine, which is covered by cementum on its root surface where it is held in the alveolar bone. The part projecting above the gum, the crown of the tooth, is covered by enamel. Dentine is about the same yellowish colour in all teeth. It consists of hundreds of thousands of fine tubules radiating out from the pulp, which is the vascular

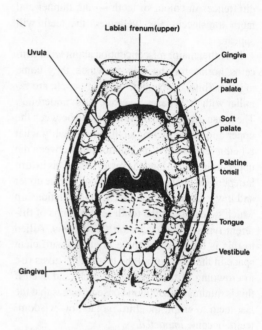

Fig. 29.1   Cross-section of the oral cavity

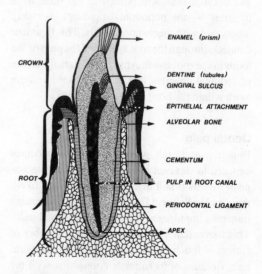

Fig. 29.2   Structure of a normal incisor tooth, longitudinal section

and nervous tissue core of the tooth. Dentine is about 33% organic and 67% inorganic matter. Enamel, however, is about 96% inorganic, and is the hardest substance in the body. Dentine is opaque; enamel is translucent. The relative thickness of the enamel and its translucency cause the differences in colour of teeth — the thinner and more translucent, the 'yellower' the teeth will appear.

The other major misconception about teeth concerns norms for the way in which they come together (bite, or 'occlude'). Most people are familiar with the phrases 'overbite' and 'underbite'. These usually refer to the relationship between the upper and lower incisor teeth, but in reality what is being referred to is the relationship between the upper arch of teeth, and the lower arch. This in turn is dependent on the relationship between the upper and lower jaws, and it is this skeletal relationship which gives rise to the tooth relationships of different types of *malocclusion (see below)*. Allied to this is the fact that there is often insufficient space in the jaws for all the teeth. This gives rise to crowding of the teeth in the arch, and even if this is minimal, a common consequence is that the last teeth to erupt, the third molars, or 'wisdom' teeth, become *impacted*.

Teeth are sensitive because the enamel fits tightly onto the more elastic, but sensitive, dentine, and because the tooth is held in the bone by a ligament — the periodontal ligament — richly innervated with mechanoreceptors. This ligament connects through the root apex with the pulp of the tooth in the root canal. Any loss or damage to the periodontal ligament will lead to looseness of the tooth within the bone.

Dental pain

Dental pain is felt when the dentine becomes exposed to noxious stimuli. The precise mechanism for this is still unknown, but it seems likely that fluid movement in the tubules of the dentine transmits impulses to the innervated dental pulp. This movement may be initiated by a number of factors — touch, chemicals (e.g., sugar), temperature. Because of its intimate connection with the pulp, dentine should really be considered the calcified portion of the pulp tissue.

Oral mucosa

The healthy mucosa of the oral cavity *(see Fig. 29.3)* is either unkeratinized or para-keratinized, and this accounts for its variety of appearance and colour. The oral cavity is an area where various manifestations of systemic disease occur. It has been claimed that there are up to 70 systemic diseases which can be diagnosed by, or at least manifest in, changes in the oral mucosa. Often these changes provide useful warning signs, e.g., Koplik's spots in pre-eruptive measles.

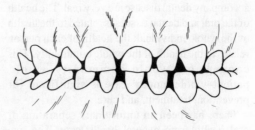

Fig. 29.3 *Normal appearance of teeth and gingiva of a 6-year-old child*

Gingivae

The gingivae are important indicators of localized disease and inflammation. They contain a complex series of fibres which pass to and from the crest of the alveolar bone surrounding the tooth. These attachment fibres give the gingivae their characteristic stippled appearance, a bit like that of orange or lemon skin. Absence of this stippling indicates underlying oedema and inflammation. The gingiva forms a cuff, or collar, around each tooth by folding under it, rather like the skin over the bottom of a finger nail. This creates a gingival crevice, the lining of which is very permeable and consists in places of only one or two layers of cells. Gingival fluid or exudate flowing through the crevice contains secretory products such as antibodies. Unfortunately the permeability works both ways, and toxins enter easily, causing inflammation and oedema. Normal healthy mucosa and gums appear pale pink in colour, and any variation may indicate local or systemic disease processes.

Dental caries

Tooth decay is primarily a disease of children. It is an infection, caused by the action of micro-organisms on fermentable carbohydrates. This action results in the production of acid which demineralizes the dental hard tissues, thereby softening them. Caries usually begins as a small area in the enamel, often hidden from sight in between the teeth or in the fissures (grooves) on the biting (occlusal) surfaces. Continued demineralization of the enamel causes the destruction to spread to the dentine. This undermines the softened enamel, which breaks away to form a cavity, and the tooth tissues continue to be progressively destroyed.

Causes

A clean enamel surface exposed to the oral environment, quickly becomes coated with an amorphous organic film of glycoprotein, precipitated from saliva. This *pellicle* is very tenacious, and unfortunately very attractive for bacteria. The organisms which colonize this pellicle are largely streptococci initially, but become mixed as more organisms are attracted into what is now dental plaque.

Some of the plaque bacteria are capable of fermenting dietary carbohydrate. Sugar is quickly converted to acid, which is consequently held within the plaque. The longer or more frequently sugar is in contact with plaque, the longer the acid contacts the tooth surface, and the greater the likelihood of the enamel being demineralized. This opens up the tooth for bacterial invasion. Thus there are four essential factors which must be present to cause caries: micro-organisms, a substrate rich in fermentable sugars, a susceptible tooth (and host), and time. All four must interact for demineralization to occur *(see Fig. 29.4)*.

Appearance and progression

The early lesion in the enamel is a white spot. This appearance is due to the increasing opacity of the enamel as a result of its demineralization. It is easy to detect on the smooth surfaces of teeth which are visible, and with a mirror and a strong light it is also possible to detect in between the teeth. On the biting surfaces it is more difficult to see, but starts on the sides of the fissures, eventually extending into them.

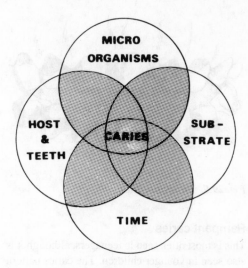

Fig. 29.4 Principal factors in decay process

As demineralization progresses, the lesion takes on a brown colour. This is again easy to detect on visible surfaces of the teeth; but on the biting surfaces the discoloration of the fissures may not reveal the true extent of the lesion, as the caries can and does spread out below the surface. The cavity is often much larger than it appears.

Once the enamel cavitates, bacteria are able to penetrate the dentine. Here the spread is more rapid, both because of the lower mineral content and because the tubules provide easy pathways for invasion. Dentinal caries expands circumferentially, undermining the enamel. A mirror and a bright light will reveal a shadow beneath an enamel surface that has been undermined in this manner but which is still largely intact.

Eventually the undermined enamel fractures away, revealing an obvious cavity in the tooth, varying in colour from yellowish-tan to dark brown. The variation in colour can often give an indication of the rate of progression of the lesion. Most lesions progress slowly and have time to accumulate deposits of bacterial pigmentation. As will be dealt with in a later section, dental caries is a dynamic process, with periods of demineralization and remineralization. In some children, however, two types of rapidly advancing caries, known as rampant caries and nursing-bottle caries, are often encountered *(see Fig. 29.5)*.

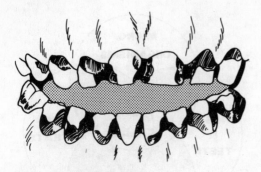

Fig. 29.5   Rampant caries

Rampant caries

This is most often seen in teenagers, although it is also seen in younger children. The caries pattern is very destructive, and is characterized by the widespread attack of a number of sites, but especially those not normally susceptible to decay. These include areas between the lower incisors, the outer surfaces of upper incisors, and the inner surfaces of posterior teeth. The caries progresses rapidly, and patients often present with dental abscesses *(see below)*.

Nursing caries

This is differentiated from rampant caries by the absence of decay in the lower incisors. It has been called nursing-bottle caries, milk-bottle syndrome, and baby-bottle caries. The term 'nursing caries' is more accurate, for it is caused not only by sucrose-containing liquids in the bottle, but also by the use of sweetened pacifiers (dummies) in babies who are breast-fed. The bottle contents responsible for nursing caries can include milk (either with or without added sugar), sugared water, fruit juices, and carbonated or non-carbonated beverages. Baby formula powders are also potential promoters of nursing caries: some contain lactose, and others — such as soya-based formula — are lactose-free, but contain sucrose or other sugars.

Epidemiology

Although many factors have been incriminated in various societies — race, religion, culture, economy, diet, hygiene practices, etc. — dental caries remains a problem for large numbers of children.

Many industrialized countries have seen a marked reduction in the prevalence of caries in the last two decades, to an extent which has led to the closure of some dental schools. What is often forgotten, though, is that the reduction is not universal: in Britain about 20% of the child population still suffer fairly high levels of the disease, and some still experience rampant caries. In general, in industrialized countries the disease appears to be confined to the lower socio-economic groups, which generally also display lower educational levels.

In developing countries the pattern is different: children from the higher socio-economic groups tend to have more caries than their counterparts in the lower socio-economic groups. Children in the latter groups tend to live in the rural areas, whilst the higher socio-economic groups tend to live in the urban, more affluent parts of the country. This situation is very similar to that which existed in industrialized countries about 60 years ago.

In South Africa there seems to be a tendency amongst epidemiologists to seek racial and cultural reasons for disease patterns. However, such studies have largely been discredited, and it is now almost universally accepted that caries patterns observed in any community in any society are linked to the consumption of refined sugars. Factors such as race, culture, and religion have much to do with communication and education, and little — if anything — to do with any kind of predisposition to dental caries. People in developing countries are as susceptible to caries as anyone else.

The relationship between sugar and caries will account for the differences seen in the socio-economic patterns of caries, and explains the caries rates in the poor groups (by economy and education) in industrialized countries, and in the more affluent groups in developing countries. Both groups have access to sugar, but lack knowledge of its effects. A further characteristic of developing countries is that as access to sugar products increases, there is no concomitant increase in resources to deal with its effects, and so the caries rate continues to increase. *(See Figs. 29.6–29.9.)*

This is James. He is 9 years old. Both his parents have their own teeth, but his father has had some crowns on his front teeth and his mother has some bridge-work at the back of her mouth. James' mother first took him to see the family dentist when he was 2 years old. The dentist did not need to do anything to James' teeth; he just gave him a ride in his chair and talked to his mother. His mother was told she had been quite right to give James fluoride tablets, as they lived in an area without natural fluoride in the water supply, and where the water was not artificially fluoridated. James may soon have some fissure sealants put onto the biting surfaces of his back teeth by the dentist's oral hygienist.

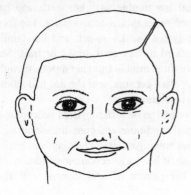

James eats sweets, but only after meals, and his parents refuse him sticky sweets and let him eat chocolate instead. James brushes his teeth after breakfast, and last thing at night. He is unlikely ever to have dental caries or periodontal disease, unless his oral hygiene practices and dietary behaviour change in the future.

Fig. 29.6

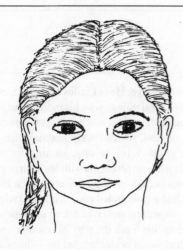

Fig. 29.7

This is Maggie. She is 8 years old. Both her parents wear false teeth. Maggie has been taken twice to the dental clinic run by the local authority. The first time was because she had a swelling on her gum discharging yellowish pus with an unpleasant taste. She had had toothache before the swelling, but no one had been able to take her to the clinic; both her parents work, and the clinic is only open during the day. Her grandmother put some oil of cloves onto the bad tooth and that helped until the pain went away. At the clinic they gave her some gas and extracted her tooth.

The next time she went to the clinic because every time she ate or drank something hot or cold, her teeth hurt. She was very scared, and wouldn't let the dentist look in her mouth. Her parents had to take time off work to take her back to the clinic, where a dentist took out five of her baby teeth under general anaesthetic. All five of these teeth had cavities in them. Maggie will go to the clinic for the third time soon, in the school holidays. She is going with a friend who is going to have a filling, and Maggie wants to see what happens because she has heard her parents say that fillings are 'no good as they fall out and give you more toothache'. Maggie's parents earn enough money to buy some small luxuries, and there are always sweets in the house. Her mother often bakes cakes and confectionery. Maggie especially likes the jam tarts her mother makes, though sometimes when they stick in her teeth she feels her teeth get a bit sore.

Maggie's parents will probably buy her a set of false teeth for her 21st birthday.

This is Lindiwe. She is 6 years old. She lives with her mother and two sisters in a shack in a squatter settlement. Her mother gets occasional work as a domestic. Lindiwe plays with the other children in the area where they live, and does not go to school because there is not one nearby. She has never had any trouble with her teeth, and has only tasted sweet things occasionally. The food she eats is not usually sweet, and her family cannot afford to buy cool-drinks or fruit. She does have some trouble from her mouth, though: her gums often get sore, and she has had mouth ulcers several times.

Lindiwe will go on suffering from malnutrition-related oral conditions and gum disease because she knows nothing of teeth-cleaning, and has no toothbrush. If her socio-economic condition improves, her pattern of oral disease will also change.

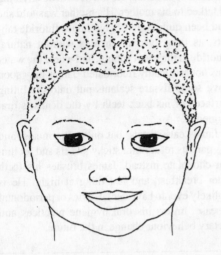

Fig. 29.8

This is Simpiwe. He is Lindiwe's cousin, and he lives in a rural village with his mother and brothers and sisters. His mother works their small patch of land, which barely sustains them. His father is away in the city, looking for work. Simpiwe has no problems with his teeth or gums, but does occasionally get mouth ulcers. He has never had a carbonated cool-drink, and when he wants something sweet, he chews on sugar-cane. He cleans his teeth the way his mother and the local traditional healer taught him — he bites the end of a green stick until it is well frayed and soft, and then uses that as a brush. He occasionally dips it in a little charcoal, the way his grandmother told him.

Simpiwe will not experience gum disease or caries unless his mother starts to use refined sugars in the bread and porridge she gives to her family.

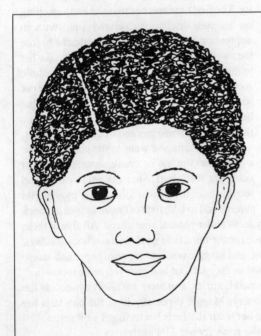

Fig. 29.9

Documentation of dental problems

Caries prevalence is measured in a number of ways, and expressed either as a percentage of teeth carious or a percentage of tooth surfaces carious. Early enamel lesions should be differentiated from later stages of caries progression. Usually, the number of decayed (D), missing (M), and filled (F) teeth (T) are used to make up a composite DMFT score.

The consequences of dental caries

The obvious consequences of caries are pain and sepsis. The less obvious consequences are those that follow the treatment of the pain and sepsis.

Pain is initially felt when the carious process reaches the sensitive dentine, and the stimuli most often eliciting pain will be contact with heat, cold, or sweet drinks and foodstuffs. As the lesion progresses and the pulp becomes involved, hyperaemia causes the pain to be less transient and more intense, especially on contact with heat. Soon the pain persists, can be throbbing, and the tooth is painful to bite on. The bacterial invasion of the pulp causes death and necrosis of the tissues, and the resultant pus accumulates under and around the roots of the tooth, causing severe pain. The pus may track through the bone to the soft tissues. Initially this presents as a swelling on the gum (a 'gum boil' or 'gum bubble'), which in children often spontaneously ruptures, or points to drain the pus (*see Fig. 29.10*). This is very convenient, as it relieves the pain, but dangerous in that treatment may not be sought promptly. A persistent infection

will cause damage to the developing tooth below an infected primary tooth, and will be dangerous in a malnourished child. Pus may continue to accumulate without the formation of a track or sinus to the outside, and invade the soft tissues of the cheek to present as an obvious swelling. These can reach surprisingly large proportions before help is sought. Untreated, the danger is spread via fascial planes to cause asphyxiation or, in rare cases, cavernous sinus infection.

Less obvious consequences of dental sepsis are damage to underlying structures (such as the developing teeth, mentioned above), but also disruption to the developing tooth arch as a result of premature extraction of primary teeth. Teeth on either side of a gap tend to drift towards that gap, and teeth opposite a gap continue to erupt into it. Primary teeth that do this carry with them the developing tooth germ of their permanent successors, and this means that those permanent teeth will erupt out of position, causing problems with crowding (*see malocclusion, below*).

Treatment

It is beyond the scope of this chapter to discuss the specific dental treatment of caries and its consequences. Where there are no dentally-trained personnel available, however, there is still much that can be done to treat pain and sepsis, at least until other arrangements can be made.

Cavities that are obvious and have not progressed to form an abscess should be cleaned out as much as possible with a spoon excavator (*see Fig. 29.11*). A local anaesthetic may be required to do this satisfactorily, but if not available, it is still helpful to clean out as much as possible. Then a temporary filling material can be put in, which is essentially a mixture of zinc oxide powder and oil of cloves. Analgesics can be given if available. Patients should then be referred for dental treatment, where more permanent restorations can be carried out.

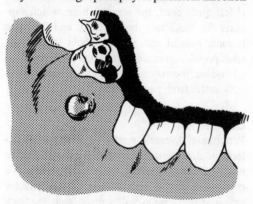

Fig. 29.10   Gum boil of lower right second primary molar

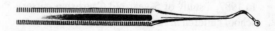

Fig. 29.11   A spoon excavator

A tooth with an abscess should be extracted unless there are dental personnel available who can carry out a root canal treatment. This procedure involves cleaning out the infected and necrotic pulp in the root canals and then filling all the canals as well as the tooth itself. Extraction will require a local anaesthetic, but sometimes the presence of inflammation contraindicates this and a local anaesthetic will not work. Then adequate suppression of the abscess must be obtained either by antibiotic therapy alone, or by a combination of antibiotics and incision and drainage (usually intra-orally, but large facial swellings should be drained extra-orally, especially if there is danger of asphyxiation). Penicillin or erythromycin are the drugs of choice. Only rarely will it be necessary to inject an antibiotic. Moist heat applied to the swelling will also help, and analgesics can be given.

▶ WHO Goals for oral and dental health

Whilst a score of zero is obviously the goal, this is unrealistic for almost all populations, so the WHO has set certain goals which help in planning oral health programmes. The following are the proposed global goals for the year 2000:

Goal 1: 50% of 5–6 year olds to be caries-free.

Goal 2: No more than 3 DMF teeth at 12 years of age (global average).

Goal 3: 85% of the population to retain all their teeth at 18 years of age.

Goal 4: A 50% reduction in present levels of edentulousness (having no teeth) by the age of 35 – 44 years.

Goal 5: A 25% reduction in present levels of edentulousness at the age of 65 years.

Goal 6: Establishment of a data-based system for monitoring changes in oral health.

Some S.A. statistics

In 1987, a study of 5-year-old Caucasian nursery school children in Pretoria showed that 51% were caries-free, and the mean DMFT was 1.97.

In 1988, a study of children living in the village of Mamre (a rural 'coloured' community) showed that 41% of the primary teeth of 6-year-olds were carious.

In 1990, a study of 5-year-old 'black' children attending pre-schools in Cape Town revealed a mean DMFT of 5.2. Rampant caries was found in 54% of both 4-and 5-year-old children.

Sinus infection

(Also see Chapter 14, Ear, Nose, and Throat Disorders.)

This is mentioned here because infection of the maxillary sinuses can give rise to symptoms in the teeth that are strongly suggestive of a dental abscess. It is more difficult to diagnose this when the teeth have fillings (because one may suspect something having gone wrong under a filling), but pain in several upper back teeth should always be regarded suspiciously. Sinus infection is fairly characteristic, as usually there are or have been signs of a recent cold, and pain can be elicited by pressing against the maxilla below the orbit. Several teeth may hurt when tapped, and usually there is no sign of decay or gum disease in the teeth. If in any doubt, treat for the sinus first for at least 3 days — the toothache will disappear as the sinus infection clears up.

Periodontal disease

Periodontal disease is an inflammatory condition which affects the gum and bone supporting the teeth — the periodontal tissues. It is a condition which usually begins in childhood and increases in severity through early childhood to middle age. If left unchecked, the alveolar bone which supports the tooth may be attacked, and the teeth become painful and mobile. About 95% of the adult population exhibit some degree of periodontal disease; the majority have gingivitis, and about 20% suffer from periodontitis.

Cause

Periodontal disease is caused by a variety of bacterial toxins contained in dental plaque. Plaque itself is inherently sticky, and attaches easily as a continuous layer to smooth surfaces, so any factor aiding that retention will worsen matters. Such factors commonly encountered are crowded and irregular teeth, mouth-breathing (because of the reduction in salivary flow), and any roughness created by artificial substances such as tooth fillings and dentures. Calculus ('tartar') is plaque which has become calcified and hence has a rough surface which is ideal for attracting more plaque. This additional plaque in turn becomes calcified, and so on.

The reaction of the periodontal tissues themselves also affects the severity of the disease process, and this is a very variable factor. Certainly hormonal and metabolic changes are involved (pregnancy often results in an exaggerated response to plaque), but the cause of the variation remains unknown.

Gingivitis

Appearance
Gingivitis is the initial form of periodontal disease, and begins as inflammation of the gum margin, which may bleed on brushing, and appear shiny and swollen. A blunt probe inserted between the margin and tooth will induce bleeding if gingivitis is present, and is indicative of the need for mechanical removal of the plaque. In moderate to severe gingivitis the oedema is more pronounced, and the gingiva may be easily deflected from the teeth. The child may complain of spontaneous bleeding, or bleeding when eating or brushing. There is always plaque present to a greater or lesser extent. Gingivitis is painless; the only complaint will be the bleeding, and bad breath in many cases.

Treatment
The clinical management of gingivitis is related to its prevention *(see section on prevention)*. Where plaque has built up to the extent of becoming calcified, as calculus deposits, these must be removed by instrumentation. In children and even adolescents, the calculus is usually found above the level of the gum, and is easily removed using hand scalers and curettes. These should be used with care, using good finger-rests to avoid damage to adjacent soft tissues. When the gingiva bleed very easily, it is often better to wait for a week before scaling, and advise use of a warm salt-water mouth rinse and more frequent brushing by the child and/or parent in the meantime. This in itself will do much to reduce the gingival inflammation.

Periodontitis

Appearance and treatment
Chronic gingivitis may persist for many years, and possibly for life in some patients. In many, however, it may slowly give way to chronic periodontitis, as the plaque accumulates below the gum, between gingiva and tooth. This creates a large pocket between gum and tooth — ideal conditions for the accumulation of more bacterial plaque. The toxins cause a progressive destruction of the periodontal tissues, including the bone, eventually leading to loosening and then loss of the tooth *(see Fig. 29.12)*.

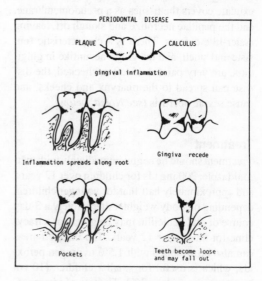

Fig. 29.12 Periodontal disease

Advanced periodontal disease in children is usually a manifestation of an underlying systemic disorder (e.g., diabetes, leukaemia).

Periodontitis can be arrested, although any bone destruction cannot be reversed without specialized treatment. Chemical control of plaque has been shown to be effective: the solution of choice is 0.2% chlorhexidine gluconate, but this does cause staining of the teeth and should not be used for long periods.

Teeth with poor prognosis will have to be extracted. *Increasing* looseness (mobility) of the teeth is a better indication for extraction than just looseness *per se*.

Acute necrotizing ulcerative gingivitis (ANUG)

Appearance

Also known as Vincent's infection or 'trench mouth', this is an infectious but non-communicable disease, caused by micro-organisms which invade the gingival tissue. It occurs in under- and malnourished children, but in later adolescence in some normal individuals, when it is often related to smoking.

The disease initially presents at the tips of the interdental papillae as acute inflammation and redness, progressing to ulceration and spontaneous bleeding involving all the gingivae. A necrotic exudate covers the tissues as a pseudomembrane, and the papillae necrotize and slough off, leaving crater-like defects. There is a characteristic foul taste and smell, and the gingivae, unlike in gingivitis, are very painful. If left unchecked, the disease can spread to the pharynx and cheeks, and cause severe necrosis *(see Noma, below)*.

Treatment

Treatment should be begun immediately with metronidazole: 200 mg tds for children over 12 years, and approximately half that for younger children, depending on body weight. Alternatively a 3-day course of oral penicillin may be given, or tetracycline for those over 12 years. The infected areas can also be swabbed with 1.5% hydrogen peroxide, which is useful for smaller children (10 vol hydrogen peroxide = 3%). The use of vitamin C 500 mg bd has also been advocated.

The plaque and calculus must be removed, but this can be very difficult, and painful for the child. It should therefore be done very gently, first removing the gross calculus, and using warm water to rinse. If a topical anaesthetic spray is available, this can be used to great effect. Home care involves rinsing the mouth with a warm 3% solution of hydrogen peroxide, or application of this solution with cotton gauze by the parent, if the child cannot rinse. Brushing should be done with a soft brush, further softened in warm water prior to use. The diet should be of a soft consistency and spices should be avoided; nutrient supplements should be prescribed.

The scaling of the teeth should be continued until all traces of calculus are removed, and the parents and child should be encouraged to continue a preventive regime. It is, however, a sad fact that many patients must return to the same socio-economic conditions that contributed to the development of the disease in the first place, and the health professional must be aware of the urgent need for improvement of those conditions.

Acute herpetic gingivostomatitis

See Chapter 8, Infectious Disorders.

Juvenile periodontitis

Appearance and treatment

This has its onset around the time of puberty and is characterized by bone loss and deep pocketing around the permanent first molars and incisors. The tissues frequently appear normal, and usually very little plaque or calculus is seen. Progression is often rapid, and the disease may only be detected when the bone loss is such that the teeth become mobile.

Many different **treatment** regimes have been proposed for juvenile periodontitis, but when detected, it should be treated as for any localized and severe periodontitis. Tetracycline has been shown to be beneficial (250 mg qid for 2–3 weeks). The pocketing can be irrigated with a 0.2% solution of chlorhexidine gluconate.

Diabetic periodontitis

In children with uncontrolled diabetes, the resistance to plaque is diminished, and a severe periodontitis can result, often leading to loss of many of the teeth. Besides management of the diabetes, treatment is as for severe periodontitis.

Epidemiology of periodontal diseases

Chronic marginal gingivitis in young people is very common, and endemic in some population groups. Bleeding on probing the gums has been found to be common in adolescents in a number of surveys. Global data suggests that only a relatively small minority of the population is at risk of developing destructive periodontal disease. Prevalence is often inferred from the levels of loss of teeth in adult populations, but for developing communities oral health can be expected to im-

Flossing

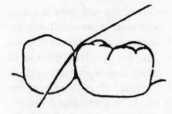

1. Guide floss between teeth.

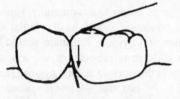

2. Run floss down just beneath the gum line.

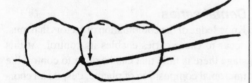

3. Curve floss into a 'C' and move in an up-and-down scraping motion.

Tooth brushing

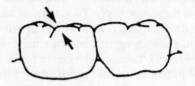

1. Brush both inside and out-side of teeth.

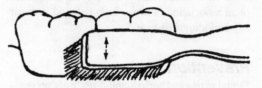

2. Place brush at gum line moving gently in short strokes.

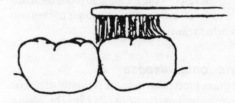

3. Brush top surface of teeth.

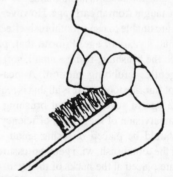

4. Brush behind upper and lower front teeth.

Fig. 29.13 Brushing and flossing technique

prove with advances in general health, hygiene, and living conditions.

There is evidence that underprivileged, lower socio-economic communities suffer more severe periodontal destruction than more affluent communities in the same country. Poor nutrition has been linked to increased prevalence and severity of acute ulcerative gingivitis and cancrum oris *(Noma, see below)*. There is a well-known familial and racial pattern to juvenile periodontitis: it is inherited as an autosomal recessive with full penetrance, and the global prevalence varies from 0.8% in negroids to 0.2% in Asians and 0.1% or less in white Caucasians. This is the only firm evidence of an association between high risk and race for any periodontal disease.

Prevention

Dental caries and periodontal disease are preventable, being diseases of 'diet and dirt'. The main means of limiting periodontal disease is by plaque control, and as plaque contains the microorganisms responsible for the acid production that initiates dental caries, adequate plaque control will also help to prevent that disease.

Periodontal disease

The prime prevention measure is control of plaque by teeth-brushing *(see Fig. 29.13)*. The plaque must be removed effectively without causing damage, and the teeth-brushing skills to do this should be taught from an early age. However, most children are unable to use a toothbrush effectively until about 7 years of age. Prior to that, parents should do the brushing, using a small, soft brush and a gentle scrubbing motion. A pea-sized amount of fluoride toothpaste is all that is required. After the age of seven, parental brushing gives way to supervision of the child's efficiency. Emphasis should be placed on using small movements of the toothbrush, with gentle pressure. The bristles are placed at the necks of the teeth. Older children, adolescents and adults should also be encouraged to use dental floss at least once daily. There is a decreased salivary flow during sleep, so the most important time for cleaning is just before retiring. It has been mentioned that chlorhexidine can act as a chemical suppressant of plaque activity, and is available in more developed countries

as a mouthwash and in toothpastes. However, it can cause staining of teeth, and for a variety of reasons its long-term unsupervised use is not recommended.

Where resources are scarce and teeth-brushing and toothpaste unobtainable or unaffordable, other methods of plaque removal must be resorted to. Traditionally, this has involved the use of chewsticks and various cleaning agents such as salt and charcoal. Too much abrasive material can be damaging and should be discouraged, but traditional practices such as chewsticks should be encouraged in areas where their use is effective and customary.

If oral hygiene is new to a community, general oral health education should be the initial approach. Then oral hygiene education should be directed at children in pre-schools and schools, and at adults in the workplace. Oral hygiene practices need to be just that — practice sessions should be encouraged, with follow-ups, as instruction alone is not adequate.

Dental caries

Knowledge of the combination of factors that must occur to cause caries enables its control. At this stage there is little that can be done to control the microbial composition of plaque, despite an enormous amount of research that has been directed to the development of a vaccine against *Streptococcus mutans,* which plays a key role in the development of caries. The control of caries therefore takes two main forms. First, the reduction or elimination of dietary sugar and plaque. Second, the tooth's resistance to acid attack can be increased by the incorporation of fluoride into the developing enamel, and by lifetime contact of the teeth with fluoride.

Plaque control

The control of plaque has been mentioned in relation to periodontal disease. However, there is no clear association between tooth brushing and caries incidence, so this measure on its own will be insufficient. One reason is that normal brushing inevitably leaves some plaque in the fissures of the teeth and other stagnation sites where caries occurs. In fact for caries prevention, the real value of brushing is that it is a means of applying fluoride via the toothpaste. This will not help those communities who cannot afford toothpaste; hence the value of fluoridating the water supply *(see below)*. There is, though, some hope in recent research into substances which will aid the remineralization process: one such is casein phosphopeptide, which can be used as an additive in a variety of foodstuffs, but especially in confectionary such as chocolates. Its absolute efficiency and use has still to be proved, but it is promising.

Dietary control

Control of dietary sugars is one main factor in the control of caries. Acid is generated in the plaque within seconds of its contact with sugar, and in 1–2 minutes is at a pH below that necessary to dissolve enamel. The effect lasts for 20–40 minutes *(see Figs 29.14a and b)*.

During this time there is an outflow of mineral from the tooth, subsequently reversed if there is

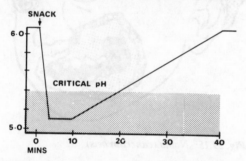

Fig. 29.14a   Change of plaque pH after a sugar drink

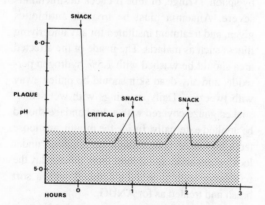

Fig. 29.14b   Effect of frequency of sugar consumption

no further contact with sugar, and especially if there is contact with fluoride. Demineralization, however, will be the net result if sugar is consumed *frequently*. Hence dietary control is directed at limiting the amount, and especially the frequency, of sugar intake. Health professionals need to give advice on sugar-containing foods and drinks and contrast them with sugar-free foods that could be used for between-meal snacks. Mothers of infants, particularly, should be informed of the dangers of putting sugar-sweetened drinks and fruit juices into feeding bottles, especially at night. It should be noted that there are hidden sugars in many preparations, especially in infant 'health drinks' and medicines, and the addition of this sugar should be condemned by all health workers. It should also be noted that whilst sucrose is the most cariogenic of all sugars, both glucose and fructose will also induce acid formation in plaque.

Fluoride

Fluoride promotes remineralization and, when incorporated into the enamel during development, increases the enamel's resistance to acid attack. It is the most effective measure for reducing dental caries. The safest and most efficient way of getting fluoride to the entire population, irrespective of social status, is via the public drinking water. More than 95 surveys in 21 countries have shown that at a concentration of about 1 part per million (ppm), the caries incidence is reduced to about half that in a non-fluoridated area. Furthermore, *all* studies have shown that there is no adverse effect on general health at the level of 1 ppm. There are, however, adverse effects on the appearance and formation of enamel at concentrations much higher than this.

In many parts of the world, however, either local authorities have resisted fluoridation or large sectors of the population do not have access to treated drinking water. In the absence of water-borne fluoride, dietary supplementation is advocated. This requires the ability to pay for these supplements, and they must be readily available. Fluoride supplements take the form of drops or tablets, to be given daily throughout the period of tooth development from shortly after birth to adolescence. Obviously this requires a high degree of commitment on the part of the parents to buy and apply these supplements.

There is no good evidence that fluoride supplementation during pregnancy benefits the child.

Table 29.1 Fluoride supplementation with tablets or drops

For an area with less than 0.3 ppm in the water supply:

Age	Daily dosages
0 – 2 years	0.25 mg F (0.55 mg sodium fluoride)
2 – 4 years	0.5 mg F (1.1 mg sodium fluoride)
4 – 12 years	1.0 mg F (2.2 mg sodium fluoride)

Note: For an area with a supply of 0.3 – 0.7 ppm, these dosages should be halved. Older children should chew, and allow tablets to be dissolved slowly in the mouth, to obtain a topical effect on the erupted teeth.

The most cost-effective topical agent is fluoride toothpaste. The most cost-effective measure on a public health basis is fluoride mouth rinses for home use by people at high risk of caries, but this is not advocated for the pre-school child because of the risk of swallowing. Weekly fluoride rinses can be organized for school children: the children can brush together first, and on the same day each week rinse with a mouthful of fluoride mouth rinse for one minute, then spit it out (they are not to swallow). They should not have anything to eat or drink for 30 minutes. If commercial rinses are not available, mix 2 grams of sodium fluoride powder in 1 litre of water. This can be diluted ten times for a daily mouth rinse.

Oral mucosal diseases

Some conditions are briefly described here. The oral manifestations of the more common systemic diseases will be found elsewhere in this book.

Noma (cancrum oris)

This is a complication of ANUG *(see page above)*, which develops when the child's resistance is low, usually as a result of malnutrition and anaemia. Often the child may have TB, or may recently have had a serious illness such as measles or malaria. The original infection spreads to the jaw if untreated, destroying alveolar bone and therefore

loosening the teeth; often loose pieces of bone are seen around the teeth. Finally it reaches the cheek, appearing as a tight, dark red swelling on the inside and a black spot externally, which breaks open, leaving a hole into the mouth. If left unchecked, the destruction can become severe and disfiguring, ultimately requiring plastic surgery for correction, and intra-oral appliances to prevent tightening of the scar *(see Fig. 29.15)*.

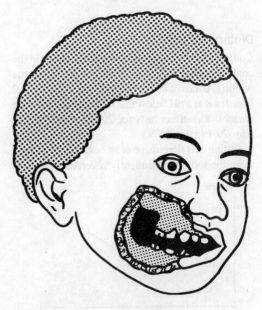

Fig. 29.15 Noma (cancrum oris)

The child requires fluids and supplements fed by spoon, syringe, or tube if cheek destruction is severe. Anaemia must be treated, antibiotics given, and treatment instituted for any underlying illness such as malaria. The inside of the affected area should be washed with 1.5% hydrogen peroxide, and any dead skin should be pulled away with tweezers. Daily dressings with wet saline-soaked gauze covered with a dry bandage should be applied externally. Inside the mouth, any loose teeth and dead bone should be removed under local anaesthetic, and at least three times a day the remaining teeth should be brushed with a soft brush and treated as for ANUG.

It is important to stress once again that Noma is preventable: sick, undernourished children require special attention to their oral condition.

Oral candidiasis
See Chapter 8, Infectious Disorders.

Leukaemia
This disease may manifest initially in the oral cavity with gingival haemorrhage, swelling, and ulceration of the oral mucous membrane and cervical lymphadenopathy. Oral care is important during the treatment of the disease, and chemical plaque control has been useful, using a 0.2% chlorhexidine gluconate mouthwash twice daily.

Histiocytosis X
Oral lesions are found in patients with eosinophilic granuloma, a destructive lesion of the mandible being the most common. The lesion causes a marked gingivitis and swelling of the tissues in the area, with ulceration and bleeding on touch. The teeth become extremely loose and are often exfoliated.

Phenytoin hyperplasia
A common condition in the past, this has become infrequent in patients when serum blood levels of phenytoin are carefully monitored. In extreme cases the tissue may cover the crowns of the teeth *(see Fig. 29.16)*. There is a significant correlation between the degree of hyperplasia and inflammation, which means that excellent oral hygiene will help to control the condition. Surgical excision of the hyperplasia may be necessary in some cases.

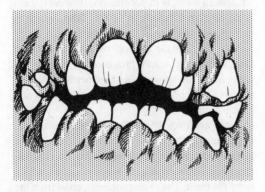

Fig. 29.16 Phenytoin hyperplasia in a teenager (the teeth are crowded)

Other conditions
There are some fairly common oral conditions which are relatively harmless and of unknown cause. Two of these are aphthous ulcers and geographic tongue.

Aphthous ulcers
Aphthae may start in childhood and continue throughout life. They have a tan-yellow base and an erythematous halo. They vary in size quite considerably, and can occur anywhere on the oral mucosa. Treatment is limited to symptomatic relief of the ulcers, usually by applying a protective ointment (e.g., Orabase®) which may carry a steroid, triamcinolone (e.g., Kenalog® in Orabase®). Vitamin A supplements have had anecdotal success, but overdosage should of course be avoided.

Geographic tongue
Migratory glossitis, or geographic tongue, may be alarming to the child or parent because of its appearance — red areas with an irregular circinate pattern appear and disappear on the tongue. The borders of these areas are often outlined by a thin white or yellowish line. The condition, however, is usually symptomless, and only reassurance of its benign nature is required.

Developmental aspects
Eruption times of the teeth are very variable. Some babies are born with teeth, others may have none until a year of age or later. Average times of eruption are tabulated below.

Teething
The first primary teeth erupt at about 6–8 months of age and all are present by 3 years. At about 6 months, the maternal antibodies present in the baby's circulation start to diminish, and the baby's own immune system starts to develop. This does not reach maturity until about 3 years of age. It is an unfortunate coincidence that the symptoms resulting from an immature immune system coincide with teething. As a result, teething has been associated with fever, flu, colds, skin eruptions, and especially gastrointestinal disturbances. Even though there is no scientific correlation between these symptoms and teething, it has been the

Table 29.2 Approximate average eruption times of the teeth

Note that there is a variation around each of these times.

Primary teeth

Lower central (first two) incisors	8 months
Upper central incisors	10 months
Upper lateral incisors	11 months
Lower lateral incisors	13 months
Upper and lower first molars	16 months
Upper canines	19 months
Lower canines	20 months
Lower second molars	27 months
Upper second molars	29 months

Permanent teeth

Upper and lower first molars	6 years
Lower incisors	6–7 years
Upper incisors	7–8 years
Upper and lower first premolars	10 years
Lower canines	10 years
Upper and lower second premolars	11 years
Upper canines	11 years
Second molars	12 years
Third molars	20 years

author's experience that a scientific explanation does not help to alleviate anxiety caused by commonly-held beliefs. Medication prescribed for the underlying illness may ease the symptoms, and so convince the parents that the medication really was for the teething, thus perpetuating the myth. There is little that can be done about this unless the general educational levels of the community are high. What may help the teething process is to give the child something hard to bite on, such as a hard, dry biscuit.

There are, however, some complications and associated symptoms when teeth erupt. The presence of something new in the mouth will cause a reflex and excess salivation for a while, and when the primary molars erupt there may be a local increase in temperature so that the cheek may feel hot.

Sometimes an eruption cyst may form: the follicular sac which surrounds the developing tooth may become filled with fluid or blood if traumatized. It appears as a fluctuant blue or purple swelling on the crest of the ridge, nearly always painless. No treatment is indicated.

Occasionally as a molar tooth erupts, a flap of gum tissue is left over the distal half of the biting surface for a while. This can cause problems in two ways: first, if the opposing tooth has already erupted, it will bite down onto the flap, trapping it between the teeth with obviously painful results; in severe cases the flap may have to be excised. Secondly, food debris becomes trapped between the flap and the tooth, where conditions are ideal for the development of infection and inflammation. This is called *pericoronitis*. Treatment consists of cleansing the area with a saline rinse, but antibiotics may be required if there is an associated lymphadenopathy, and the flap may need to be excised.

Occlusion and malocclusion

Erupting teeth are guided into their final positions by the interaction between all the forces influencing them. They cease to erupt in a vertical direction when they meet an opposing tooth, and their horizontal position is determined by the balanced forces of tongue, lips, and cheek musculature. If the teeth all erupt into the arches without any crowding, with the opposing teeth fitting into each other when brought together, this is considered to be normal occlusion. The primary teeth should ideally have small gaps between them, as this helps to ensure sufficient room for the larger permanent teeth.

Malocclusion, on the other hand, is a term which means different things to different people. Some believe that *any* deviation from a perfect appearance of the teeth, with the uppers slightly overlapping the lowers, and no gaps between the permanent teeth, is malocclusion. However, there is no objective definition of this term, which is unfortunate because it is then difficult to determine when a malocclusion requires correction. Orthodontic treatment provision is largely dependent on the subjective judgements of professionals and the subjective desires of patients and their parents.

There are two types of malocclusion: dental, implying that the teeth within the jaws are out of place; and skeletal, implying that there is a discrepancy between the two bony arches which carry the teeth. The main problems, apart from the obvious effect on aesthetics, are those of maintaining good oral hygiene when teeth are crowded together or misplaced from the arch, and possible difficulties in function because of the unstable way in which the teeth occlude. Severe malocclusions, therefore, should receive expert management.

The most obvious preventive measure is to ensure that the primary teeth are retained until naturally exfoliated. When overcrowding of the permanent teeth is apparent, symmetrical extractions — most usually of the four first premolars — may be required.

Traumatic injuries
Injuries to the teeth
(See Fig. 29.17.)

A variety of injuries occur. There may be fracture of the crown of a tooth and/or its root, or a tooth may be partially or completely displaced from its socket. The consequences may be irreversible damage to the pulp, resulting in its death and leading to discoloration of the tooth and infection of the necrotic tissue. This can be treated by root canal therapy if dental personnel are available. The only alternative is extraction.

It should be noted that in all cases of trauma, the cause should be ascertained. The health professional must always bear in mind the possibility of child abuse.

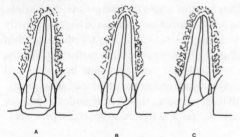

Fig. 29.17 Tooth fractures: a: in enamel b: in dentine c: involving the pulp

Primary teeth

A fracture of the root requires that the tooth be extracted. A fracture of the crown of the tooth can be left if it affects only the enamel, and if the sharp edges can be filed smooth. If the dentine is exposed, the tooth will be sensitive and painful, and if no dental personnel are available, it should be extracted. If the tooth is pushed up into its socket it can be left, but if completely displaced

(avulsed), it should not be replaced. In all cases where the tooth is not extracted it should be observed for signs of discoloration or the development of an abscess (identified by the formation of a gum boil). Again, if no dental service is available, the tooth should be extracted, to avoid damage to its permanent successor.

Permanent teeth

Fracture of the root: This can be detected by holding the crown of the tooth and pushing gently whilst also feeling the bone around the root. It may be that the root is not broken, but the bone of the socket is, in which case both tooth and bone will be felt moving together. The tooth should be immobilized by splinting it to the other teeth *(see below)*. If the tooth moves but the bone does not, the root is probably fractured. Again, it can be immobilized and watched carefully; a horizontal fracture has a good chance of healing, but a vertical fracture will not. Pain will be felt in this latter case, and swelling of the gums is likely. The tooth will have to be extracted if a vertical root fracture occurs. In all cases of root fracture, if no follow-up dental treatment is possible, it is probably better to extract the tooth.

Fracture of the crown: Management of crown fractures will depend on where the fracture line is. If in enamel only, the dentine will not be exposed (the tooth will therefore not be sensitive) and the sharp edges can be filed smooth and left, or a tooth-coloured restoration can be placed by dental personnel. If the dentine is exposed, it must be covered by a dressing such as that used for temporary fillings and, preferably, subsequently restored permanently. If the pulp is exposed, it should be assumed to have been infected, and the tooth must be extracted if root canal therapy cannot be carried out.

Partial displacement from the socket: Often the blow to a tooth results in tearing of the periodontal ligament and displacement of the tooth so that it lies at an obviously incorrect angle in its socket. The tooth should be pushed back to its correct position as soon as possible, and then immobilized by splinting, to allow the periodontal tissues to heal. This usually takes about 3 weeks, and about 3 months is required to watch and assess for pulpal damage.

Complete displacement (avulsion): When this occurs, the tooth should be reinserted (reimplanted) immediately, and immobilized. Prior to reimplantation, the displaced tooth should be washed under tap water to remove any debris, but the tissues of the root should *not* under any circumstances be rubbed or scraped. This will destroy any periodontal ligament cells still attached to the root, and these cells are vital for reimplantation to succeed. To reimplant the tooth, push it gently into the socket, using a slight turning movement, back and forth, until the incisal edge lines up with the teeth on either side. Hold it in place for about five minutes, and then immobilize with a splint.

When immediate reimplantation is not possible because the child is some distance away, the tooth should be stored in milk, because it is nearly isotonic and relatively free of bacterial contamination. If milk is not available, the tooth can be kept in saliva by holding it under the tongue. Alternative media are saline or, least effective, wrapping it in a damp tissue.

The cells of the periodontal ligament can survive for up to 60 minutes outside the mouth, but the prognosis diminishes markedly after 30 minutes, or if the cells are allowed to dry. A tooth left out for more than 60 minutes and left dry should *not* be reimplanted.

Immobilization of teeth (splinting): To allow for healing of the damaged root or periodontal ligament, a tooth should be immobilized by splinting it to at least two teeth on either side. Ideally this should be carried out by dental personnel, who can use a variety of methods, including ligature wire and tooth-coloured restorative materials. If these materials are not available, ligature wire on its own can be 'threaded' between the teeth, but taking care to avoid getting close to the gingival margins. Alternatively (or in addition), beeswax can be used. A thin strip can be softened in warm water, made into a roll, and pressed against and between the teeth. A second roll is then placed on the other side of the teeth from the inside, and again pressed over and between the teeth to connect with the outer wax through the embrasures between the teeth. The patient can then be referred, or if this is not possible, the splint will need to be replaced regularly over about a 6-week period.

Injuries to the soft tissues

These can be treated as for any other soft tissue injury: sutures may be placed, and bleeding controlled. The main difficulty is that during the initial healing phase, oral hygiene is difficult, but the patient and parents should be encouraged to use the measures already detailed.

Injuries to the jaw

If the bone is fractured around the roots of a tooth or teeth, it/they should be splinted firmly to the remaining teeth. This is necessary even if the teeth will subsequently be extracted, because the bone must heal first to allow the tooth or teeth to be extracted on their own without loss of this bone. A stronger splint than described above can be constructed using ligature wire to hold an arched piece of firmer wire placed against the outside of the teeth. An hypodermic needle can be used (cut off the point), bent to conform to the arch of the teeth. Short pieces of ligature wire are used to tie each tooth to the needle.

Fractures of the maxilla or mandible can be immobilized with ligature wire by first placing wire around two strong teeth on either side of the fracture (even if these teeth are several teeth away from the fracture site), and then twisting the two wires together across the fracture site. Prior to this, the broken part of the jaw must be aligned properly by asking the patient to bite together, and then lifting the broken part until all teeth meet. Finally, a head-and-chin bandage should be placed, and analgesics and antibiotics prescribed as necessary. All these measures should be regarded as primary measures prior to referral to specialist personnel.

Dental anomalies

There are a number of conditions affecting the teeth that are caused by hereditary, environmental, or unknown factors. Some of these are mentioned here.

Dentinogenesis imperfecta

This is an inherited defect occurring in 1 in 8 000 individuals, and affecting both primary and permanent dentitions. It may also be associated with osteogenesis imperfecta. The teeth are characteristically a reddish-brown opalescent colour, and the enamel chips away because the junction between the dentine and enamel is abnormal. This then results in rapid wear of the softer dentine, so the teeth are flattened to gum level. The permanent teeth can be treated, but referral to a dental specialist is required.

Amelogenesis imperfecta

This inherited disorder causes defective enamel formation in both dentitions. Ten variations have been described, each presenting a slightly different clinical picture, but these can be grouped into three appearance types:
♦ the enamel is thin and may be smooth or pitted
♦ it may be of normal thickness, but mottled and soft, and chips away easily
♦ it may be of normal thickness but hypocalcified and therefore very soft. In all cases it is lost very easily, leaving exposed dentine. Once again, the condition can be treated, but requires specialist dental personnel.

Systemic effects

Systemic factors such as nutritional deficiencies, childhood diseases, and fevers (especially those associated with exanthematous diseases), can cause an interference with the normal process of maturation and differentiation of the dental hard tissues. This most often results in visible defects of the enamel, appearing either as brownish mottling or white spots in the enamel. The position of these areas will depend on what part of the enamel of the crown was maturing at the time of the interference. The appearance can be improved, but referral to dental personnel is necessary.

Discoloration

Intrinsic staining of the teeth occurs when agents are taken up during their formation. Structural changes that occur in dental fluorosis can vary from white opacities to the yellowish-brown mottled appearance that occurs with concentrations of fluoride greater than 3 parts per million. Endogenous agents cause a variety of coloration (bluishgreen to yellow, brown, or black from erythroblastosis fetalis; green from biliary atresia; pinkishbrown from congenital porphyria). One of the more commonly-known stains is the yellowbrown appearance following tectracycline therapy: if taken during pregnancy or the first 3 months of life, the primary teeth will be affected. The permanent teeth will be discoloured if it is taken between birth and 8 years of age. Treatment to improve the appearance is best carried out by dental personnel.

Extrinsic staining is caused by the effects of various agents on the pellicle and plaque, and therefore can be removed (and obviously prevented) by good oral hygiene. Among the causes are the effects of chromogenic bacteria (usually staining green, but also brown, black, or orange); various foods and beverages such as tea; tobacco; and betel nut chewing.

Conclusion

For primary health care to be effective in the prevention of disease it must be available to those who need it as well as to those who demand it. Oral health care needs the support of nutritionists, water engineers, and educationists, as well as of the health and welfare sector. Such personnel need to accept certain duties in promoting oral health, even in sophisticated communities. All health personnel should have some training in oral health care and promotion.

P. Owen

30
Psychological and behavioural disorders

This chapter shows the need for child psychiatry in primary health care and outlines an approach to children presenting with psychological or behavioural problems. It goes on to give short accounts of a number of common conditions grouped according to the age ranges in which they present.

Introduction and epidemiology

Psychiatry is the branch of medical science which deals with abnormalities of behaviour, emotion, and thought which interfere with a person's capacity to function socially, at school, at work, or in leisure time. Only in the last 20 years have child psychiatry theory and practice been based on sound epidemiological research in Britain and in the United States. This has brought a new scientific respectability to child psychiatry, and an increasing number of syndromes are being clearly defined.

Prevalence rates of significant psychiatric disorders amongst children range from 6–25%: variation depends on age, geographical location, and identification criteria.

A community-based study amongst black children aged 5–15 years in Durban, South Africa, revealed a prevalence of 12% with significant behavioural disturbance. Generally boys are more frequently affected than girls.

Child psychiatry in developing countries

In most developing countries half the population is below the age of 16 years. In these communities, expertise in the field of psychological disorders is far more limited than for other health issues, leaving the majority of children with these problems undiagnosed and untreated. Qualified child psychologists tend to practise among the privileged minority and have little time or inclination to pass on their skills to less specialized workers. To meet the needs of emotionally disturbed children and adolescents, expertise must therefore be developed in the primary health care sector. A system must be devised whereby the most skilled people spend most of their time teaching and supervising rather than providing the service themselves. The system will require screening at various levels by personnel with increasing degrees of expertise, constantly upgraded by means of in-service training.

Health personnel involved in the care of children should establish what mental health expertise is available in the area, and lines of referral. Health workers suited to this type of work need to be identified, and appropriate training arranged.

The professional team

There is a logical overlap of educational, physical, and emotional problems in a school-going child. Emotional problems frequently present with physical symptoms, and educational problems may present with physical or emotional symptoms, or as behavioural problems. Whatever the problem, the first contact is usually a doctor or nurse.

Child psychiatry in its most sophisticated form depends on interdisciplinary management. In developing countries it is rarely possible to have a team of experts, such as psychiatrist, psychologist, remedial teacher, occupational therapist, and speech therapist. However, it is often possible and extremely useful to bring together a doctor, nurse, and teacher to form a basic team and to pool their information and expertise. The doctor contributes knowledge of physical illness or handicap and child development; the nurse. is frequently the co-ordinator of the team, and has a broad knowledge of physical problems and social factors; the teacher is an expert in the cognitive and emotional aspects of education, and is able to judge a child's performance in comparison with other local children.

Any member of the team may make the first contact and take a detailed history from the child's parents. Where circumstances permit, it is to everyone's advantage for the assessment to be shaped in a series of appointments. Where the family's time and the resources are limited, the team should endeavour to complete the assessment at a single attendance. This can be achieved by means of good communication and co-ordination, and a clear idea of aims. Where a fully constituted team of allied health professionals exists, there is further overlap of functions. It is helpful to be familiar with the specific expertise of the different professions:

The **child psychiatrist** is a medical doctor who has specialized in the psychological problems of children, and thus combines knowledge of physical medicine with psychological and social aspects of mental distress. The **psychologist** is skilled in the administration of specific psychological tests and in psychotherapy. The **educational psychologist** has made a special study of the psychological aspects of education and learning. The **psychiatric nurse** has special skills in history-taking, counselling and follow-up management. The **social worker** is trained to collect information from home visits and family interviews, and may undertake group and family therapy. The social worker also has a wide knowledge of the law as it applies to children and families, and is able to advise on grants, financial aid, or placement. The **occupational therapist** (OT) has detailed knowledge of the physical development of children, and is most useful in defining developmental problems of co-ordination or motor function. The OT helps to clarify specific learning problems, and performs individual and group therapy aimed at remedying deficiencies of function. The **speech therapist** defines problems in the reception and expression of language (spoken and read). Since most education is language-based. the speech therapist is a most important member of the team. The **remedial teacher** has made a special study of learning disabilities, and is able to recognize and treat specific problems.

All team members should have knowledge of the emotional and social development of the children in the community they serve. Team members should be prepared to communicate with and learn from each other. The team may work within an existing organization, and may be able to enlist the help of other willing and able members of the community to extend their services, e.g., helping children with study skills, counselling parents, and providing ongoing support and follow-up.

In summary, the team should comprise the most skilled and suitable people available, be it a primary care nurse with a community worker, or the multi-professional group.

Approach to the problem

The problem-solving approach outlined in *Chapter 1* is admirably suited for the child with a psychological/emotional problem. However, particular attention will have to be paid to:
♦ developmental milestones, including possible regression
♦ child's level of function, e.g., toilet training, peer relationships
♦ academic and social performance at school, including a report from the teacher
♦ family history, including a three-generation genogram
♦ cognitive and education-related tests.

In developing countries, educational difficulties are a common cause of psychological or emotional problems. The patient is either failing at school, or is referred by the teacher because of a behaviour problem. Parents tend to attribute failure to poor memory, laziness, or naughtiness, so the child has often already been punished. Furthermore, failure at school evokes great stress in the child and the family because of the considerable sacrifices made for the child's education.

Less commonly, children present with developmental delay or regression (slow speech, faecal soiling, enuresis), other physical symptoms, or unacceptable behaviour. The physical symptoms may have been investigated and no organic cause found: children under stress commonly complain of headaches, sore eyes, abdominal pain, diarrhoea, or pains in the legs. Behaviour problems present as aggression, running away, and stealing. It is important to clarify the time-span over which the patient has had the presenting problem. A sudden deterioration in school performance would point to a physical illness, depression, or interpersonal problems either at school or at home. On the other hand, a mentally retarded child will have a long history of failure at school.

The World Health Organization list of questions *(see Table 30.1)* is a useful screening device to help professionals and care-givers outline the problem area.

The majority of children experience minor emotional and behavioural difficulties which need not be regarded as significant unless they elicit severe disapproval and are multiple, persistent, or socially handicapping.

Table 30.1   WHO list of questions, suitable for 5 to 15-year-olds

1   Is the child's speech in any way abnormal (retarded, incomprehensible, stammering)?
2   Does the child sleep badly?
3   Did the child have a fit or fall to the ground for no reason?
4   Does the child suffer from frequent headaches?
5   Does the child run away from home frequently?
6   Does the child steal things from home?
7   Does the child get scared and nervous for no good reason?
8   Does the child appear in any way backward or slow to learn as compared with other children of about the same age?
9   Does the child hardly ever play with other children?
10 Does the child wet or soil herself/himself?

Assessment procedure

Comprehensive assessment

The following aspects require particular attention in the assessment of the child with a possible psychological or emotional problem:

◆ development
◆ family environment
◆ cultural environment.

Child development

A knowledge of the expected normal physical, social, and emotional development of the child is fundamental in the assessment of a patient. In the absence of standardized psychological and other tests, the *estimated level of function* (ELOF) is a useful concept. This is a rough estimate of the overall level of function of the child, based on the history provided by the care-giver. The comparison should be made with other children in the family, class, or community, in terms of speech, social interaction, play, tasks in the home,

performance at school, level of responsibility given to the child, and the care-giver's and family's expectations of the child. The ELOF given by the care-giver should correspond broadly to the objective observations *(see Testing basic cognitive tasks, below)*. If, for example, the patient is 10 years old and the ELOF is five, a very approximate indication of the level of functional performance can be arrived at: $(5/10 \times 100 = 50\%)$ which is roughly equal to the Intelligence Quotient.

Where there are inconsistencies, the patient needs more careful evaluation, bearing in mind that some children are advanced in some tasks and slow in others. A report from the school teacher is most useful in this regard.

The family environment

Apart from physical needs, the child has fundamental social and emotional needs which must be met to enable development into a balanced and mature person *(see Table 30.2)*.

Table 30.2   The needs of the child

Physical care
Love, acceptance, and security
Continuity and consistency of care-giving
Behaviour controls
Cultural identity
Appropriate cognitive stimulation

Children can be reared successfully within a nuclear or an extended family, provided that there is consistency of primary care-givers. Permanent psychological and emotional scars are sustained by children who suffer disruption by frequent change of care-givers and by exposure to family violence.

However, children differ widely in temperament: some successfully withstand great social and emotional deprivation, while others are much more vulnerable to bad parenting and poor quality of family life.

Cultural environment

Many families are in a state of transition, moving away from the cultural and religious norms of their parents. High mobility between towns and rural areas, migration from rural to informal periurban settlements, high social upward mobility, and pressures of employment and unemployment are among factors which influence this transition. These in turn alter the language, religion, family structure, and acceptable standards of behaviour. Such external stresses have a marked bearing on child-rearing practices and family life. An analysis of the effect of these stresses on a specific family is recommended for every assessment, but at the same time attempts should be made to identify the strengths and positive features on which one will have to build.

Examination
Physical examination
A routine but thorough examination is essential, with specific emphasis on the neurological system, hearing, and vision.

Testing basic cognitive tasks
This can be an extension of the physical examination, and is intended to confirm the ELOF *(see above)*, estimating the child's intellectual ability and screening for possible specific learning disorders.

Reading, calculations, writing, and drawing are screened, and age-appropriate responses measured. More ingenuity is required to test children who have had little exposure to Western culture. Bearing this in mind, an appropriate test kit could be put together *(see Table 30.3)*. The art of assessment is to use a few test items and gain experience

---

Table 30.3   Test kit for assessment of cognitive tasks

Books
- a simple picture book with good illustrations of familiar objects
- pages taken from 3 or 4 different graded reading books in English and local vernacular languages
- sets of maths calculations from 3 or 4 graded books

Pencil, paper, and eraser for writing and drawing

Tennis ball

Toys: a few cars, doll, and animals

Large beads and strings

Set of basic blocks in various colours

---

by observing the responses of a number of children. Where available, the clinical or educational psychologist can verify test results if there is uncertainty. In most cases problems can be clearly identified and may be acted upon.

Tests for laterality and co-ordination
As a child matures, awareness of left- and right-sidedness and motor co-ordination develop. This is tested by observing which eye, hand, or foot the child prefers. Immaturity in these areas may indicate a specific learning disorder *(see below)* which can benefit from early remedial training. Exercises can be prescribed with the help of an OT, which can be supervised by a lay assistant or parent.

Drawing
Children usually love to draw. Both the way they draw and the content of the drawings can be most informative. The patient may be given drawing materials while the history is being taken. Subsequently the child is asked to draw a person. This should be done in pencil on plain paper for scoring by the OT or psychologist where appropriate. This 'Draw a Person' (DAP) test gives a good indication of intelligence, but culture and possible deprivation have to be considered. The example of a DAP shown in *Fig. 30.1* was done by a child who presented disruptive behaviour at school and who was not coping. This was at the time of the 1986 school boycotts. The disturbance and distress is not difficult to diagnose — he is standing on an army personnel carrier. There is also evidence of a major learning problem in letter formation. This child was not mentally retarded.

Play
A play assessment is done by observing the child at play, which is especially useful in very young or grossly disturbed children. Even in the brief assessment which is being advocated, observations of the child's interaction with people, objects, and toys are very useful. Some children are anxious, afraid, and totally inhibited; some will not use equipment appropriately at all, others are uninhibited and explore everything in a very short time. The interaction between care-giver and child, the encouragement given, and the control exercised are all useful observations.

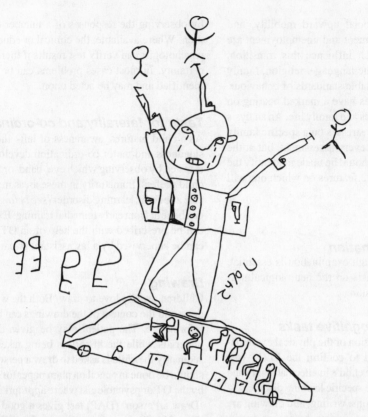

Fig. 30.1 Example of a person drawn by a disturbed school boy

Family interaction

The 'family' in this case is broadly defined as the system in which the child is cared for. The patient is ideally brought by both parents, but this does not occur often. The assessor constructs a picture of the family, with positive and negative relationships. The annotated genogram includes the patient, siblings, parents, and grandparents, and is useful in showing relationships. The older child may be asked to draw the members of the family and each person doing something — a Kinetic Family Drawing. This may help to confirm or refute hypotheses about the family which have been made, and provides an important illustration of how the child sees the family.

Problem analysis

The science and art of assessment lie in being able to collate a great deal of information and give

priority to the main problem areas. The various aspects of the case should be discussed and correlated by the team before feedback is given. All findings are grouped under the following headings:

- Problems in the child
  - physical
  - psychological: intelligence
  - mental disorders
  - educational
- Problems in the family
- Problems in the environment (including school).

The strengths of the patient, the family, and school (if appropriate) should be outlined. The team should discuss with the parents the problems considered to be most important. The presenting problem should be the starting point for this discussion. Correctly 'labelling' the child's problem often brings great relief to the family. The parents'

Table 30.4   Factors influencing the outcome of childhood psychosocial disorders

Risk factors	Ameliorating factors
	Parent and/or child
Family	Stable temperament
Unstable	Good coping skills
Socio-economically	Positive experience
deprived	outside home
Parent	**Child**
Single	Good relationship with one or
Immature	both parents
Mildly retarded	
Displays conduct/	
behaviour disorder	
Rejects child	
In discord with	
other parent	
Other	**Other**
Unstable environment	Isolated nature of stress
Inadequate school and	Improving socio-economic
recreational activities	circumstances

expectations need to be analysed, and time must be given for parents to question and discuss the team's findings, especially if these findings differ from those of the parents. Authoritarian pronouncements should be avoided, since these make the parents feel belittled, and they may withdraw their child before help can be provided.

Treatment

The team should decide whether treatment is really essential.

Factors which determine the choice of treatment include accessibility and affordability in terms of time and cost, as well as the severity of the problem. A careful evaluation of the factors listed in *Table 30.4* is recommended. Possible treatment modalities may include medical treatment, psychotherapy or special educational intervention (home programme), information or counselling for the parents, and family therapy.

A report to the school is usually necessary, especially if the child was referred by the school. Where the child is not being seen on a regular

basis, organized follow-up is essential to monitor progress and to review the intervention.

Assessment in itself should be recognized as a major intervention, which frequently leads to great improvement in the child's problem through insights gained by both parents and child.

Prevention

The WHO recommendations on the prevention of childhood mental disorders and the fostering of healthy psychosocial development include the following:
- striving for the improvement of the general health of mothers and children
- continuity of parent figures
- maintaining family cohesions
- unlimited access by parents to hospitalized children
- avoiding unwanted children.

Professionals dealing with children should endeavour to further these objectives.

All health workers with expertise in these fields need to consider means of disseminating knowledge and skills to the community, aimed at effective parenthood and prevention of maladjustment in the face of cultural disruption and deprivation. High quality care of children who are removed from their parents is of utmost importance.

Common psychological and behavioural problems

In this section problems are grouped according to the age groups in which they generally occur. Only a few of the most common problems can be presented.

0–5 years

Mental retardation (MR)
(Also see Chapter 3, Genetics and Congenital Disorders.)
This is a common disorder, with a prevalence in the Third World of 8–12 per 1 000 children aged 3–10 years.

Mild degrees of retardation are frequently unrecognized. Causes include birth asphyxia, intrauterine infections, intracranial infections, congenital abnormalities, and brain damage due to status epilepticus. MR results in a global delay in achieving milestones. Regression of development is an indication of a progressive disorder, e.g., lipid storage disease.

The subtypes are: Mild (IQ 50–70), Moderate (IQ 35–49), Severe (IQ 20–34), and Profound (IQ below 20).

Examination: Apart from establishing the ELOF *(see above),* a thorough clinical examination is essential. Dysmorphic features might suggest a chromosomal abnormality or hypothyroidism. It is imperative that hearing is assessed, as many a deaf child has been erroneously labelled as retarded. Common associated features of global developmental delay are cerebral palsy and epilepsy.

It may be difficult to be sure of the degree of MR in a young child, and a firm prognosis should be avoided.

Management:

◆ Treat the child for any physical problems (e.g., epilepsy, contractures).

u Counsel parents about the condition, and about social benefits available. The need for genetic counselling may be of particular relevance here.

◆ Encourage appropriate stimulation of the child.

◆ Discuss education, where appropriate.

◆ Follow up.

It is important to dispel unrealistic expectations, which many parents have, but at the same time to provide a step-by-step programme that challenges the child to achieve. Toilet training, personal care, and basic social skills are amongst the most important achievements for which to aim. Such a programme involves reinforcement of the positive aspects of intellect and behaviour to provide guidance towards these modest yet rewarding achievements. Community workers specifically trained in this field can be of tremendous support to the family. The younger the child, the more effective the therapy will be. It must be emphasized that mentally retarded girls require protection against sexual exploitation. Behaviour problems may require special behaviour modification therapy or medication. Anxiolytics or antipsychotics used for short periods can be useful. Anti-epileptic drugs must be prescribed where appropriate.

Temper tantrums

This is a common problem amongst toddlers in some communities. Severity ranges from an occasional outburst following extreme frustration to daily episodes associated with breath-holding attacks, cyanosis, and even minor seizures. Usually this is a passing phase, with good response to counselling where parents are reassured and helped to cope with the tantrum. This becomes difficult where parental control is lacking and the life-style is chaotic. The underlying principles of counselling are:

◆ avoid frustrating situations by offering alternatives to the 'forbidden fruit'

◆ ignore the tantrum by walking away from the child

◆ avoid punishing the child for the tantrum

◆ give full attention and approval when behaviour is acceptable

◆ be consistent.

Reassurance and encouragement may have to be given on subsequent visits.

Sleep disorders

The establishment of a good routine can be difficult with some children. Failing to sleep and excessive crying are common during the first years, and night terrors, nightmares, and sleep-walking may be additional problems in the young child.

Management:

◆ Exclude any physical abnormality.

◆ Consider possible covert child abuse.

◆ Take a detailed history, looking at feeding patterns, routine in the family, stresses on the child, and parents' attempts at coping with the problem.

◆ Reassurance is of paramount importance, particularly where the child is otherwise well and thriving.

◆ Find a way of getting the mother a few good nights' sleep to help her to cope.

◆ Involve the father or other members of the family.

◆ Assist in developing a bed-time routine.

◆ Family therapy for chaotic and violent families.

◆ Hypnotics for the child are generally *not* useful.

Pervasive developmental disorders (PDD)

This group of disorders includes children who have major impairment of social interaction, impairment of communication, and are markedly restricted in their activities and interests. The age of onset is during the first 3 years. Although some have normal intelligence, the majority are below average. These children are particularly severely handicapped — more than can be attributed to the mental retardation alone. The prevalence rate is about 2–4 per 10 000 children.

PDD is subdivided into infantile autism and nonspecific PDD.

The former is characterized by autistic aloneness (autism = lack of responsiveness to other people), delayed or abnormal speech, an obsessive desire for sameness, and unusual repetitive and sometimes inappropriate patterns of play.

Management: If the condition is suspected, the child should be referred to a psychologist, psychiatrist, or paediatrician for diagnosis. These children can benefit from special intensive educational programmes which should start early. Regrettably these are unattainable in all but the most privileged sectors. The prognosis for independence in later life is not good.

6–10 years

School failure

School failure is a very common presenting problem. There are many causes for a child failing or performing badly at school. A detailed history is essential. When a child's performance has suddenly deteriorated, the cause is most likely to be physical or emotional. Consistently poor performance is more likely to indicate mental retardation or specific learning problems.

In a study of 2 190 pupils in Zululand who had failed to pass their first year at school, 20% were found to have visual or hearing problems, and only 2.5% were found to be mentally retarded. Further testing revealed that 81% were quick or normal learners.

Specific learning disorders (SLD)

These disorders must be seen as maturational and developmental problems, and may occur despite a good educational foundation in a child with normal intelligence. They may occur as discrete disorders limited to one or more learning modalities: arithmetic, reading, expressive or receptive language co-ordination, and others. Developmental reading disorder (so-called dyslexia) was found in some 4% of 10-year-olds in a First World study. These disorders are missed unless a careful history is taken and assessment performed. Teachers should suspect SLD when a child has very poor performance in certain areas but in general appears intelligent. The diagnosis should be considered in any pre-school child with a specific developmental delay. An unrecognized SLD may cause profound emotional difficulties, which in turn aggravate the problem. Early intervention is essential.

Management:

◆ Be on the alert for SLD.

◆ Preferably have the problem defined by a remedial teacher or psychologist.

◆ Explain to parents and class teacher.

◆ Introduce a remedial programme — preferably home-based.

◆ Support the child emotionally.

◆ Follow up and monitor.

Hyperkinetic and attention deficit disorders

This is a confusing and controversial group of disorders, and debate is still continuing. Prevalence figures vary greatly. The main problem is an inability to give sustained attention appropriate for the child's age. The lack of attention (attention deficit) may occur with greatly increased activity (i.e., hyperkinetic syndrome, or hyperactivity). The child presents with a short attention span, and is distractable, uninhibited, and poorly organized, with extreme overactivity.

Hyperactivity is not always present, particularly when the child is in a strange environment. The attention deficit disorder without hyperactivity can easily be missed, since the child is usually not troublesome in the class or at home. Children in these latter groups do badly at school, like their hyperactive counterparts, but they tend to be withdrawn, anxious, socially isolated, and poor at sport.

Management:

◆ Early diagnosis, including identification of possible SLD.

◆ Special education, allowing for short attention and gross distractability.

◆ Behaviour modification techniques.

◆ Medication with methylphenidate is sometimes useful.

Hyperactivity following brain damage may improve with behaviour modification techniques and/or haloperidol or diazepam.

School refusal (school phobia)

The main feature of school refusal is reluctance to attend school, associated with anxiety, and often depressed mood. The child appears frightened to go to school (hence *phobia*). In a Western European setting it was found to occur in some 3% of 10- to 11-year-olds. The anxious school-refusing child must be distinguished from the delinquent child not attending school.

Management:

◆ Full assessment of the child, with parents and teacher co-operating.

◆ Establish areas of stress which may be remedied (at school, in the home, or within the child — physical, emotional, or educational factors).

◆ Get the child to school again with support and as soon as possible *(see note below)*.

◆ Treat for ongoing problems.

◆ Medication is rarely necessary.

▶ The longer the child stays away from school, the more difficult it may be to treat, and the poorer the general prognosis. It may be necessary for someone to accompany the child to school each day in the early stages of treatment.

Bedwetting (enuresis)

Most children achieve day and night control of the bladder by 4 years of age. Bed-wetting at night (nocturnal enuresis) is considered a problem after the child has reached a mental age of 4 – 5 years. It may be an isolated developmental problem. It can also be a very disturbing symptom to the child and the family, often resulting in punishment. **Primary enuresis** implies that a child has never had total bladder control. **Secondary enuresis**

occurs when a child starts bed-wetting again after attaining bladder control for several months. Secondary enuresis is often the result of emotional stress or a physical problem. Enuresis tends to run in families. Approximately 10% of 5-year-olds wet their beds, 5% of 10-year-olds, and 1–2% of children continue into their teens. The older the child, the more active the intervention has to be to achieve bladder control.

Management: Enuresis can be assumed to be non-organic if it is nocturnal and there are no other urinary symptoms (frequency, urgency, dysuria). There is a tendency to spontaneous cure. When enuresis is a symptom of a disturbed family setting or underlying psychopathology, symptomatic treatment is unlikely to be successful if the root cause does not receive attention.

Informing the parents of the nature of the problem often relieves the tension appreciably. Coercion and a punitive attitude must be replaced with an understanding and systematic approach. A simple home programme has been shown to have considerable success.

The home programme is based on two principles:

◆ *Increasing bladder capacity:* Bladder capacity can be readily assessed by holding back the urine for as long as possible and then voiding into a container (30 ml per year of age is a good guide). The bladder capacity can be increased by drinking large quantities of fluids during the early part of the day and holding in the urine as long as possible. Other than an occasional word of encouragement, this is best left to the child.

◆ *Self-training to wake up when there is an urge to urinate:* A firm decision must be made by the child when he or she goes to bed, to wake up should the bladder be full. Initially it may help if the parents wake the child, provided that he or she is fully conscious of what is happening and has recall of the event the following day.

Reduction of fluid intake during the evening is advisable. A simple reward system such as a star chart will be an additional inducement. A bell-and-pad system has been successful, but is not always readily available.

Imipramine is the only useful drug. A dose of 25 mg on retiring usually suffices, though this can be doubled in the older child. It must be stressed that drug therapy in isolation is unlikely to have a lasting cure. It may have to be continued for several months, then gradually tailed off, and preferably replaced with a placebo before discontinuation.

Encopresis

Encopresis involves voluntary or involuntary passage of faeces in places that are inappropriate for the social and cultural background of the child. This distressing symptom may be primary or secondary. It may be intermittent, or there may be a constant dribbling of offensive liquid stool. A detailed history is necessary to obtain a clear picture. In each instance a careful clinical examination must be undertaken to rule out organic causes such as megacolon, which causes chronic constipation with 'overflow' incontinence. A rectal examination is obviously essential. Primary neurological deficits such as spina bifida or cord lesions must be excluded.

Encopresis of late onset with no neurological lesion is a feature of emotional stress. It is often accompanied by enuresis, and infrequently by other psychopathology.

Management: Where possible, correct the stressful situation, at the same time as introducing behaviour modification techniques (*see Enuresis, above*).

Stereotyped movement disorders

These include transient tics, chronic motor tics, Tourette's syndrome, and atypical tics and stereotyped movement disorder. The presenting features are rapid movements of a group of functionally related skeletal muscles, or an involuntary production of noises or words. These characteristics distinguish them from other movement disturbances, such as choreiform movements. In some instances there may be an association with emotional disturbances.

Management: If the tic is of short duration, a trial with anxiolytics may be useful. Focus on the tic should be minimized, to prevent it from becoming worse. Parental counselling is important. A comprehensive biopsychosocial assessment is indicated in assessing tics. The more severe form of this disorder requires specialist attention.

Atypical stereotyped movement disorders include conditions such as head-banging, rocking, and repetitive hand movements. They are distinguished from tics in that they involve voluntary or non-spasmodic movement and the patient is not usually distressed by the symptoms. Incidence is high in children with mental retardation or pervasive developmental disorder, and in children with markedly inadequate social stimulation. It may also occur in the absence of mental disorder.

Management involves a detailed assessment of the interaction between parents and child. Increased contact between mother and child, and parent counselling are often indicated. Increased stimulation may help the child. Parents require reassurance about the favourable outcome of treatment. A useful technique for controlling rocking and hand movements is to try to make these rhythmic motor habits purposeful by using music, dancing, hobby-horses, see-saws, swings, and so on. Problems may arise if rocking occurs in a profoundly mentally retarded child, but even here increased stimulation and the introduction of some purpose into the movements may help.

Stuttering

Stuttering or stammering may be accompanied by jerks, blinks, or tremors. The onset is usually before the age of 12 years, and there may be a family history. Over 50% of milder cases make a spontaneous and complete recovery. The child is distressed because of teasing and social ostracism by peers, a reluctance to speak in class, and academic difficulties.

Management: As there is no consensus on the long-term efficacy of the various treatment modalities, management remains controversial. Modern approaches are based on the concept that the disorder is a learned form of behaviour. Most patients can be helped significantly through use of techniques such as speech therapy, and behaviour and individual therapy directed at reducing fears, pressures, and feelings of inadequacy.

Childhood sexuality and masturbation

Sex roles in the young child are acquired with the understanding that males and females differ, and are reinforced by differences between the sexes in appearance, dress, behaviour, and attitudes, and by parental expectations. Parents are generally the main models of appropriate sexual roles. Although cultural influences play a major role in this process, most pre-school children experience a period of sexual curiosity, when interest in the genitalia of siblings and friends is common. In some cultures children tend to be open and spontaneous in their sexual behaviour, whereas in others their sexual activity or curiosity is suppressed by parents.

Children quickly discover the gratification which results from stimulation of the well-innervated external genitalia. Touching the penis — with consequent erection — and rubbing the vulva against a firm object are common practices in young children. Masturbation should be viewed with concern only if it becomes a persistent habit. In most children it is a passing phase.

Precocious and/or persistent aberrant sexual behaviour must raise the suspicion of sexual abuse *(see Chapter 4, Community Paediatrics).*

Management: This must take into account the developmental level of the child. In the very young it tends to be effective, because the habit is not well established. Spontaneous remission is common in infants, most of whom grow up to be normal unless the situation is mismanaged. Parents' attitudes need to be assessed, and they should be assured of the innocuousness of the habit. Boredom must be considered a contributory factor, as must the possibility of irritations such as tight clothing.

In young children, opportunities for masturbation should be reduced, and the child's energy channelled into physical exercise. Sex education for the child may be necessary, during which it is useful to mention that masturbation is an infantile habit. Urethral irritation, urinary frequency, and pruritus may be present and require attention. With correct handling, masturbation can be discouraged, particularly if a constructive pastime can be suggested.

Masturbation may become a frequent preoccupation in the deprived or seriously retarded child, or when harsh punitive measures have overemphasised the undesirability of this practice. Whenever it is a presenting symptom, careful enquiry should be made into any contributory emotional factors. A simple explanation of the harmless nature of this habit, with appropriate parental guidance, is all that is required in the vast majority of cases.

The pre-school child often develops a natural interest in the genitalia of the opposite sex, but parents are inclined to over-react and interpret this normal development as perversion or deviation. A matter-of-fact approach is sometimes all that is required. Emotional deprivation occasionally leads to an uninhibited and affectionate attitude towards relative strangers, which may be interpreted as sexual precocity, and has resulted in sexual abuse.

During adolescence, sexual feelings go through a period of renewed awareness and heterosexual interest. Many parents and children find it difficult to discuss these within the confines of the family, with the result that guidance and support are often not obtained. Lack of appropriate education in a community, particularly during cultural change, has often resulted in a wave of adolescent pregnancies, giving rise to large numbers of unwanted infants.

Anxiety disorders (neurotic and emotional disorders)

These are common disorders even amongst children. Heightened anxiety varies according to the age of the child. Symptoms include fearfulness, misery, unhappiness, sensitivity, shyness, relationship problems, and separation anxiety. In adolescence, somatic disorders with physical symptoms are quite common. Anxiety may be severe and affect the child's performance socially and at school.

Management:
◆ Detailed assessment, with careful exclusion of physical pathology.
◆ Therapy usually must involve both parents and the child.
◆ Specific treatment of physical or educational problems.
◆ Medication may prove useful — short-term with anxiolytics or long-term with antidepressants.
◆ Refer the child to a specialist for review if no improvement is seen in a few months.

Depression

This is part of the group of mood disorders (affective disorders) not unlike those seen in adults. However, children may present with different

594

symptoms and signs from adults. Mania is less common in young children than in adolescence.

Before puberty the prevalence of depressive disorder ranges from about 2–4%. After puberty it approaches the prevalence in adults, where 20–30% will suffer a depressive episode sometime in life. The cause may be hereditary, with a biological vulnerability. Depression may be precipitated by bereavement, or by environmental stress such as family breakup due to divorce. On the other hand there may be underlying emotional problems such as anxiety.

The essential features are depressed mood, sadness, tearfulness, loss of energy, self-blame, and feelings of guilt. There are often changes in the sleep and appetite pattern, which may be increased or decreased. Misery may be expressed as physical symptoms. In adolescents, psychotic symptoms such as auditory hallucinations may occur.

Management:

◆ Detailed assessment as previously outlined.
◆ Treat the child for specific areas of stress.
◆ Family counselling.
◆ Antidepressant medication may be useful, and should be maintained for several months.

Caution: Tricyclic antidepressants taken in overdose can be lethal.

◆ Referral is imperative where there is suicidal behaviour, or if there is no significant response within 5–6 weeks.

Child abuse and neglect
See Chapter 4, Community Paediatrics.

11–14 years
Conduct disorders
Conduct disorders are characterized by antisocial behaviour. There is a persistent pattern of conduct in which the basic rights of others are violated or major age-appropriate societal norms or rules transgressed. The problems must have existed for 6 months or longer to constitute a 'disorder'. Conduct disorders are the commonest psychiatric disorders in older children. British figures show the prevalence to be 4–12% of young adolescents, with the condition being twice as common in boys.

Common features are aggressive behaviour, theft, vandalism, arson, truancy, drug abuse, and aberrant sexual behaviour. Conduct problems may occur as a group activity or as solitary physical aggression.

Management: The only really useful forms of treatment are family and behaviour therapy, which call for expert guidance. The intervention will be long, trying, and arduous, but the prognosis is not hopeless. Conduct disorders frequently occur together with other problems such as SLD or attention deficit disorders *(see above)*, which must be treated at the same time. Medication has a small place, as for instance in attention deficit disorder. Enforced institutionalization should be only a last resort.

Suicidal behaviour
Suicide threats or behaviour should never be taken lightly as just 'attention seeking' or 'a cry for help'. Depression and conduct disorders each account for approximately 50% of children and adolescents with suicidal behaviour problems. The presentation ranges from a well-planned, potentially-lethal, failed suicide attempt, through impulsive acts of low potential danger, to threats of suicide.

The assessment should always include an evaluation of the risk of a repeat, and possibly successful, attempt. Disorders such as depression, psychosis, and drug abuse should be identified and attended to. In the evaluation, predisposing, precipitating, perpetuating, and protective factors must be identified, for which an interview with the parents is essential. A common scenario is a disagreement between the teenager and parent, followed by the impulsive taking of tablets or a household cleaner. Simply facilitating communication may go a long way to restoring a positive relationship. Good supportive work can be done by lay people in this field, and societal structures should be used.

Psychotic disorders
'Psychotic' means that a patient is out of touch with reality. The main features are disorientation, memory loss, and inability to do simple intellectual tasks. It is important to exclude organic causes such as typhoid and other infections, brain tumours, substance abuse, and epilepsy. Apart from therapy for these specific causes, management of

psychotic disorders is in the realm of specialists and calls for referral.

Substance abuse

See Chapter 4, Community Paediatrics.

Teenage pregnancy and abortion

See Chapter 4, Community Paediatrics.

Violence, children, and mental health

This chapter would be incomplete without putting the emotional problems of children into the context of this violent era in the history of South Africa. Children who started school in 1976 are now 20 years and over. Violence has therefore been a constant partner for members of this generation throughout their development. It is inconceivable that it has left them unscathed.

Initially many children and adults were the victims of the 'security forces'. This was followed by the 'necklace' murders — reflected in nursery school children playing 'necklace necklace' instead of 'cops and robbers'. Then there have been the most brutal, ruthless, and unpredictable mass murders by unidentified terrorists killing indiscriminately in trains and public places.

Children are unavoidably a part of all this, and in no way can it be called a 'normal society'. The evil effects of racism, educational deprivation, and more recently the 15 years of sporadic violence, have taken a tragic toll on the mental health of a generation. These factors may contribute to every disorder covered in this chapter, and should be taken into account in the treatment of many of them.

There is an urgent need to establish community-based, easily accessible, walk-in Child and Family Help Centres, where preventive and rehabilitative mental health principles will be applied; where educational problems can be addressed, and where help can be given to people to restore stable family life, and to maintain the integrity of the family. The church and concerned members of the community could possibly meet this need. Professionals of all kinds can join with lay people and youth groups in mass action to provide dignity and hope.

C. Allwood
W.E.K. Loening

31

Procedures

Overview

This chapter addresses important aspects and hazards of procedures used in paediatrics. For brevity, restraint of the child, preparation, and anaesthesia have not been repeated for each procedure. Common procedures only are outlined.

Preparation

Preparation of the child and family

Explanations to the child depend on the age, developmental status, and ability to understand. Parents should be informed about the need for and risks of a painful procedure, but should not assist in its performance.

Preparation of the assistant

The auxiliary staff who assist need guidance about the procedure — the equipment, position, and restraint required. Adequate restraint and correct positioning are important for speed and safety. The assistant must prevent movement that could make the procedure more difficult or hazardous.

Sedation

Sedation should be adequate. Parenteral diazepam or midazolam (Dormicum®) are frequently used in a titrated dose because they have rapid onset and are short-acting. Midazolam is sometimes chosen because of its amnesic effect. Ketamine (2 mg/kg IV) is also useful, but laryngospasm may necessitate respiratory support. Oral trimeprazine (Vallergan®) 3 mg/kg in older children, and chloral hydrate (Tricloryl®) 30 mg/kg in infants, may be given 1 hour before the procedure.

Local anaesthesia

Lignocaine is the recommended local anaesthetic for most minor procedures, in a dose not exceeding 3 mg/kg. The two main solutions available are 1% (10 mg/ml) and 2% (20 mg/ml). Preparations with adrenaline are useful to reduce bleeding, but should never be used on extremities (digits, ears, penis). Occasionally regional anaesthesia may be required. Injections into inflamed or infected tissues, periosteum, or liver capsule, may be followed by rapid systemic absorption with toxic side-effects such as restlessness, convulsions, and cardiac arrhythmias. Control of the convulsion should initially be with diazepam given rectally. Temporary respiratory support may be required.

Technique

Aseptic technique should be followed. Hazards to the persons performing the procedure should be minimized by use of gloves and judicious use of gowns, caps, masks, and goggles. The risk of needle-stick injury is reduced if used needles are not re-sheathed and are appropriately discarded immediately after use.

Injections

Intramuscular injections

It is useful to assess the depth of subcutaneous fat by pinching the skin over the injection site. Before injecting withdraw the plunger to ensure that the needle tip is not in a vein. For thigh injections (see Fig. 31.1), the area chosen is on the lateral aspect, one-third of the way down from the hip, and into the belly of the quadriceps femoris. For buttock injections (see Fig. 31.2), the upper outer quadrant is chosen, in order to avoid the sciatic nerve. Injections into the deltoid are given into the proximal muscle belly on the lateral aspect of the shoulder.

Subcutaneous injections

These are performed by pinching a fold of skin between the thumb and forefinger and aiming for the subcutaneous fat layer. Sites are the lower abdomen, axilla, and deltoid (see Fig. 31.3).

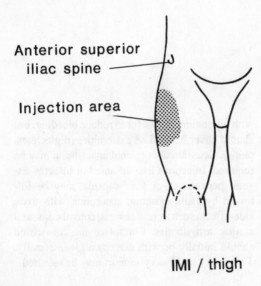

Fig. 31.1 Intramuscular injection into the thigh

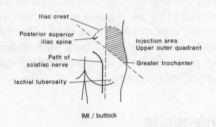

Fig. 31.2 Intramuscular injection into the buttock

Intradermal injections

These are used for vaccinations, Mantoux, etc., and are performed by piercing the dermal layer of the skin at an oblique angle *(see Fig. 31.4)*. Avoid going through into subcutaneous tissue. On injection a wheal is raised, which has the typical *peau d'orange* (orange peel) appearance.

Vascular access

The superficial veins commonly used for blood sampling are the veins of the upper limbs, and in infants of 1–2 years of age the external jugular vein. Other sites include scalp veins (infants), internal jugular, femoral, and saphenous veins. Tourniquets should be tight enough to occlude veins but not to prevent arterial perfusion. It is easier to penetrate veins where they emerge through fascia or at a confluence. Puncture of the internal jugular, subclavian, and femoral veins, which are the larger vessels, should be avoided when there is a bleeding disorder.

External jugular puncture

This is performed with the infant held supine with the occiput at the edge and the head tilted 15–20 ° down. The assistant holds the ipsilateral shoulder down and turns the head toward the opposite shoulder. Crying, or having the vein occluded with the operator's fingers on the clavicle, helps to distend the vessel. The external jugular runs from the angle of the mandible to behind the middle of the clavicle over the sternomastoid muscle. *See after-puncture procedure given for internal jugular vein, below.*

The internal jugular vein

This structure runs close to the lateral border of the carotid artery, behind the sternomastoid, between the sternal and clavicular heads. The positioning is similar to that for external jugular puncture. In children the high approach *(see Fig. 31.5)* is used. The needle is inserted deep to the posterior border of the sternomastoid at its midpoint, and directed to just above the sternal notch. Negative pressure is applied while advancing the needle.

Firm pressure is required over the puncture site for 3–5 minutes with the child in the sitting position after internal and external jugular punctures. Complications include deep-neck bleeding, damage to local structures, and pneumothorax.

The femoral vein

(See Fig. 31.6.)

The vein runs anterior to the hip joint, medial to the femoral artery. The femoral artery runs deep to the inguinal ligament, midway between the anterior superior iliac spine and the pubic symphysis. Lateral to the artery is the femoral nerve. The artery is palpated 1–2 cm distal to the flexion crease of the thigh, and the needle is advanced almost vertically 0.5 cm medial to the pulsation with negative pressure applied to the syringe.

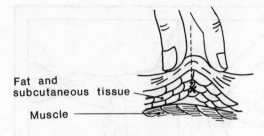

Fat and subcutaneous tissue

Muscle

Fig. 31.3   Subcutaneous injection

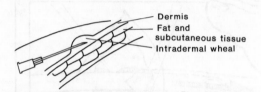

Dermis
Fat and subcutaneous tissue
Intradermal wheal

Fig. 31.4   Intradermal injection

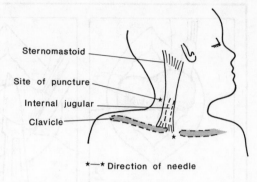

Sternomastoid
Site of puncture
Internal jugular
Clavicle

★—★ Direction of needle

Fig. 31.5   Internal jugular puncture

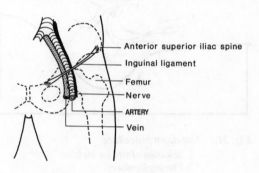

Anterior superior iliac spine
Inguinal ligament
Femur
Nerve
ARTERY
Vein

Fig. 31.6   Femoral vessel puncture

Femoral arterial puncture

This procedure is identical to femoral vein puncture except that the needle is directed more laterally into the pulsating vessel, and gentle or no negative pressure may be required. *Pressure over the puncture site for 10 minutes is essential.* Complications include arthritis of the hip, osteomyelitis of the femur, and compromised circulation to the leg. If the procedure is done too high up, bowel or bladder puncture may occur.

The radial artery

This vessel is preferred for arterial blood sampling, but the brachial or temporal arteries may also be used. The artery is located by careful palpation, and the needle is directed at a 30–60° angle from the horizontal into the vessel.

Saphenous vein cut-down

(See Fig. 31.7.)

A cut-down is performed when venous access is necessary but percutaneous venipuncture is not possible. The patient is kept supine with the foot restrained in an externally rotated position. The saphenous vein is palpated just anterior to and above the medial malleolus. After infiltrating local anaesthetic, a 1.5–2 cm incision is made over the vein, and the vein, which lies fairly deep and just superficial to the periosteum, is exposed by blunt dissection using artery forceps. A length of the vessel is freed for a distance of 1 cm, and two ligatures placed underneath the vessel. The distal ligature is tied and the other is loosely knotted. While applying tension to the distal ligature, the vein is incised with a small blade. A catheter filled with saline or other infusion fluid is carefully inserted into the vein via the incision. The loose proximal ligature is then tightened over the catheter, and the infusion commenced. The skin incision is sutured with silk and the catheter secured with a suture and adhesive plaster.

A subclavian vein

A catheter may be used for vascular access as well as for monitoring central venous pressure. The

599

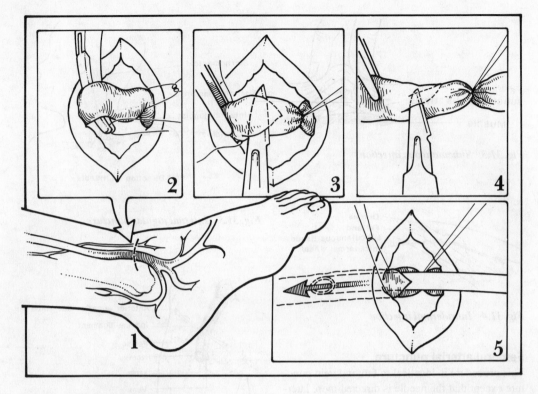

Fig. 31.7 Cut-down procedure
    1. Selection of site for incision
    2. Placing ligatures
    3. Incision of vein with distal ligature tied
    4. Preparation of flap
    5. Insertion of catheter

subclavian vein *(see Fig. 31.8)* crosses over the first rib in front of the anterior scalene muscle and continues behind the medial third of the clavicle to join the internal jugular vein and to form the innominate vein on that side. The patient is supine in a $10-20°$ Trendelenburg position, with the head turned to the opposite side. A towel roll under the shoulders may be needed to hyperextend the back. Either side may be used, although the right is preferred. Using aseptic techniques, local anaesthesia is injected at the entry site and the intended track, including periosteum of adjacent clavicle and first rib. The puncture site is under the distal third of the clavicle in the depression bordered by the deltoid and pectoralis major muscles. The needle is directed under the clavicle at its midpoint, toward the junction of the first rib and clavicle. Aspirate gently while advancing the needle with the bevel upward. When

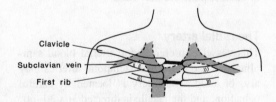

Fig. 31.8 Subclavian vein puncture

blood is aspirated, advance the needle a few millimetres further. Placement of the catheter could be through the needle or over a guidewire (Seldinger's technique). Keep the catheter patent using heparin (10 IU per ml). Take care to avoid air embolism, and attach the IV infusion with an in-line manometer. Fix the cannula securely in place and check that blood flows back under the influence of gravity. The position of the catheter tip should be confirmed with a chest X-ray. Complications include pneumothorax, haemothorax, arterial puncture, damage to the thoracic duct, air embolism, infection, and thrombosis.

Umbilical vessels

In the newborn, umbilical catheterization is possible via the vein or arteries. Secure fixation of the catheter is required. The umbilical vessels comprise two white, thick-walled arteries on the one side, and a larger thin-walled vein on the other. To facilitate cannulation, cut the umbilical stump 1.5–2 cm above the abdominal wall. Place a silk tie (3-0 or 4-0) or cord ligature around the base of the umbilical stump, but leave a purse-string knot untied. Locate the umbilical vessels. The vein is grasped with a pair of toothed forceps and the lumen opened with a curved probe. A catheter of appropriate size is inserted into it until there is free flow of blood (approximately half the distance between shoulder and umbilicus).

The procedure is similar for the arterial catheterization, and the lumen is gently dilated to a depth of 1 cm. If the vessel is tortuous, the stump is cut shorter. Blood should flow after passing the resistance of the bend which marks entry into the iliac artery. The knot in the ligature at the base is then tied and the catheter is securely fixed to the abdominal wall.

Intra-cardiac injection

This approach is used during resuscitation. The needle is inserted perpendicularly at the left sternal border in the 4th or 5th interspace and advanced while continually aspirating.

Intra-osseous infusion

This is indicated only when intravenous access is not available and immediate access is required on a temporary basis for infusion of crystalloid. A bone marrow aspiration needle is inserted into the marrow, usually of the tibia immediately distal to tubercle. Hypertonic and strongly alkaline fluid should be avoided.

Urine collection

Specimens may be obtained by collection bag over the genitalia, by mid-stream urine collection during voiding, by catheterization, or suprapubic puncture. The prepuce is retracted sufficiently to expose the urethral meatus, which is then cleaned with soap, saline, or antiseptic solution. In the female the perineum and vulva are cleaned and the labia widely separated. The sample of urine can then be collected during voiding or in the collection bag. Any specimen obtained should be sent for culture immediately or refrigerated.

Despite aseptic technique and use of sterile equipment, catheterization still carries the risk of introducing bacteria into the bladder and causing bacteraemia; this risk is increased with indwelling catheters.

Suprapubic puncture

Suprapubic puncture of the bladder *(see Fig. 31.9)* is a safe method to collect uncontaminated urine from infants and children less than 2 years old. The distended bladder at this age is primarily intra-abdominal. For children over 2 years catheterization is required. The bladder must be full — about

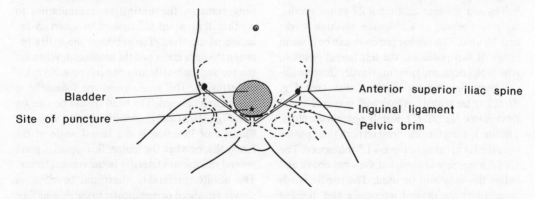

Bladder
Site of puncture
Anterior superior iliac spine
Inguinal ligament
Pelvic brim

Fig. 31.9 Suprapubic bladder aspiration

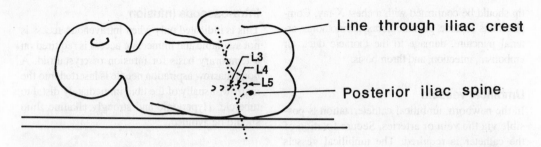

Fig. 31.10   Lumbar puncture: lying in the left lateral position

1 hour after the last voiding. Have a specimen bottle at hand to collect urine if the infant voids during the preparation. Position the child supine and restrain firmly. Insert a 22-gauge needle in the midline 1–2 cm above the symphysis with the needle directed 10–20° cephalad. Advance the needle under negative pressure. If no urine is obtained, do not remove the needle completely, but re-insert it at an angle further away from or towards the pelvic brim. If still no urine is obtained, try again after 1 hour. Microscopic haematuria virtually always occurs. Complications include gross haematuria, bowel puncture, or infection of the abdominal wall. Peritonitis is uncommon.

Lumbar puncture

This is usually done to confirm meningitis. Increased intracranial pressure, focal neurological signs with suspicion of a mass or cord compression, and a bleeding tendency or anticoagulant therapy are contra-indications to lumbar puncture. A lumbar puncture needle with a stylet is used. In babies and younger children a 22-gauge needle, scalp vein needle, or a 21-gauge injection needle may be used. The lumbar puncture can be done in either of two positions: the left lateral position, with hips, knees, and spine maximally flexed without compromising the upper airway *(see Fig. 31.10),* or the seated position with maximal spinal flexion *(see Fig. 31.11).* Firmly restrain the child. The line joining the iliac crest on both sides passes over the L4 vertebra or the L4-L5 interspace. The L3-L4 interspace is used, but the ones above and below this may also be used. The needle is advanced into the desired interspace and directed toward the umbilicus. A 'give' is felt in older

patients once the dura is pierced *(see Fig. 31.12).* The needle is rotated to maximize CSF flow and the opening pressure is recorded. The foramen magnum is zero point in the sitting position, and the needle level is zero point in the lateral position. Normal CSF pressure is between 50 and 180 mm. If no CSF is obtained initially, advance the needle another millimetre or so. Should this fail, then re-insert. Aspiration of CSF with a syringe must be avoided. If blood is obtained, serial samples are taken. If the subsequent samples become clear, then a traumatic tap is likely (usually because the needle has been advanced too far). Complications include headache, back pain, transient limping, radicular pain, dural leak, bleeding into the cord, infection, and in the presence of increased intracranial pressure, herniation of the brainstem or cerebellum ('coning').

Subdural and ventricular tap

Subdural tap

Cold light transillumination of the skull may reveal subdural fluid collection. Although CT scanning remains the definitive examination to confirm this, a tap is required to ascertain the nature of the fluid. The subdural space lies between the dura mater and the arachnoid. When the sutures and fontanelle are open it is possible to tap the effusion. The area around the fontanelle is shaved and cleaned. The head should be face up *(see Fig. 31.13)* and immobilized by an assistant. The site of insertion is the lateral angle of the fontanelle, or when the fontanelle is small, a point several millimetres laterally in the coronal suture. The needle, preferably short and bevelled, is slowly advanced perpendicular to the skin surface until there is a drop in resistance. The needle

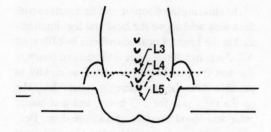

Fig. 31.11   Lumbar punture: sitting position

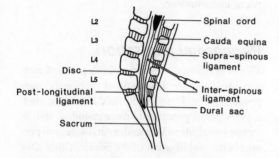

L2 — Spinal cord
L3 — Cauda equina
L4 — Supra-spinous ligament
Disc
L5
Post-longitudinal ligament — Inter-spinous ligament
Dural sac
Sacrum

Fig. 31.12   Lumbar puncture anatomy

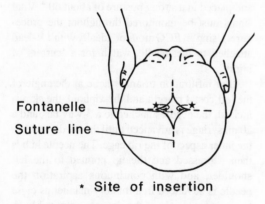

Fontanelle
Suture line

* Site of insertion

Fig. 31.13   Subdural and ventricular tap

normally need not be advanced more than 5–8 mm. It is quite safe to evacuate 15–20 mls of fluid from each side. The fluid should be cultured and have microscopy and chemistry checked as for routine CSF. Some infants require bilateral taps, and with chronic effusions daily taps are needed (*see Chapter 15, Neurological Disorders*). Complications include infection, subgaleal fluid

collection, laceration of the superior sagittal sinus (insertion too medial), and trauma to the cerebral cortex.

Ventricular puncture

This is performed with suspected ventriculitis or for relieving non-communicating hydrocephalus. Ultrasound examination helps to confirm the thickness of the cerebral cortex and the degree of ventricular dilatation. The child is prepared as for subdural tap. The needle is inserted at the lateral angle of the anterior fontanelle and directed toward the medial canthus of the opposite eye. Ventricular fluid is usually obtained at a depth of less than 3 cm. A short bevel needle with stylet is least traumatic, and care should be taken not to change direction or rotate the needle in the skull, to minimize damage to brain tissue. Whenever possible the right side is used in order to spare the left hemisphere (more commonly dominant and involved in speech). Normal ventricular pressure is less than 10 mm CSF. Porencephalic cyst formation along the puncture track, trauma to brain, and puncture of the superior sagittal sinus are the major complications. Repeated ventricular punctures, preferably by the same operator, should attempt to follow the previous track.

Liver biopsy

A full blood count and coagulation tests should be checked, and a specimen for cross-match be available prior to the procedure. Prolonged coagulation or bleeding times, an unco-operative patient, local infection, cholangitis, marked anaemia, or gross ascites are contra-indications. Whenever possible the patient should practise holding the breath for about 10 seconds (full inspiration for subcostal approach and full expiration for intercostal approach). A Tru-cut® biopsy needle is used, and the technique used for breast biopsy is recommended (*see Fig 31.14*). The operator must be familiar with the mechanics of the needle prior to the procedure. With enlarged livers the biopsy is performed in the midclavicular line, just below the costal margin or to the right of the epigastrium (in the direction of the lower right axilla). The intercostal approach is used when the liver is not palpable below the costal margin. Maximal liver dullness is pin-pointed between the anterior and

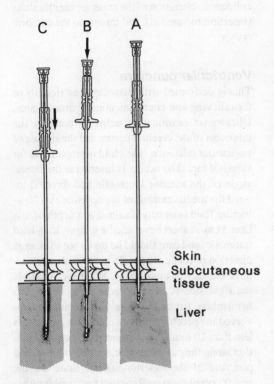

Fig. 31.14 Trucut® needle technique

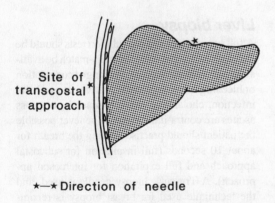

★—★ **Direction of needle**

Fig. 31.15 Liver biopsy: intercostal approach

mid-axillary lines at end-expiration, and a site chosen one or two intercostal spaces below this *(see Fig.31.15).* The needle is inserted close to the superior ridge of the rib to avoid injury to the neurovascular bundle.

The child is placed supine on a firm surface with the hands held above the head and legs immobilized at the knees. Local anaesthetic is infiltrated. A 2–3 mm incision is made at the desired puncture site and the procedure completed as rapidly as possible. After the procedure the patient should lie on the right side for 2–3 hours, and half-hourly pulse and blood pressure checks are done. Bedrest for 24 hours is recommended. Complications include pain, bleeding, cholangitis, bile peritonitis, puncture of adjacent viscera, and pneumothorax or haemothorax.

Pericardial aspiration

This is performed to remove fluid, purulent exudate, or blood for diagnostic or therapeutic purposes *(see Fig. 31.16).* If the fluid is not loculated, a sub-xiphoid puncture is recommended, as it is extra-pleural, allows dependent drainage, and permits better stabilization of the needle. Other sites for puncture include the apical site, or the 5th or 6th interspace at the left sternal margin. The patient should be well sedated prior to the procedure and placed in a sitting posture of about 60°. Vital signs must be monitored throughout the procedure. Using an ECG monitor, ideally with a V-lead attached to the needle, watch for a 'current of injury'.

After infiltration of anaesthetic at the angle of the left costal margin and the xiphoid, the skin is incised, the needle attached to a 3-way tap, and a 20 ml syringe is advanced until the needle reaches the inner aspect of the rib cage. The needle hub is then depressed and the tip pointed to the left shoulder, and with continuous aspiration the needle is advanced in a rotatory manner as close to the inner aspect of the rib cage as possible. A 'give' may be felt with pericardial puncture. Fluid must be aspirated slowly to avoid pericardial shock. If no fluid is obtained, withdraw the needle and re-direct the needle to the head or right shoulder.

A 'ventricular' ECG complex or a 'current of injury' (ST segment change and T waves) suggest myocardial penetration. Withdraw the needle and wait for return to baseline before resuming. Other complications include arrhythmias, damage to the coronary arteries, haemopericardium, pneumothorax, and infection. Following the procedure there should be close observation (BP, pulse, and general condition) every 15 minutes for 2 hours. Any complication of the procedure is unlikely to occur after this period. A follow-up chest X-ray is useful to assess size of the effusion and to exclude pneumothorax.

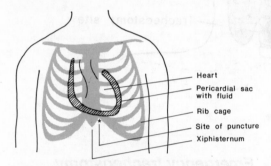

Fig. 31.16   Pericardial aspiration

Paracentesis

Adequate restraint and sometimes sedation is required.

Thoracic paracentesis

Thoracic paracentesis (diagnostic or therapeutic) is performed with the patient seated. With the arms elevated, the puncture site is just below the lower tip of the scapula (7th intercostal space) in the posterior axillary line.

Peritoneal tap

This is performed after clinically confirming the presence of ascites. The patient is placed in a sitting or a lateral decubitus position. The puncture site could be in the midline or at a point two-thirds of the way along a line between the umbilicus and the anterior superior iliac spine.

For insertion of a peritoneal dialysis catheter a site halfway between the umbilicus and the symphysis pubis is selected.

Bone marrow

Both the anterior and posterior portions of the iliac crest are suitable sites, and contain cellular marrow at any age. In neonates and young infants the tibia is preferred, with the puncture site being 1 cm medial and 1 cm distal to the tibial tubercle. Local

anaesthetic is injected into the subcutaneous tissue down to and including the underlying periosteum.

For aspiration, the needle with obturator in place is advanced through a skin incision into the cortex of the bone with increased force and a slight to and fro rotation. A 'give' is felt on entry into marrow. The obturator is removed and an aspirate specimen obtained by sustained suction on a syringe. Prolonged aspiration will dilute the specimen. A 'dry tap' may be the result of faulty technique, or abnormal marrow (hyperplasia/myelofibrosis).

For a trephine biopsy the Jamshidi® needle is used. The site selected is usually the posterior iliac crest or spine. After advancing the needle and obturator through the bony cortex, the obturator is removed, and using smooth, rotatory, to-and-fro motions the needle is advanced for 1–2 cm. The needle is rotated several times and moved from side to side to separate the core of marrow, and then slowly removed using slight rotatory motions. The specimen is removed through the proximal end of the needle by using the probe, and after touch imprints have been made, placed into appropriate fixative.

Endotracheal intubation

The patient is positioned supine with the head extended and resting on the occiput in a 'sniffing position'. Hyperextension must be avoided. Preoxygenation by mask or bag is imperative. Adequate suction must always be at hand.

Suggested sizes (inner diameters) for paediatric endotracheal tubes are: premature 2.5–3.5 mm, term newborn 3.5mm, 3 – 12 months 4.0 mm, 1–2 years 4.5 mm, and for children over 2 years 4.5 mm + 0.5 mm for every 2 years of age.

Using the left hand, insert the appropriate laryngoscope (straight blade in infants) in the right corner of the mouth; by pulling the blade to the centre the tongue is lifted out of the way to obtain a view of the cords. The cords are attached to the cricoid cartilage, and cricoid pressure will push the larynx down into view. Cricoid pressure also occludes the oesophagus, thereby reducing the risk of aspiration. The tube is passed through the cords for an appropriate distance (usually 2–3 cm) into the trachea. The trachea of an infant is very short, and it is easy to intubate the mainstem bronchus, especially with further flexion of the

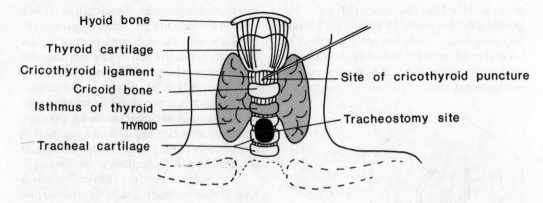

Hyoid bone

Thyroid cartilage

Cricothyroid ligament

Cricoid bone

Isthmus of thyroid

THYROID

Tracheal cartilage

Site of cricothyroid puncture

Tracheostomy site

Fig. 31.17 Tracheostomy and cricothyroid puncture

head. The airways of infants are small and delicate, and even minimal trauma can cause oedema which may be life-threatening. Direct pressure of the laryngoscope blade onto the dento-alveolar ridge must be avoided, and one must be wary of dislodging any teeth.

Note that adequate vetilation is more important than intubation, and when difficulty is encountered, ventilate via an oral/nasal airway and mask.

The position of the tube should be checked clinically and by a chest X-ray.

Cricothyroidotomy

This is performed as an emergency procedure in order to maintain an airway. The patient is placed supine with the neck extended. The gap between the thyroid and cricoid cartilages is palpated. The thyroid cartilage is grasped with thumb and middle finger, and using the tip of the index finger as a guide, a large bore needle or scalpel blade is inserted through the cricothyroid membrane into the larynx *(see Fig. 31.17)*. Any makeshift tube can be used, but must be fixed in place to prevent it slipping through into the trachea.

Emergency tracheostomy

The patient is placed supine with support below the shoulders in order to hyperextend the head. The chin, thyroid cartilage, and suprasternal notch are kept in a straight line. The operator's left thumb and second and third fingers are arched over the trachea to immobilize it, pushing the great vessels of the neck back under the sternomastoid and also keeping the skin taut. A vertical incision 2–3 cm long is made midway between the cricoid and the suprasternal notch. By blunt dissection the trachea is exposed over a distance of 2 or 3 rings. The isthmus of the thyroid should be mobilized and retracted upward if encountered. A vertical incision is made through the 2nd and 3rd tracheal rings. An appropriate-sized tube is inserted, and secured firmly but not tightly. The skin edges are loosely sutured together. Suctioning the tube in a sterile manner is important; this is done every 15 minutes for the first hour, and then hourly, or more frequently when required.

Complications include mediastinal or subcutaneous emphysema, pneumothorax, haemorrhage, and infection, and in the long term, ulceration of the trachea, and laryngeal or tracheal stenosis.

R. Thejpal

Select Bibliography

1 HISTORY-TAKING AND PHYSICAL EXAMINATION
Athreya, B.H. 1980. *Clinical Methods in Pediatric Diagnosis.* New York: Van Nostrand Reinhold Co.

Schneiderman, H. 1990. The Problem-oriented Medical Record. In Oski, F.A. (Ed.) *Principles and Practice of Pediatrics.* Philadelphia: J.B. Lippincott Co., (pp. 44–6).

2 GROWTH AND DEVELOPMENT
Behrman, R.E., and Kliegman, R. 1990. *Essentials of Pediatrics.* Philadelphia: W.B. Saunders and Co.

Kibel, M.A., and Wagstaff, L.A. 1991. *Child Health for All: A Manual for Southern Africa.* Cape Town: Oxford University Press.

Walker, D., Gugenheims Downs, M.P., and Northern, J.L. 1989. Early Language Milestone Scale and Language Screening of Young Children. In *Pediatrics* 83: 2, (pp. 284–8).

3 GENETICS AND CONGENITAL DISORDERS
Harper, P.S. 1988. *Practical Genetic Counselling* (3rd edition). London: Butterworth.

Connor, J.M. and Ferguson-Smith, M.A. 1984. *Essential Medical Genetics* (3rd edition). Oxford: Blackwell.

4 COMMUNITY PAEDIATRICS
Morley, D. 1973. *Paediatric Priorities in Developing Countries.* London: Butterworth.

Morley, D., Rohde, J., and Williams, G. 1983. *Practising Health for All.* Oxford: Oxford University Press.

Walker, C.E., Bower, B.L., and Kaufman, K.L. 1988. *The Physically and Sexually Abused Child: Evaluation and Treatment.* New York: Pergamon Press.

Werner, D.B., and Bower, B.L. 1982. *Helping Health Workers Learn.* Palo Alto: Hesperian Foundation.

5 NEWBORNS
Avery, G.B. 1987. *Neonatology, Pathophysiology and Management of the Newborn* (3rd edition). Philadelphia: J.P. Lippincott Co.

Robertson, W.R.C. 1986. *Textbook of Neonatology.* London: Churchill Livingstone.

Volpe, J.J. 1987. *Neurology of the Newborn* (2nd edition). Vol. 22 in the series 'Major Problems in Clinical Paediatrics'. London: W.B. Saunders and Co.

6 FEEDING OF INFANTS AND TODDLERS
Grant, J.P. 1989. *The State of The World's Children.* Oxford: Oxford University Press.

Hansen, M. *et al.* 1989. Weaning Foods with Improved Energy and Nutrient Density prepared from Germinated Cereals. In *Food and Nutrition Bulletin* 11: 2 (pp. 40–52).

Helsing, E., and Savage King, F. 1982. *Breastfeeding in Practise: A Manual for Health Workers.* Oxford: Oxford Medical Publications.

Priyani, S. 1988. The Introduction of Semi-solid and Solid Foods to Feeding Infants. In *Food and Nutrition Bulletin* 10: 1 (pp. 49–51).

Rubin, D.S. 1990. Women's Work and Children's Nutrition in Southern-western Kenya. In *Food and Nutrition Bulletin* 12: 4 (pp. 268–72).

7 NUTRITIONAL DISORDERS
Hansen, J.D.L. 1990. *Malnutrition Review.* Paediatric Reviews and Communications, Vol. 4 (pp. 201–12).

McLaren, D.S., *et al.* 1991. *Textbook of Paediatric Nutrition* (3rd edition). London: Churchill Livingstone.

8 INFECTIOUS DISORDERS

Brown, H.W., and Neva, F.A. 1983. *Basic Clinical Parasitology* (5th edition). Norwalk, Connecticut: Appleton-Century-Crofts.

Christie, A.B. 1987. *Infectious Diseases: Epidemiology and Clinical Practice* (4th edition). Edinburgh: Churchill Livingstone.

Fripp, P.J. 1983. *An Introduction to Human Parasitology with Reference to South Africa* (2nd edition). Johannesburg: Macmillan.

Krugman, S., Ward, R., and Katz, S.L. 1985. *Infectious Diseases of Children* (8th edition). Saint Louis: The C.V. Mosby Co.

Manson-Bahr, P.E.C., and Bell, D.R. 1987. *Manson's Tropical Diseases* (19th edition). London: Ballière Tindall.

9 TUBERCULOSIS

Coovadia, H.M. and Benatar, S.R. 1991. *A Century of Tuberculosis: South African Perspectives*. Cape Town: Oxford University Press.

Dubos, R. and Dubos, J. 1953. *The White Plague*. London: Victor Gollancz.

Miller, F.J.W. 1982. Tuberculosis in Children. In *Medicine in the Tropics*. New York: Longman.

10 AIDS

Stein, Z., and Zwi, A. 1990. *Action on AIDS in Southern Africa*. Maputo Conference on Health in Transition in Southern Africa.

Thomas, C. *et al.* 1986. AIDS in Africa: An Epidemiologic Paradigm. In *Science* Vol. 234.

Various authors. 1991. *Childhood AIDS. The Pediatric Clinics of North America*. Vol. 38: 1. Philadelphia: W.B. Saunders and Co.

11 GASTROINTESTINAL DISORDERS

Bowie, M.D. & Hill, I.D. 1987. Management of Persistent Diarrhoea in Infants. In *Indian Journal of Paediatrics* 54: 475–80.

Diarrhoea: Acute and Chronic. In Gryboski, J., and Walker, W.A. (eds). 1983. *Gastrointestinal Problems in the Infant* (2nd edition). Philadelphia: W.B. Saunders and Co. (pp. 541–86).

Lebenthal, E. (ed.) 1989. *Textbook of Gastroenterology and Nutrition in Infancy* (2nd edition). New York: Raven Press Ltd.

Milla, P.J., and Muller, D.P. (eds). 1988. *Harries' Paediatric Gastroenterology* (2nd edition). London: Churchill Livingstone.

12 LIVER DISORDERS

Milla, P.J., and Muller, D.P.R. 1988. *Harries' Paediatric Gastroenterology* (2nd edition). Edinburgh: Churchill Livingstone.

Mowat, A.P 1987. *Liver Disorders in Childhood* (2nd edition). London: Butterworths.

Tripp, J.H., and Candy, D.C.A. 1985. *Manual of Paediatric Gastroenterology*. London: Churchill Livingstone.

13 RESPIRATORY DISEASES IN CHILDREN

Kendig, E.L., and Chernick, V. 1990. *Disorders of the Respiratory Tract in Children* (5th edition). Philadelphia: W.B. Saunders and Co.

Phelan, P.D., Landau, L.I., and Olinsky, A. 1990. *Respiratory Illness in Children* (3rd edition). Oxford: Blackwell Scientific Publications.

14 EAR, NOSE, AND THROAT DISORDERS

Groves, J., and Gray, R.F. 1985. *Synopsis of Otorhinolaryngology* (4th edition). Bristol: Wright.

Paparella, M.M., and Shumrick, D.A. 1991. *Otolaryngology* (3rd edition). Philadelphia: W.B. Saunders and Co.

Scott-Brown W.G. 1987. *Otolaryngology* (5th edition). London: Butterworths.

15 NEUROLOGICAL DISORDERS
Dubowitz, V. 1978. *Muscle Disorders in Childhood.* London: W.B. Saunders and Co.
Gordon, N., and McKinlay, I. 1986. *Children with Neurological Disorders, Vols 1 and 2.* Oxford: Blackwell Scientific Publications.
O'Donohoe, N.V. 1985. *Epilepsies of Childhood.* London: Butterworths.

16 RENAL DISORDERS
Holliday, M.A., Barratt, T.M. and Vernier, R.L. 1987. *Pediatric Nephrology* (2nd edition). Baltimore: The Williams and Wilkins Company.
Houston, I.B. and Hendrikse, R.G. 1991. The Genito-urinary System. In Hendrickse, R.G., Barr, D.G., and Matthews, T.S. *Paediatrics in the Tropics.* Oxford: Blackwell Scientific Publications (pp. 373–409).
Kibukamusoke, J.W. 1984. *Tropical Nephrology.* Canberra: Citjonge Pty. Ltd.
Kim Yap Hui, 1991. Disorders of the Kidney and Urinary Tract, in Stanfield, P. *et al. Diseases of Children in the Subtropics and Tropics* (4th edition). London: Edward Arnold (pp. 784–805).

17 CARDIAC DISORDERS
Fink, B.W. 1991. *Congenital Heart Disease: A Deductive Approach to its Diagnosis* (3rd edition). St. Louis: Mosby, Year Book Medical Publishers Inc.
Gillette, P.C. 1978. Symposium on Pediatric Cardiology. In *The Pediatric Clinics of North America* Vol. 37: 1. Philadelphia: W.B. Saunders and Co.
Taranta, A., and Markowitz, M. 1981. *Rheumatic Fever: A Guide to its Recognition, Prevention, and Cure with Special Reference to Developing Countries.* Boston: M.T.P. Press.

18 BLOOD DISORDERS
Bachmer, R.L. 1980. Symposium on Pediatric Haematology. In *Pediatric Clinics of North America* Vol. 27. Philadelphia: W.B. Saunders and Co. (pp. 217– 489).
Kernoff, L. 1980. Purpura: A Review. In *Modern Medicine* Vol. 4 (pp. 5–19).
Machim, S.J.M. 1980. The Bleeding Patient. In *British Journal of Hospital Medicine* Vol. 24: 2 (pp. 152–6).

19 COMMON NEOPLASTIC DISORDERS
Malpas, J.S. 1982. Lymphomas in Children. In *Seminars in Haematology* Vol. 19. (pp. 301–14).
Morris Jones, P. 1979. Cancer in Children. In *The Practitoner* Vol. 222 (pp. 221–8).
Pochedly, C. 1976. *Clinical Management of Cancer in Children.* London: Edward Arnold.

20 ENDOCRINE AND METABOLIC DISORDERS
Brook, C.G.D. (ed.) 1989. *Clinical Paediatric Endocrinology* (2nd edition). Oxford: Blackwell Scientific Publications.

21 METABOLIC BONE DISORDERS
Castells, S., and Fineberg, L. 1990. *Metabolic Bone Disease in Children.* New York: Marcell Dekker.
Glorieux, F.H. 1991. *Rickets.* Nestlé Nutrition Workshop Series, Vol. 21. New York: Raven Press.
Harrison, H.E., and Harrison, H.C. 1979. *Disorders of Calcium and Phosphate Metabolism in Childhood and Adolescence.* Philadelphia: W.B. Saunders and Co.
Pettifor, J.M. 1988. Rickets and Osteomalacia. In *South African Journal of Continuing Medical Education* Vol. 6 (pp. 27–37).

22 COMMON ALLERGY PROBLEMS
Mygind, N. 1986. *Essential Allergy.* Oxford: Blackwells.
Mygind, N. 1978. *Nasal Allergy.* Oxford: Blackwells.
South African Childhood Working Group Consensus, 1991. Childhood and Adolescent Asthma. In *South African Medical Journal* Vol. 81 (pp. 38-41).

23 JUVENILE CHRONIC ARTHRITIS AND VASCULITIDES

Brewer, E.J. 1986. Pitfalls in the Diagnosis of Juvenile Rheumatoid Arthritis. In *Pediatric Clinics of North America* Vol. 35 (pp. 1 015–32).

Emery, H. 1986. Clinical Aspects of Systemic Lupus Erthematosus in Childhood. In *Pediatric Clinics of North America* Vol. 33 (pp. 1 177–90).

Fink, C.W. 1986. Vasculitis. In *Pediatric Clinics of North America* Vol. 33 (pp. 1 203–20).

Shackelford, P.G., and Strauss, A.W. 1991. Kawasaki Syndrome. Editorial in *New England Journal of Medicine* Vol. 324 (pp. 1 664–6).

24 DERMATOLOGICAL DISORDERS

Canizares, O.A. 1982. *A Manual of Dermatology for Developing Countries.* Oxford: Oxford University Press.

Hurwitz, S. 1981. *Clinical Paediatric Dermatology.* Philadelphia: W.B. Saunders and Co.

Verbov, J. 1979. *Modern Topics in Paediatric Dermatology.* London: Heinemann.

25 DISORDERS OF THE EYE

Kanski, J. 1989. *Clinical Ophthalmology* (2nd edition). London: Butterworth and Co.

Nelson, L.B., Calhoun, J.H., and Harley, R.D. 1991. *Pediatric Ophthalmology* (3rd edition). Philadelphia: W.B. Saunders and Co.

Schwab, L. 1987. *Primary Eye Care in Developing Nations.* New York: Oxford University Press.

Taylor, D., *et al.* 1990. *Paediatric Ophthalmology.* Oxford: Blackwell Scientific Publications.

26 ORTHOPAEDIC PROBLEMS

Huckstep, R.L. 1975. *Poliomyelitis.* Edinburgh: Churchill Livingstone.

Sharrard, W.J.W. 1979. *Paediatric Orthopaedic Fractures* (2nd edition). London: Blackwell Scientifc Publications.

27 POISONING

Sommers, De K. 1992. *The Treatment of Acute Poisoning.* Durban: Butterworths.

28 SURGICAL PROBLEMS

Lister, J., and Irving, I.M. 1990. *Neonatal Surgery* (3rd edition). London: Butterworths.

MacMahon, R.A. 1990. *An Aid to Paediatric Surgery* (2nd edition). Melbourne: Churchill Livingstone.

Raffensprenger, J.G. 1990. *Swenson's Pediatric Surgery* (5th edition). Norwalk, Connecticut: Appleton and Lange.

29 ORAL HEALTH

Dickson, M. 1983. *Where There is No Dentist.* Palo Alto: The Hesperian Foundation.

Elderton, R.J. 1990. *Evolution in Dental Care.* Bristol: Clinical Press.

World Health Organization. 1987. *Prevention of Oral Diseases.* WHO offset publication No. 103. Geneva: WHO.

30 PSYCHOLOGICAL AND BEHAVIOURAL DISORDERS

Barker, P. 1988. *Basic Child Psychiatry* (5th edition). Oxford: Blackwell Scientific Publications.

Kibel, M.A., and Wagstaff, L.A. 1991. *Child Health for All.* Cape Town: Oxford University Press.

Nikapota, A.D. 1991. Child Psychiatry in Developing Countries. Review article in *British Journal of Psychiatry* Vol. 158 (pp. 743–51).

Rutter, M., and Hersov, L. 1985. *Child and Adolescent Psychiatry* (2nd edition). Oxford: Blackwell Scientific Publications.

31 PROCEDURES

Barkin, R. 1987. *Emergency Pediatrics.* C.V. Mosby Company.

Hughes, W.T., and Buescher, E.S. 1980. *Pediatric Procedures.* London: W.B. Saunders and Company.

— 1989. *Practical Procedures in Medicine and Surgery.* Heinemann Medical Books.

Index